HEALTHCARE

FINANCE

An Introduction to

Accounting and

Financial Management

HEALTHCARE FINANCE

An Introduction to

Accounting and

Financial Management

Louis C. Gapenski

AUPHA
HAP

Health Administration Press, Chicago, Illinois
AUPHA Press, Washington, D.C.

02 01   5 4 3 2

Library of Congress Cataloging-in-Publication Data

Gapenski, Louis C.
    Introduction to healthcare finance / Louis C. Gapenski.
        p.   cm.
    Includes bibliographical references and index.
    ISBN 1-56793-090-5
    1. Health facilities—Finance.   2. Health facilities—Accounting.
    I. Title.
    RA971.3.G3695   1998
    362.1'068'1—dc21   98-8639
                                                                            CIP

The paper used in this publication meets the minimum requirements of American National Standards for Information Sciences—Permanente of Paper for Printed Library Materials, ANSI Z39.48–1984. ⊚ ™

Health Administration Press
A division of the Foundation
   of the American College of
   Healthcare Executives
One North Franklin Street
Chicago, IL 60606
(312) 424–2800

Association of University Programs
   in Health Administration
1911 North Fort Meyer Drive
Suite 503
Arlington, VA 22209
(703) 524–5500

CONTENTS

PREFACE

Some ten years ago, after years of teaching corporate finance and writing related textbooks and casebooks, I began teaching healthcare financial management in the University of Florida's joint MBA/MHA program. The move prompted me to write my first healthcare finance textbook, *Understanding Health Care Financial Management*. The book was designed for use in health services administration finance courses in which students had prerequisite courses in both accounting and corporate finance.

In recent years, I expanded my healthcare teaching to include courses in nontraditional and clinician-oriented programs in which students do not have a formal background in financial issues. Finance courses in these programs require a text that starts from scratch. Furthermore, these courses often were part of programs that contained just one healthcare finance course, so the course had to cover both accounting and financial management. In reviewing the texts available for use in such courses, I found some that were strong in accounting and others that were strong in financial management, however, I could not find one that gave equal emphasis to both components of healthcare finance. This situation prompted me to write *Healthcare Finance: An Introduction to Accounting and Financial Management*.

Concept of the Book

My goal in writing this book was to create a text that introduces students to the most important principles and applications of healthcare finance including both accounting and financial management. Thus, it contains almost equal coverage of the two primary components of healthcare finance. Furthermore, because the book is intended for use primarily in clinical and health services administration programs, in which students are trained primarily for professional positions within healthcare providers, its focus is on healthcare finance as practiced within such organizations. The examples within the book are based on such organizations as hospitals, physician practices, clinics, home health agencies, nursing homes, and managed care organizations.

Another consideration in writing the book was that most readers would be seeing the material for the first time. Thus, it is very important that the material be explained as clearly and succinctly as possible. I have tried very hard to create a book that readers will find user-friendly—one that they will enjoy reading and can learn from on their own. If students don't find a text interesting, understandable, and useful, they won't read it.

The book begins with an introduction to the field of healthcare finance and a description of the financial environment in which providers operate today. From there, it takes students through the basics of financial and managerial accounting. Here, my goal was not to turn clinicians or generalist managers into accountants, but rather to present those accounting concepts that are most critical to managerial decision making. The book then discusses the basic foundations of financial management before progressing to demonstrate how health services managers can apply financial management theory and principles to help make better decisions, where *better* is defined as decisions that promote the financial well-being of the organization. Finally, the book was written under the premise that managed care is changing the way providers operate, and hence the way that finance principles are applied by managers. Thus, the emphasis is on financial decision making within a managed care environment.

Intended Market and Use

The text is not targeted for specific types of educational programs. Rather, it is designed to teach students, in one course, the fundamental concepts of healthcare finance including both accounting and financial management, with emphasis on provider organizations. Thus, the text can be used in a wide variety of settings: undergraduate and graduate programs, traditional and executive programs, on-campus and distance learning programs, and even independently for self-improvement. The key to its usefulness is not the educational program, but rather the focus of the course. If the course is a stand-alone course designed to cover both accounting and financial management, the book will fit. In fact, the book can be easily used across a two-course healthcare finance sequence, especially in modular programs where each course is two hours. Typically, such a sequence begins with an accounting course and ends with a financial management course. This book, supplemented by readings and cases, would be ideal for such a sequence. (Health Administration Press is planning to introduce a new book, *Cases in Healthcare Finance*, in the fall of 1999. This book will contain 25–30 cases that could be used in conjunction with the text, *Healthcare Finance: An Introduction to Accounting and Financial Management*.)

The book should also be useful to practicing healthcare professionals who, for one reason or another, must increase their understanding of healthcare finance. Such professionals include clinicians who have some management responsibilities, as well as line managers who now require additional finance skills. Finally, many members of financial staffs, especially those working exclusively in a single area such as patient accounts, would benefit from having a broader understanding of finance principles, and hence would find this book useful.

Ancillary Materials

Two important teaching aids were developed to accompany the text:

- *Instructor's Manual:* A comprehensive manual is available to instructors who adopt the book. The manual includes a sample course outline and solutions to the end-of-chapter questions and problems.
- *Lecture Presentation Software:* I have developed a set of PowerPoint slides that cover all the essential issues contained in each chapter. Concepts, graphs, tables, lists, and calculations are presented in about 40 slides per chapter, much as an instructor might do on a blackboard. However, the slides are more crisp, clear, and colorful, and can be displayed on a screen almost instantaneously. Furthermore, hard copies of the slides can be provided to students for use as lecture notes. Many instructors will find these slides useful, either as is or as customized to best meet the situation at hand.

Acknowledgments

This book reflects the efforts of many people. First and foremost, I would like to thank Mark Covaleski of the University of Wisconsin who made significant contributions to the accounting content of the book. In fact, without his materials, advice, and counsel, the book could not have been written.

Colleagues, students, and staff at the University of Florida provided inspirational support, as well as more tangible support, during the development and class testing of the text. Last, but certainly not least, the Health Administration Press staff was instrumental in ensuring the quality and usefulness of the text.

Errors in the Text

In spite of the significant effort that has been expended by many individuals on this book, it is safe to say that some errors exist. In an attempt to create the most error-free and useful text possible, I strongly encourage both instructors and students to write me at the address below with comments and suggestions for improving the text. I certainly welcome your input.

Conclusion

In the environment faced by healthcare providers today, good finance is more important than ever to the economic well-being of the enterprise. Because of its importance, managers of all types and at all levels should be thoroughly grounded in finance principles and applications, but this is easier said than done. I hope that *Healthcare Finance: An Introduction to Accounting and Financial Management* will help you understand the finance problems currently faced by healthcare providers and, more importantly, that it will provide guidance on how best to solve them.

Louis C. Gapenski, Ph.D.
Box 100195
Health Science Center
University of Florida
Gainesville, Florida 32610–0195
September 1998

The Healthcare Environment

INTRODUCTION TO HEALTHCARE FINANCE

Learning Objectives

After studying this chapter, readers will be able to:

- Define the term *healthcare finance* as it is used in this book.
- Discuss the role of finance in health services organizations and how this role has changed over time.
- Describe the major players in the health services industry.
- Describe the organization of this text and the learning aids contained in each chapter.

Introduction

What is *healthcare finance*? Surprisingly, there is no single answer to that question because the definition of healthcare finance depends, for the most part, on the context in which the term is used. To a healthcare policymaker, healthcare finance encompasses how society chooses to finance the health services required by its members. To a manager in the health insurance industry, healthcare finance consists of the collection of premiums from payors and the payment of these funds to a panel, or group, of healthcare providers for services rendered. To a faculty member or student in a college of business, healthcare finance probably would be defined as the application of corporate finance to health services organizations. Thus, in writing this book, the first step was to decide how to define healthcare finance.

The *healthcare sector* of the economy, which is second in size only to the real estate sector, is a diverse collection of industries that involve, either directly or indirectly, the healthcare of the population. The major industries in the healthcare sector include:

1. the *health services industry*, which consists of providers such as medical (physician) practices, hospitals, clinics, nursing homes, and home health care agencies;
2. the *health insurance industry*, including both government programs and commercial insurers;
3. the *managed care industry*, which includes organizations such as health maintenance organizations (HMOs) that incorporate both insurance and provider functions;

4. the *medical equipment* and *supplies industries,* which include the makers of durable medical equipment such as diagnostic equipment and wheel chairs, and expendable medical supplies such as disposable surgical instruments and bandages;
5. the *pharmaceutical* and *biotechnology industries,* which develop and market drugs and other medications; and
6. a diverse collection of *other entities,* ranging from consulting firms to educational institutions to government and private research agencies.

Most students who use this book will become managers at health services organizations, or at companies such as managed care organizations and consulting firms that deal directly with such organizations. Thus, to create a text having the most value for its primary users, the focus of this book is on finance as it is applied within the health services industry. Of course, the principles and practices of finance cannot be applied in a vacuum, but must be based on the realities of the current healthcare environment, including how health services are financed. Furthermore, much of managed care involves the management of healthcare providers, either directly or through contracts, and much of the consulting work is done for providers, so the material in this book is also relevant for managers in these two industries.

Now that a better picture of the healthcare focus of this book has been painted, the term *finance* must be defined. Finance, as the term is used within the health services industry, and as defined in this text, consists both of the accounting and financial management functions. (In many settings, accounting and financial management are separate disciplines.) *Accounting,* as its name implies, concerns the counting, in financial terms, of economic events that reflect the operations, resources, and financing of an organization. In general, the purpose of accounting is to create and provide to interested parties, both internal and external, useful information about an organization's financial status and operations.

Whereas accounting provides a rational means by which to measure a business' financial performance and assess operations, *financial management (corporate finance)* provides the theory, concepts, and tools necessary to help managers make better financial decisions. Of course, the boundary between accounting and financial management is blurred; certain aspects of accounting involve decision making, and much of the application of financial management theory and concepts requires accounting data.

Many texts cover the general topics of accounting and financial management, so why is a text that focuses on health services organizations needed? The reason is that while all industries have certain individual characteristics, the health services industry is truly unique. For example, the provision of health services is dominated by *not-for-profit* organizations, both private and governmental, and such entities are inherently different from *investor-owned* businesses.[1] Also, the majority of payments made to healthcare providers are not made by the individuals that use the services, but rather by *third-party payors* (e.g., a commercial insurance company or a government program). Indeed, employers, rather than the individuals who receive the benefits of such coverage, dominate the purchase of health insurance. Throughout the text, ways in which the unique features of the health services industry influence the application of finance principles and practices are emphasized.

This book is designed to **introduce** students to healthcare finance, which has two important implications. First, the text assumes no prior knowledge of the subject matter. Thus, the text is totally self-contained, with each topic explained from the beginning in basic terms. Furthermore, because clarity is so important when concepts are first introduced, the chapters have been written in an easy-to-read fashion. None of the topics are inherently difficult, but new concepts often take some effort to understand. This process is made easier by the writing style used.

Second, because this book is introductory, it contains a broad overview of healthcare finance. The good news here is that the book presents virtually all the important healthcare finance principles that are used by managers in health services organizations. The bad news is that the large number of topics prevent covering principles in great depth or including a wide variety of application illustrations. Thus, students that use this book are not expected to fully understand every nuance of every finance principle and practice that pertains to every type of health services organization, nor are students expected to become experts in quantitative analysis. Nevertheless, this book provides a sufficient knowledge of healthcare finance so that readers will be able to function better as managers, judge the quality of financial analyses performed by others, and incorporate sound principles and practices into personal finance decisions.

Naturally, an introductory book does not contain everything that a healthcare financial manager must know to perform his or her job in a competent manner. Nevertheless, the book is useful even for those working in financial positions because it presents an overview of the finance function. Often, when working in specific areas of finance, it is too easy to lose sight of the context of one's work. This book will help provide that context.

The Role of Finance in Health Services Organizations

The primary role of finance in health services organizations, as in all businesses, is to plan for, acquire, and utilize resources to maximize the efficiency and value of the enterprise. The specific goals of finance depend on the nature of the firm, so that discussion is postponed until Chapter 2. The two broad areas of finance—accounting and financial management—are separate functions at larger organizations, although the accounting function usually is carried out under the direction of the organization's chief financial officer (CFO), and hence falls under the overall category of finance.

In general, finance activities include:

1. *Planning and Budgeting.* First and foremost, finance is used to assess the financial effectiveness of current operations and to plan for the future. Nonfinancial managers generally are most involved in this facet of finance, particularly that portion of planning and budgeting that is part of managerial accounting.
2. *Long-Term Investment Decisions.* Although more important to senior management, managers at all levels must be concerned with the capital investment decision process. Such decisions, which focus on the acquisition of new plant and equipment (i.e., fixed assets), are the primary determinants of a business' strategic direction, and hence financial future.
3. *Financing Decisions.* All organizations must raise funds to buy the assets necessary to support operations. Such decisions involve the choice between internal and external funds, the use of debt versus equity capital, and the use of long-term versus short-term debt. Although senior managers typically make financing decisions, these decisions have ramifications for managers at all levels.
4. *Short-Term Asset Management.* An organization's current, or short-term, assets, such as cash, marketable securities, receivables, and inventories, must be properly managed both to ensure operational effectiveness and to reduce costs. Generally, managers at all levels are involved to some extent in short-term asset management.
5. *Contract Management.* In today's healthcare environment, health services organizations must negotiate, sign, and monitor contracts with managed care organizations and third-party payors. The financial staff typically has primary responsibility for these tasks, but managers at all levels are involved in these activities and must be aware of their effect on operating decisions.

In times of high profitability and abundant financial resources, the role of finance tends to decline in importance. Thus, when most healthcare providers were reimbursed on the basis of costs incurred, the role of finance was minimal. At that time, the most critical finance function was cost accounting because it was more important to account for costs than it was to control them. Today, however, healthcare providers are facing an increasingly hostile environment, and any firm that ignores the finance function runs the risk of financial deterioration, which ultimately could lead to bankruptcy and closure.

In recent years, providers have been redesigning their finance functions to recognize the changes that have been occurring in the health services industry. For the most part, the practice of finance had been driven by the Medicare program, which demanded that providers (primarily hospitals) churn out a multitude of reports both to comply with regulations and to maximize Medicare revenues. Third-party reimbursement complexities meant that a large amount of time had to be spent on cumbersome accounting, billing, and collection procedures. Thus, instead of focusing on value-adding activities, most finance work was spent on bureaucratic functions. Today, to be of maximum value to the enterprise, the finance function must support cost-containment efforts, managed care and other payor contract negotiations, joint venture decisions, and integrated delivery system participation. In essence, finance must help lead organizations into the future, rather than account for what has happened in the past.

In this text, the emphasis is on finance, but there are no unimportant functions in health services organizations. Managers must understand a multitude of functions such as marketing and human resource management in addition to finance. Still, all business decisions have financial implications, so all managers—whether in operations, marketing, personnel, or facilities—must know enough about finance to incorporate financial implications in decisions made within their own specialized areas. Thus, all managers must understand the principles and practices of finance because this knowledge will make them even more effective at their own specialized work.

1. What is the role of finance in today's health services organizations?
2. How has this role changed over time?

Self-Test Questions

Health Services Settings

Healthcare services are provided by numerous types of organizations in many different settings including: hospitals, ambulatory care facilities, long-term care facilities, and at home. Prior to the 1980s, most health services organizations were freestanding and not formally linked with other organizations. Those that were linked tended to be part of horizontally integrated systems that controlled a single type of healthcare facility, such as hospitals or nursing homes. Recently, however, many health services organizations have diversified and become vertically integrated. Because our study of healthcare finance focuses on provider organizations, a brief overview of the most important health services settings is useful.

Hospitals

Hospitals provide diagnostic and therapeutic services to individuals who require more than several hours of care, although most hospitals also are actively engaged in ambulatory services, including emergency services. To ensure a minimum standard of safety and quality, hospitals must be licensed by the state and undergo inspections for compliance with state regulations. In addition, most hospitals are accredited by the Joint Commission on Accreditation of Healthcare Organizations (JCAHO). JCAHO accreditation is a voluntary process that is intended to promote high standards of care. Although the cost to achieve and maintain compliance with standards can be substantial, accreditation provides eligibility for participation in the Medicare program, and hence most general, acute care hospitals seek accreditation.

Recent changes in the healthcare environment have created significant challenges for hospital managers. For example, hospitals, on average, have experienced decreased admission rates and shorter average stays, which resulted in reduced revenues and lower occupancy rates. At the same time, hospitals have been under pressure to give discounts to managed care plans, to limit the growth in patient charges, and to assume greater risk in their contracts with third-party payors. The net effect of these factors has been a decline in the number of hospitals (and beds) in the United States. Furthermore, increasing cost-containment pressures are likely to accelerate this trend, with the end result being fewer, but more efficient, hospitals.

Hospitals differ in function, patient length of stay, size, and ownership. *General, acute care hospitals*, which provide general medical and surgical services and selected acute specialty services, are short-stay facilities that account for the majority of hospitals. *Specialty hospitals*, such as psychiatric, children's, women's, rehabilitation, and cancer hospitals, limit admission of patients to specific ages, sexes, illnesses, or conditions. The number of psychiatric and rehabilitation hospitals has grown substantially in recent years because of increased needs created by substance abuse, as well as increased government reimbursement for such services. Hospitals vary in size from fewer than 25 beds to more than 1,000 beds. General, acute care hospitals tend to be larger than specialty hospitals.

Hospitals are organized as governmental, private not-for-profit, and investor-owned entities.[2] *Governmental hospitals* constitute about 30 percent of all hospitals. They include both *federal hospitals*, which are funded by the federal government, and *public hospitals*, which are funded wholly or in part by state, county, or city governments. In general, federal hospitals serve special purposes, such as those administered by the military services or the Department of Veterans Affairs (VA), whereas *public hospitals* often provide either special services, such as mental health services, or are located in areas where there are substantial numbers of indigent patients. In recent years, many public hospitals have converted to other ownership categories—primarily private not for profits. This trend is caused by the financial burdens placed on state and local governments, which limit the amount of public funds available for hospital care, as well as the inherent inability of bureaucratic organizations to respond effectively to the massive changes that are occurring in the healthcare environment.

Private, not-for-profit hospitals, which make up about 50 percent of all hospitals, are nongovernment entities organized for the sole purpose of providing healthcare services. These hospitals historically have provided a significant amount of indigent care because of the charitable origins of hospitals in the United States and their long tradition of community service. In return for charitable service, private, not-for-profit hospitals receive numerous benefits, including exemption from federal and state income taxes, exemption from property and sales taxes, eligibility to receive tax-deductible charitable contributions, and access to tax-exempt (lower cost) debt financing.

The remaining 20 percent of hospitals are *investor owned*. This means that they have shareholders who benefit directly from any profits generated by the hospital, and that they do not share the charitable mission of not-for-profit hospitals. Historically, physicians have owned most investor-owned hospitals. Now, large corporations such as Columbia/HCA and Tenet Healthcare, which together own over 400 hospitals across the United States, own most investor-owned hospitals. Unlike not-for-profit hospitals, investor-owned hospitals pay taxes and forgo the other benefits of not-for-profit status.

Despite the expressed differences in mission between investor-owned and not-for-profit hospitals (discussed in detail in Chapter 2), not-for-profit hospitals are being forced to place greater emphasis on the financial implications of operating decisions than in the past. This trend has raised concerns in certain quarters that many not-for-profit hospitals are now failing to meet their charitable mission, and hence should lose some, if not all, of the benefits associated with such status.

Hospitals are labor intensive because of the necessity of providing continuous nursing supervision to patients, in addition to the other services provided by professional and semiprofessional staffs. Physicians petition for privileges to practice in hospitals. While they admit and provide care to hospitalized patients, physicians generally are not hospital employees, and hence are not directly accountable to hospital management. However, physicians retain a major responsibility for determining which services will be provided to patients, so physicians play a critical role in determining a hospital's costs and revenues, and hence financial condition.

Ambulatory Care

Ambulatory care, also known as *outpatient care*, encompasses services provided to noninstitutionalized patients in a healthcare facility, as opposed to at home. Traditional outpatient settings include medical (physician) practices, hospital outpatient departments, and emergency rooms. In addition, the 1980s and 1990s witnessed substantial growth in nontraditional ambulatory care settings such as ambulatory surgery centers, urgent care centers (walk-in clinics), diagnostic imaging centers, rehabilitation/sports medicine centers, and clinical laboratories. In general, the new settings offer patients increased amenities and convenience (e.g., atmosphere, parking, scheduling, waiting times, and privacy) compared to hospital-based services, and, in many situations, provide services at a lower cost than hospitals.

Many factors have contributed to the expansion of ambulatory services, but technology has been a leading factor. Patients who once required hospitalization because of the complexity, intensity, invasiveness, or risk associated with certain procedures often now can be treated in outpatient settings. In addition, third-party payors have encouraged providers to expand their outpatient services through mandatory authorization for inpatient services and by payment mechanisms that provide incentives to perform services on an outpatient basis. Finally, fewer entry barriers exist to outpatient services than to institutional care. For example, ambulatory care facilities ordinarily are less costly, less often subject to licensure and certificate-of-need regulations (with exceptions of hospital outpatient units and ambulatory surgery centers), and generally are not accredited.

As outpatient care consumes an increasing portion of the healthcare dollar and as efforts to control outpatient spending are enhanced, the traditional role of the ambulatory care manager is changing. Ambulatory care managers have typically met the needs of physician owners, specifically ensuring adequate billing, collections, staffing, scheduling, and patient relations, while physicians have tended to make the more important business decisions. However, reimbursement changes, including managed care affiliations, are requiring a higher level of management expertise. Increasing competition, as well as the increasing complexity of the environment, is forcing managers of ambulatory care facilities to become more sophisticated in making business decisions, including finance decisions.

Home Health Care

Home health care brings many of the same services provided in ambulatory care settings into the patient's home. In addition to meeting purely medical needs such as infusion therapy, ventilator care, pregnancy monitoring, and pain management, home health care often involves assistance with daily living activities such as eating, bathing, and locomotion.

The provision of home health care services has expanded rapidly over the last two decades for several reasons. First, the segment of the population that is most suitable for home health care—the elderly—is growing at a faster rate than other segments. Second, home health care is viewed by many as a lower-cost alternative to other, more traditional settings. Third, most patients and their families prefer home health care to other settings, especially for treatments that extend over long periods of time. Finally, advances in medical technology have created therapies that can be provided in a home setting that formerly only were available in clinics and offices.

As home health care services expand and use an increasing portion of the healthcare dollar, payors are beginning to examine reimbursement levels with a sharper eye than in the past. Thus, managers of home health care services will bear many of the financial pressures that their colleagues in other health services organizations have already experienced.

Long-Term Care

Long-term care, which encompasses healthcare services that must be provided over an extended period (generally considered to be more than 30 days), includes inpatient, outpatient, and home health care services, often with a focus on mental health, rehabilitation, and nursing home care. Although the greatest use is among the elderly, long-term care services are used by individuals of all ages.

As discussed in connection with home health care, long-term care often is concerned more with daily living activities than with medical services. Individuals become candidates for long-term care when they become too mentally or physically incapacitated to perform tasks necessary to function in their environment, and their family members are unable to provide the services needed. Although long-term care is a hybrid of health services and social services, perhaps the most prominent setting for such care is the *nursing home.*

Three levels of nursing home care exist: skilled nursing facilities, intermediate care facilities, and residential care facilities. *Skilled nursing facilities (SNFs)* provide the level of care closest to hospital care. Services must be under the supervision of a physician and must include 24-hour daily nursing care. *Intermediate care facilities (ICFs)* are intended for individuals who do not require hospital or SNF care, but whose mental or physical conditions require the daily continuity of one or more medical services. *Residential care facilities (RCFs)* are sheltered environments that do not provide professional healthcare services, and for which most insurance programs including Medicare and Medicaid do not provide coverage.

Nursing homes are more abundant, but smaller than hospitals, and have an average bed size of about 100 beds, compared to about 170 beds for hospitals. About 75 percent of nursing homes are investor owned; their occupancy rate is a high 92 percent; and their average patient length of stay is 2.9 years. Nursing homes and nursing home administrators are licensed by states. Although the JCAHO accredits nursing homes, only a small percentage participate because accreditation is not required for reimbursement and the standards to achieve accreditation are much higher than licensure requirements.

Although long-term care often is perceived as nursing home care, many new services are now being offered to meet society's needs in less institutional surroundings, such as adult day care, life care centers, or hospice programs. Furthermore, home health care, when provided for an extended period, can be an alternative to nursing home care in many situations.

Integrated Delivery Systems

Hospitals and physicians currently are developing new organizations that, instead of providing a single healthcare service, provide a coordinated continuum of services. Although these organizations can be structured in many different ways, they all fall under the broad category of *integrated delivery systems* (IDS). The defining characteristic of an IDS is that the organization assumes full clinical and, in certain cases, financial responsibility for the healthcare needs of the members of a managed care plan or the employees of a major company or government unit.

The benefits of providing hospital care, ambulatory care, long-term care, and other healthcare services through an IDS can be considerable. Some of the more obvious benefits include the following:

1. Patients are kept in the organizational network of services (*patient capture*).
2. Providers have access to managerial and functional specialists (e.g., reimbursement and marketing professionals).
3. Information systems that track all aspects of patient care, including both insurance and clinical data, can be developed more easily.
4. Larger, more diversified organizations have better access to capital.

5. The ability to recruit and retain management and professional staff is enhanced.
6. IDSs are able to offer insurers a complete package of services (sometimes called *one-stop shopping*).
7. Incentives can be created that encourage all providers in the system to work in common for the good of the system; this has the potential both to improve quality of care and control costs.

To be an effective competitor in today's healthcare environment, IDSs must minimize the provision of unnecessary services because more services mean higher costs. Thus, the objective of most IDSs is to provide all needed services to the covered population in the lowest-cost setting, using the lowest-cost treatment regimen, without hurting quality of care. To achieve this goal, IDSs must invest heavily in primary care services including prevention, early intervention, and wellness programs. The *gatekeeper* concept, in which the primary care physician must pre-authorize all services, is frequently used to control costs. Also, IDSs tend to be more aggressive in developing *critical pathways*, which identify low-cost treatment patterns. While hospitals continue to be centers of technology, the primary strategies of IDSs are to shift patients toward lower-cost outpatient settings and provide the clinical integration necessary to achieve lower costs, higher quality, greater efficiency, and better patient satisfaction.

Self-Test Questions

1. What are some different types of hospitals, and what trends are occurring in the hospital industry?
2. What trends are occurring in outpatient and long-term care?
3. What is an integrated delivery system?
4. Will integrated delivery systems be more or less prevalent in the future? Explain your answer.

Organization of the Text

In *Alice in Wonderland*, Lewis Carroll wrote, "Any road will do if you don't know where you are going." Therefore, the destination of this book has been carefully charted: the readers of this text need to learn those finance principles and practices that are most important to managers in the health services industry. The organization of the book paves the road to this destination.

Part I (The Healthcare Environment) contains fundamental background materials essential to the practice of healthcare finance. Chapter 1 introduces the text, while Chapter 2 provides additional insights into the uniqueness of the health services industry. Healthcare finance cannot be studied in a vacuum because the practice of finance is profoundly influenced by the economic and social environment of the industry, including alternative types of ownership, taxes, and reimbursement methods.

Part II (Financial Accounting) begins the actual discussion of healthcare finance principles and practices. Financial accounting, which involves the creation of statements that summarize a business' financial status, is most useful for managing at the organizational (aggregate) level. In Chapter 3, financial accounting concepts and the income statement are discussed, while in Chapter 4 the balance sheet and statement of cash flows are reviewed. Part III (Managerial Accounting), which consists of Chapters 5 through 8, focuses on the creation of data used in the day-to-day management and control of a business. Here, the focus changes from the aggregate organization to sub-unit (department) level management. The key topics in Part III include cost behavior, profit planning, cost allocation, pricing and service decisions, and planning and budgeting.

In Part IV (Basic Financial Analysis Concepts), the focus moves from accounting to financial management. Chapter 9 covers time value analysis, which provides techniques for valuing future cash flows, and Chapter 10 presents financial risk and return, one of the most important concepts in financial decision making. Part V (Long-Term Financing) turns to the capital acquisition process. Businesses need capital, or funds, to purchase assets, and in Chapters 11 and 12, the two primary types of long-term financing—long-term debt and equity—are examined. These chapters not only provide descriptive information about securities and the markets in which they are traded, but discuss security valuation. Chapter 13 provides the framework for analyzing the appropriate mix of capital financing and assessing its cost to the business.

In Part VI (Capital Investment Decisions), the vital topic of how businesses analyze new capital investment opportunities (or capital budgeting) is considered. Because major capital projects take years to plan and execute, and because these decisions generally are not easily reversed and will affect operations for many years, their impact on the future of an organization is profound. Chapter 14 focuses on basic concepts, while Chapter 15 discusses risk assessment and incorporation.

Part VII (Other Topics) contains two unrelated chapters. In Chapter 16, the management of short-term assets is reviewed, including cash, receivables, and inventories, as well as how such assets are financed. The techniques used to analyze a business' financial and operating condition are discussed in Chapter 17. Healthcare managers must be able to assess the current financial condition of their organizations. Even more important, managers must be able to monitor and control current operations, and to assess ways in which alternative courses of action will affect the organization's future financial condition.

1. Briefly, what is the organization of this book?

Self-Test Question

How to Use This Text

As mentioned earlier, the overriding goal in creating this book is to provide an easy-to-read, content-filled introductory text on healthcare finance. This book contains several features designed to assist in learning the material.

First, pay particular attention to the *learning objectives* listed at the beginning of each chapter. These objectives provide a feel for the most important topics in each chapter and what readers should set as learning goals for that chapter. After each major section, except the introduction, one or more *self-test questions* are included. Try to provide reasonable answers to these questions. They do not need to be expert answers, so after answering the question with a fairly accurate response, it is safe to move on to the next section. If a fairly accurate response cannot be provided, it would be best to reread that section before proceeding. Answers are not provided for the self-test questions, so review the section preceding the question to obtain the answer when necessary.

Within the text, italics and boldface are used to indicate importance. *Italics* are used whenever a key term is introduced. Thus, italics alert readers that a new and important concept is being presented. **Boldface** is solely used for emphasis. Thus, the meaning of a boldfaced phrase has unusual significance to the point under discussion.

In addition to in-chapter learning aids, materials designed to help readers learn healthcare finance are included at the end of each chapter. First, each chapter ends with a summary section titled "Key Concepts." These sections very briefly summarize the most important principles and practices covered in the chapter. If the meaning of the key concepts is not apparent, readers may find it useful to review the applicable sections. Each chapter also contains a series of questions designed to assess the understanding of the conceptual, qualitative material in the chapter. The questions are followed by a set of problems designed to assess understanding of the quantitative material.

Finally, each chapter ends with a set of references. The books and articles cited here can provide a more in-depth understanding of the material covered in the chapter. Taken together, the pedagogic structure of the text is designed to make the learning of healthcare finance as easy and enjoyable as possible.

Key Concepts

This chapter provided an introduction to healthcare finance. The key concepts of this chapter are:

- The term *healthcare finance*, as it is used in this book, means the accounting and financial management principles and practices used within health services organizations to ensure the financial well-being of the enterprise.
- The *primary role of finance* in health services organizations, as in all businesses, is to plan for, acquire, and utilize resources to maximize the efficiency and value of the enterprise.
- Finance activities generally include the following: (1) *planning and budgeting,* (2) *long-term investment decisions,* (3) *financing decisions,* (4) *short-term asset management,* and (5) *contract management.*

- All business decisions have *financial implications,* so all managers—whether in operations, marketing, personnel, or facilities—must know enough about finance to incorporate its implications into their own specialized decision making processes.
- Healthcare services are provided in numerous settings, including hospitals, ambulatory care facilities, long-term care facilities, and even at home.
- *Hospitals* differ in function (*general, acute care* versus *specialty*), patient length of stay, size, and ownership (*governmental* versus *private* and, within the private sector, *for profit* versus *not for profit*).
- *Ambulatory care,* also known as *outpatient care,* encompasses services provided to noninstitutionalized patients. Outpatient settings include medical (physician) practices, hospital outpatient departments, ambulatory surgery centers, urgent care centers, diagnostic imaging centers, rehabilitation/sports medicine centers, and clinical laboratories.
- *Home health care* brings many of the same services provided in ambulatory care settings into the patient's home.
- *Long-term care* entails healthcare services that cover an extended period of time, including inpatient, outpatient, and home health care, often with a focus on mental health, rehabilitation, or nursing home care.
- The defining characteristic of an *integrated delivery system* is that the organization assumes full clinical, and in certain cases financial, responsibility for the healthcare needs of the covered population.

In the next chapter, the discussion of the healthcare environment is continued, moving to more finance-related topics such as forms of organization, reimbursement, and taxes.

Questions

1.1 a. What are some of the industries in the healthcare sector?
   b. What is meant by the term *healthcare finance* as used in this book?
   c. What are the two broad areas of healthcare finance?
   d. Why is it necessary to have a book on healthcare finance as opposed to using a generic text?

1.2 a. Briefly discuss the role of finance in the health services industry.
   b. Has this role increased or decreased in importance in recent years?

1.3 a. Briefly describe the following health services settings:
     (1) Hospitals
     (2) Ambulatory care
     (3) Home health care
     (4) Long-term care
     (5) Integrated delivery systems
   b. What are the benefits attributed to integrated delivery systems?

1.4 Describe the organization of the text and the learning tools embedded in each chapter.

Notes

1. Not-for-profit organizations are also called *nonprofit* organizations, but the former designation is becoming dominant within the health services industry. Also, investor-owned firms are sometimes called *proprietary*, or *for-profit*, firms. The differences in these forms of ownership are discussed in detail in Chapter 2.
2. Hospital ownership is briefly overviewed here. The effect of ownership on finance goals is considered in greater detail in Chapter 2.

References

For a general introduction to the healthcare system in the United States, see

Lee, P. R. and C. L. Estes. 1997. *The Nation's Health.* Sudbury, MA: Jones and Bartlett.

Raffel, M. W. and N. K. Raffel. 1989. *The U.S. Health System.* New York: John Wiley & Sons.

Williams, S. J. and P. R. Torrens. 1999. *Introduction to Health Services.* Albany, NY: Delmar Publishers.

For the latest information on events that affect healthcare organizations, see

Medical Benefits, published semimonthly by Kelly Communications, Inc., Charlottesville, VA.

Modern Healthcare, published weekly by Crain Communications Inc., Chicago.

For ideas on the future of healthcare in the United States, see

Kajander, J. and M. Samuels. 1996. "Future Trends in the Health Care Economy." *Journal of Health Care Finance* (Fall): 17–22.

National Coalition on Health Care. 1997. "How Americans Perceive the Health Care System: A Report on a National Survey." *Journal of Health Care Finance* (Summer): 12–20.

Sullivan, J. M. 1992. "Health Care Reform: Towards a Healthier Society." *Hospital & Health Services Administration* (Winter): 519–532.

Taylor, R. and L. Lessin. 1996. "Restructuring the Health Care Delivery System in the United States." *Journal of Health Care Finance* (Summer): 33–60.

THE FINANCIAL ENVIRONMENT

Learning Objectives

After studying this chapter, readers will be able to:

- Describe the alternative forms of business organization and ownership.
- Explain why taxes are important to healthcare finance.
- Briefly describe the third-party payor system.
- Explain the different types of payment methods used by payors.
- Describe the major trends in the healthcare sector influencing health services organizations.

Introduction

Fortunately, most of the basic concepts of accounting and financial management are independent of the industry and organizational setting. However, some aspects of healthcare finance are influenced by industry setting, while the unique ownership structure of healthcare providers influences specific applications of finance concepts.

In this chapter, some background material is presented that creates the context in which finance is practiced in health services organizations. The fact that many healthcare businesses are organized as not-for-profit corporations has a significant impact on the practice of finance. Thus, the chapter begins with a discussion of alternative forms of business organization and ownership. Because ownership affects taxes, tax laws also are briefly introduced. Third-party payors and the reimbursement methods that they use are then examined. The chapter ends with a broad discussion of how managed care is changing the financial environment of health services organizations.

Alternative Forms of Business Organization

Throughout the text, the focus is on business finance—that is, the practice of accounting and financial management within business organizations. There are three primary forms of *business organization*: proprietorship, partnership, and corporation. Because most health services managers work for corporations and because not-for-profit businesses are organized as corporations, this form of organization is emphasized. However, many individual physician practices are organized as proprietorships, and partnerships are common in group practices and joint ventures. Health services managers must therefore be familiar with all forms of business organization.

Proprietorship

A *proprietorship*, sometimes called a *sole proprietorship*, is a business owned by one individual. Going into business as a proprietor is easy—the owner merely begins business operations. However, most cities require even the smallest businesses to be licensed, and state licensure is required for most healthcare professionals.

The proprietorship form of organization is easily and inexpensively formed, is subject to few governmental regulations, and pays no corporate income taxes. All earnings of the business, whether reinvested in the business or withdrawn by the owner, are taxed as personal income to the proprietor. In general, a sole proprietorship will pay lower total taxes than a comparable taxable corporation because corporate profits are taxed twice—once at the corporate level and again by stockholders at the personal level when profits are distributed as dividends or when capital gains are realized.

Partnership

A *partnership* is formed when two or more persons associate to conduct a non-incorporated business. Partnerships may operate under different degrees of formality, ranging from informal, oral understandings to formal agreements filed with the state in which the partnership does business. Like a proprietorship, the major advantage of the partnership form of organization is its low cost and ease of formation. In addition, the tax treatment of a partnership is similar to that of a proprietorship; the partnership's earnings are allocated to the partners and taxed as personal income regardless of whether the earnings are actually paid out to the partners or retained in the business.[1]

Proprietorships and partnerships have three important limitations:

1. Selling their interest in the business is difficult for owners.
2. The owners have unlimited personal liability for the debts of the business, which can result in losses greater than the amount invested in the business. In a proprietorship, unlimited liability means that the owner is personally responsible for the debts of the business. In a partnership, it means that if any partner is unable to meet his or her pro rata obligation in the event of bankruptcy, the remaining partners are responsible for the unsatisfied claims and must draw on their personal assets if necessary.
3. The life of the business is limited to the life of the owners.

For these reasons, proprietorships and most partnerships are restricted primarily to small businesses.[2]

These three disadvantages—difficulty in transferring ownership, unlimited liability, and impermanence of the business—lead to the fourth, and perhaps the most important, disadvantage from a finance perspective—the difficulty that proprietorships and partnerships have in attracting substantial amounts of capital. This is no particular problem for a slow-growing business or when the owners are very wealthy, but for most businesses, the difficulty of attracting capital becomes a real handicap if the business needs to expand rapidly to take advantage of market opportunities. Thus, many growth companies start out as sole proprietorships or partnerships, but then ultimately convert to the corporate form of organization.

Corporation

A *corporation* is a legal entity that is separate and distinct from its owners and managers. The creation of a separate business entity gives the corporation three main advantages:

1. A corporation has unlimited life and can continue in existence after its original owners and managers have died or left the company.
2. It is easy to transfer ownership in a corporation because ownership is divided into shares of stock that can be easily sold.
3. Owners of a corporation have limited liability.

To illustrate limited liability, suppose that one person made an investment of $10,000 in a partnership that subsequently went bankrupt, owing $100,000. Because the partners are liable for the debts of the partnership, that partner could be assessed for a share of the partnership's debt in addition to the initial $10,000 contribution. In fact, if the other partners were unable to pay their shares of the indebtedness, one partner would be held liable for the entire $100,000. However, if the $10,000 had been invested in a corporation that went bankrupt, the potential loss for the investor would be limited to the $10,000 investment. (However, in the case of small, financially weak corporations, the limited liability feature of ownership is often fictitious because bankers and other lenders will require personal guarantees from the stockholders.) With these three factors—unlimited life, ease of ownership transfer, and limited liability—corporations can more easily raise money in the financial markets than sole proprietorships or partnerships can.[3]

The corporate form of organization has two primary disadvantages. First, corporate earnings of taxable entities are subject to double taxation; once at the corporate level and again at the personal level when dividends are paid to stockholders or capital gains are realized. Second, setting up a corporation and then filing the required periodic state and federal reports is more costly and time-consuming than what is required to establish a proprietorship or partnership.

Although a proprietorship or partnership can begin operations without much legal paperwork, setting up a corporation requires that the founders, or their attorney, prepare a charter and a set of bylaws. Today, attorneys have standard forms for charters and bylaws on their computers, so they can set up a "no frills" corporation with much less work than what would have been required in the past. However, setting up a corporation remains relatively difficult when compared to a proprietorship or partnership, and still more difficult if the corporation has nonstandard features.

The *charter* includes the name of the corporation, its proposed activities, the amount of stock to be issued (if investor owned), and the number and names of the initial set of directors. The charter is filed with the appropriate official of the state in which the business will be incorporated, and when approved, the corporation is officially in existence.[4] After the corporation has been officially formed, it must file quarterly and annual financial and tax reports with state and federal agencies.

The *bylaws* are a set of rules drawn up by the founders to provide guidance for the governing and internal management of the corporation. Bylaws include features such as how directors are to be elected, whether the existing shareholders have the first right to buy any new shares that the firm issues, and the procedures for changing the charter or bylaws.

The value of any investor-owned business, other than a very small one, generally will be maximized if it is organized as a corporation for the following three reasons:

1. Limited liability reduces the risks borne by equity investors (the owners); with all else the same, the lower the risk, the higher the value of the investment.
2. A business' value is dependent on growth opportunities, which in turn are dependent on the business' ability to attract capital. Because corporations can obtain capital more easily than can other forms of business, they are better able to take advantage of growth opportunities.
3. The value of any investment depends on its *liquidity*, which means the ease at which it can be sold for a fair price. Because an equity investment in a corporation is much more liquid than a similar investment in a proprietorship or partnership, the corporate form of organization creates more value for its owners.

Hybrid Forms of Organization

Although the three basic forms of organization—proprietorship, partnership, and corporation—dominate the overall business scene, several hybrid forms of organization also are used by businesses. Some of these forms are found in the health services industry.

Several specialized types of partnerships have characteristics somewhat different than a standard form of partnership. First, limiting some of the partners' liabilities is possible by establishing a *limited partnership*, wherein certain partners are designated *general partners* and others *limited partners*. The limited partners, like the owners of a corporation, are liable only for the amount of their investment in the partnership, while the general partners have unlimited liability. However, the limited partners typically have no control, which rests solely with the general partners. Limited partnerships are quite common in real estate and mineral investments; they are not as common in the health services industry, however, because in this setting finding one partner that is willing to accept all of the business' risk and a second partner that is willing to relinquish control is difficult.

The *limited liability partnership* (*LLP*) is a relatively new type of partnership that is available in many states. In a limited liability partnership, the general partners have joint liability for all actions of the partnership, including professional malpractice and indebtedness. However, all partners enjoy limited liability regarding professional malpractice because partners are only liable for their own individual malpractice actions, not those of the other partners. In spite of limited malpractice liability, the partners are jointly liable for the partnership's debts. Menomonee Falls Ambulatory Surgery Center, in Wisconsin, is an example of a LLP.

The *limited liability company* (*LLC*) is another new type of business organization. It has some characteristics of both a partnership and a corporation. The owners of a LLC are called *members*, and they are taxed as if they are partners in a partnership. However, a member's liability is like that of a stockholder of a corporation because liability is limited to the member's initial contribution in the business. Personal assets are only at risk if the member assumes specific liability, such as by signing a personal loan guarantee. Both the LLP and LLC are new and complex forms of organizations, so setting them up can be time consuming and costly. Charter Behavioral Health Systems, the nation's largest behavioral health system, is an example of a LLC.

The *professional corporation (PC)*, which is called a *professional association (PA)* in some states, is a form of organization that is common among physicians and other individual and group practice healthcare professionals. All 50 states have statutes that prescribe the requirements for such corporations, which provide the usual benefits of incorporation, but do not relieve the participants of professional liability. Indeed, the primary motivation behind the professional corporation, which is a relatively old business form compared to the LLP and LLC, was to provide a way for professionals to incorporate, yet still be held liable for professional malpractice.

PCs have tight restrictions, however. First, one or more owners must be licensed in the profession of the PC. Second, PCs are taxed as corporations; they cannot be designated as an S corporation for tax purposes (see the following paragraph). The Atlanta Cardiology Group, comprising 20 physicians who provide a full range of cardiac services at multiple sites, typifies a PC.

For tax purposes, standard for-profit corporations are called *C corporations*. If certain requirements are met, either one or a few individuals can incorporate, but, for tax purposes only, elect to be treated as if the business were a proprietorship or partnership. Such corporations, which differ only in how the owners are taxed, are called *S corporations*. Although S corporations are similar to LLPs and LLCs regarding taxes, LLPs and LLCs provide more flexibility and benefits to owners. Many businesses, especially group practices, are therefore converting to the newer forms.

Self-Test Questions

1. What are the three major forms of business organization, and how do they differ?
2. What are some different types of partnerships?
3. What are some different types of corporations?

Alternative Forms of Ownership

Unlike other sectors in the economy, not-for-profit corporations play a major role in the healthcare sector, especially among providers. For example, about half of the hospitals in the United States are private, not-for-profit hospitals. Only 20 percent of all hospitals are investor owned; the remaining 30 percent are governmental. Furthermore, not-for-profit ownership is common in the nursing home, home health care, and managed care industries.

Investor-Owned Corporations

When the average person thinks of a corporation, he or she probably thinks of an *investor-owned*, or *for-profit, corporation*. Larger businesses (e.g., Ford, IBM, and General Electric) are investor-owned corporations.

Investors become owners of such businesses by buying shares of *common stock* in the company. Investors may buy common stock when it is first sold by the company. Such sales are called *primary market transactions*. In a primary market transaction, the funds raised from the sale generally go to the corporation.[5] After the shares have been initially sold by the corporation, they are traded in the *secondary market*. These sales may take place on *exchanges* such as the New York Stock Exchange (NYSE) and the American Stock Exchange (AMEX). They may also take place in the *over-the-counter (OTC) market*, which is composed of a large number of dealer/brokers connected by a sophisticated electronic trading system. When shares are bought and sold in the secondary market, the corporations whose stocks are traded receive no funds from the trades (corporations receive funds only when shares are first sold to investors).

Investor-owned corporations may be either publicly held or privately held. The shares of *publicly held* companies are owned by a large number of investors and are widely traded. For example, Columbia/HCA Healthcare, which owns and operates over 300 hospitals and has over 500 million shares outstanding, is owned by some 50,000 individual and institutional stockholders. Another example is Beverly Enterprises, which owns and operates about 775 nursing homes and has over 80 million shares outstanding owned by about 8,000 stockholders. Drug companies such as Merck and Pfizer, and medical equipment manufacturers such as St. Jude Medical, which makes heart valves, and U.S. Surgical, which makes surgical stapling instruments, are all publicly held corporations.

Conversely, the shares of *privately held* (also called *closely held*) companies are owned by just a handful of investors and are not publicly traded. In general, the managers of privately held companies are major stockholders. In regards to ownership and control, therefore, privately held companies are more similar to partnerships than to publicly held companies. Often, the privately held corporation is a transitional form of organization that exists for a short time between a proprietorship and a publicly owned corporation in which the motivation to go public is driven by capital needs. Community Health Systems, a Tennessee company that owns or manages over 35 hospitals in 14 states, is an example of a closely held company in the health services industry.

The *stockholders* (also called *shareholders*) are the owners of investor-owned companies. As owners, they have three basic rights:

1. *The right of control.* Common stockholders have the right to vote for the corporation's board of directors, which oversees the management of the company. Each year, a company's stockholders receive a *proxy* ballot, which they use to vote for directors and to vote on other issues that are proposed by management or stockholders. In this way, stockholders exercise control. In the voting process, stockholders cast one vote for each common share held.
2. *A claim on the residual earnings of the firm.* A corporation sells products or services and realizes revenues from the sales. To produce these revenues, the corporation must incur expenses for materials, labor, insurance, debt capital, and so on. Any excess of revenues over expenses—the residual earnings—belong to the shareholders of the business. Often, a portion of these earnings is paid out in the form of *dividends*, which are merely cash payments to stockholders, or *stock repurchases,* in which the company buys back shares held by stockholders. However, management typically elects to reinvest some (or all) of the residual earnings in the business, which presumably will produce even higher payouts to stockholders in the future.
3. *A claim on liquidation proceeds.* In the event of bankruptcy and liquidation, shareholders are entitled to any proceeds that remain after all other claimants have been satisfied.

In summary, there are three key features of investor-owned corporations. First, the owners (the stockholders) of the business are well defined and exercise control of the firm by voting for directors. Second, the residual earnings of the business belong to the owners, so management is responsible only to the stockholders for the profitability of the firm. Finally, investor-owned corporations are subject to taxation at the local, state, and federal levels.

Not-For-Profit Corporations

If an organization meets a set of stringent requirements, it can qualify for incorporation as a *tax-exempt*, or *not-for-profit, corporation.* Tax-exempt corporations are sometimes called *nonprofit corporations.* Because nonprofit **businesses** (as opposed to pure charities) need profits to sustain operations, and because it is hard to explain why nonprofit corporations should earn profits, the term "not-for-profit" is more descriptive of such health services corporations.

Tax-exempt status is granted to businesses that meet the tax definition of a charitable corporation, as defined by Internal Revenue Service (IRS) Tax Code Section 501(c)(3) or (4). Hence, such corporations are also known as *501(c)(3) or (4) corporations.*[6] The tax code defines a charitable organization as, " . . . any corporation, community chest, fund, or foundation that is organized and operated exclusively for religious, charitable, scientific, public safety, literary, or educational purposes." Because the promotion of health is commonly considered a charitable activity, a corporation that provides healthcare services can qualify for tax-exempt status provided that it meets other requirements.

In addition to the charitable purpose, a not-for-profit corporation must be organized and operated so that it operates exclusively for the public, rather than private, interest. Thus, no profits can be used for private gain and no political activity can be conducted. Also, if the corporation is liquidated or if sold to an investor-owned firm, the proceeds from the liquidation or sale must be used for a charitable purpose. Because individuals cannot benefit from the profits of not-for-profit corporations, such organizations cannot pay dividends. However, prohibition of private gain from profits does not prevent parties, such as managers and physicians, of not-for-profit corporations from benefiting through salaries, perquisites, contracts, and so on.

Not-for-profit corporations differ significantly from investor-owned corporations. Because not-for-profit firms have no shareholders, no single body of individuals has ownership rights to the firm's residual earnings or exercises control of the firm. Rather, control is exercised by a board of trustees that is not constrained by outside oversight. Also, not-for-profit corporations are generally exempt from taxation, including both property and income taxes, and have the right to issue tax-exempt debt (municipal bonds). Finally, individual contributions to not-for-profit organizations can be deducted from taxable income by the donor, so not-for-profit firms have access to tax-subsidized contribution capital. (The tax benefits enjoyed by not-for-profit corporations are reviewed in a later section on tax laws.)

The financial problems facing most federal, state, and local governments have caused politicians to take a closer look at the tax subsidies provided to not-for-profit hospitals. For example, several bills have been introduced in Congress that require hospitals to meet minimum standards for care to the indigent to retain tax-exempt status. Also, officials in several states have been fighting to restrict or strip tax exemptions to hospitals, or to specify mandatory levels of charity care. For example, Texas has established minimum requirements for charity care, which in effect hold not-for-profit hospitals accountable to the public for the tax exemptions they receive. The Texas law specifies four tests and each hospital must meet at least one of them. The test that most hospitals use to comply with the law requires that four percent of net patient service revenue be spent for charity care.

Finally, money-starved municipalities in several states have attacked the property tax exemption of not-for-profit hospitals that have "neglected" their charitable missions. For example, tax assessors are fighting to remove property tax exemptions from not-for-profit hospitals in several Pennsylvania cities after a recent appellate court ruling supported the Erie school district's authority to tax a local hospital that had strayed too far from its charitable purpose. According to one estimate, if all not-for-profit hospitals had to pay taxes comparable to their investor-owned counterparts, local, state, and federal governments would garner an additional $3.5 billion in tax revenues. This explains why tax authorities in some jurisdictions are pursuing not-for-profit hospitals as a source of revenue.[7]

The inherent differences between investor-owned and not-for-profit organizations have profound implications for many elements of healthcare finance, including organizational goals, financing decisions (i.e., the choice between debt and equity financing and the specific types of securities to issue), and capital investment decisions. How ownership affects the application of healthcare finance concepts will be addressed throughout the book.

Self-Test Questions

1. What are the major differences between investor-owned and not-for-profit corporations?
2. What pressures recently have been placed on not-for-profit hospitals to ensure that they meet their charitable mission?

Organizational Goals

Financial decisions are not made in a vacuum, but with an objective in mind. Finance goals within an organization clearly must be consistent with and in support of the overall goals of the business. Thus, by discussing organizational goals, a framework for financial decision making within health services organizations is provided.

In a proprietorship or partnership, the owners of the business generally are also its managers. In theory, the business can be operated for the exclusive benefit of the owners. If the owners want to work very hard to maximize wealth, they can. On the other hand, if every Wednesday is devoted to golf, no one is hurt by such actions. (Of course, the business still has to cater to its customers or else it will not survive.) It is in corporations, in which owners and managers are separate parties, that organizational goals become very important to finance.

Investor-Owned Corporations

From a finance perspective, the primary goal of investor-owned corporations is generally assumed to be *shareholder wealth maximization*, which translates to stock price maximization. Investor-owned firms do, of course, have other goals. Managers who make the actual decisions are interested in their own personal welfare, in their employees' welfare, and in the good of the community and of society at large. Still, the goal of stock price maximization is a reasonable operating objective upon which to build financial decision rules.

The primary obstacle to shareholder wealth maximization as the goal of investor-owned firms is the *agency problem*. An agency problem exists when one or more individuals (the *principals*) hire another individual or group of individuals (the *agents*) to perform a service on their behalf, and then delegate a decision-making authority to those agents. Within the healthcare finance framework, the agency problem exists between stockholders and managers, and between debtholders and stockholders. (The stockholder/manager problem is reviewed in this chapter, but the review of the debtholder/stockholder problem is deferred until Chapter 11).

The agency problem between stockholders and managers occurs because the managers of large, investor-owned firms hold only a very small proportion of the firm's stock, so they benefit very little from stock price increases. On the other hand, managers benefit substantially from such actions as increasing the size of the firm to justify higher salaries and more fringe benefits; awarding themselves generous retirement plans; and spending too much on office space, personal staff, and travel—actions often detrimental to shareholders' wealth. Clearly, many situations can arise in which managers are motivated to take actions that are in their best interests, rather than in the best interests of the firm's stockholders.

Shareholders recognize the agency problem and counter it by creating compensation incentives, such as stock options and performance-based bonus plans, that encourage managers to act in shareholders' interests. Additionally, other factors, such as the threat of takeover or removal, are at work to keep managers focused on shareholder wealth maximization.

Clearly, managers of investor-owned corporations can have motivations that are inconsistent with shareholder wealth maximization. Still, sufficient incentives are in place to force managers to view shareholder wealth maximization as their primary goal. Thus, shareholder wealth maximization is a reasonable goal for financial decision making within investor-owned corporations.

Not-for-Profit Corporations

Because not-for-profit corporations do not have shareholders, shareholder wealth maximization is not an appropriate goal for such organizations. Not-for-profit firms consist of a number of classes of *stakeholders* who are directly affected by the organization. Stakeholders include all parties that have an interest, usually of a financial nature, in the organization. For example, a not-for-profit hospital's stakeholders include the board of trustees, managers, employees, physicians, creditors, suppliers, patients, and even potential patients, which may include the entire community. An investor-owned hospital has the same set of stakeholders, plus one additional class—stockholders. While managers of investor-owned companies have to please only one class of stakeholders—the shareholders—to keep their jobs, managers of not-for-profit firms face a different situation. They have to try to please all of the organization's stakeholders because no single, well-defined group exercises control.

Many people argue that managers of not-for-profit firms do not have to please anyone at all, because they tend to dominate the board of trustees who are supposed to exercise oversight. Others argue that managers of not-for-profit firms have to please all of the firm's stakeholders to a greater or lesser extent because all are necessary to the successful performance of the business. Of course, even managers of investor-owned firms should not attempt to enhance shareholder wealth by treating any of their firm's other stakeholders unfairly because such actions ultimately will be detrimental to shareholders.

Typically, the goal of not-for-profit firms is stated in terms of a mission. An example is the current mission statement of Riverside Memorial Hospital, a 450-bed, not-for-profit, acute care hospital:

> Riverside Memorial Hospital, along with its medical staff, is a recognized, innovative healthcare leader dedicated to meeting the needs of the community. We strive to be the best comprehensive healthcare provider through our commitment to excellence.

Although this mission statement provides Riverside's managers and employees with a framework for developing specific goals and objectives, it does not provide much insight into the goal of the hospital's finance function. For Riverside to accomplish its mission, its managers have identified five financial goals:

1. The hospital must maintain its financial viability.
2. The hospital must generate sufficient profits to continue to provide the current range of healthcare services to the community. This means that current buildings and equipment must be replaced as they become obsolete.
3. The hospital must generate sufficient profits to invest in new medical technologies and services as they are developed and needed.
4. Although the hospital has an aggressive philanthropy program in place, it does not want to rely upon this program or government grants to fund its operations.
5. The hospital will strive to provide services to the community as inexpensively as possible, given the above financial requirements.

In effect, Riverside's managers are saying that to achieve the hospital's commitment to excellence as stated in its mission statement, the hospital must remain financially strong and profitable. Financially weak organizations cannot continue to accomplish their stated missions over the long run. What is interesting is that Riverside's five financial goals are probably not much different from the finance goals of Jefferson Regional Medical Center (JRMC), a for-profit competitor. Of course, JRMC has to worry about providing a return to its shareholders, and it receives only a very small amount of contributions and grants. However, to maximize shareholder wealth, JRMC also must retain its financial viability and have the financial resources necessary to offer new services and technologies. Furthermore, competition in the market for hospital services will not permit JRMC to charge appreciably more for services than its not-for-profit competitors.

Self-Test Questions

1. What is the difference in goals between investor-owned and not-for-profit firms?
2. What is the agency problem, and how does it apply to investor-owned firms?
3. What factors tend to reduce the agency problem?

Tax Laws

The value of any investment—whether the investment is a stock, a bond, or an entire business—depends on the **usable** cash flows (i.e., the cash flows after all taxes have been paid) that the investment is expected to provide to the owner. Thus, a book on healthcare finance has to be concerned about taxes, at least for those businesses that must pay them.

Tax laws are very complicated and are constantly changing. Consequently, covering even the most basic features of our tax laws in an introductory finance text is impossible. However, what is important is to recognize that individuals must pay *personal* (*individual*) *taxes* to federal and state (in most states) authorities that can exceed 50 percent of income. Thus, income from proprietorships and partnerships, as well as dividends and capital gains on stock investments, will be reduced by up to half when personal taxes are taken into account.

To illustrate the effect of personal taxes, assume that a person's tax rate is 40 percent and he or she receives $100 in dividends on HEALTHSOUTH stock. Using the letter T to represent tax rate, that person must pay T × $100 = 0.40 × $100 = $40 in taxes on the dividend, which leaves him or her with only $100 − $40 = $60 on an after-tax basis. This tax analysis leads to the following useful equation:

$$AT = BT - (T \times BT)$$

$$= BT \times (1 - T)$$

where AT = after tax, and BT = before tax. To illustrate, the after-tax dividend amount for the preceding example is AT = BT × (1 − T) = $100 × (1 − 0.40) = $100 × 0.60 = $60. (This equation can be applied to interest rates as well as dollar amounts. See Problem 2.3 as an example.) Clearly, taxes will influence investment decisions, so any differential tax implications on investment alternatives must be considered in the decision process.

In addition to personal taxes paid by individuals, investor-owned (for-profit) corporations must pay both federal and state *corporate taxes*, which can exceed 40 percent of the corporation's taxable income. Corporate taxes are paid on earnings before dividends are distributed, so corporate income is really subject to double taxation—once at the corporate level and again when stockholders receive dividends.

Not-for-profit corporations, for the most part, are not subject to taxation. Also, such organizations benefit from being able to issue debt with interest payments that are exempt from personal taxes. To illustrate the advantage of being able to issue tax-exempt debt, first consider the bonds issued by Jefferson Regional Medical Center (JRMC), an investor-owned hospital. Its debt carries an interest rate of 10 percent, so bond investors receive 0.10 × $100 = $10 in interest for every $100 worth of bonds that they own. For a bond investor that pays 40 percent in federal and state income taxes, each $10 of interest requires 0.40 × $10 = $4 in taxes, so the investor is left with $6 of after-tax interest. However, if the bonds had been issued by Riverside Memorial Hospital, a not-for-profit corporation, the investor would have to pay no taxes on the interest, and hence would keep the entire $10. If investors are satisfied with a $6 after-tax return, Riverside can issue debt with an interest rate of only 6 percent and, with all else the same, investors in the 40 percent tax bracket would be as willing to buy these bonds as they are the JRMC 10 percent bonds. Thus, the interest rate that Riverside must set on its debt issues to sell them to investors is lower than the rate that JRMC must set because of the tax exemption on debt issued by not-for-profit corporations.

Finally, contributions that individuals make to not-for-profit corporations are tax deductible to the donor. If John Brooks is in the 40 percent tax bracket and he donates $1,000 to Riverside Memorial Hospital, his taxable income would be reduced by $1,000. A reduction in taxable income of this amount would save John $T \times \$1,000 = 0.40 \times \$1,000 = \$400$ in taxes. Thus, the effective cost of his contribution would only be $600. In effect, the government will pay John 40 cents for every dollar he contributes. Thus, not-for-profit corporations have access to a source of income that, for all practical purposes, is not available to investor-owned firms.

Because of the impact that taxes have on usable earnings of investor-owned businesses and because not-for-profit ownership has important tax consequences, tax implications are highlighted and explained as necessary throughout the book. Still, what is important now is to recognize that taxes will play an important role in many topics to be discussed.

1. Why does a finance text have to consider taxes?
2. Why is the ability to issue tax-exempt debt an advantage for not-for-profit corporations?
3. What advantage accrues to businesses that can accept tax-exempt contributions?

Self-Test Questions

Third-Party Payors

Up to this point in the chapter, basic concepts about the form and ownership of healthcare businesses have been considered. A large proportion of the health services industry receives its revenues not directly from the users of their services—the patients—but rather from insurers known collectively as *third-party payors*. Because an organization's revenues are key to its financial viability, a brief examination of the source of most revenues in the health services industry is provided. In the next section, the types of reimbursement methods employed by payors is reviewed in more detail.

Health insurance originated in Europe in the early 1800s when mutual benefit societies were formed to reduce the financial burden associated with illness or injury. Today, health insurers fall into two broad categories: private insurers and public programs.[8]

Private Insurers

In the United States, the concept of public, or government, health insurance is relatively new, while private health insurance has been in existence since the turn of the century. In this section, the major private insurers are discussed: Blue Cross/Blue Shield, commercial insurers, and self-insurers.

Blue Cross/
Blue Shield

Blue Cross/Blue Shield organizations trace their roots to the Great Depression, when both hospitals and physicians were concerned about their patients' abilities to pay healthcare bills.

Blue Cross originated as a number of separate insurance programs offered by individual hospitals. At that time, many patients were unable to pay their hospital bills, but most people, except the very poorest, could afford to purchase some type of hospitalization insurance. Thus, the programs were initially designed to benefit hospitals as well as patients. The programs were all similar in structure: hospitals agreed to provide a certain amount of services to program members who made periodic payments of fixed amounts to the hospitals whether services were used or not. In a short time, these programs were expanded from single hospital programs to community-wide, multi-hospital plans that were called *hospital service plans*. The American Hospital Association (AHA) recognized the benefits of such plans to hospitals, so a close relationship was formed between the AHA and the organizations that offered hospital service plans.

In the early years, several states ruled that the sale of hospital services by prepayment did not constitute insurance, so the plans were exempt from regulations governing insurance companies. However, the legal status of hospital service plans clearly would be subject to future scrutiny unless their status was formalized. The states, one by one, passed enabling legislation that provided for the founding of not-for-profit hospital service corporations that were exempt both from taxes and from the capital requirements mandated for other insurers. However, state insurance departments had—and continue to have—oversight over most aspects of the plans' operations. The Blue Cross name was officially adopted by most of these plans in 1939.

Blue Shield plans developed in a manner similar to that of the Blue Cross plans, except that the providers were physicians instead of hospitals, and the professional organization was the American Medical Association (AMA) instead of the AHA. Today, almost 70 Blue Cross/Blue Shield (Blues) organizations exist; some offer only one of the two plans, but most offer both plans. The Blues are organized as local or statewide corporations, but all belong to a single, national association that sets standards that must be met to use the Blue Cross/Blue Shield name.

Historically, the Blues have been not-for-profit corporations that enjoyed the full benefits accorded to that status, including freedom from taxes. In 1986, however, Congress eliminated the Blues' tax exemption on the grounds that they operated commercial-type insurance activities. However, the plans were given special deductions, which resulted in taxes that are generally less than those paid by commercial insurance companies. In spite of the 1986 change in tax status, the national association continued to require all Blues to operate entirely as not-for-profit corporations, although they could establish for-profit subsidiaries. In 1994, however, the national association lifted its traditional ban on member plans becoming investor-owned companies. Since that time several plans have converted to for-profit status.

Commercial health insurance is issued by life insurance companies, by casualty insurance companies, and by companies that were formed exclusively to write health insurance. Commercial insurance companies can be organized either as stock or mutual companies. *Stock* companies are shareholder owned, and can raise capital by selling shares of stock just like any other for-profit company. Further, the stockholders assume the risks and responsibilities of ownership and management. A *mutual* company has no shareholders; its management is controlled by a board of directors elected by the company's policyholders. Regardless of the form of ownership, commercial insurance companies are taxable entities. ***Commercial Insurers***

Commercial insurers moved strongly into health insurance following World War II. At that time, the United Auto Workers (UAW) negotiated the first contract with employers in which fringe benefits were a major part of the contract. Like the Blues, the majority of individuals with commercial health insurance are covered under *group policies* with employee groups, professional and other associations, and labor unions.

The third major form of private insurance is *self-insurance*. An argument can be made that all individuals who do not have some form of health insurance are self-insurers, but this is not technically correct. Self-insurers make a conscious decision to bear the risks associated with healthcare costs, and then set aside funds to pay future costs as they occur. Individuals are not good candidates for self-insurance because they face too much uncertainty concerning healthcare expenses. On the other hand, large groups, especially employers, are good candidates for self-insurance. Today, most large groups are self-insured. For example, employees of the State of Florida are covered by health insurance that is administered by Blue Cross/Blue Shield of Florida, but the actual benefits to plan members are paid directly by the state. Blue Cross/Blue Shield is paid for administering the plan, but the state bears all risks associated with cost and utilization uncertainty. ***Self-insurers***

Many firms today are even going one or two steps further in their self-insurance programs. For example, Digital Equipment Corporation, a major computer maker, negotiates discounts directly with hospitals and physicians and self-administers its program. Others, such as Deere & Company, a farm implements manufacturer, have set up company-owned subsidiaries to provide healthcare services to their employees. These companies believe that they can lower healthcare costs by applying the kind of management attention to healthcare that they do to their core businesses.

Public Insurers

Government is a major insurer as well as a direct provider of healthcare services. For example, the government provides healthcare services directly to qualifying individuals through the Department of Veterans Affairs (VA), Department of Defense (DOD), and Public Health Service (PHS) medical facilities. In addition, the government either provides or mandates a variety of insurance programs such as worker's compensation and TRICARE/CHAMPUS (Civilian Health and Medical Program of the Uniformed Services). In this section, however, the focus is on the two major government insurance programs: Medicare and Medicaid.

Medicare   *Medicare* was established by the federal government in 1966 to provide medical benefits to individuals age 65 and older. Medicare consists of two separate coverages: Part A provides hospital and some skilled nursing home coverage; Part B covers physician services, ambulatory surgical services, outpatient services, and other miscellaneous services. Part A coverage is free to all persons eligible for social security benefits. Individuals who are not eligible for social security benefits can obtain Part A medical benefits by paying premiums into the program. Part B, which requires a monthly premium, is optional to all individuals who have Part A coverage. About 97 percent of Part A participants purchase Part B coverage.

The Medicare program falls under the *Department of Health and Human Services (DHHS)*, which creates the specific rules of the program on the basis of enabling legislation. Medicare is administered by an agency under DHHS called the *Health Care Financing Administration (HCFA)*. HCFA has eight regional offices that oversee the Medicare program and ensure that regulations are followed.

Medicare payments to providers are not made directly by HCFA, but rather by contractors at state or local level called *intermediaries* for Part A payments and *carriers* for Part B payments.[9] Part A intermediaries are all either Blue Cross associations or commercial insurers. For example, Blue Cross/Blue Shield of Florida is the HCFA intermediary for Florida, while Aetna is the intermediary for Oklahoma.

Medicaid   *Medicaid* began in 1966 as a modest program to be jointly funded and operated by the states and the federal government to provide a medical safety net for low-income mothers and children, and for elderly, blind, and disabled individuals receiving benefits from the Supplemental Security Income (SSI) program. Congress mandated that Medicaid cover hospital and physician care, but states were encouraged to expand on the basic package of benefits either by increasing the range of benefits or extending the program to cover more people. States with large tax bases were quick to expand coverage to many groups, while states with limited abilities to raise funds for Medicaid were forced to construct more limited programs. A mandatory nursing home benefit was added in 1972.

Over the years, Medicaid has provided access to healthcare services for many low-income individuals who otherwise would have no insurance coverage.

Furthermore, Medicaid has become an important source of revenue for healthcare providers, especially for nursing homes and other providers that treat large numbers of indigent patients. However, Medicaid expenditures have been growing at an alarming rate, which has forced both federal and state policymakers to search for more effective ways to improve the program's access, quality, and cost.

1. What are some different types of private insurers?
2. Briefly, what are the origins and purpose of Medicare?
3. What is Medicaid, and how is it administered?

Self-Test Questions

Managed Care Plans

Managed care plans strive to combine the provision of healthcare services and the insurance function into a single entity. Traditionally, such plans have been created by insurers, who either directly own a provider network or create one through contractual arrangements with independent providers. Recently, however, providers in some areas have banded together to form *integrated delivery systems* (*IDSs*) that are capable of offering both insurance and healthcare services.

One type of managed care plan is the *health maintenance organization* (*HMO*). HMOs are based on the premise that the traditional insurer/provider relationship creates perverse incentives that reward providers for treating patients' illnesses while offering little incentive for providing prevention and rehabilitation services. By combining the financing and delivery of comprehensive healthcare services into a single system, HMOs theoretically have as strong an incentive to prevent as to treat illnesses.

Because of the many types of organizational structures, ownership, and financial incentives provided, HMOs vary widely in cost and quality. HMOs use a variety of methods to control costs. These include: limiting patients to particular providers by using *gatekeeper* physicians who must authorize any specialized or referral services; using utilization review to ensure that services rendered are appropriate and needed; offering discounted rate schedules for providers; and using payment methods that transfer some risk to providers. In general, services are not covered if beneficiaries bypass their gatekeeper physician or use providers that are not part of the HMO. Today, about 65 percent of all HMOs are investor owned, while the remaining 35 percent are not-for-profit entities.

The federal Health Maintenance Act of 1973 encouraged the development of HMOs and created a great deal of interest in the concept by providing federal funds for HMO-operating grants and loans. In addition, the act required larger employers offering healthcare benefits to their employees to include a federally qualified HMO as a healthcare alternative, if one was available, in addition to traditional insurance plans.

Another type of managed care plan, the *preferred provider organization* (*PPO*), evolved during the early 1980s. PPOs are a hybrid of HMOs and traditional health insurance plans that use many of the cost-saving strategies developed by HMOs. PPOs do not mandate that beneficiaries use specific providers, although financial incentives are created that encourage members to use those providers that are part of the *provider panel*, which are those providers having discounted-fee contracts with the PPO. Unlike HMOs, PPOs do not require beneficiaries to use preselected gatekeeper physicians who serve as the initial contact and authorize all services received. PPOs are less likely than HMOs to provide preventive services. PPOs also do not assume any responsibility for quality assurance because the enrollees are not constrained to use only the PPO panel of providers.

HMOs and PPOs grew rapidly in numbers and size during the 1980s, and have continued to expand thus far in the 1990s. Hybrids of HMOs and PPOs continue to develop. For example, *exclusive provider organizations (EPOs)* are PPO-like plans that require members to use only participating providers, but do not designate a specific gatekeeper. Also, *point of service (POS) plans* permit enrollees to choose either to obtain services from within the HMO or to bear higher out-of-pocket costs to obtain services from providers outside the HMO.

In an effort to achieve the potential cost savings of managed care plans, insurance companies have started to apply managed care strategies to their conventional plans. Such plans, which are called *managed fee-for-service plans*, are using preadmission certification, utilization review, and second surgical opinions to control inappropriate utilization. Although the distinctions between managed care and conventional plans were once quite apparent, considerable overlap now exists in the strategies and incentives employed. Thus, the term *managed care* now describes a continuum of plans, which can vary significantly in their approaches to providing combined insurance and healthcare services. The common feature in managed care plans is that the insurer has a mechanism by which it controls, or at least influences, patients' utilization of healthcare services.

Self-Test Questions

1. What is meant by the term *managed care*?
2. What are some different types of managed care plans?

Alternative Reimbursement Methods

Regardless of the payor for a particular healthcare service, only a limited number of payment methods are used to reimburse providers. Payment methods fall into two broad classifications: fee-for-service and capitation. In *fee-for-service* payment methods, of which many variations exist, the greater the amount of services provided, the higher the amount of reimbursement. Under *capitation*, a fixed payment is made to providers for each covered life that is independent of the amount of services provided. In this section, the mechanics of alternative payment methods are first considered. The incentives created for providers under the alternative methods are then discussed. Finally, the risk implications of the alternative reimbursement methods are analyzed.

The Methods

The three primary fee-for-service methods of reimbursement are: cost based, charge based, and prospective payment. In addition to the fee-for-service methods, some payors, especially managed care plans, pay by capitation. In this section, the methods are reviewed in more detail.

Under *cost-based reimbursement*, the payor agrees to reimburse the provider for costs incurred in providing services to the insured population. Reimbursement is limited to *allowable costs*, usually defined as those costs directly related to the provision of healthcare services. Nevertheless, for all practical purposes, cost-based reimbursement guarantees that a provider's costs will be covered by payments from payors. Typically, the payor makes *periodic interim payments (PIPs)* to the provider, and a final reconciliation is made after the contract period expires and all costs have been processed through the provider's accounting system. During the early years (1966–1983), Medicare reimbursed providers on the basis of costs incurred.

Cost-based Reimbursement

When payors pay *billed charges*, they pay according to the schedule of charge rates established by the provider. To a certain extent, this reimbursement system places payors at the mercy of providers in regards to the cost of healthcare services, especially in markets where competition is limited. In the very early days of health insurance, all payors reimbursed providers on the basis of billed charges. Some insurers still reimburse providers according to billed charges, but the trend for payors is toward other, less generous reimbursement methods. If this trend continues, the only payors that will be expected to pay billed charges are self-pay, or private-pay, patients.

Charge-based Reimbursement

Some payors that historically have reimbursed providers on the basis of billed charges now pay by *negotiated*, or *discounted*, *charges*. This is especially true for insurers that have established managed care plans such as HMOs and PPOs. Because HMOs and PPOs, as well as some conventional insurers, have bargaining power because of the large number of patients that they bring to a provider, they can negotiate discounts from billed charges. Such discounts generally range from 20 to 30 percent, or even more, of billed charges.

In a *prospective payment system*, the rates paid by payors are determined before the services are provided. Furthermore, payments are not directly related to either reimbursable costs or billed charges. Four common units of payment are included in the category of prospective payment:

Prospective Payment

1. *Per procedure:* Under *per procedure* reimbursement, a separate payment is made for each procedure performed on a patient. Because of the high administrative costs associated with this method when applied to complex

diagnoses, per procedure reimbursement is more commonly used in outpatient than in inpatient settings.

2. *Per diagnosis:* In the *per diagnosis* reimbursement method, the provider is paid a rate that depends on the patient's diagnosis. Diagnoses that require higher resource utilization, and hence are more costly to treat, have higher reimbursement rates. Medicare pioneered this basis of payment in its *diagnosis related group (DRG)* system, which it first used for hospital reimbursement in 1983.

3. *Per day (per diem):* If reimbursement is based on a *per diem* rate, the provider is paid a fixed amount for each day that service is provided, regardless of the nature of the services. This type of reimbursement is applicable only to inpatient settings. Note that per diem rates can be *stratified*. For example, a hospital may be paid one rate for a medical/surgical day, a higher rate for a critical care unit day, and yet a different rate for an obstetrical day. Stratified per diems recognize that providers incur widely different daily costs for providing different types of care.

4. *Global pricing:* Under *global pricing*, payors pay a single prospective payment that covers all services delivered in a single episode, whether the services are rendered by a single or by multiple providers. For example, a global fee may be set for all obstetric services associated with a pregnancy provided by a single physician, including all prenatal and postnatal visits, as well as the delivery. For another example, a global price may be paid for all physician and hospital services associated with a cardiac bypass operation.

Capitation   Up to this point, all the reimbursement methods presented have been fee-for-service methods. That is, providers are reimbursed on the basis of the amount of services provided. The service may be defined as a visit, a diagnosis, a hospital day, or in some other manner, but the key feature is that the more services that are performed, the greater the reimbursement amount. *Capitation*, although a form of prospective payment, is an entirely different approach to reimbursement, and hence deserves to be treated as a separate category. Under capitated reimbursement, the provider is paid a fixed amount per covered life per period (usually a month) regardless of the amount of services provided.

Capitation payment, which is used primarily by managed care plans, dramatically changes the financial landscape of healthcare providers. It has implications for financial accounting, managerial accounting, and financial management. A discussion of how capitation, as opposed to fee-for-service reimbursement, affects healthcare finance is provided throughout the remainder of this book.

Provider Incentives

Providers, like individuals or businesses, react to the incentives created by the financial environment. For example, individuals can deduct mortgage interest from income for tax purposes, but they cannot deduct interest payments on personal loans. Loan companies have responded by offering home equity loans that are a type of second mortgage. The intent is not that such loans would be used to finance home ownership, as the tax laws intended, but rather the funds can be used for any purpose, including vacations, cars, and appliances. In this situation, tax laws created incentives for consumers to have mortgage debt rather than personal debt, and the mortgage loan industry responded accordingly.

In the same vein, it is interesting to briefly examine the incentives that alternative reimbursement methods have on provider behavior. Under cost-based reimbursement, providers are given a "blank check" in regards to acquiring assets and incurring operating costs. If payors reimburse providers for all costs, the incentive is to incur costs. Facilities will be lavish and conveniently located, and staff will be available to ensure that patients are given "deluxe" treatment. Furthermore, as in billed charges reimbursement, services that may not truly be required will be provided because more services lead to higher costs, which means higher revenues.

Under charge-based reimbursement, providers have the incentive to set high charge rates, which lead to high revenues. However, in competitive markets, there will be a constraint on how high providers can go. But, to the extent that insurers, rather than patients, are footing the bill, there is often considerable leeway in setting charges. Because billed charges is a fee-for-service type of reimbursement, in which more services result in higher revenue, a strong incentive exists to provide the highest possible amount of services. In essence, providers can increase utilization, and hence revenues, by *churning*—creating more visits, ordering more tests, extending inpatient stays, and so on. Although charge-based reimbursement does encourage providers to contain costs, the incentive is weak because charges can be more easily increased than costs can be reduced. Note, however, that discounted charge reimbursement places additional pressure on profitability, and hence creates increased incentive for providers to lower costs.

Under prospective payment reimbursement, provider incentives are altered. First, under per procedure reimbursement, the profitability of individual procedures will vary depending on the relationship between the actual costs incurred and the payment for that procedure. Providers, usually physicians, have the incentive to perform procedures that have the highest profit potential. Furthermore, the more procedures the better because each procedure typically generates additional profit. The incentives under per diagnosis reimbursement are similar. Providers, usually hospitals, will seek patients with those diagnoses that have the greatest profit potential and discourage (even discontinue) those services that have the least potential. Furthermore, to the extent that providers have some flexibility in assigning diagnoses to patients, an incentive exists to *upcode* diagnoses to another one that provides greater reimbursement.

In all prospective payment methods, providers have the incentive to reduce costs because the amount of reimbursement is fixed and independent of the costs actually incurred. When per diem reimbursement is used, particularly with hospitals, providers have an incentive to increase length of stay. Because the early days of a hospitalization are typically more costly to the provider than the later days, the later days are more profitable. However, as mentioned previously, hospitals have the incentive to reduce costs during each day of a patient stay.

Under global pricing, providers do not have the opportunity to be reimbursed for a series of separate services, which is called *unbundling*. For example, a physician's treatment of a fracture could be bundled, and hence billed as one episode, or it could be unbundled with separate bills submitted for diagnosis, x-rays, setting the fracture, removing the cast, and so on. The rationale for unbundling is usually to provide more detailed records of treatments rendered, but often the result is higher total charges for the parts than would be charged for the entire package. Also, global pricing, when applied to multiple providers for a single episode of care, forces involved providers (e.g., physicians and a hospital) to jointly offer the most cost-effective treatment. Such a joint view of cost containment may be more effective than each provider separately attempting to minimize its treatment costs because lowering costs in one phase of treatment could increase costs in another.

Finally, capitation reimbursement totally changes the playing field by completely reversing the actions that providers must take to ensure financial success. Under all prospective payment methods, the key to provider success is to work harder, increase utilization, and hence increase profits; under capitation, the key to profitability is to work smarter and decrease utilization. As with prospective payment, capitated providers have the incentive to reduce costs, but now they also have the incentive to reduce utilization. Thus, only those procedures that are truly medically necessary should be performed, and treatment should take place in the lowest cost setting that can provide the appropriate quality of care. Furthermore, providers have the incentive to promote health, rather than just treat illness and injury, because a healthier population consumes fewer healthcare services.

Financial Risks to Providers

A key issue that providers face is the impact of various reimbursement methods on financial risk, which is a concept that is explained in detail in Chapter 10. For now, think of financial risk in terms of the effect that the reimbursement methods have on profit uncertainty—the greater the chances of losing money, the higher the risk. Cost-based and charge-based reimbursement are the least risky for providers because payors more or less ensure that costs will be covered, and hence profits will be earned. In cost-based systems, costs are automatically covered. In charge-based systems, providers typically can set charges high enough to ensure that costs are covered, although discounts introduce uncertainty into the reimbursement process.

Regardless of the reimbursement method (except cost-based), providers bear the cost-of-service risk in that costs can exceed revenues. However, a primary difference among the reimbursement types is the ability of the provider to influence the revenue/cost ratio. If providers set charge rates for each type of service provided, they can most easily ensure that revenues exceed costs. Furthermore, if providers have the power to set rates above those that would exist in a truly competitive market, charge-based reimbursement could result in higher profits than cost-based reimbursement.

Prospective payment adds a second dimension of risk to reimbursement contracts because the bundle of services needed to treat a particular patient may be more extensive than that assumed in the payment. However, when the prospective payment is made on a per procedure basis, risk is minimal because each procedure will produce its own revenue. When prospective payment is made on a per diagnosis basis, provider risk is increased. If, on average, patients require more intensive treatments, and for inpatients, a longer length of stay (LOS) than assumed in the prospective payment amount, the provider must bear the added costs.[10]

When prospective payment is made on a per diem basis, even when stratified, one daily rate usually covers a large number of diagnoses. Because the nature of the services provided could vary widely, both because of varying diagnoses as well as intensity differences within a single diagnosis, the provider bears the risk that costs associated with the services provided on any day exceed the per diem rate. However, patients with complex diagnoses and greater intensity tend to remain hospitalized longer, and per diem reimbursement does differentiate among different LOS. However, the additional days of stay may be insufficient to make up for the increased resources consumed. In addition, providers bear the risk that the payor, through the utilization review process, will constrain LOS, and hence increase intensity during the days that a patient is hospitalized. Thus, under per diem, compression of services and shortened LOS can put significant pressure on providers' profitability.

Under global pricing, a more inclusive set of procedures, or providers, are included in one fixed payment. Clearly, the more services that must be rendered for a single payment—or the more providers that have to share a single payment—the more providers are at risk for intensity of services.

Finally, under capitation, providers assume all utilization and actuarial risks along with the risks assumed under the other reimbursement methods. The assumption of utilization risk has traditionally been an insurance, rather than a provider, function. In the traditional fee-for-service system, the financial risk of providing healthcare is shared between purchasers and insurers. Hospitals, physicians, and other providers bear negligible risk because they are paid on the basis of the amount of services provided. Insurers bear short-term risk in that payments to providers in any year can exceed the amount of premiums collected. However, poor profitability by insurers in one year usually can be offset by premium increases to purchasers the next year, so the long-term risk of financing the healthcare system is borne by purchasers. Capitation, however, places the burden of short-term utilization risk on providers.

When provider risk under different reimbursement methods is discussed in this descriptive fashion, an easy conclusion to make is that capitation is by far the riskiest to providers, while cost-based and charge-based reimbursement are by far the least risky. Although this conclusion is not a bad starting point for analysis, financial risk is a complex subject and its surface has just been scratched. One of the key issues throughout the remainder of this book is financial risk, so readers will see this topic over and over. For now, keep in mind that different payors use different reimbursement methods. Thus, providers can face conflicting incentives and differing risk, depending on the predominant method of reimbursement.

In closing, note that all prospective payment methods involve a transfer of risk from insurers to providers that increases as the payment unit moves from per procedure to capitation. The added risk does not mean that providers should avoid such reimbursement methods; indeed, refusing to accept contracts with prospective payment provisions would be tantamount to organizational suicide for most providers. However, providers must understand the risks involved in prospective payment arrangements, especially the effect on profitability, and make every effort to negotiate a level of payment that is consistent with the risk incurred.

Self-Test Questions

1. Briefly, describe the following payment methodologies:
   a. Cost based
   b. Charge based and discounted charges
   c. Per procedure
   d. Per diagnosis
   e. Per diem
   f. Global
   g. Capitation
2. What is the major difference between fee-for-service reimbursement and capitation?
3. What provider incentives are created under each of the payment methods previously listed?
4. Which of these payment methods carries the least risk for providers? The most risk? Explain.

The Changing Market for Healthcare Services

So far in this chapter, a diverse collection of background material has been introduced about the healthcare finance environment; however, perhaps the most interesting environmental factor is the change that is currently taking place in the healthcare sector. This chapter closes with an analysis of the changing market for healthcare services. In this section, many of the concepts that were introduced in earlier sections are reinforced.

Healthcare reform is indeed taking place, but purchasers, not politicians, are driving it. The motivating factor has been healthcare costs, which have been rising at twice the rate of general inflation. To illustrate, the "big three" auto makers estimate that about $700 of the cost of each car and truck produced is attributable to employee healthcare benefits, compared to about half that amount only a decade ago. The same story applies to government healthcare programs. Medicare and Medicaid costs have risen at such high rates that every few years there is a new "crisis," with some pundits even predicting the collapse of these programs.

The first major market trend is that both private and government purchasers of healthcare services are taking cost-containment matters into their own hands. Rather than simply leave cost containment to the insurers, who have found it much easier to pass costs on to purchasers than to control them, purchasers are now taking a proactive role. Today, buyers are asserting themselves to increase their financial leverage in negotiating with providers. The predominant purchasers of healthcare services—managed care plans, business coalitions, insurance companies, and federal and state governments—have sent notice that market forces will now play an important role in determining prices. The impact of the newly exercised power of buyers has been compounded by the fact that some healthcare providers, especially hospitals, entered the 1990s with excess capacity.

A potential problem with the emerging market for healthcare services is that purchasers may be more concerned with price than with quality. However, as the new healthcare market matures, the purchase decision is becoming increasingly complex. Factors other than price, such as quality, patient satisfaction, and accessibility, are being factored into the buying decision. Many purchasers are now demanding that providers measure and report the value and quality of healthcare services provided.

The dynamics between purchasers and providers of healthcare services are increasingly revolving around managed care relationships. As previously mentioned, many forms of managed care plans exist, with no consistent philosophy regarding payment method. Typically, a purchasing group, which usually consists of one or more employers, signs a contract with a *managed care organization (MCO)*. The MCO may be an IDS (Integrated Delivery System) established by the providers or it may be a loosely structured panel of providers that is created by contractual relationships between an insurer and providers. In a typical MCO arrangement, the purchaser agrees to pay the MCO a fixed monthly fee per covered life. For these payments, the MCO agrees to provide all necessary care for the covered population.

Even though MCOs receive capitated payments from purchasers, the method of payment from the MCO to the individual providers does not have to be capitation. Providers can be paid on a fee-for-service basis such as per diem or per procedure. However, the managed care relationship, even if based on fee-for-service payment, changes the way providers do business in two important ways. First is an active intervention in the provision of healthcare services by the insurer (the MCO). The focus of this intervention is utilization, both in terms of whether the services are needed, and if they are needed, ensuring that they are being delivered in the lowest cost setting. The second factor that makes managed care relationships somewhat different from traditional insurance relationships pertains to pricing. The purchaser expects, and often receives, sizeable discounts from the MCO in recognition of the volume of business created by the contract. In turn, the

MCO uses the same logic and leverage to demand discounts from the dominant providers serving the covered population.

A major implication of managed care for health services organizations is the need for the investment in, and development of, better information systems. The shift of risk from purchasers to providers necessitates that health services organizations must have better cost and utilization data, which are critical for any organization paid under capitation. Both MCOs and providers must know the expected utilization of each type of service for each covered life. Such estimates require actuarial expertise—a skill set not commonly found at providers or at IDSs formed by providers. Without such information, MCOs and providers will not be able to assess the costs and risks that they face in their contracts, and hence will not be able to rationally price the services provided.

The second major trend in the healthcare environment is the changing role of health insurance. Traditionally, purchasers contracted with insurers, who then contracted with—or merely agreed to pay—providers. MCOs, which initially were created by insurers, tightened the relationship between insurers and providers, either through creating a single insurer/provider organization or through contracts. Now, insurers are coming under siege as employers take on the insurance function (self-insurance) and providers create IDSs that are capable of contracting directly with employers. In either case, insurers are being bypassed. The argument for those supporting this trend is that independent insurance companies add no value to the provision of healthcare services. Providers can do everything that insurers can do, so why should providers not deal directly with large purchasers of healthcare services? Direct contracting between purchasers and providers would cut out the middlemen—the insurance companies. Conversely, insurers argue that they add value by both assuming some risk for the costs of services and by administering healthcare programs in a more cost-efficient manner.

While IDSs may desire to take on the insurance function, states have laws that prohibit providers from taking on insurance risk without first having an insurance license. To obtain a license, providers must meet the *reserve requirements* established for healthcare insurers. The theory is that insurers should maintain a certain level of financial strength to weather the periodic losses that the industry typically encounters. For the most part, provider networks do not meet these requirements, so IDSs have been barred from contracting directly with purchasers. However, federal legislation appears to be on the horizon that would make it easier for providers to assume the insurance function.

At the same time that providers are moving into the insurance side of healthcare, insurers are moving into the provider side. This is most evident at Blue Cross/Blue Shield organizations, which recognize that their strongest competition is not other insurance companies, but rather employers who are moving into self-insurance and providers who are taking on the insurance function. One result is that some Blues are acquiring hospital systems and physician groups to solidify their managed care networks. To raise the vast amount of capital required for such acquisitions, these Blues are giving up their not-for-profit status to gain the ability to sell stock publicly to raise capital; when they were not-for-profit corporations, they were denied access to this source of capital.

The third major trend is added complexity in the financing and provision of healthcare services. At one time a more or less standard approach to healthcare services existed. Now, geographical markets are evolving differently because of unique buyer, insurer, and provider characteristics. Power struggles have broken out in certain markets as purchasers shop among provider networks for the best prices, standardized benefits, and superior customer satisfaction and outcomes. To be successful, providers in today's financial environment require more than just recognizing that the health services industry has moved from an environment in which costs were merely passed on to purchasers to an environment in which costs must be controlled. Furthermore, efforts to provide healthcare at lower cost must not come at the expense of choice, quality, and access.

Finally, today's healthcare environment is being redefined by capitation, or in many cases, the mere threat of capitation. As discussed previously, MCOs accept the risk for the cost of the care provided to the covered population. The plan may choose to bear all of the utilization risk and to purchase healthcare services as needed from providers on the basis of billed or discounted charges. However, more plans are seeking one or more classes of providers that will share the financial risk of care in the form of prospective payments, particularly capitated payments. Some services may still be purchased as needed on a fee-for-service basis, but more often, some providers in the network will share utilization risk with the MCO.

In this capitated mode of managed care, the factor that is driving revenue is the number of covered lives, not the amount of services provided. Profit moves up and down with the number of lives covered by the plan and the ability of providers to control costs. In the aggregate, the newer payment methods with incentives for controlling costs are dictating massive changes in patient treatment patterns. To illustrate, hospital average LOS has dropped from 5.8 days in 1992 to 4.5 days in 1997. At the same time, hospital occupancy has fallen from 52 percent filled beds to 43 percent. Providers, especially IDSs, are responding to these forces by emphasizing case management and the ability to offer a continuum of care to patients. Essentially, the premium dollar is moving away from hospital inpatient services and toward prevention, wellness, and primary care. In addition, outpatient services, chronic care (i.e., nursing home and home health care), rehabilitation care (i.e., occupational and physical therapy), and support care (i.e., hospice and home health care) are playing increasingly important roles in the provision of healthcare services.

1. Briefly, what are the current trends in the delivery of healthcare services?
2. What effect do these trends have on health services organizations?

Self-Test Questions

Key Concepts

In this chapter, important background material was presented that will be used throughout the remainder of the book. The key concepts of this chapter are:

- The three main forms of business organization are the *proprietorship*, *partnership*, and *corporation*. Although each form of organization has its own unique advantages and disadvantages, most large organizations, and all not-for-profit entities, are organized as *corporations*.
- *Investor-owned corporations* have *stockholders* who are the owners of the corporation. Stockholders exercise control through the *proxy* process, in which they elect the corporation's board of directors and vote on matters of major consequence to the firm. As owners, the stockholders have claim on the residual earnings of the corporation. Investor-owned corporations are fully taxable.
- Charitable organizations that meet certain criteria can be organized as *not-for-profit corporations*. Rather than having a well-defined set of owners, such organizations have a large number of *stakeholders* who have an interest in the organization. Not-for-profit corporations do not pay taxes; they can accept tax-deductible contributions, and they can issue tax-exempt debt.
- From a financial management perspective, the primary goal of investor-owned corporations is *shareholder wealth maximization*, which translates to stock price maximization. For not-for-profit corporations, a reasonable goal for financial management is to *ensure that the organization can fulfill its mission*, which translates to maintaining the corporation's financial viability.
- An *agency problem* is a potential conflict of interests that can arise between principals and agents. One type of agency problem in financial management is the conflict between the owners of a firm and its managers.
- The value of any income stream depends on the amount of *usable*, or *after-tax, income*. Thus, tax laws play an important role in financial management decisions.
- Most provider revenue is not obtained directly from patients, but rather from healthcare insurers that are known collectively as *third-party payors*.
- Third-party payors are classified as *private insurers* (Blue Cross/Blue Shield, commercial, and self-insurers) and *public insurers* (Medicare and Medicaid).
- *Managed care plans*, such as *health maintenance organizations (HMOs)*, strive to combine both the insurance function and the provision of healthcare services.
- Third-party payors use many different payment methods that fall into two broad classifications: *fee-for-service* and *capitation*. Each payment method creates a unique set of incentives and risk for providers.
- The market for healthcare services is undergoing significant change as a result of purchasers taking more aggressive actions to control spiraling healthcare costs.

These background concepts will be used over and over throughout the remainder of the book.

Questions

2.1 What are the three primary forms of business organization? Describe their advantages and disadvantages.

2.2 What are the primary differences between investor-owned and not-for-profit corporations?

2.3 a. What is the primary goal of investor-owned corporations?
  b. What is the primary goal of most not-for-profit health services corporations?
  c. Are there substantial differences between the finance goals of investor-owned and not-for-profit corporations? Explain.
  d. What is the agency problem?

2.4 a. Why are tax laws important to healthcare finance?
  b. What three major advantages do tax laws give to not-for-profit corporations?

2.5 Briefly describe the major third-party payors.

2.6 a. What are the primary characteristics of managed care plans?
  b. Describe different types of managed care plans.

2.7 What is the difference between fee-for-service reimbursement and capitation?

2.8 Describe provider incentives and risks under each of the following reimbursement methods:
  a. Cost based
  b. Charge based (including discounted charges)
  c. Per procedure
  d. Per diagnosis
  e. Per diem
  f. Global pricing
  g. Capitation

2.9 Briefly describe current trends in the market for healthcare services.

Problems

2.1 Assume that Provident Health System, a for-profit hospital, has $1 million in taxable income for 1999, and its tax rate is 30 percent.
  a. Given this information, what is the firm's net income? (Hint: net income is what remains after taxes have been paid.)
  b. Suppose the hospital pays out $300 thousand in dividends. A stockholder receives $10 thousand. If the stockholder's tax rate is 40 percent, what is the after-tax dividend?

2.2 A firm that owns the stock of another corporation does not have to pay taxes on the entire amount of dividends received. In general, only 30 percent of the dividends received by one corporation from another are taxable. The reason for this tax law feature is to mitigate the effect of triple taxation, which occurs when earnings are first taxed at one firm, then its dividends paid to a second firm are taxed again, and finally the dividends paid to stockholders by the second firm are taxed yet again. Assume that a firm with a 35 percent tax rate receives $100 thousand in dividends from another corporation. What taxes must be paid on this dividend and what is the after-tax amount of the dividend?

2.3 John Doe is in the 40 percent personal tax bracket. He is considering investing in Columbia/HCA bonds that carry a 12 percent interest rate.
   a. What is his after-tax yield (interest rate) on the bonds?
   b. Suppose Twin Cities Memorial Hospital has issued tax-exempt bonds having an interest rate of 6 percent. With all else the same, should John buy the Columbia/HCA or the Twin Cities bonds?
   c. With all else the same, what interest rate on the tax-exempt Twin Cities bonds would make John indifferent between these bonds and the Columbia/HCA bonds?

2.4 Jane Smith currently holds tax-exempt bonds of Good Samaritan Healthcare that pay 7 percent interest. She is in the 40 percent tax bracket. Her broker wants her to buy some Beverly Enterprises taxable bonds that will be issued next week. With all else the same, what rate must be set on the Beverly bonds to make Jane interested in making a switch?

2.5 George and Margaret Wealthy are in the 48 percent tax bracket, considering both federal and state personal taxes. Norman Briggs, the CEO of Community General Hospital, has been aggressively pursuing the couple to contribute $500 thousand to the hospital's soon-to-be-built Cancer Care Center. Without the contribution, the Wealthy's taxable income for 1999 would be $2 million. What impact would the contribution have on the Wealthy's 1999 tax bill?

Notes

1. A tax-exempt corporation (discussed later in the chapter) can be one partner of a partnership. In this situation, profits allocated to the tax-exempt partner are not taxed, but those allocated to taxable partners are subject to taxation.
2. Although most partnerships are small, there are some very large businesses that are organized as partnerships or as hybrid organizations (which will be discussed in a later section). Examples include the major public accounting firms and many large law firms.
3. *Financial markets* bring together people and businesses that need money with other people and businesses that have funds to invest. In a developed country such as the United States, a great many financial markets exist. Some markets deal with debt capital and others with equity capital; some deal with short-term capital and others with long-term capital, and so on. How financial markets operate and their benefit to health services organizations are discussed throughout the book.
4. Over 60 percent of corporations in the United States are chartered in Delaware, which over the years has provided a favorable governmental and legal environment

for corporations. A firm does not have to be headquartered or conduct business operations in its state of incorporation.

5. In certain situations, shares can be sold to the public for the first time by the company's original owners, rather than by the company itself. In this case, the proceeds from the sale go the original owners, not to the company. Stock sales are discussed in much more detail in Chapter 12.

6. This entire chapter could easily be filled with the details of obtaining and maintaining tax-exempt status. However, that is not the purpose of this book. Therefore, enough information is provided to show the ways in which not-for-profit status has an impact on financial decisions, but the details concerning tax-exempt status are left to outside readings or other courses. For additional information, see the Summer 1988 issue of *Topics in Health Care Financing*, titled "Tax Management for Exempt Providers."

7. For more information on the challenges to tax exemption, see the January 1991 issue of *Healthcare Financial Management*.

8. The following sections include only a brief introduction to the major third-party payors. For more information, see Section E, titled "Payment," in *Handbook of Health Care Accounting and Finance*, Volume II, edited by W. O. Cleverley (Rockville, MD: Aspen, 1989), or H. J. Berman, S. F. Kukla, and L. E. Weeks, *The Financial Management of Hospitals* (Chicago: Health Administration Press, 1993).

9. HCFA had planned to consolidate the processing of Medicare claims at regional processing centers beginning in the fall of 1997. The new system, called the *Medicare Transaction System*, was designed to standardize claims processing by creating one national system. The intent was to permit hospitals to file Medicare claims—mostly in electronic format—directly to HCFA. Other functions such as audits, customer service, and medical reviews would continue to be performed by intermediaries. However, the initial contract for the system was terminated in September of 1997 because of gigantic cost overruns, and HCFA had to go back to the drawing board.

10. Most per procedure payment systems contain *outlier clauses*, whereby providers receive additional reimbursement when costs are far above average for a particular patient. However, such extra payments typically do not cover the full amount of the cost differential.

References

For the latest information on events that affect the healthcare sector, see

Medical Benefits, published semimonthly by Kelly Communications, Inc., Charlottesville, VA.

Modern Healthcare, published weekly by Crain Communications Inc., Chicago.

Other references pertaining to this chapter include the following:

Blair, J. D., G. T. Savage, and C. J. Whitehead. 1989. "A Strategic Approach for Negotiating with Hospital Stakeholders." *Health Care Management Review* (Winter): 13–23.

Clement, J. P., D. G. Smith, and J. R. C. Wheeler. 1994. "What Do We Want and What Do We Get from Not-for-Profit Hospitals?" *Hospital & Health Services Administration* (Summer): 159–178.

Coddington, D. C., D. J. Keene, K. D. Moore, and R. L. Clarke. 1991. "Factors Driving

Costs Must Figure into Reform." *Healthcare Financial Management* (July): 44–62.

Fallon, R. P. 1991. "Not-For-Profit ≠ No Profit: Profitability Planning in Not-For-Profit Organizations." *Health Care Management Review* (Summer): 47–59.

Fottler, M. D., J. D. Blair, C. J. Whitehead, M. D. Laus, and G. T. Savage. 1989. "Assessing Key Stakeholders: Who Matters to Hospitals and Why?" *Hospital & Health Services Administration* (Winter): 525–546.

Healthcare Financial Management. The July 1997 issue has several articles related to the tax sanctions imposed on not-for-profit corporations when excess benefits accrue to individuals.

Herzlinger, R. E. and W. S. Krasker. 1987. "Who Profits From Nonprofits." *Harvard Business Review* (January–February): 93–105.

Hill, J. F. 1986. "Third Party Payment Strategies." *Topics in Health Care Financing* (Winter): 1–88.

Lamm, R. D. 1990. "High-Tech Health Care and Society's Ability to Pay." *Healthcare Financial Management* (September): 20–30.

McLean, R. A. 1989. "Agency Costs and Complex Contracts in Health Care Organizations." *Health Care Management Review* (Winter): 65–71.

Nauert, R. C., A. B. Sanborn, II, C. F. MacKelvie, and J. L. Harvitt. 1988. "Hospitals Face Loss of Federal Tax-Exempt Status." *Healthcare Financial Management* (September): 48–60.

Pink, G. H. and P. Leatt. 1991. "Are Managers Compensated for Hospital Financial Performance." *Health Care Management Review* (Summer): 37–45.

Umbdenstock, R. J., W. M. Hageman, and B. Amundson. 1990. "The Five Critical Areas for Effective Governance of Not-for-Profit Hospitals." *Hospital & Health Services Administration* (Winter): 481–492.

Walker, C. L. and L. W. Humphreys. 1993. "Hospital Control and Decision Making: A Financial Perspective." *Healthcare Financial Management* (June): 90–96.

Wolfson, J. and S. L. Hopes. 1994. "What Makes Tax-Exempt Hospitals Special?" *Healthcare Financial Management* (July): 57–60.

FINANCIAL ACCOUNTING

THE INCOME STATEMENT

Learning Objectives

After studying this chapter, readers will be able to:

- Explain why financial accounting statements are so important both to managers and to outside parties.
- Describe the standard setting process under which financial accounting information is created and reported, as well as the underlying principles applied.
- Describe the components of the income statement—revenues, expenses, and net income—and the relationships within and between these components.
- Explain the difference between net income and cash flow.

Introduction

Financial accounting involves identifying, measuring, recording, and communicating the economic events and status of an organization to interested parties that are both internal and external to the organization. This information is summarized and presented in three important *financial statements*: the income statement, the balance sheet, and the statement of cash flows. Because these statements communicate financial information about an organization, financial accounting is often called "the language of business." Managers of health services organizations must understand the basics of financial accounting because the organization's financial statements, more than anything else, describe the financial performance of the business.

The coverage of financial accounting extends over several chapters. This chapter includes an introduction to basic financial accounting concepts and an explanation of how organizations report revenues, costs, and profits. In Chapter 4, the discussion is extended to include the reporting of assets, liabilities, equity, and cash flows. In Chapter 17, the focus again is on financial statements, including a description of how managers and other parties use financial statements to assess the financial condition of an organization. That chapter has purposely been placed at the end of the book because the nuances of financial statement analysis can be better understood after learning more about the financial workings of a business. These three chapters will provide you with a basic understanding of how financial statements are created and used to make judgments regarding the financial condition of a health services organization.

Historical Foundations of Financial Accounting

Students often think of accounting statements as pieces of paper with numbers written on them, and they do not think about the *physical assets*—such as land, buildings, and equipment—that underlie the numbers. However, if readers understand how and why financial accounting began and how financial statements are used, they can better visualize what is happening within a health services organization and why financial accounting information is so important.

Thousands of years ago, individuals or families were self-contained in the sense that they gathered their own food, made their own clothes, and built their own shelters. When specialization began, some individuals or families became good at hunting, others at making arrowheads, others at making clothing, and so on. With specialization came trade, initially by bartering one type of goods for another. At first, each producer worked alone and trade was strictly local. Over time, some people set up production shops that employed workers, simple forms of money were used, and trade expanded beyond the local area. As these simple economies expanded, more formal forms of money developed and a primitive form of banking began, with wealthy merchants lending profits from past dealings to enterprising shop owners and traders who needed money to expand their operations.

When the first loans were made, lenders could physically inspect borrowers' assets and judge the likelihood of repayment. Eventually, though, lending became much more complex. Industrial borrowers were developing large factories, merchants were acquiring fleets of ships and wagons, and loans were being made to finance business activities at distant locations. At that point, lenders could no longer easily inspect the assets that backed their loans, and they needed a practical way of summarizing the value of those assets. Also, certain loans were made on the basis of a share of the profits of the business, so a uniform, widely accepted method for expressing income was required. In addition, owners required reports to see how effectively their own enterprises were being operated, and governments needed information for use in assessing taxes. For all these reasons, a need arose for financial statements, for accountants to prepare the statements, and for auditors to verify the accuracy of the accountants' work.

The economic systems of the industrialized countries have grown enormously since the beginning, and financial accounting has become much more complex. However, the original reasons for accounting statements still apply: bankers and other investors need accounting information to make intelligent investment decisions, managers need it to operate their organizations efficiently, and taxing authorities need it to assess taxes in an equitable manner.

It should be no surprise that problems can arise when translating physical assets and economic events into accounting numbers. Nevertheless, that is what accountants must do when they construct financial statements. To illustrate the translation problem, the numbers shown on the balance sheet to reflect a business' assets and liabilities generally reflect historical costs and prices. However, inventories may be spoiled, obsolete, or even missing; land, buildings, and equipment may have a current value that is much higher or lower than their historical costs; and money owed to the business may be uncollectible. Also, some liabilities, such as obligations to make lease payments, may not even show up in the numbers. Similarly, costs reported on an income statement may be understated or overstated, and some costs, such as depreciation, do not even represent current cash expenses. When examining a set of financial statements, it is best to keep in mind the physical reality that underlies the numbers, and also to recognize that problems can occur in the translation process.

1. What are the historical foundations of financial accounting statements?
2. Do any problems arise when translating physical assets and economic events into monetary units? Give one or two illustrations to support your answer.

Self-Test Questions

The Users of Financial Accounting Information

The predominant users of financial accounting information are those parties who have a *financial interest* in the organization, and hence are concerned with its economic status. All organizations, whether not-for-profit or investor owned, have *stakeholders* who have an interest in the business. In a not-for-profit organization, such as a community hospital, the stakeholders include managers, staff physicians, employees, suppliers, creditors, patients, and even the community at large. Investor-owned organizations have essentially the same set of stakeholders, with the addition of stockholders—the owners. Because all stakeholders, by definition, have an interest in the organization, all stakeholders have an interest in its financial condition.

Of all the outside stakeholders, *investors* typically have the greatest **financial** interest in health services organizations. These parties, who supply *capital* (money) to businesses, include both stockholders, who supply equity capital to investor-owned businesses, and *creditors* (or *lenders*), who supply debt capital to both investor-owned and not-for-profit businesses. In general, only one category of stockholders exists. However, creditors constitute a diverse group of investors including banks, suppliers granting trade credit, and bondholders. Because of their direct financial interest in healthcare businesses, investors are the primary outside users of financial accounting information. They use the information to make judgments pertaining to whether or not to make a particular investment, as well as in setting the return required on the investment. (Investor-supplied capital is covered in greater detail in Chapters 11, 12, and 13.)

Although financial accounting developed primarily to meet the information needs of outside parties, the managers of an organization, including its board of directors (trustees), also are important users of the information. After all, managers are charged with ensuring that the organization has the financial strength to accomplish its mission, whether that mission is to maximize the wealth of its shareholders or to provide healthcare services to the community at large. Thus, an organization's managers are not only involved with creating financial statements, but they are also primary users of the statements, both to assess current financial condition and to formulate plans to ensure that the future financial condition of the organization will support its goals.

In summary, investors and managers are the predominant users of financial accounting information as a result of their direct financial interest in the organization. Furthermore, investors are not merely important users of financial accounting information; they do more than just read and interpret the statements. Often, they actively pressure management to meet certain financial targets that are based on the numbers reported in the financial statements. Indeed, many debt agreements require borrowers to maintain financial standards, such as a minimum earnings level, to keep the debt in force. If the standards are not met, the lender can demand that the borrower immediately repay the full amount of the loan.

Self-Test Questions

1. Who are the primary users of financial accounting information?
2. Are investors passive users of this information?

Regulation and Standards in Financial Accounting

As a consequence of the Great Depression of the 1930s, which caused many businesses to fail and almost brought down the entire securities industry, the federal government began regulating the form and disclosure of information related to publicly traded securities. The regulation is based on the theory that financial information constructed and presented according to standardized rules allows stockholders, creditors, and other interested parties to make the best informed decisions. The newly formed *Securities and Exchange Commission (SEC)*, an independent regulatory agency of the U.S. government, was given the authority to establish and enforce the form and content of financial statements. Nonconforming companies are prohibited from selling securities to the public, so most businesses of any size must comply. In addition, most businesses that do not sell securities to the public are willing to follow the SEC-established guidelines to ensure uniformity of presentation of financial data.

The SEC does not create the standards, but rather allows other organizations to create and implement the standard system. For the most part, the SEC has delegated the responsibility for establishing standards to the *Financial Accounting Standards Board (FASB)*, a private organization whose mission is to establish and improve standards of financial accounting and reporting for private businesses. (The *Government Accounting Standards Board [GASB]* has the identical responsibility for public businesses.) The FASB and its predecessor organization (the *Accounting Principles Board [APB]*) promulgate guidelines in pronouncements with various names such as *statements* or *opinions*. Taken together, these pronouncements, along with guidance issued by other organizations, constitute a set of guidelines called *generally accepted accounting principles (GAAP)*. GAAP can be thought of as a set of objectives, conventions, and principles that have evolved through the years to guide the preparation and presentation of financial statements. The GAAP only apply to the area of financial accounting, as distinct from other areas of accounting such as managerial accounting (discussed in later chapters) and tax accounting.

Typically, the guidelines established by the FASB apply across a wide range of industries and, by design, are somewhat general in nature. Yet another organization is needed to provide more specific implementation rules, especially when industry-unique guidance is required. This task is accomplished by the *American Institute of Certified Public Accountants (AICPA)*, which is the professional association of public (financial) accountants. The AICPA has substantial influence with its membership, much like the influence that the American Medical Association (AMA) has on its member physicians. The AICPA, through its *industry committees*, promulgates the actual rules that accountants follow when preparing and auditing an organization's financial statements. For example, financial statements in the health services industry are based on the AICPA Audit and Accounting Guide titled *Health Care Organizations* (May 1, 1997).

Finally, when even more specific guidance is required, other professional organizations may participate in the standard-setting process, although such work does not have the same degree of influence as the FASB or the AICPA. For example, the *Healthcare Financial Management Association (HFMA)* has established a *Principles and Practices Board*, which develops position statements on issues that require further guidance, such as its statement on August 11, 1997 regarding the handling of mergers, acquisitions, and collaborations.

For most organizations, the final link in the financial statement quality assurance process is the external audit, which is performed by an independent (outside) *auditor*, usually one of the large accounting firms. The results of the external audit are reported in the *auditor's opinion*, which is a letter attached to the financial statements stating whether or not the statements are a fair presentation of the organization's operations, cash flows, and financial position as specified by the GAAP. The entire auditing process, which is performed both by the organization's internal auditors and the external auditor, is a means of verifying and validating the organization's financial statements.[1] Of course, the audit process gives users, especially those external to the organization, more confidence that the statements truly represent the organization's current financial condition.

The field of financial accounting is typically classified as a social science rather than a physical science. Financial accounting is as much an art as a science, and the end result represents negotiation, compromise, and interpretation. The organizations involved in setting standards are continuously reviewing and revising the GAAP to ensure the best possible development and presentation of financial data. This task, which is essential to economic prosperity, is motivated by the fact that the U.S. economy is constantly evolving, with new types of business arrangements and securities being created almost daily.[2]

1. What entities are involved in regulating the development and presentation of financial accounting information?

Self-Test Questions

2. What does GAAP stand for?
3. What is the primary purpose of the GAAP?
4. What is the purpose of the auditor's opinion?

Measurement and Recording of Economic Events

To better understand the content of financial statements, it is useful to discuss some of the basic concepts that accountants use when they prepare an organization's financial statements. Because the actual preparation of financial statements is done by accountants, a detailed presentation of accounting theory is not required. Still, a better understanding of the content of the financial statements will be possible with an understanding of the measurement and recording processes that underlie their preparation.

The Time Period

One of the purposes of financial statements is to identify an organization's revenues, expenses, and profitability during a specific period of time. For financial reporting purposes, this time period is called an *accounting period*. It can be any length of time—a week or month or year—during which an organization's managers, or outside parties, want to evaluate operational results. Most health services organizations use calendar periods—months, quarters, and years—as their accounting periods. However, occasionally an organization will use a *fiscal year* (financial year) that does not coincide with the calendar year. For example, Access Health, a provider of management services for health maintenance organizations (HMOs), has a fiscal year that runs from October 1 to September 30. In this book, an annual accounting period is used in the illustrations. However, financial statement information typically is also prepared for periods shorter than one year.[3]

Cash Versus Accrual Accounting

Perhaps the most important concept used in the preparation of financial statements is the *accrual concept*, which is primarily applied to revenues and expenses. When applied to revenues, the accrual concept implies that revenue earned does not necessarily correspond to the receipt of cash. Why? Earned revenue is recognized in financial statements when a service has been provided **that creates a payment obligation** on the part of the purchaser, rather than when the payment is actually made.

For healthcare providers, the payment obligation typically falls on the patient, a third-party payor, or both. If the obligation is satisfied immediately, such as when a patient makes full payment at the time the services are rendered, the revenue is in the form of cash. However, in most cases, the bulk of the payment for services is not received until later, perhaps several months after the services are provided. In this situation, the revenue created by the service does not create an immediate cash payment. If the payment is received within an accounting period, one year for our purposes, the conversion of revenues to cash will be completed, and, as far as the financial statements are concerned, the reported revenue is cash. However, when the revenue is recorded (i.e., services are provided) in one accounting period and payment does not occur until the next period, the revenue reported is not cash.

To illustrate, suppose Sunnyvale Clinic, a large multi-specialty group practice, provided services to a patient in December 1998. At that time, the clinic billed the insurer—Blue Cross/Blue Shield of Florida—$700, the full amount that the insurer is obligated to pay. However, Sunnyvale did not receive payment from the insurer until February 1999. Sunnyvale's accounting year ends on December 31, so the clinic's books are closed after the revenue has been recorded, but before the cash is received. Thus, Sunnyvale reported this $700 of revenue on its 1998 income statement, even though no cash was collected.

The *cash basis* of accounting takes a different approach to recording revenues. The cash basis requires that the clinic report a service as revenue when the cash is actually received. The core argument is that the most important event to record is the receipt of cash, not the provision of the service (i.e., the obligation to pay). Supporters of accrual accounting argue that the cash basis of accounting fails to portray the true economic status of the organization—the primary goal of financial accounting—because it is the provision of the service that actually creates the revenue. In rebuttal, the supporters of cash accounting argue that accrual accounting is misleading because readers of financial statements logically expect revenues to represent cash inflows to the reporting organization.

If accrual accounting is followed, it becomes necessary to provide information indicating that not all reported revenues represent cash. In essence, those revenues that have not been collected will appear in an asset account on the balance sheet called *receivables*. When examining an organization's financial statements, it will be clear that this account represents revenues that have been reported, but for which payment has not been received. In reality, some portion of the aggregate amount shown on an organization's balance sheet as receivables may never be collected, and hence become a bad debt loss. This possibility is also reported, however. The point here is that the accounting profession is comfortable enough with the benefits of accrual accounting to recommend in the GAAP that it be used, rather than cash accounting, when financial statements are prepared.

The accrual accounting concept also applies to expenses. To illustrate, assume that Sunnyvale had payroll obligations of $400 for employees' work during the last two weeks of 1998 that would not be paid until the first payday in 1999. Because the employees actually performed the work, the obligation to pay the salaries was created in 1998. However, because the payment will not be made until the next accounting period, an expense will be recorded, even though no cash payment was made. (Under the cash basis of accounting, Sunnyvale would not recognize the expense until it was paid, in this case in 1999.) Under accrual accounting, the $400 will be shown as an expense on the income statement in 1998 and, at the same time, the balance sheet will show a $400 liability, or obligation to pay. This obligation will appear as a short-term liability called *accrued expense*, which means that Sunnyvale will have to make this cash payment sometime in 1999.

The Matching Principle

The *matching principle* has two components. First, it requires that the revenues of an organization be *matched* with the accounting period during which they are earned. Although this terminology was not introduced in the last section, the matching principle underlies the preference that accountants have for accrual accounting over cash accounting. Second, the matching principle requires that an organization's expenses be matched, to the extent possible, with the revenues to which they are related. In essence, after the revenues have been allocated to a particular accounting period, all expenses associated with producing those revenues should be matched to the same period.

The matching principle applies regardless of the reimbursement method used by payors, but its consequences are particularly obvious under capitation. If a clinic is paid under fee-for-service, both revenues and costs more or less accrue when the services are provided. However, under capitation, revenues are received up-front, while much of the expense associated with providing services to the covered population occurs later, perhaps much later. As explained in Chapter 4, providers with significant capitation revenues must forecast what the associated costs will be and, according to the matching principle, record them in the same accounting period that the revenues are reported.

Materiality

The final basic concept of measurement and reporting is *materiality*, which recognizes that an almost infinite number of economic events could be reported in an organization's financial statements. If statements were created that contain all relevant information, they would be so long and detailed that making inferences about the organization's economic status would be very difficult without a great deal of analysis. Thus, to keep financial statements manageable, only entries that are material to the financial condition of an organization need be separately categorized.

The materiality principle affects the detailed presentation of the financial statements rather than their aggregate financial content (i.e., the final numbers). For example, medical equipment manufacturers carry large inventories of materials that are both substantial in dollar value relative to other assets and instrumental to their core business. Medical equipment manufacturers should, therefore, report inventories as a separate asset item on the balance sheet. Hospitals, on the other hand, carry a relatively small amount of inventories. Thus, many hospitals, and other healthcare providers, do not report inventories separately, but rather combine them into an asset account called "other assets." Clearly, leeway exists for interpretation as to what is and is not material, so different organizations in the same industry may have somewhat different looking financial statements. Nonetheless, the GAAP, as formulated on the basis of the principles discussed here, ensure that sufficient uniformity exists to permit rational comparisons across firms.

1. Why are widely accepted principles important for the measurement and recording of economic events?
2. Briefly explain the following principles:
   a. Time period
   b. Cash accounting
   c. Accrual accounting
   d. Matching
   e. Materiality
3. How does the matching principle apply to providers under capitation?

The Annual Report

When people think of financial accounting, the first thing that usually comes to mind is the *annual report,* which is the most important report that an organization provides to outsiders. Two types of information are given in the report: verbal and numerical. The verbal section, often presented as a letter from the chairman, describes in general terms the organization's operating results during the past year, and then discusses developments that will affect future operations. The numerical section contains three important financial statements: the income statement, the balance sheet, and the statement of cash flows.[4] This chapter provides a detailed discussion of the contents and logic behind the income statement. In Chapter 4, the remaining two important statements—the balance sheet and the statement of cash flows—are discussed.

Because the three primary financial statements cannot possibly contain all the information that can affect an organization's financial condition, additional information is provided in the *footnotes.* For health services organizations, these footnotes contain information on such topics as inventory accounting practices, the composition of long-term debt, pension plan status, amount of charity care provided, and malpractice insurance coverage. Pertinent footnote information is discussed as needed.

The primary purpose in the financial accounting chapters is to provide a basic understanding of the content and interpretation of the three most important financial statements. Note that the financial statements of large organizations can be complex. Furthermore, there is significant leeway regarding the format of the statements, and readers of this text come from a wide variety of health services organizations. Key issues are, therefore, presented using generic format statements. This is the best way to learn the basics; the nuances must be left to other books that focus exclusively on accounting issues.

1. What is an annual report?
2. What three primary financial statements are contained in the annual report?
3. Why are the footnotes to the financial statements important?

Income Statement Basics

Perhaps the most frequently asked, and the most important, question about a business is this: Is the business making money? The *income statement* summarizes the operations (i.e., the activities) of an organization with a focus on its revenues, expenses, and profitability. Thus, the income statement is often called the *statement of operations* or the *statement of activities*.

The 1998 and 1997 income statements of Sunnyvale Clinic are presented in Table 3.1. Most financial statements contain two years of data, with the most recent year presented first. The title section of the income statement shows that these are annual statements for the years 1998 and 1997, ending on December 31. Whereas the balance sheet, which is covered in Chapter 4, reports an organization's financial position at a single point in time, the income statement contains operational results **over a specified period of time**. Because the assumption here is that the financial statements are part of Sunnyvale's annual report, the time period for the illustrative income statements is one year. Also, the dollar amounts reported in Table 3.1 are listed in **thousands** of dollars, so the $169,013 reported as net patient service revenue for 1998 is actually $169,013,**000**.

The core components of the income statement are straightforward: revenues, expenses, and profitability (i.e., net income). *Revenues*, as discussed previously in the section on cash versus accrual accounting, represent both cash and the obligations of payors for services provided during the period. For healthcare providers, the revenues result mostly from the provision of patient services. To produce revenues, organizations must incur *costs*, or *expenses*, which are classified as operating or financial. *Operating costs* consist of salaries, supply costs, equipment costs, and other costs directly related with providing services. *Financial costs* are the costs associated with obtaining the funds needed to buy the organization's assets. Expenses decrease the profitability of a business, so expenses are subtracted from revenues to determine an organization's profitability:

$$\text{Revenues} - \text{Expenses} = \text{Net income.}$$

Note that net income may be positive or negative. When revenues exceed expenses, the resulting profit is called *net income*. When expenses exceed revenues, a negative net income (or *net loss*) results.

Net income is an important measure of a business' profitability. (Several other measures of profitability are discussed in later chapters.) The greater the net income, the greater the accounting profitability of the business and, with all else the same, the better its financial position.

The income statement, then, summarizes the ability of an organization to generate profits. Basically, it lists the organization's income (revenues), the costs that must be incurred to produce the revenues (expenses), and the difference between the two (net income). In the following sections, the major components of the income statement are discussed in detail.

	1998	1997
Revenues:		
Net patient service revenue	$ 169,013	$ 140,896
Other revenue	7,079	5,704
Total revenues	$ 176,092	$ 146,600
Expenses:		
Salaries and benefits	$ 109,693	$ 89,953
Medical supplies	20,568	18,673
Purchased medical services	9,863	7,448
Research and education	4,518	3,710
Lease expense	3,189	2,603
Depreciation and amortization	6,405	5,798
Provision for bad debts	2,000	1,800
Interest	5,329	3,476
Other	6,667	4,933
Total expenses	$ 168,232	$ 138,394
Net income	$ 7,860	$ 8,206

TABLE 3.1
Sunnyvale Clinic:
Income Statements,
Years Ended
December 31, 1998
and 1997
(in thousands)

1. What is the primary purpose of the income statement?
2. In regards to time, how do the income statement and balance sheet differ?
3. What are the major components of the income statement?

**Self-Test
Questions**

Revenues

Revenues can be shown on the income statement in several different formats. In fact, there is more latitude in the construction of the income statement than there is in the balance sheet, so the income statements for different types of healthcare providers tend to differ more in presentation than their balance sheets. (See Problems 3.2 and 3.3, as well Table 17.1, for examples of income statements of other types of providers.)

Sunnyvale reported *net patient service revenue* of $169,013,000 for 1998. The key terms here are *net* and *patient service*. This line contains revenues that stem from patient services, as opposed to revenues stemming from other activities such as contributions or returns on securities investments. However, patient service can be rather broadly defined, so revenues associated with such activities as parking garages and visitor food services often are categorized as patient service revenue.

The term *net* signifies that the amount shown is less than the clinic's gross charges for the services provided. Sunnyvale, like most healthcare providers, has a *fee schedule* that contains the *list price* of each service that it provides. However, this price does not always represent the amount the clinic expects to be paid for a particular service. Some services are provided to patients enrolled in managed care plans that have contracts with Sunnyvale that specify a discount from charges. For these services, the clinic expects to be paid less than the amount shown on the fee schedule, so the amount to be paid is the listed charge less the negotiated discount. Such discounts are incorporated before the revenue is recorded on the net patient service revenue line, so the amounts recorded are charges **net of discounts**.

Furthermore, some services have been provided as *charity care* to indigent patients. (*Indigent patients* are those who presumably are willing to pay for services provided, but do not have the ability to pay.) Sunnyvale has no expectation of ever collecting for these services, so, like discounts, charges for such services are **not** reflected in the $169,013,000 net patient service revenue reported for 1998. Finally, some revenues that are expected, and hence reported, will never be realized and ultimately will become *bad debt losses*. To recognize that Sunnyvale does not really expect to collect the entire $169,013,000 net patient service revenue reported, the clinic lists as an expense a $2,000,000 provision for bad debts. (This expense item is discussed in more detail in the next section.)

Note the distinction between charity care and bad debt losses. Charity care represents services that are provided to patients that **do not have** the capacity to pay. Bad debt losses result from the failure to collect for services provided to patients or third-party payors that **do have** the capacity to pay.

A description of policies regarding discounts and charity care will often appear in the footnotes to the financial statements. To illustrate, the Sunnyvale financial statements include the following two footnotes:

> **Revenues.** Sunnyvale has entered into agreements with third-party payors, including government programs and managed care plans, under which it is paid for services on the basis of established charges, the cost of providing services, predetermined rates per diagnosis, or discounts from established charges. Revenues are recorded at estimated amounts due from patients and third-party payors for the services provided. Settlements under reimbursement agreements with third-party payors are estimated and recorded in the period the related services are rendered, and are adjusted in future periods as final settlements are determined. The adjustments to estimated settlements for prior years are not considered material, and thus are not shown in the financial statements or footnotes.

> **Charity care.** Sunnyvale has a policy of providing charity care to indigent patients in emergency situations. These services, which are subtracted from gross revenues, amounted to $67,541 in 1998 and $51,344 in 1997.

Even though Sunnyvale ultimately expects to collect all of its reported net patient service revenue not yet received, less realized bad debt losses, the clinic did not actually receive $169,013,000 in cash payments in 1998. Rather, some of the revenue have not yet been collected. As readers will learn in Chapter 4, the yet-to-be-collected portion of the patient service revenue, $28,509,000, appears on the balance sheet (Table 4.1) as net patient accounts receivable.

In a fee-for-service environment, providers offer healthcare services that are paid for on the basis of utilization (i.e., the volume of services provided). That is, revenues stem from reimbursement made on a per diem, per test, per procedure, or per ancillary service basis, and so on, so revenues are tied to the amount of services provided. Sunnyvale operates primarily as a fee-for-service provider, so its patient service revenue is reported as shown in Table 3.1.

Revenue associated with capitation contracts is often called *premium revenue* when reported on the income statement. If the provider has almost all capitated revenue, it may replace the patient service revenue category as reported by Sunnyvale by the premium revenue category. Other providers, with significant amounts of both fee-for-service and capitation revenue may report both patient service revenue and premium revenue on the income statement. The key difference is that patient service revenue is reported when services are provided, but premium revenue is reported when contractual coverage begins, typically at the beginning of each month. Thus, premium revenue implies an obligation on the part of the reporting organization to provide future services, while patient service revenue represents an obligation on the part of payors to pay the reporting organization for services already provided. Also, different types of providers may use different terminology for revenues; for example, nursing homes report resident service revenue.

Most health services organizations have revenue besides that which arises from patient services, and Sunnyvale is no exception. In 1998, Sunnyvale reported *other revenue* of $7,079,000. One major source of other revenue is *interest earned* on securities investments. Although not shown directly on the income statement, the footnotes to the financial statements indicated that the clinic earned $3,543,000 in interest income during 1998. In Chapter 4, readers will see that Sunnyvale had $10,000,000 in marketable securities (short-term investments) at the end of 1998, as well as $42,889,000 in long-term securities, for a total of $52,889,000. Also, the footnotes indicated that all the clinic's securities holdings were debt securities, so all the return came in the form of interest. With $3,543,000 in interest earned on a total investment of $52,889,000, Sunnyvale earned roughly $3,543,000 / $52,889,000 = 0.067 = 6.7% on its financial investments, assuming that the investment amount was relatively stable throughout 1998. Interest earnings, financial returns, and debt investments all are discussed in more detail in future chapters.

Contributions represent the second major component of the other revenue category. Some not-for-profit organizations, especially those with large, well-endowed, and active foundations, rely heavily on contributions, as well as earnings on securities investments, as a revenue source. However, health services managers must recognize that such revenue is not central to the core business, which is providing healthcare services. Over-reliance on other revenues could mask serious operational inefficiencies that, if not corrected, could lead to financial problems later.

Additional sources of other revenues include revenue from such activities as consulting services, renting of space, educational activities, and sales of pharmaceuticals to employees, staff, and visitors. A unique problem facing not-for-profit providers is that a large amount of revenues associated with tangential activities, which is good financially, may be perceived by others, especially tax authorities, as evidence that the provider has strayed from its charitable purpose. This could lead to either explicit or implicit taxation. An interesting example of this problem involved a not-for-profit hospital in Buffalo, New York that generated substantial revenue from a yacht cruise business on Lake Erie. The Internal Revenue Service (IRS), which does not take such activities lightly, revoked the hospital's not-for-profit status. In hindsight, the hospital would have been much better off had it created a for-profit subsidiary for the cruise business and paid taxes on these revenues like any other cruise operator. By doing so, it would have protected the tax-exempt status for its patient service revenue.

At this point, it is worthwhile to spend some time on historical perspective. Until recently, healthcare providers reported *gross patient service revenue*, deductions for contractual allowances and charity care, and net patient service revenue directly on the income statement. The advantage to this presentation was that it allowed providers to very explicitly account for the amount of resources devoted to charity care. The disadvantage was that it made the income statements of healthcare providers different from businesses in virtually every other industry. For example, airlines have a set of full fares, such as $750 for a one-way coach ticket from New York to Chicago. Most travelers in coach do not pay this fare, however. Rather, they pay restricted, excursion fares that could be even less than $99. When an airline prepares its income statement, it does not list revenues at full fares, and then subtract an allowance for discount fares. What it shows on the income statement are those revenues that it actually expects to collect. Thus, the rest of the "world" reports only those revenues that businesses truly expect to receive, except for bad debt losses, which are accounted for by other means. In the early 1990s, healthcare providers were forced to report revenues in the same way as everyone else.

The charity care issue is a bit more controversial. Again, the charity care given by a healthcare provider historically was reported as a deduction in the revenue section of the income statement. That is, if $500 worth of charity services were provided, the income statement included this $500 in gross patient service revenue, then deducted the $500 as charity care, resulting in $0 net patient service revenue for those services. Now, charity care is not reported at all on the income statement. The logic is basically the same as that just discussed regarding discounts. That is, if no expectation of being paid for the services provided exists, no revenue is attributable to those services. Furthermore, no widely accepted methodology exists for setting the value of charity care that should be reported as revenue. Is it the charge on the provider's fee schedule, the charge less some discount, the provider's cost of providing the service, the societal value for the service, or some other amount? Reporting charity care directly on the income statement would make it more difficult to compare one organization's income statement to another.

The problem with not acknowledging charity care directly on the income statement stems from the fact that many not-for-profit organizations are under attack to defend their tax-exempt status. Such attacks occur for a variety of reasons, including the increasing pressure that local governments are under to increase their tax revenues. One way to defend an organization's charitable status is to prominently display the value of charity care provided. The logic is that instead of paying taxes, the organization pays back the community by providing charity care. By highlighting the amount of charity care provided, the old income statement format did that. (An argument may be that the prominent display of the amount of charity care provided encouraged not-for-profit organizations to provide such care.) Of course, healthcare providers still track and report the amount of charity care provided, but it is no longer shown directly on the income statement, and hence no longer subject to an external audit process that provides some validity of the reported numbers. As previously illustrated, however, a broad description of the organization's charity care policy, and perhaps an estimate of the value of such care provided, usually is contained in the footnotes to the financial statements.

Self-Test Questions

1. What categories of revenue are reported on the income statement?
2. Briefly, what is the difference between gross patient service revenue and net patient service revenue?
3. Describe how the following types of revenue are reported in the annual report:
   a. Discounts from charges
   b. Charity care
   c. Bad debt losses

Expenses

Expenses are the costs of doing business. As shown in Table 3.1, Sunnyvale reports its expenses in categories such as salaries and benefits, medical supplies, purchased medical services, and so on. According to the GAAP, expenses may be reported using either a *natural classification*, which classifies expenses by the nature of the expense, as Sunnyvale does, or a *functional classification*, which classifies expenses by purpose, such as inpatient services, outpatient services, and administrative. The number and nature of expense items reported on the income statement can vary widely, and depend on the nature and complexity of the organization. For example, some organizations, typically smaller ones, may report only two categories of expenses: health services, and general and administrative. Others may report a whole host of categories. Sunnyvale takes a middle-of-the-road approach to the number of expense categories. Most users of financial statements would prefer more, as well as a mixing of categories, rather than less because more insights can be gleaned if an organization reports revenues and expenses both by service breakdown (e.g., inpatient versus outpatient) and by type (e.g., salaries versus supplies).

Sunnyvale is typical of most healthcare providers in that the dominant portion of its cost structure is related to labor. The clinic reported *salaries and benefits* of $109,693,000 for 1998. The detail of how these costs are broken down by department or contract, or the relationship of these expenses to volume, is not part of the financial accounting information system. However, such information, which is very important to managers, is provided by the Sunnyvale managerial accounting system. Chapters 5 through 8 focus on managerial accounting matters.

The expense item titled *medical supplies* represents the cost of supplies used in providing patient services. Sunnyvale does not order supplies when a particular patient service requires them. Rather, the clinic's managers estimate the usage of individual items, orders them beforehand, and then maintains a medical supplies inventory. As readers will see in Chapter 4, the amount of supplies on hand is reported on the balance sheet. The income statement expense reported by Sunnyvale represents the cost of the supplies **actually consumed** in providing patient services. The expense reported for medical supplies does **not** reflect the actual cash spent by Sunnyvale on supplies purchases. In theory, Sunnyvale could have several years worth of supplies in its inventories at the beginning of 1998, could have used some (or all) of these supplies without replenishing the stocks, and hence not have spent one dime on supplies in 1998.

Purchased medical services represent the costs associated with services provided by outside contractors on behalf of the clinic. For example, rather than possess every piece of diagnostic equipment needed by its patients, Sunnyvale uses an independent diagnostic center for some of the tests. Sunnyvale charges its patients for these tests, even though they are performed by another organization. Sunnyvale then pays the diagnostic center for its services on the basis of a contract for services. Purchased medical services often arise when providers have capitated contracts. In such situations, it is not uncommon for major providers to accept responsibilities (and premium payment) for some services that they can not provide. Then, when patients covered by the capitated contract require such services, they are sent to other providers that have contracts to provide the services.

Sunnyvale conducts a small research program, typically clinical trials. Furthermore, the clinic conducts several educational programs for the community. The $9,863,000 reported as a *research and education* expense for 1998 reflects the costs associated with these programs.

Sunnyvale owns all of its property (i.e., land and buildings), but leases much of its diagnostic equipment. The total amount of lease expense, $3,189,000 for 1998, is reported as an expense on the income statement. Furthermore, some leased assets are reported directly on Sunnyvale's balance sheet, while other leased assets are reported in a footnote to the financial statements.[5] To assist users, the Sunnyvale financial statements contain this footnote:

> **Operating leases.** The clinic leases various equipment under operating leases expiring at various dates through December 2002. The following is a schedule by year of future minimum lease payments under operating leases in force as of December 31, 1998, that have initial or remaining lease terms in excess of one year.
>
> | | |
> |------|-------------|
> | 1999 | $2,989,135 |
> | 2000 | 2,668,000 |
> | 2001 | 1,875,000 |
> | 2002 | 1,223,000 |

The next expense category, *depreciation and amortization*, requires more extensive explanation. Businesses require *fixed assets* (i.e., long-term assets such as land, buildings, and equipment) to provide goods and services. Although some of these assets are leased, Sunnyvale owns most of the fixed assets necessary to support its mission. When the fixed assets were initially purchased, Sunnyvale did not report their purchase price as an expense on the income statement. Once acquired, the fixed assets were listed on the balance sheet as property owned by the clinic, but no expense was associated with their initial cost. The logic is that it would be improper to allocate fixed asset acquisition costs to a single accounting period because these assets are used to produce revenues over a long period of time, certainly longer than one accounting period. A more pragmatic reason for not reporting the costs of fixed assets when they are acquired is that such outlays would have a severe impact on reported profitability in years when large amounts are purchased. Furthermore, reported earnings would fluctuate widely from year to year on the basis of the amount of fixed assets acquired.

To match the cost of fixed assets to the services supported by those assets, accountants use the concept of *depreciation*, which spreads the cost of a fixed asset over many years. In essence, *depreciation expense* recognizes that fixed assets, which are not free, are required to provide the services that generate revenues. However, because fixed assets often can be used for long periods and hence generate revenues over many years, the costs associated with such assets should also be spread over long periods.

Note that most people use the terms "cost" and "expense" interchangeably. To accountants, however, the terms can have different meanings. Depreciation expense is a good example. Here the term "cost" is applied to the actual cash outlay for a fixed asset, while the term expense is used to describe the allocation of that cost over time.

The calculation of depreciation expense is somewhat arbitrary, so its amount generally is not closely related to the actual usage of a fixed asset nor its loss in market value. To illustrate, Sunnyvale owns a piece of diagnostic equipment that it uses infrequently. In 1997 it was used 23 times, while in 1998 it was used only nine times. Still, the depreciation expense associated with this equipment was the same $7,725 in both 1998 and 1997. Also, the clinic owns another piece of equipment that could be sold today for about the same price that Sunnyvale paid for it four years ago, yet each year the clinic reports a depreciation expense for that equipment, which implies loss of value.

Depreciation expense, like all other financial statement entries, is calculated in accordance with the GAAP. The calculation typically uses the *straight-line method;* that is, the depreciation expense is obtained by dividing the historical cost of the asset, less its estimated *salvage value*, by the number of years of its estimated useful life. (Salvage value is the amount, if any, expected to be received when final disposition occurs at the end of an asset's useful life.) The result is the asset's annual depreciation expense, which is the charge that is reflected in each year's income statement over the estimated life of the asset and, as readers will discover in Chapter 4, accumulated over time on the organization's balance sheet.[6] (The term *straight-line* stems from the fact that the depreciation expense is constant in each year, and hence the implied value of the asset declines evenly—like a straight line—over time.)

Amortization expense, which Sunnyvale combines with depreciation expense for income statement reporting, is related to mergers and acquisitions. In essence, when the clinic purchased some physician practices in the past, it was required to report a portion of the purchase price on its balance sheet as an asset called *goodwill*. Like fixed assets, goodwill is "depreciated" over time, but rather than called depreciation, this allocation of value is called *amortization*. Amortization is discussed in greater detail in Chapter 4.

Sunnyvale's depreciation and amortization expense totaled $6,405,000 for 1998. The footnotes to the financial statements disclosed that of this amount, $5,955,000 was for depreciation of fixed assets and $450,000 was for amortization of goodwill.

The next expense category on Sunnyvale's income statement is *provision for bad debts*. As discussed previously, the clinic reports as revenue in each year the charges for services provided minus discounts and charity care. Thus, it either collected, or expects to collect, a total of $169,013,000 for services provided in 1998. However, past experience indicates that the clinic will not collect every dollar that it expects to collect, even though payors are assumed to have the ability to pay. Of the reported $169,013,000 in net patient service revenue, Sunnyvale expects that $2,000,000 will never be collected. Thus, the clinic either has already collected, or expects to collect, $167,013,000 for services provided in 1998. With bad debt losses running at about $2,000 / $169,013 = 0.012 = 1.2% of patient service revenue, Sunnyvale is not losing a high percentage to deadbeat payors. Still, $2,000,000 is a great deal of money, and managers should review the clinic's collection policy to ensure that its efforts are effective. Finally, accountants must reconcile actual realized bad debt losses (which will not be known for some time) with past estimates. The details of this reconciliation are not discussed here, but rather best left to accounting books.

The next expense line reports *interest expense*. Sunnyvale owes or paid its lenders $5,329,000 in interest expense for debt capital supplied during 1998. The amount of interest expense reported by an organization is influenced primarily by its *capital structure*, which reflects the amount of debt that it uses. Also, interest expense is affected by the borrower's creditworthiness, its mix of long-term versus short-term debt, and the general level of interest rates. (These factors are discussed in detail at different points in later chapters.)

As readers will discover in Chapter 4, Sunnyvale reported roughly $88 million in long-term debt, including debt coming due in one year, at the end of 1998. Thus, the implied interest cost on its debt capital is $5,329 / $88,000 = 0.061 = 6.1%. This is just a rough estimate of the clinic's true cost of debt capital because the amount of debt outstanding fluctuated over the year from the $88,000,000 end-of-year value reported on the balance sheet. In fact, as we will see in Table 4.1, Sunnyvale began 1998 with $56 million of debt, so the clinic added considerable debt during the year. The average amount of long-term debt outstanding was ($56 + $88) / 2 = $72 million. Using this amount, the implied interest cost is $5,329 / $72,000 = 0.074 = 7.4%.

Under certain circumstances, Sunnyvale, like all not-for-profit organizations, may earn more on its debt investments than it pays for debt capital. The implication of this situation is that the clinic could borrow large amounts of debt capital, reinvest it in securities, and make a killing. However, the primary factor that creates this positive *spread* between borrowing costs and investment returns is that not-for-profit organizations can issue tax-exempt debt on which lenders are willing to accept a relatively low return. On the other hand, Sunnyvale and other not-for-profit organizations do not have to pay taxes on their interest earnings, so they keep the entire amount. Although not-for-profit organizations can engage in this type of *tax arbitrage* in support of operations, tax laws prohibit them from issuing tax-exempt debt for the sole purpose of investing in securities.

Finally, Sunnyvale reported $6,667,000 in expenses for 1998 in the catchall category of "other." Listed here are general and administrative expenses that individually are too small to list separately, including items such as marketing expenses and independent auditor's fees. Although organizations cannot possibly report every expense item separately, it is frustrating for users of financial statement information to come across a large, unexplained expense item. Thus, some financial statements include a footnote that provides additional detail regarding other expenses.

Self-Test Questions

1. What is an expense?
2. Briefly, what are some of the commonly reported expense categories?
3. What is the logic behind depreciation expense?
4. What is the logic behind the provision for bad losses?

Net Income

Although the reporting of revenues and expenses is clearly important, the most important single piece of information on the income statement is profitability, as captured in Table 3.1 by the line titled *net income*. As discussed earlier, net income is merely the difference between total revenues and total expenses. To illustrate, Sunnyvale reported net income of $7,860,000 for 1998: $176,092,000 − $168,232,000 = $7,860,000.

Because of its location on the income statement and its importance, net income is often referred to as the *bottom line*. The income statements of not-for-profit organizations often call the profit line *revenues over expenses, excess of revenues over expenses, change in net assets,* or something else. Regardless of the terminology used, not-for-profit organizations are required by the GAAP to include a *performance indicator* on their income statements that reports the financial results of operations. Throughout this book, this performance indicator is referred to as net income because this terminology, which is used on for-profit income statements, has universal recognition.

In spite of the fact that Sunnyvale is a not-for-profit organization, **it still has to make a profit**. If the clinic is to offer new services in the future, it must earn a profit today to produce the funds needed for new assets. Because of inflation, the clinic could not even replace its current fixed asset base as needed without the funds generated by profitable operations. Thus, turning a profit is essential for all businesses, including those having not-for-profit status. The logic behind this statement is examined in more detail in the next section.

What happens to an organization's net income? For the most part, it is reinvested in the organization. Not-for-profit businesses **must** reinvest all earnings in the business. An investor-owned business, on the other hand, may use a portion, or all, of its net income to make *dividend payments* to shareholders. The amount of profits reinvested in an investor-owned business, therefore, is net income minus the amount of dividends paid out to stockholders.

The proportion of net income paid out as dividends is called the *payout ratio,* while the proportion that is retained within the business is called the *retention ratio.* Thus, if Sunnyvale were an investor-owned clinic and if it paid $2,000,000 in dividends in 1998, its payout ratio would be $2,000 / $7,860 = 0.254 = 25.4% and its retention ratio would be ($7,860 − $2,000) / $7,860 = $5,860 / $7,860 = 0.746 = 74.6%. Also, net income only has two places to go—dividends and retained earnings—so the retention ratio is equal to 1 − Payout ratio, and the payout ratio is equal to 1 − Retention ratio.

Net income represents profitability **as defined by the GAAP**. In establishing the GAAP, accountants have created guidelines that attempt to measure the *economic income* of a business, which, honestly, is a very difficult task because economic gains and losses often are not matched by easy to identify financial events. Thus, the fact that Sunnyvale reported net income of $7,860,000 for 1998 does not mean that the clinic, on net, experienced a cash inflow of that amount. This point is discussed in greater detail in the next section.

Before moving on, note that some not-for-profit income statements contain a section below the net income entry that reconciles the reported net income with the net assets (i.e., equity) reported on the balance sheet. In essence, the entire amount of net income of not-for-profit organizations must be reinvested in the business, so the amount of net assets reported on the balance sheet, after various adjustments, must increase over the year by the amount of net income. The important relationships between the income statement and the balance sheet are considered in more depth in Chapter 4.

1. How is net income calculated?
2. Why is net income called the bottom line?
3. What happens to net income?
4. What is the payout ratio?
5. What is the retention ratio?
6. What are the payout and retention ratios of a not-for-profit organization?

Net Income Versus Cash Flow

As stated previously, the income statement reports profitability as net income, which is determined in accordance with the GAAP. Although net income is an important measure of profitability, an organization's financial condition, at least in the short run, depends more on the actual cash that flows into and out of the business than it does on reported net income. Thus, occasionally a business will go bankrupt even though its net income has historically been positive. More commonly, many businesses that have reported negative net incomes (i.e., net losses) have survived with little or no financial damage. How can these things happen?

The problem is that the income statement is like a mixture of apples and oranges. Consider Table 3.1. Sunnyvale reported total revenues of $176,092,000 for 1998, yet this is not the amount of cash that was actually collected during the year. Furthermore, some revenues reported for 1997 were actually collected in 1998, but these do not appear on the 1998 income statement. Thus, because of accrual accounting, reported revenue is not the same as cash revenue. The same logic applies to expenses; few of the values reported as expenses on the income statement are the same as the actual cash outflows. To make matters worse, not one cent of depreciation and amortization expense was paid out as cash. Depreciation expense, as well as amortization, is an accounting reflection of asset use, but Sunnyvale did not actually pay out $6,405,000 in cash to someone called the *collector of depreciation and amortization*. Sunnyvale actually paid out $88,549,000 sometime in the past to purchase the clinic's total fixed assets, as well as some additional amount to purchase physician practices, of which $6,405,000 was recognized in 1998 as a cost of doing business, just as salaries and benefits were a cost of doing business.

How can net income be converted to cash flow, the actual amount of cash generated during the year? As a rough estimate, cash flow can be thought of as net income plus the major categories of noncash expenses. Thus, the actual cash flow generated by Sunnyvale in 1998 is not merely the $7,860,000 reported net income, but this amount plus the $6,405,000 shown for depreciation and amortization, for a total of $14,265,000.[7] The depreciation and amortization expense must be added back to net income to get cash flow because depreciation and amortization is a noncash expense. That is, on the income statement this amount was subtracted from revenues to obtain net income, even though there was no cash outlay.

Here is another way of looking at cash flow versus accounting income. If Sunnyvale showed no net income for 1998, it would still be generating cash of $6,405,000 because that amount was listed as an expense but not actually paid out in cash. The idea behind the income statement treatment is that Sunnyvale would be able to set aside this amount, which is above and beyond its operating expenses, this year and in future years. Eventually, the accumulated total of depreciation and amortization would be used by Sunnyvale to replace its fixed assets as they wear out or become obsolete. Thus, the incorporation of depreciation expense into the cost, and ultimately the price structure, is designed to ensure the ability of an organization to replenish its investment in fixed assets, assuming that the assets could be purchased in the future at their historical cost. To be more realistic, businesses must plan to generate net income in addition to the accumulated funds sufficient to replace existing fixed assets in the future at inflated costs, or even to expand the asset base. It appears that Sunnyvale does have such capabilities as reflected in its $7,860,000 net income and $14,265,000 cash flow for 1998.[8]

It is important to understand that the $14,265,000 cash flow calculated here is only an **estimate** of actual cash flow for 1998. The problem again is accrual accounting. Although the major category of noncash expenses was recognized in estimating cash flow, almost every item of revenues and expenses listed on the income statement does not equal its cash flow counterpart. The greater the difference between the reported values and cash values, the less reliable the rough estimate of cash flow as defined here. The value of knowing the precise amount of cash generated or lost during an accounting period has not gone unnoticed by accountants. In Chapter 4, readers will learn about the statement of cash flows, which can be thought of as an income statement that is recast totally to focus on cash flow.

Self-Test Questions

1. What is the difference between net income and cash flow?
2. How can income statement data be used to estimate cash flow?
3. Why do not-for-profit businesses need to make profits?

Income Statements of Investor-Owned Firms

Our income statement discussion focused on a not-for-profit organization: Sunnyvale Clinic. What do the income statements for investor-owned firms such as Columbia/HCA and Beverly Enterprises look like? According to the FASB, the financial statements of investor-owned firms and not-for-profit businesses are generally similar, except for transactions that are clearly only applicable to one form of ownership. Because the transactions of all health services organizations in the same core business are similar, ownership plays only a minor role in the presentation of financial statement data. In reality, more differences exist in financial statements because of lines of business (e.g., hospitals versus nursing homes versus managed care plans) than differences because of ownership.

1. Are there appreciable differences in the financial statements of not-for-profit businesses and investor-owned businesses?

Self-Test Question

A Look Ahead: Using Income Statement Data in Financial Statement Analysis

Chapter 17 discusses in some detail the techniques used to analyze financial statements. The purpose of such an analysis is to gain an appreciation of a business' financial condition. At this point, however, it would be worthwhile to introduce *ratio analysis*, one of the techniques used in financial statement analysis. In ratio analysis, values found on the financial statements are combined into ratios that have economic meaning, and hence that help managers and investors interpret the numbers.

To illustrate, *total profit margin*, sometimes just called *profit margin*, is defined as net income divided by total revenues. For Sunnyvale Clinic, the profit margin for 1998 was $7,860,000 / $176,092,000 = 0.045 = 4.5\%$. Thus, each dollar of revenues generated by the clinic produced 4.5 cents of profit (i.e., net income). By implication, each dollar of revenues required 95.5 cents of expenses. The profit margin is a measure of expense control; for a given amount of revenues, the higher the net income, and hence the profit margin, the lower the expenses. If the profit margin for other clinics were known, judgments about how well Sunnyvale is doing in the area of expense control, relative to its peers, could be made.

The Sunnyvale profit margin for 1997 was $8,206,000 / $146,600,000 = 0.060 = 6.0\%$, so the clinic's profit margin slipped from 1997 to 1998. This finding should alert managers to examine carefully the increase in expenses in 1998. In effect, Sunnyvale's expenses increased faster than its revenues, which resulted in falling profitability as measured by the profit margin. If this trend continues, it would not take the clinic long to be operating in the red (i.e., losing money). A complete discussion of ratio analysis can be found in Chapter 17. The discussion here, along with a brief visit in Chapter 4, is merely intended to give readers a preview of how financial statement data can be used to make judgments about a business' financial condition.

1. Explain how ratio analysis can be used to help interpret income statement data.
2. What is the total profit margin, and what does it measure?

Self-Test Questions

Key Concepts

Financial accounting information is the result of a process of identifying, measuring, recording, and communicating the economic events and status of an organization to interested parties. This information is summarized and presented in three primary financial statements: the income statement, the balance sheet, and the statement of cash flows. The key concepts of this chapter are:

- The predominant *users of financial accounting information* are parties who have a direct financial interest in the economic status of a health services organization, primarily its managers and investors.
- *Generally accepted accounting principles* (*GAAP*) establish the standards for financial accounting measurement and reporting. These principles have been sanctioned by the *Securities and Exchange Commission* (*SEC*); developed by the *Financial Accounting Standards Board* (*FASB*) and its predecessor, the *Accounting Principles Board* (*APB*); and refined by the *American Institute of Certified Public Accountants* (*AICPA*) and other organizations.
- The preparation and presentation of financial accounting data is based on several principles, the most important being (1) *time period*, (2) *accrual accounting*, (3) *matching*, and (4) *materiality*.
- An organization's *annual report* contains both qualitative information (the verbal discussion) and quantitative information (the financial statements).
- The *income statement* reports on an organization's operations over a period of time. Its basic structure consists of *revenues*, *expenses*, and *profit* (i.e., *net income*), which equals revenues minus expenses.
- *Revenues*, for the most part, are monies collected or expected to be collected as a result of providing services.
- *Expenses* are the economic costs associated with the provision of services.
- *Net income* represents the economic profitability of a business as defined by the GAAP.
- Because the income statement is constructed using accrual accounting, net income does not represent the actual amount of cash that has been earned or lost during the reporting period. To estimate *cash flow*, the most important noncash expenses, typically depreciation and amortization, must be added back to net income.
- The financial statements of investor-owned and not-for-profit businesses tend to look very much alike. However, the statements of health services organizations in different lines of business can vary. The good news is that all financial statements have essentially the same economic content.
- *Ratio analysis*, which combines values that are found in the financial statements, helps managers and investors interpret the data with the goal of making judgments about the financial condition of the business.

In this chapter, the focus is on financial accounting basics and the income statement. In Chapter 4, the discussion of financial accounting continues with the remaining two primary statements: the balance sheet and statement of cash flows.

Questions

3.1 a. What is a stakeholder?
    b. What stakeholders are most interested in the financial condition of a healthcare provider?

3.2 a. What are the generally acceptable accounting principles (GAAP)?
    b. What is the purpose of the GAAP?
    c. What organizations are involved in establishing the GAAP?

3.3 Briefly describe the following concepts as they apply to the preparation of financial statements:
    a. Time period
    b. Cash versus accrual accounting
    c. Matching principle
    d. Materiality

3.4 What is an annual report?

3.5 Briefly describe the format of the income statement.

3.6 a. What is the difference between gross revenues and net revenues? (Hint: Think about discounts and charity care.)
    b. What is the difference between patient service revenue and other revenue?
    c. What is the difference between charity care and bad debt losses? How is each handled on the income statement?

3.7 a. What is meant by the term *expense*?
    b. What is depreciation expense and what is its purpose?
    c. What are other categories of expenses?

3.8 a. What is net income?
    b. Why is net income called the bottom line?
    c. What is the difference between net income and cash flow?
    d. Is financial condition more closely related to net income or to cash flow?

Problems

3.1 Entries for Warren Clinic's 1998 income statement are listed below in alphabetical order. Reorder the data in proper format.

Bad debt expense	$ 40,000
Depreciation expense	90,000
General/administrative expenses	70,000
Interest expense	20,000
Interest income	40,000
Net income	30,000
Other revenue	10,000
Patient service revenue	440,000
Purchased clinic services	90,000
Salaries and benefits	150,000
Total revenues	490,000
Total expenses	460,000

3.2 Consider the following 1998 income statement:

BestCare HMO
Statement of Operations
Year Ended June 30, 1998
(in thousands)

Revenue:
Premiums earned	$26,682
Coinsurance	1,689
Interest and other income	242
Total revenues	$28,613

Expenses:
Salaries and benefits	$15,154
Medical supplies and drugs	7,507
Insurance	3,963
Provision for bad debts	19
Depreciation	367
Interest	385
Total expenses	$27,395
Net income	$ 1,218

a. How does this income statement differ from the one presented in Table 3.1?
b. Did BestCare spend $367,000 on new fixed assets during fiscal year 1998? If not, what is the economic rationale behind its reported depreciation expense?
c. Explain the provision for bad debts entry.
d. What is BestCare's total profit margin? How can it be interpreted?

3.3 Consider this 1998 income statement:

Green Valley Nursing Home, Inc.
Statement of Income
Year Ended December 31, 1998

Revenue:
Net patient service revenue	$3,163,258
Other revenue	106,146
Total revenues	$3,269,404

Expenses:	
Salaries and benefits	$1,515,438
Medical supplies and drugs	966,781
Insurance and other	296,357
Provision for bad debts	110,000
Depreciation	85,000
Interest	206,780
Total expenses	$3,180,356
Operating income	$ 89,048
Provision for income taxes	31,167
Net income	$ 57,881

a. How does this income statement differ from the ones presented in Table 3.1 and Problem 3.2?

b. Why does Green Valley show a provision for income taxes while the other two income statements did not?

c. What is Green Valley's total profit margin? How does this value compare with the values for Sunnyvale Clinic and BestCare?

d. The before-tax profit margin for Green Valley is operating income divided by total revenues. Calculate Green Valley's before-tax profit margin. Why may this be a better measure of expense control when comparing an investor-owned business with a not-for-profit business?

3.4 Great Forks Hospital reported net income for 1998 of $2.4 million on total revenues of $30 million. Depreciation expense totaled $1 million.

a. What were total expenses for 1998?

b. What were total cash expenses for 1998? (Hint: Assume that all expenses except depreciation were cash expenses.)

c. What was the hospital's 1998 cash flow?

3.5 Brandywine Homecare, a not-for-profit business, had revenues of $12 million in 1998. Expenses other than depreciation totaled 75 percent of revenues, and depreciation expense was $1.5 million. All revenues were collected in cash during the year and all expenses other than depreciation were paid in cash.

a. Construct Brandywine's 1998 income statement.

b. What were Brandywine's net income, total profit margin, and cash flow?

c. Now, suppose the company changed its depreciation calculation procedures (still within the GAAP) such that its depreciation expense doubled. How would this change affect Brandywine's net income, total profit margin, and cash flow?

d. Suppose the change had halved, rather than doubled, the firm's depreciation expense. Now, what would be the impact on net income, total profit margin, and cash flow?

3.6 Assume that Mainline Homecare, a for-profit corporation, had exactly the same situation as reported in Problem 3.5. However, Mainline must pay taxes at a rate of 40 percent of pre-tax income. Assuming that the same revenues and expenses reported for financial accounting purposes would be reported for tax purposes, redo Problem 3.5 for Mainline.

Notes

1. Historically, external auditors were mostly concerned with the letter of the law. Their work was relatively narrow in scope—primarily ensuring that financial statements were prepared and presented in accordance with the GAAP. However, this approach seldom identified problems, especially fraud, which affected the organization's financial condition. After several large lawsuits found major accounting firms negligent in failing to identify problem areas, auditors are now paying much more attention to the activities behind the numbers.

2. Each year, the FASB must deal with very difficult and controversial matters. At this time, the FASB is grappling with how to measure and report dealings in very complex derivative securities, such as options and swaps, that are used by businesses to help manage risk.

3. Investor-owned health services organizations with publicly traded securities are required by the Securities and Exchange Commission (SEC) to file both annual and quarterly financial statements. Many of these statements are available for free at various Internet web sites.

4. Four basic financial statements exist; the focus in this book is on the three statements that are most important. The fourth statement, titled the *statement of changes in net assets* or the *statement of changes in equity*, focuses on changes in the owners' position from one year to the next. Because this statement is relatively short, not-for-profit organizations have the option to include it at the end of the income statement.

5. *Operating leases* are relatively short-term leases that have a term that is less than the useful life of the leased property. For example, automobile leases are operating leases. Conversely, *financial*, or *capital*, *leases* have a term that roughly equals the life of the leased property. As readers will see in Chapter 4, the balance sheet consequences of operating leases are reported in the footnotes to the financial statements; the consequences of financial leases must be reported directly on the statement.

6. For-profit firms have to be concerned with both *book depreciation*, which is calculated according to the GAAP and reported on the firm's income statement, and *tax depreciation*, which is calculated according to Internal Revenue Service (IRS) regulations and used to determine the firm's income for tax purposes. Also, note that land is not depreciated for financial accounting or tax purposes.

7. Why not add back the provision for bad debts when converting accounting income to cash flow because it too is a noncash expense? It could be added, but typically this amount is small relative to the other values. Furthermore, this calculation is just a rough estimate. Finally, bad losses, to the extent that estimates are met, actually reduce cash flow, as these revenues will never be collected.

8. Indeed, the need to generate revenues to replenish fixed assets at inflated prices and to grow assets is a very important reason that so-called not-for-profit organizations **must** make a profit.

References

AICPA. 1997a. *Audit and Accounting Guide.* New York: American Institute of Certified Public Accountants.

———. 1997b. *Checklists and Illustrative Financial Statements for Health Care Organizations.* New York: American Institute of Certified Public Accountants.

Bitter, M. E. and J. Cassidy. 1992. "Perceptions of New AICPA Audit Guide." *Healthcare Financial Management* (November): 38–48.

Duis, T. E. 1993. "The Need for Consistency in Healthcare Reporting." *Healthcare Financial Management* (July): 40–44.

———. 1994. "Unravelling the Confusion Caused by GASB, FASB Accounting Rules." *Healthcare Financial Management* (November): 66–69.

Robbins, W. A. and R. Turpin. 1993. "Accounting Practice Diversity in the Healthcare Industry." *Healthcare Financial Management* (May): 111–114.

THE BALANCE SHEET AND STATEMENT OF CASH FLOWS

Learning Objectives

After studying this chapter, readers will be able to:

- Explain the purpose of the balance sheet.
- Describe the contents of the balance sheet and its interrelationship with the income statement.
- Explain the purpose of the statement of cash flows.
- Describe the contents of the statement of cash flows and how it differs from the income statement.
- Describe how a business' transactions affect its income statement and balance sheet.

Introduction

Although the income statement, which was covered in Chapter 3, contains information about an organization's operations, it does not provide information about the resources needed to produce the revenues or how those resources were financed. Another primary financial statement, the *balance sheet*, contains information about an organization's assets and the financing used to acquire those assets.

Over the years, accountants and managers have become increasingly aware that net income is not the most important determinant of financial condition. Although net income, which reflects an organization's profitability according to the GAAP, is an important profitability measure, financial condition is more closely related to the actual flow of cash into and out of a business. The second financial statement discussed in this chapter, the *statement of cash flows*, focuses on this important determinant of financial condition.

In addition to understanding the composition of these two financial statements, it is very important that managers understand the relationships among all three primary financial statements. Thus, emphasis is placed on the interrelationships among the statements throughout the chapter. Finally, the end of the chapter contains a brief introduction on how actual business transactions work their way into an organization's financial statements; this provides readers with a feel for how financial statements actually are created.

Balance Sheet Basics

Whereas the income statement reports the results of operations **over a period of time**, the *balance sheet* presents a snapshot of the financial position of an organization **at a given point in time**. For this reason, the balance sheet is also called the *statement of financial position*. The balance sheet changes every day as a business increases or decreases its assets or changes its financing. The important point is that the balance sheet, unlike the income statement, reflects a business' financial position as of a given date; the data in it typically become invalid one day later, even when both dates are in the same accounting period. Healthcare providers with seasonal demand, such as a walk-in clinic in Fort Lauderdale, Florida, have especially large changes in their balance sheets during the year. For such businesses, a balance sheet constructed in February can look quite different from one prepared in August. Also, businesses that are growing very rapidly will have significant changes in their balance sheets over relatively short periods of time.

The balance sheet lists, as of the end of the reporting period, the resources of an organization and the claims against those resources. In other words, the balance sheet reports the assets of an organization and how those assets were financed. The balance sheet has the following basic structure:

Assets	Liabilities and Equity
Current assets	Current liabilities
Long-term assets	Long-term liabilities
	Equity
Total assets	Total liabilities and equity.

The *assets side* (left side) of the balance sheet lists all the resources, or assets, owned by the organization in dollar terms. In general, assets are broken down into categories that distinguish short-lived assets from long-lived assets. The *liabilities and equity side* (claims side or right side) lists the claims against these resources, again in dollar terms. In essence, the right side reports the sources of financing used to acquire the assets listed on the left side. The claims of creditors (the suppliers of debt capital) are the liabilities of an organization, while the owners (the suppliers of equity capital) have a residual claim (after that of the creditors) against the assets. In other words, the dollar amounts of liability claims are fixed by contract, whereas the dollar amount of equity depends both on asset values and the amount of liabilities.

Perhaps the most important characteristic of the balance sheet is simply that it must balance: the left side must equal the right side. This relationship, which is called the *accounting identity* or *basic accounting equation*, is expressed in equation form as:

$$A = L + E,$$

where A = Total assets, L = Total liabilities, and E = Total equity. Because creditor claims are paid before equity claims if a health services organization is liquidated, liabilities are shown before equity both on the balance sheet and in the basic accounting equation.

Table 4.1 contains Sunnyvale's balance sheet, which follows the basic structure explained above. The title of the balance sheet reinforces the fact that the data are presented for the clinic as a whole. The balance sheet is not going to provide much information, if any, about the subparts of an organization such as product or service lines. Rather, the balance sheet will provide an overview of the economic position of the organization as a whole. The timing of the balance sheet is also apparent in the title. The data are reported for 1998 and 1997 as of December 31. Whereas the income statement indicated the data were for the years ended, the balance merely indicates a closing date. This minor difference in terminology reinforces the point that the income statement reports operational results over a period of time, while the balance sheet reports financial position at a single point in time. Finally, the amounts reported on Sunnyvale's balance sheet, just as on income statement, are expressed in thousands of dollars.

The format of the balance sheet emphasizes the basic accounting equation. For example, as of December 31, 1998, Sunnyvale had a total of $154,815,000 in assets that were financed by a total of $154,815,000 of liabilities and equity. Besides this obvious confirmation that the balance sheet balances, this statement indicates that the total assets of Sunnyvale were valued, according to the GAAP, at $154,815,000. Liabilities and equity represent claims of various classes of creditors and "owners" against these assets, with creditors having first priority in claims for $100,747,000 and "owners" following with a residual claim of $54,068,000. The right side of the balance sheet (liabilities and equity, which are in the bottom section of Table 4.1) reflects the manner in which Sunnyvale raised the capital needed to acquire its assets.

1. What is the purpose of the balance sheet?
2. What are the three major sections of the balance sheet?
3. What is the accounting identity, and what information does it provide?

**Self-Test
Questions**

Assets

All *assets* either possess or create economic benefit for the organization. The asset section of the balance sheet is organized in a very logical way. Table 4.1 contains four major categories of assets: current assets, long-term investments, property and equipment (fixed assets), and other assets. The following sections describe the asset categories in detail.

Current Assets

Current assets include cash and other assets that are expected to be converted into cash **within a year**. For Sunnyvale, current assets totaled $54,306,000 at the end

TABLE 4.1
Sunnyvale Clinic:
Balance Sheets
December 31, 1998
and 1997
(in thousands)

ASSETS	1998	1997
Current Assets:		
Cash	$ 12,102	$ 6,486
Marketable securities	10,000	5,000
Net patient accounts receivable	28,509	25,927
Inventories	3,695	2,302
Total current assets	$ 54,306	$ 39,715
Long-term investments	$ 42,889	$ 20,667
Property and Equipment (Fixed Assets):		
Land	$ 2,954	$ 2,035
Buildings and equipment	85,595	77,208
Gross fixed assets	$ 88,549	$ 79,243
Less: Accumulated depreciation	36,099	30,144
Net fixed assets	$ 52,450	$ 49,099
Other Assets:		
Goodwill	$ 5,170	$ 5,620
Total assets	$ 154,815	$ 115,101

LIABILITIES AND EQUITY	1998	1997
Current Liabilities:		
Current maturities of long-term debt	$ 2,834	$ 2,345
Accounts payable	6,522	7,933
Accrued expenses:		
Wages and benefits	4,344	3,523
Taxes	844	996
Interest payable	881	518
Total current liabilities	$ 15,425	$ 15,315
Long-term debt	$ 85,322	$ 53,578
Total liabilities	$ 100,747	$ 68,893
Net assets (Equity)	$ 54,068	$ 46,208
Total liabilities and equity	$ 154,815	$ 115,101

of 1998. Suppose that the marketable securities on the books at that time were converted into cash as they matured, and the receivables were collected and the inventories billed to patients and collected at their stated values. With all else the same, Sunnyvale would have $54,306,000 in cash at the end of 1999. Of course, all else will not be the same, so Sunnyvale's 1999 reported cash balance will likely be different from $54,306,000.

In general, current assets are expected to provide the cash that will be used to pay off the $15,425,000 in current liabilities outstanding at the end of 1998 as they become due in 1999. Thus, current assets are a reflection of the *liquidity* of the organization. A business is *liquid* if it has the cash available to pay its bills as they become due. The difference between total current assets and total current liabilities is called *net working capital*. Thus, at the end of 1998, Sunnyvale had net working capital of $54,306,000 − $15,425,000 = $38,881,000. From a pure liquidity standpoint, the greater an organization's net working capital, the better. However, as will be pointed out in this and subsequent chapters, there are costs to carrying current assets, so health services organizations have to balance the need for liquidity against the associated costs of maintaining liquidity.

Within Sunnyvale's current assets, there is $12,102,000 in *cash*, which represent actual cash in hand and money held in commercial checking accounts (demand deposits). There is also $10,000,000 of short-term *marketable securities*, which represent short-term investments in highly liquid, low-risk securities such as U.S. Treasury bills or prime commercial paper.[1] Organizations hold marketable securities because cash and commercial checking accounts typically pay no interest. Thus, businesses should hold only enough cash and checking account balances to pay their reoccurring operating expenses; any funds on hand in excess of immediate needs should be invested in safe, short-term, highly liquid (but interest bearing) securities. Additionally, marketable securities are built up periodically to meet projected nonoperating cash outlays such as tax payments, investments in property and equipment, and legal judgments. Even though marketable securities pay relatively low interest, any return is better than none, so marketable securities are preferable to cash holdings.

Marketable securities normally are reported on the balance sheet *at cost*, which is the amount initially paid for the securities. However, because of changing interest rates and other factors, the marketable securities may actually be worth more or less than their purchase price. The current market value of the securities is listed in the notes to the financial statements.

Net patient accounts receivable represents money that is owed to Sunnyvale for services that the clinic has already provided. As discussed in Chapter 2, and reiterated in Chapter 3, third-party payors make most payments for healthcare services, and these payments often take weeks or months to be billed, processed, and ultimately paid. The patient accounts receivable amount of $28,509,000 at the end of 1998 is listed on the balance sheet *net* of allowances for discounts, charity care, and bad debt losses. Thus, the presentation on the balance sheet is consistent with the Chapter 3 discussion concerning patient service revenue.

The $28,509,000 net receivable amount seen on the balance sheet is a subset of the income statement's net patient service revenue of $169,013,000 for

1998. (See Table 3.1 in Chapter 3.) The logic is as follows. A total of $169,013,000 was billed (roughly) to payors during 1998. This is also a "net" number as there is a higher gross amount of charges in Sunnyvale's managerial accounting system that reflects charges before deductions for discounts and charity care. Of this $169,013,000 of patient service revenue, $2,000,000 was shown as a bad debt loss expense on the income statement. This bad debt expense represents Sunnyvale's estimate, based on past experience, of the total dollar amount of net patient service revenue that will never be collected.

The fact that $28,509,000 of the 1999 net patient service revenue remains to be collected and that another $2,000,000 has been written off as bad debt losses, suggest that the difference between $169,013,000 − $2,000,000 = $167,013,000 and $28,509,000, which totals $138,504,000, was collected during 1998. Where is this collected cash? It could be anywhere. Most of it went right out the door to pay operating expenses. Some of the collected cash may have been used to purchase assets (e.g., new equipment), and hence may be sitting in one of the asset accounts on the balance sheet. If the clinic were to close its doors on the last day of 1998, its patient accounts receivable balance of $28,509,000 would fall to zero when the entire amount was collected (except for any errors in the bad debt forecast). However, if Sunnyvale continues as an ongoing enterprise, the receivables balance really never does fall to zero because while Sunnyvale's collections are lowering it, new services are constantly being provided that create new billings, and hence new receivables that are added to it.

The final current asset on Table 4.1, *inventories,* primarily reflects Sunnyvale's investment in medical supplies. The value of supplies on hand at the end of 1998 was $3,695,000. As with the cash account, it is not in a business' best interest to maximize the amount of inventories that it holds. There is a certain level of supplies that is necessary to meet medical needs and to maintain a safety stock to guard against unexpected surges in usage. However, many health services organizations are trying to drive their investment in inventories toward zero through aggressive inventory management. One technique being used is the *just-in-time* system, in which suppliers are expected to manage the inventory and, as the term suggests, deliver the inventory to providers when needed.

Businesses that hold large amounts of inventories, such as medical supply companies, typically include a footnote that discusses the specific accounting practices used to value those inventories. However, most healthcare providers hold relatively small levels of inventories, and hence footnote information often is not provided. In fact, because of the materiality principle discussed in Chapter 2, many providers do not break out inventories as a separate item on their balance sheets, but rather include the value of inventories in a catchall account called *other current assets.*

Again, the primary purposes served by the current asset accounts are to support the operations of the organization and to provide liquidity. However, current assets do not generate high returns. For example, cash earns no return and marketable securities generally earn relatively low returns. The receivables account does not earn interest income nor generate new patient service revenue; inventories represent dollar amounts invested in items sitting on shelves, which earn no return until patients are billed for their use. Because of the low return on current assets, organizations try to minimize these accounts, yet ensure that the levels maintained are sufficient to support the organization's operations. (Readers will learn much more about current asset management in Chapter 16.)

Notice that the current assets section of the balance sheet is listed in order of liquidity or nearness to cash. Cash, as the most liquid asset, is listed first, while the least liquid of current assets, inventories, is listed last. Dollars invested in inventories will first move into patient accounts receivable as the patients are billed for the supplies utilized. Accounts receivable will eventually be converted into cash when they are collected, and then perhaps shifted to marketable securities if the cash is not needed to pay current bills.

Finally, the importance of converting current assets into marketable securities as quickly as possible (and ultimately converting zero-return assets into some-return assets) cannot be overemphasized. Under most reimbursement methods, providers must first build the current assets necessary to provide the services, then actually do the work, and finally, some time later (often 60 to 70 days), get paid. Providers that operate under capitation have a significant advantage as compared to those that primarily receive fee-for-service revenue. As discussed in Chapter 2, payment for capitated services occurs upfront, before the services are actually provided. Various incentive withholds exist and some managed care plans are very slow in making the payments, but generally, there are liquidity advantages to capitation. Health services organizations that work in a predominantly capitated environment will have much smaller accounts receivable balances and much larger cash and marketable securities balances than do providers, such as Sunnyvale, that operate in a predominantly fee-for-service environment.

Long-Term Investments

The second major asset category (after current assets) is *long-term investments*, which is the money Sunnyvale has invested in various forms of long-term (maturities that exceed one year) securities. This account represents investments in long-term *financial assets*, as opposed to investments in long-term *real assets*, which are listed next on the balance sheet as property and equipment (fixed assets). The $42,889,000 reported at the end of 1998 represent the amount that the clinic has invested in stocks, bonds, and other investments that have a longer maturity than marketable securities and that hopefully will provide Sunnyvale with a higher return.

Long-term securities investments are reported on the balance sheet at *fair market value*, rather than initial cost, so changes in market conditions over time will cause the value of this account to change even if the securities held remain unchanged. Also, changes in market values of long-term investments result in unrealized gains or losses on the investments, which must be incorporated into the income statement. A footnote will usually reveal the details of the types of security investments held by the organization and the resulting gains and losses. The income produced by the long-term investments, as well as the income earned on marketable securities, is reported on the income statement. As discussed in Chapter 3, Sunnyvale reported other revenue of $7,079,000 for 1998. According to the footnotes, this amount included interest income of $3,543,000.

The discussion of current assets contained a suggestion that organizations try to minimize the amounts held, maintaining only the amounts necessary to support operations. One of the benefits of prudent management of *working capital* (current assets) is that more money can be moved into long-term investments, both financial and real, which generate greater returns than those provided by current assets. The ultimate rewards for minimizing an organization's working capital are both the reduction in carrying costs (current assets costs money because each dollar in assets has to be matched by a dollar of financing) and the increased return available on long-term investments.

Sunnyvale is not in the financial services business; it is in the business of providing healthcare services. Thus, what is expected is that the funds currently invested in long-term investments will eventually be invested in real assets that provide new or improved services to Sunnyvale's patients. If Sunnyvale were investor owned rather than not for profit, the business likely would not show such a large investment in long-term securities. Most profits that are earned above the amount needed for near-term reinvestment in the business would likely be returned to the capital suppliers, either by debt repurchases or, more typically, by dividends or stock repurchases. When additional capital is needed for long-term asset investment, an investor-owned business would go to the capital markets for additional debt financing, and if necessary, equity financing.

Property and Equipment (Fixed Assets)

The third major asset category is *property and equipment,* often called *fixed assets.* Fixed assets, as compared to current assets (and even compared to long-term securities investments), are highly illiquid and are used over long periods of time by the organization. Whereas current assets rise and fall spontaneously with the organization's level of operations, fixed assets are normally set, and maintained, at a level sufficient to handle peak patient demand.

Fixed assets are listed at *historical cost* (the purchase price) minus accumulated depreciation as of the date of the balance sheet. *Accumulated depreciation* represents the total dollars of depreciation that have been expensed against the historical cost of the organization's fixed assets. Numerically, the amounts of depreciation expense reported on the income statement each year are accumulated over time to create the accumulated depreciation account on the balance sheet.[2] Note that the accumulated depreciation account is called a *contra-asset* account because it is a **negative** asset. The greater the value of this account, the smaller an organization's total assets. Contra accounts reduce the value of "parent" accounts; in this case, the parent account is gross fixed assets.

For Sunnyvale, the net balance of property and equipment (*net fixed assets*) was $52,450,000 at the end of 1998. The historical cost of these assets (*gross fixed assets*) is $88,549,000. Some of the fixed assets were purchased in 1998, some in 1988, some in 1978, and some in other years; but the total purchase price of all the fixed assets ever purchased by Sunnyvale from its inception through December 31, 1998 is $88,549,000. The accumulated depreciation through December 31, 1998 is $36,099,000, which accounts for that portion of the value of these assets that was "spent" in producing income since Sunnyvale's inception. The difference, or net, of $52,450,000, reflects the remaining *book value* of the clinic's fixed assets. Often, a more detailed explanation of the fixed asset accounts will be found in the footnotes.

As mentioned earlier, the connection of the balance sheet net fixed assets account to the income statement is through depreciation expense. The accumulated depreciation of $36,099,000 reported at the end of 1998 is $5,955,000 greater than the 1997 amount of $30,144,000. This increase in accumulated depreciation on the balance sheet reflects the $5,995,000 in depreciation expense reported on the 1998 income statement. (A footnote indicated that $5,995,000 of the $6,400,000 reported as depreciation and amortization was due to depreciation.)

If Sunnyvale were to stop purchasing fixed assets, its net fixed assets account (with the exception of land, which is not depreciated) would eventually be run down to zero as each individual asset is fully depreciated. Sunnyvale would still have some physical assets (property and equipment), and these assets may have a positive operational value as well as resale (market) value, but the book value of these assets calculated according to the GAAP would be zero.

Note that depreciation, even though it may not reflect the true change in value of an asset over time, at least ensures an orderly recognition of value loss. Occasionally, assets experience a sudden, unexpected loss of value. One example is when changing technology instantly makes a piece of diagnostic equipment obsolete, and hence worthless. When this occurs, the asset that has experienced the decline in value is *written off*, which means that its value on the balance sheet is reduced (perhaps to zero) and the amount of the reduction is taken as an expense on the income statement.

Other Assets

The fourth major asset category is *other assets*. This is really a catchall category of miscellaneous items, which may or may not be very significant. Sunnyvale showed a total of $5,170,000 of other assets at the end of 1998 in the form of *goodwill*. Goodwill is an intangible asset, in contrast to the three other major asset categories of tangible assets. *Tangible assets* have physical form and substance: cash, inventories, fixed assets, and so on can be held in the hand, or at least touched. *Intangible assets,* such as good credit standing, skilled employees, and unique products and services, do not have physical form. Typically, they are not valued and recorded on the balance sheet primarily because of the difficulty in precisely measuring the values of such assets.

However, goodwill, which is the one type of intangible asset that is recorded, is particularly relevant to the health services industry because it is born out of mergers and acquisitions, which are a common occurrence in today's healthcare world. To illustrate, assume a hospital purchases a physician group practice. The price paid for that practice establishes a fair market value for the assets of the practice. Any difference between the price paid to the owners of the practice (its fair market value) and the balance sheet value of the owner's equity (its book value) is presumed to be because of intangible factors. The value of these intangible factors, or goodwill, is then recorded as an asset on the balance sheet of the hospital that makes the purchase. The logic is that the hospital would pay more than what the tangible assets are "worth" only if the practice has valuable intangible assets. Otherwise, the hospital would simply purchase fixed assets, inventories, and so on (similar to what the practice owned), and create a duplicate operation at lower cost than the amount paid for the practice.

Sunnyvale's 1998 value of $5,170,000 for goodwill tells readers that the various businesses that the clinic has acquired over the years were, according to the prices paid, worth substantially more than the book value of the specific tangible assets acquired. However, given the problems both in setting fair market values and in interpreting book values, too much significance should not be placed on the actual dollar value of the goodwill account.

Goodwill, like fixed assets, is assumed to lose value over time, and hence is expensed on the income statement over time through an allocation process analogous to depreciation. In the case of intangible assets, however, this charge is called *amortization expense*. Amortization expense is calculated using the straight-line method, generally over periods up to 40 years for hospital acquisitions and up to 20 years for physician practice acquisitions. For example, Sunnyvale's 1998 income statement contains $450,000 in amortization expense (which is found in the footnotes of the financial statements). Notice that the goodwill asset account was $5,620,000 in 1997, which is $450,000 greater than the 1998 amount, thus reflecting the allocation of the value of this intangible asset to the income statement over time.

Self-Test Questions

1. What are the four major categories of asset accounts?
2. What is the primary difference between current assets and the remainder of the asset side of the balance sheet?
3. What is accumulated depreciation, and how does it tie in to the income statement?
4. What is goodwill, and how does it tie in to the income statement?

Liabilities

Liabilities and equity, which comprise the right side of the balance sheet, are shown in the lower section of Table 4.1. Together, they represent the *capital* (the money) that has been raised by an organization to acquire the assets shown on the left side.

Again, by definition, total capital (the sum of liabilities and equity) must equal total assets.

Liabilities represent claims against the assets of an organization that are **fixed by contract**. Some of the claims are by workers for unpaid wages and salaries and some of the claims are by tax authorities for unpaid taxes, but most of the claims are by *creditors* (lenders) who have contributed debt capital to the business. (Even not-for-profit organizations, which do not pay income taxes, typically have unpaid payroll and withholding taxes on their employees.) Of the creditor's claims, most are against the total assets of the organization (unsecured), so are not tied to specific assets that were used as collateral for the loan. In the event of *default* (nonpayment of interest or principal) by the borrower, creditors have the right to force the business into bankruptcy, with *liquidation* as a possible consequence. If liquidation occurs, the law requires that any proceeds be used first to satisfy creditor claims before any funds can be paid to equityholders or used for charitable purposes. Furthermore, the dollar value of each creditor claim, along with all other liabilities, is fixed by the value shown on the balance sheet, while the equityholders—including the community at large for not-for-profit organizations—have a claim to the residual proceeds of a liquidation rather than to a fixed amount.

Like assets, the balance sheet presentation of liabilities follows a logical format. Current liabilities, which are those liabilities that will fall due (must be paid) within one year, are listed first. Long-term debt, distinguished from short-term debt by having maturities greater than one year, is listed second. As shown in Table 4.1, Sunnyvale had total liabilities at the end of 1998 of $100,747,000. This total consisted of two parts: total current liabilities of $15,425,000 and total long-term debt of $85,322,000. The following sections describe the liabilities accounts in detail.

Current Liabilities

Current liabilities include such items as that portion of long-term debt (which is discussed in the next section) coming due during the next year, money owed to suppliers (accounts payable), and various categories of accrued expenses. Accounts payable and accrued expenses represent expenses that have been incurred as of the balance sheet date, but that have not yet been paid in cash. Although Sunnyvale has no short-term debt outstanding—other than the current maturities of long-term debt—many healthcare firms do use short-term debt. Typically, such debt is used to finance seasonal or cyclical working capital (current asset) needs. On the balance sheet, short-term debt is often called *notes payable*.

Accounts payable generally pertains to amounts due to vendors for supplies. Often, suppliers offer their customers *credit terms*, which allow payment sometime after the purchase is made. For example, one of Sunnyvale's suppliers offers credit terms of 2/10, net 30. This means that if Sunnyvale pays the invoice in ten days, it will receive a 2 percent discount off the list price; otherwise, the total amount of the invoice is due in 30 days. In effect, suppliers are offering Sunnyvale *trade credit*, the outstanding amount of which is reported on the balance sheet.[3]

Wages and benefits due to employees, interest due on loans, accrued utilities expenses, and similar items are included on the balance sheet as *accrued expenses*. Sunnyvale's employees are used to illustrate the logic behind accruals. Sunnyvale's staff earns its wages and benefits on a daily basis as the work is performed. However, the clinic pays its workers only every two weeks. Therefore, other than on paydays, the clinic owes its staff for work performed. Whenever the obligation to pay wages extends into the next accounting period, an *accrual* is created on the balance sheet. This obligation, as well as similar obligations to tax authorities and lenders, appears on Sunnyvale's balance sheet as an accrual.

Trade credit (accounts payable) and accruals are examples of *spontaneous financing* accounts. This means that, for the most part, their balances rise and fall with a business' level of operations. When operations expand because of increased patient utilization, Sunnyvale must purchase and hold more supplies, which leads to a higher level of payables. For example, suppose Sunnyvale makes purchases of $100 a day from a medical supplier having terms of net 30 (no discount), and the clinic pays the invoices in 30 days. On average, it will owe this supplier 30 × $100 = $3,000, which would be part of Sunnyvale's $6,522,000 in accounts payable at the end of 1998.[4] If operations expand by 50 percent, and now Sunnyvale must order $150 in supplies per day from the supplier to support this new higher level of operations, then the contribution to payables would also increase by 50 percent, to 30 × $150 = $4,500. Accruals rise and fall with the level of operations in a similar manner.

An important current liability account for providers with a high percentage of capitated contracts is *incurred but not reported* (IBNR) *expense*. This account is not present on Sunnyvale's balance sheet because its payor mix is dominated by fee-for-service reimbursement. Under capitation, providers receive payment before the services are rendered. At the end of an accounting period when the books are closed, there may still be a large number of expenses related to services for the capitated enrollees that have not yet been reported in the accounting system. Many of the expenses will have occurred and been reported, but the costs of services provided near the end of the period may still be in the accounting pipeline. If the provider subcontracts out for some services, these services may have been performed by subcontractors but not yet billed.

Even if the services are provided in-house, the episode of care may straddle into the next accounting period, thus resulting in a need to estimate the cost of those services. One of the last accounting entries typically done by capitated providers is to record IBNR expense both as a current liability on the balance sheet and as an operating expense on the income statement. This procedure properly matches the timing of the costs of services to be provided with the revenue for those services, which was received up-front.

Long-Term Debt

The *long-term debt* section of the balance sheet represents debt financing (loans) to the organization with remaining maturities of more than one year, and hence repayment is not required during the coming accounting period. The long-term debt section lists any debt owed to banks and other creditors such as bondholders as well as obligations under certain types of lease arrangements.[5] Usually, detailed information relative to the specific characteristics of the long-term debt is disclosed in the footnotes to the financial statements.

Although long-term debt has a maturity of more than one year, many long-term debt issues have provisions mandating that a portion of the borrowed amount (*principal*) be repaid in each year. Furthermore, some long-term debt may mature in any given year. (The features of long-term debt are discussed in detail in Chapter 11.) The portion of long-term debt that must be paid in the coming year is recorded on the balance sheet as a current asset titled *current maturities of long-term debt*. For Sunnyvale, the total long-term debt outstanding at the end of 1998 was $85,322,000. In addition, another $2,834,000 of debt originally classified as long term on earlier balance sheets is due in 1999.

Sunnyvale had *total liabilities*, combined current liabilities and long-term debt, of $100,747,000 at the end of 1998. As discussed in the next section, Sunnyvale reported $54,068,000 in equity, for total financing (which must equal total assets) of $154,815,000. Thus, based on the values recorded on the balance sheet, or *book values*, Sunnyvale uses much more debt financing than equity financing. The choice between debt and equity financing is discussed in Chapter 13. Also, Chapter 17 includes coverage of alternative ways to measure the amount of debt financing that an organization uses and its effect on the business' financial condition.

Self-Test Questions

1. What are liabilities?
2. What are some of the accounts that would be classified as current liabilities?
3. Use an example to explain the logic behind accruals.
4. What are spontaneous liabilities?
5. What is the difference between long-term debt and current maturities of long-term debt?

Equity

On the balance sheet, the equity (ownership) claim on an organization's assets is called *net assets* when the organization has not-for-profit status. As the term *net* implies, net assets represent the dollar value of assets remaining when a business' liabilities are stripped out. However, as readers learned in Chapter 2, there are a wide variety of ownership types in the health services industry, which results in an almost bewildering difference in terminology used for the equity portion of the balance sheet. For example, depending on the type of business organization, the equity section of the balance sheet may be called stockholders' equity, owner's net worth, net worth, proprietor's worth, partners' worth, or even something else. To keep things manageable in this book, the term *equity* typically will be used, but the various terms all indicate the same thing: the amount of total assets financed by nonliability capital, or total assets minus total liabilities. To determine what belongs to the owners, whether explicitly recognized as stockholders in for-profit businesses or implicitly implied in not-for-profit organizations, fixed claims (liabilities) are subtracted from the value of the business' assets. The remainder, the net assets (equity), represent the residual value of the assets of the organization.

The equity section of the balance sheet is extremely important because it, more than anything else in the financial statements, reflects the ownership of the organization. Because Table 4.1 lists the equity as *net assets*, Sunnyvale is a not-for-profit corporation. Some of the equity capital could have come from charitable contributions and some from government grants, but the vast majority of Sunnyvale's equity capital was obtained by reinvesting earnings within the business. For a not-for-profit organization such as Sunnyvale, **all earnings** (net income) **must be reinvested in the business**.

Sunnyvale's equity increased by $7,860,000 from 1997 to 1998, which is the same amount that the clinic reported as net income for 1998. It is important to recognize that this connection between the bottom line of the income statement and the equity section of the balance sheet is a mathematical necessity. In the case of not-for-profit businesses, there is simply nowhere else for those earnings to go. This highlights yet another connection between the balance sheet and the income statement.

Sunnyvale's balance sheet balances because the increase in equity of $7,860,000 was offset by a like increase in assets, along with asset increases because of other financing. The increase might be in cash, receivables, fixed assets, or in another asset account. The key point is that the equity (net asset) balance is **not** a store of cash. As Sunnyvale earned profits over the years, they were invested in supplies, property and equipment, and other assets to provide future services that would likely generate even larger profits in the future. Sunnyvale's total assets grew by $154,815,000 − $115,101,000 = $39,714,000 in 1998, which was supported by an increase in total liabilities of $100,747,000 − $68,893,000 = $31,854,000 and an increase in equity (net assets) of $54,068,000 − $46,208,000 = $7,860,000.

The net assets type of equity section shown in Table 4.1 is typical of not-for-profit organizations. This format would be seen on the balance sheets of most community and religious health systems, as well as such major providers as Kaiser Permanente and the Mayo Clinic. However, occasionally not-for-profit organizations do sell stock privately, and not-for-profit organizations may show a limited amount of stock outstanding. This type of stock is not sold in the open market, though, and does not convey ownership rights, as does the stock of investor-owned companies.

Thus far, the discussion of the balance sheet has focused on Sunnyvale, a not-for-profit corporation. In general, the asset and liability sections of the balance sheet are much the same regardless of ownership status. The equity section tends to differ in presentation for different types of ownership because the types have different forms of equity. That is the bad news. The good news is that the economic substance of the equity section remains the same.

Table 4.2 contains the equity section of the balance sheet assuming that Sunnyvale, with a new name (Southeast Healthcare), was an investor-owned (for-profit) corporation. This is the type of presentation that would be seen on the balance sheets of for-profit health services organizations such as Columbia/HCA, Beverly Enterprises, and PacifiCare. The first major difference is the title of the section, "Stockholders' Equity." This title, or a similar title such as "Shareholders' Equity," provides explicit recognition that there are stockholders (shareholders) who own the business.

The stockholders' equity section of the balance sheet consists of two parts: contributed capital and accumulated earnings. The *contributed capital* section, which is not typically identified as such, is the sum of the common stock and capital in excess of par accounts. This represents the amount of capital contributed directly, or paid out-of-pocket, by stockholders of corporations or by proprietors or partners of unincorporated businesses. The *retained earnings* account represents the accumulated earnings of the organization that have been reinvested in the business, as opposed to paid out to owners in the form of dividends. Not-for-profit organizations cannot pay dividends, so all earnings must be retained in the business.

Southeast Healthcare was incorporated in 1975, with the by-laws authorizing issuance of 1.5 million shares of common stock. At that time, one million shares were sold at a price of $10 per share, so $10 million was collected. The *par value* of the stock is $1. Par value is a somewhat antiquated legal concept that specifies the minimum liability of shareholders in the event of bankruptcy. Today, it has limited economic relevance, but accountants continue to separate contributed capital into two separate accounts. Because one million shares were sold at a par value of $1, the *common stock* account shows a balance of $1 million.

	1998	1997
Stockholders' Equity:		
Common stock ($1 par value, 1,500,000 shares authorized, 1,000,000 shares outstanding)	$ 1,000	$ 1,000
Capital in excess of par	9,000	9,000
Retained earnings	44,068	36,208
Total equity	$ 54,068	$ 46,208
Total liabilities and equity	$ 154,815	$ 115,101

TABLE 4.2
Southeast Healthcare: Balance Sheet Equity Section December 31, 1998 and 1997 (in thousands)

Any proceeds collected from the sale of common stock at a price above par value are listed in the *capital in excess of par* account. Because Southeast Healthcare collected $10 per share or $9 above par value for each of the one million shares sold, this account shows a balance of $9 million.

The *retained earnings* account represents the accumulation of earnings over time that have been reinvested in the business. Each year, the amount of net income shown on the income statement, less the amount paid out to stockholders as dividends, is transferred from the income statement to the balance sheet. Suppose that, as with Sunnyvale, Southeast Healthcare had actually earned $7,860,000 in 1998. Because the firm's retained earnings account increased by a like amount, no dividends were paid to stockholders during the year.

Retained earnings, like all equity accounts, represent a claim against assets, and they are not available to buy new equipment, to pay dividends, or for any other purpose. The financing represented by retained earnings has already been used within the organization to buy property and equipment, to buy supplies, and yes, to increase the cash, marketable securities, and long-term investment accounts. Only the portion of retained earnings that is sitting in the cash account is available to the business for immediate use.

Although Table 4.2 shows only the equity section, it is likely that there would be significant differences in the values of other balance sheet accounts between investor-owned and not-for-profit businesses. For example, it is unlikely that a for-profit healthcare business would be able to amass such a large amount of long-term investments (securities) unless the funds were earmarked for a particular use in the next few years. (In fact, the money is being accumulated by Sunnyvale to fund a large acquisition.) Southeast's stockholders would question why the company had over $42 million in long-term securities because they would prefer to have all of the business' capital invested in operating assets, which as indicated earlier, usually earn a higher return than do securities investments. Thus, there would be stockholder pressure on management to return this capital to stockholders (as dividends or stock repurchases), so that they could, themselves, make the decision on how to invest these funds. Stockholders have invested in Southeast Healthcare because it is a healthcare provider—if they had wanted to own a bank, they would have bought bank stock. If and when Southeast requires more capital for asset acquisitions, it can always issue new debt and common stock.

Access to the capital markets is seen as a real economic advantage that for-profit providers—whether they are hospitals, physician groups, or managed care plans—have over not-for-profit providers. The ability to "open the faucet" to acquire more capital has certain advantages in today's highly competitive health services industry, which is reflected in the number of not-for-profit organizations that have converted to for-profit status.[6]

1. What is equity (net assets)?
2. What are the differences in the equity sections of not-for-profit and investor-owned providers?
3. What is the relationship between the retained earnings account on the balance sheet and earnings on the income statement?

Fund Accounting

One unique feature of many not-for-profit healthcare balance sheets is that they classify certain asset and equity (net asset) accounts as being *restricted*. When a not-for-profit organization receives contributions that donors have indicated must be used for a specific purpose, the organization must create multiple funds to account for its assets and equity (net assets). A *fund* is defined as a self-contained pool set up to account for a specific activity or project. Each fund has assets, perhaps claims against those assets, and an equity (net asset) balance. Because the assets and claims of an organization that receives restricted contributions are separated into funds, this form of accounting is called *fund accounting*. Only contributions to not-for-profit organizations are tax deductible to the donor, and hence few contributions are made to investor-owned healthcare businesses. Thus, fund accounting is only applicable to not-for-profit organizations.

Here is a brief overview of how fund accounting works. *Unrestricted assets* represent all assets not restricted to specific purposes. Thus, the organization can use such assets in any way that its managers deem appropriate. The *unrestricted fund*, or *general fund*, therefore, would have the same characteristics of assets, liabilities, and equity as discussed in the Sunnyvale example. Note that the board of directors (trustees) can designate some assets as *limited use assets*. For example, funds set aside to repay a loan. Such assets, from an accounting perspective, are classified as unrestricted.

Conversely, *restricted assets* are assets whose use is restricted by law or contractual agreement to be used only for specific purposes. *Temporarily restricted assets* have restrictions that ultimately expire, while *permanently restricted assets* typically involve endowments in which the contributed capital cannot be spent; only the return on investments made with endowment capital can be used. Restricted assets must have separate funds established for each category of restriction: temporary or permanent.

Restricted contributions and gifts impose legal and fiduciary responsibilities on health services organizations to carry out the written wishes of donors. Thus, numerous rules are associated with fund accounting that go well beyond the scope of this book. The good news is that organizations required to use fund accounting are encouraged to present balance sheets to outside parties that are roughly similar to that shown in Table 4.1. Thus, with the exception of further breakdown into unrestricted, temporarily restricted, and permanently restricted accounts, such balance sheets have the same economic content as those prepared by nonfund-account health services organizations.

1. What is fund accounting?
2. What type of a health services organization is most likely to use fund accounting?
3. Is there a significant difference in the economic content of balance sheets created by investor-owned and not-for-profit health services organizations?

The Statement of Cash Flows

The balance sheet and income statement are traditional financial statements that have been required in annual reports for many years. In contrast, the *statement of cash flows* has only been required since the late 1980s.[7] This relatively new financial statement has been added to the annual report in response to demands by users for better information about a firm's cash inflows and outflows.

While the balance sheet reports the cash balance on hand at the end of the period, it does not provide details on why the cash account is smaller or greater than the previous year's value. Furthermore, the income statement does not give detailed information on cash flows. In addition to the problems of accrual accounting and noncash expenses discussed in Chapter 3, there may be cash raised by means other than operations that does not even appear on the income statement. For example, Sunnyvale may have raised cash during 1998 by taking on more debt or by selling some fixed assets. Such flows, which are not shown on the income statement, affect a firm's cash balance. Finally, the cash coming into a firm does not sit in the cash account forever. Most of it is spent on other assets or for investor-owned firms, some may be paid out as dividends. Thus, the cash account does not increase by the gross amount of cash generated, and it would be useful to know how the difference was spent.

The statement of cash flows, which considers both income statement and balance sheet events, details where cash resources come from and how they are used. Sunnyvale's 1998 and 1997 statements are presented in Table 4.3. To develop the cash flows, many adjustments must be made to the underlying income statement and balance sheet data. These adjustments are often complicated, so it is necessary to be well-versed in financial accounting to prepare a complete statement of cash flows. The statements shown in Table 4.3 have been simplified; they are somewhat shorter and easier to comprehend than most "real world" statements. Nevertheless, an understanding of the composition and presentation of Table 4.3 will give readers and excellent appreciation of the value of the statement of cash flows.

The statement of cash flows is formatted to make it easy to understand why and how Sunnyvale's cash position increased by $5,616,000 during 1998. In other words, what were Sunnyvale's sources of cash and how was this cash used? The statement is divided into three major sections: cash flows from operating activities, cash flows from investing activities, and cash flows from financing activities.

The first section, *cash flows from operating activities*, focuses on the sources and uses of cash **tied directly to operations**. Of course, the most important

	1998	1997	TABLE 4.3
			Sunnyvale Clinic:
			Statements of
Cash Flows from Operating Activities:			Cash Flows
Net income	$ 7,860	$ 8,206	Years Ended
Adjustments:			December 31, 1998
Depreciation and amortization	6,405	5,798	and 1997
Change in accounts receivable	(2,582)	(1,423)	(in thousands)
Change in inventories	(1,393)	(673)	
Change in accounts payable	(1,411)	(966)	
Change in accruals	1,032	865	
Net cash from operations	$ 9,911	$ 11,807	
Cash Flows from Investing Activities:			
Capital expenditures	($ 9,306)	($ 1,953)	
Cash Flows from Financing Activities:			
Change in marketable securities	($ 5,000)	$ 0	
Change in long-term investments	(22,222)	(20,667)	
Change in long-term debt	32,233	0	
Net cash from financing	$ 5,011	($ 20,667)	
Net increase (decrease) in cash	$ 5,616	($ 10,813)	
Cash, beginning of year	$ 6,486	$ 17,299	
Cash, end of year	$ 12,102	$ 6,486	

source is net income so it is listed first. However, net income does not equal cash flow, so various adjustments must be made. The first adjustment is to add back the noncash expenses that appear on the income statement. Adjustments are then made for changes in current assets and liabilities (net working capital). The theory for these adjustments is that accounts such as inventories and accruals stem directly from operations, and hence any cash that either stems from or is used for these accounts should be included as part of operations. To illustrate, consider accounts receivable. Sunnyvale's net patient accounts receivable increased from $25,927,000 to $28,509,000, or by $2,582,000, during 1998. Cash had to be used to provide the services that created these receivables, so this amount is shown as a deduction (negative adjustment). As another illustration, total accruals increased by $1,032,000 in 1998. Because an increase in accruals creates financing for the clinic, this change is shown as an addition to operating cash flow.[8]

Sunnyvale reported $9,911,000 in net cash from operations for 1998. For a business, whether investor owned or not for profit, to be financially sustainable, it must generate a positive cash flow from operations. Thus, at least for 1998 and 1997, Sunnyvale's operations are doing what they should be doing—generating cash. However, the clinic's cash flow from operations has decreased from 1997 to 1998, so its managers should be identifying why this happened and then taking appropriate action.

The second major category on the statement of cash flows is *cash flows from investing activities*. The emphasis here is on *capital investing*, which is investment in fixed assets, as opposed to financial investing (investing in securities). As evidenced by the 1997 to 1998 change in gross fixed assets derived from the balance sheets, Sunnyvale spent $9,306,000 to acquire additional property and equipment. Thus, virtually all the clinic's operating cash flow was spent on new fixed assets.

The final major category is *cash flows from financing activities*. The changes in balance sheet accounts from 1997 to 1998 indicate that the clinic invested $5,000,000 in marketable securities, invested $22,222,000 in long-term securities, and took on an additional $32,233,000 in long-term debt. On net, Sunnyvale generated a $5,011,000 cash inflow from financing activities. This section shows that Sunnyvale used the vast majority of new debt to purchase securities. In general, new debt would be used to acquire real assets rather than financial assets. However, Sunnyvale is planning to acquire a large group practice in 1999, and the financing activities undertaken in 1998 are in preparation for this purchase.

The next line of the statement of cash flows is the *net increase (decrease) in cash*. Unlike the "bottom line" of the income statement, the change in cash has limited value in assessing an organization's financial condition because it can be manipulated by financing activities. If an organization is losing cash on operations, but its managers want to increase its cash account, usually they simply can borrow the funds necessary to show a net cash increase on the statement of cash flows. Thus, the net cash from operations line is much more important than the net increase (decrease) in cash line. The value of the net increase (decrease) in cash line is that it is used to verify the correctness of the entries on the statement of cash flows. As shown in Table 4.3, the $5,616,000 increase in cash reported by Sunnyvale for 1998 is added to the beginning of year cash balance, $6,486,000, to get an end of year total of $12,102,000. A check of the end-of-1998 cash balance shown in Table 4.1 confirms the amount calculated on the statement of cash flows.

In summary, the income statement focuses on accounting profitability, while the statement of cash flows focuses on the movement of cash: Where did the money come from and how did the organization spend it? While the major concern of the income statement is economic profitability as defined by the GAAP, the statement of cash flows is concerned with cash viability. Is the organization generating, and will it continue to generate, sufficient cash to meet both short-term and long-term needs?

Self-Test Questions

1. How does the statement of cash flows differ from the income statement?
2. Briefly explain the three major categories shown on the statement.
3. In your view, what is the most important piece of information reported on the statement?

Transactions

Transactions are the economic events of the enterprise as recorded by accountants. Transactions begin on *ledgers,* often referred to as *T accounts* because of the way the entries are formatted, and then work their way to the financial statements. Understanding how T account entries are made is not important to most managers, but understanding how transactions ultimately affect the financial statements will help managers better understand and interpret their content.

The transactions that flow to the income statement are relatively apparent. For example, net patient service revenue stems directly from the provision of patient services and the expectation of receiving payment. However, the transactions that flow to the balance sheet are more difficult to understand. In this section, ten typical balance sheet transactions are presented. Understanding these transactions will help readers understand how an organization's economic events are transformed into financial statement data.

The primary concept behind all balance sheet transactions is that the basic accounting equation must be preserved (i.e., the balance sheet must balance). Thus, each transaction must have a dual effect, either one on the left side and one on the right side, or offsetting effects on the same side. Here are the transactions:

1. **Investment by owners.** Suppose five radiologists decide to open a diagnostic center that they incorporate as an investor-owned business called Bayshore Radiology Center. They each invest $200,000 cash in the business in exchange for $200,000 of common stock. The transaction results in an equal increase in both assets and equity. In this case, there is an increase in the cash account of $1,000,000 and an increase in the common stock account of $1,000,000. The effect of this transaction looks like this:

Cash	$1,000,000	Common stock	$1,000,000
Total assets	$1,000,000	Total claims	$1,000,000

2. **Purchase of equipment for cash.** To support operations, the business needs diagnostic equipment. Assume that the first piece of equipment purchased costs $200,000. This transaction results in an equal increase and decrease in total assets. The composition of assets is changed, however:

Cash	$ 800,000	Common stock	$1,000,000
Gross fixed assets	200,000		
Total assets	$1,000,000	Total claims	$1,000,000

   Total assets and total claims still amount to $1,000,000 because no new capital was acquired by the business.

3. **Purchase of supplies on credit.** Assume that Bayshore purchases medical supplies for $20,000. The supplier's terms give the clinic 60 days to pay the

bill. Assets are increased by this transaction because of the expected benefit of using these supplies to provide services. Also, liabilities (accounts payable) are increased by the amount due the supplier:

Cash	$ 800,000	Accounts payable	$ 20,000
Supplies	20,000	Common stock	1,000,000
Gross fixed assets	200,000		
Total assets	$1,020,000	Total claims	$1,020,000

4. **Services rendered for credit.** Assume that Bayshore provides $50,000 of services (at net prices) that are billed to third-party payors. This transaction will increase assets (accounts receivable) and the retained earnings portion of equity. The $50,000 would also show up on the income statement as revenue, which, after expenses and dividends are deducted, would ultimately flow through to the balance sheet, and hence support the increase in equity:

Cash	$ 800,000	Accounts payable	$ 20,000
Accounts receivable	50,000	Common stock	1,000,000
Supplies	20,000	Retained earnings	50,000
Gross fixed assets	200,000		
Total assets	$1,070,000	Total claims	$1,070,000

Retained earnings (equity) is increased when revenues are earned, even though no cash has been generated. When accounts receivable are collected at a later date, cash will be increased and receivables will be decreased (see Transaction 10).

5. **Purchase of advertising on credit.** Bayshore receives a bill for $10,000 from the *Daily News* for advertising its grand opening, but it does not have to pay the newspaper for 30 days. The transaction results in an increase in liabilities and a decrease in equity; specifically, accounts payable is increased and retained earnings is decreased. The decrease in equity will work its way through the income statement as $10,000 in advertising expense:

Cash	$ 800,000	Accounts payable	$ 30,000
Accounts receivable	50,000	Common stock	1,000,000
Supplies	20,000	Retained earnings	40,000
Gross fixed assets	200,000		
Total assets	$1,070,000	Total claims	$1,070,000

Equity is reduced when expenses are incurred. When payment is made at a later date, both payables and cash will decrease (see Transaction 8). Advertising is an expense as opposed to an asset (like supplies) because the benefits of the outlay have been immediately consumed.

6. **Payment of expenses.** Assume that the center paid $50,000 in cash for rent, salaries, and utilities. These payments result in an equal decrease in cash and

equity. The decrease in equity will be matched by a reduction in net income on the income statement:

Cash	$ 750,000	Accounts payable	$ 30,000
Accounts receivable	50,000	Common stock	1,000,000
Supplies	20,000	Retained earnings	(10,000)
Gross fixed assets	200,000		
Total assets	$1,020,000	Total claims	$1,020,000

Note that Bayshore's retained earnings have been driven negative by this transaction. In essence, the net assets of the clinic ($1,020,000 − $30,000 = $990,000) are now worth less than the total capital supplied by the clinic's stockholders.

7. **Recognition of supplies used.** Assume that $2,000 of supplies were used in providing healthcare services to Bayshore's patients. The cost of supplies used is an expense that decreases assets and equity. The expense is also shown on the income statement, and hence net income is reduced by a like amount:

Cash	$ 750,000	Accounts payable	$ 30,000
Accounts receivable	50,000	Common stock	1,000,000
Supplies	8,000	Retained earnings	(12,000)
Gross fixed assets	200,000		
Total assets	$1,018,000	Total claims	$1,018,000

8. **Payment of accounts payable (advertising bill).** Assume that the center paid its $10,000 advertising bill, which was due in 30 days. (The supplies bill is not due for 60 days.) The advertising bill was previously recorded in Transaction 5 as a payable. This payment on an account for an expense already recognized decreases both assets (cash) and liabilities (payables):

Cash	$ 740,000	Accounts payable	$ 20,000
Accounts receivable	50,000	Common stock	1,000,000
Supplies	18,000	Retained earnings	(12,000)
Gross fixed assets	200,000		
Total assets	$1,008,000	Total claims	$1,008,000

Payment of a liability related to an expense that has previously been incurred does not affect equity.

9. **Payment of accounts payable (supplies bill).** One month later, assume that Bayshore paid its $20,000 supplies bill. Recall that the supplies bill was previously recorded in Transaction 3 as an increase in both assets (supplies) and liabilities (accounts payable). Furthermore, part of the supplies were used and recorded in Transaction 7 as a decrease in assets (supplies) and equity:

Cash	$720,000	Common stock	$1,000,000
Accounts receivable	50,000	Retained earnings	(12,000)
Supplies	18,000		
Gross fixed assets	200,000		
Total assets	$988,000	Total claims	$ 988,000

A payment of a liability related to an asset that has previously been booked does not affect equity. Equity is not affected until the asset has been used.

10. **Receipt of cash from a third-party payor.** Assume that $5,000 is received in payment for patient services rendered from one of the center's third-party payors. This transaction does not change Bayshore's total assets or, because of the accounting identity, total claims. It does change the composition of the business' assets:

Cash	$725,000	Common stock	$1,000,000
Accounts receivable	45,000	Retained earnings	(12,000)
Supplies	18,000		
Gross fixed assets	200,000		
Total assets	$988,000	Total claims	$ 988,000

A collection on account for services previously billed and recorded does not affect equity. Revenue was already recorded in Transaction 4 and cannot be recorded again.

Of course, there are an almost limitless number of transactions that occur in everyday business activities. The purpose of this section was to give readers a sense of how transactions provide the foundation for a business' financial statements.

Self-Test Questions

1. What condition must be met when entering transactions on the balance sheet?
2. What is the effect on a business' equity account of a payment on a bill that has already been booked (recorded as an account payable)?
3. What is the effect of the collection of a receivable on a business' equity account?

Another Look Ahead: Using Balance Sheet Data in Financial Statement Analysis

In Chapter 3, readers were provided an introduction to ratio analysis. This subject is continued in this section using balance sheet data. The *debt ratio* (or *debt-to-assets ratio*) is defined as total debt divided by total assets. Total debt can be defined several ways, depending on the use of the ratio, but for purposes here assume that total debt includes all liabilities (i.e., all nonequity capital). (An alternative would be to include only interest-bearing debt in our definition.) Refer to Table 4.1. For Sunnyvale, the debt ratio at the end of 1998 was total debt (liabilities) divided by total assets = $100,747,000 / $154,815,000 = 0.65 = 65%. This ratio reveals that each dollar of assets was financed by 65 cents of debt and, by inference, 35 cents of equity.

Sunnyvale's debt ratio at the end of 1997 was $68,893,000 / $115,101,000 = 0.60 = 60%. Thus, the clinic increased its proportional use of debt financing by five percentage points in one year. That information is important to Sunnyvale's managers and creditors. (The consequences of increased debt utilization are discussed throughout this book.) Judgments about Sunnyvale's capital structure could not be made easily without constructing the debt ratio or other ratios; interpreting the dollar values directly is just too difficult.

Key Concepts

Chapter 3 contained a review of the first of three important financial statements—the income statement. This chapter extends the discussion to cover the balance sheet and the statement of cash flows, with emphasis on the interrelationships between the income statement and the balance sheet. A demonstration of how economic events work their way onto the balance sheet was also presented. The key concepts of this chapter are:

- The *balance sheet* may be thought of as a snapshot of the financial position of a business at a given point in time.
- The *accounting identity* specifies that assets must equal liabilities plus equity (assets must equal total claims).
- *Assets* represent the total resources owned by a health services organization in dollar terms. Assets are listed *by maturity* (i.e., by order of when the assets are expected to be converted into cash). Current assets are expected to be converted into cash during the coming year.
- *Liabilities* are fixed claims by employees, tax authorities, and lenders against a business' total assets. *Current liabilities*—those obligations that fall due within one year—are listed first. *Long-term liabilities* (typically debt with maturities greater than one year) are listed second.
- *Equity* is the ownership claim against total assets. Depending on the form of organization and ownership, this claim may be called *net assets, stockholders' equity, proprietor's net worth,* or something else.
- There are two *primary interrelationships* between the balance sheet and the income statement. First, the annual depreciation expense shown on the income statement accumulates on the balance sheet in the accumulated depreciation account. Second, any earnings from the income statement reinvested in the business accumulate on the balance sheet in the equity account. (There is also a connection for amortization.)
- The structure of the liabilities and equity side of the balance sheet (i.e., the proportions of debt and equity financing) defines the organization's *capital structure*.

- *Fund accounting* is used by organizations that have restricted contributions. This complicates internal accounting procedures and adds additional detail to the balance sheet. However, fund accounting does not alter the basic format of the balance sheet nor its economic interpretation.
- The *statement of cash flows* shows where an organization gets its cash and how it is used. It focuses strictly on cash flows, and hence combines information from both the income statement and the balance sheet.
- The statement of cash flows has three major sections: *cash flows from operating activities*; *cash flows from investing activities*; and *cash flows from financing activities*.
- The "bottom line" of the statement of cash flows is the *net increase (decrease) in cash*. Although this amount is useful in verifying the accuracy of the statement, its economic content is not as meaningful as the statement's component amounts.
- *Transactions* are the primary underpinning of the measurement and reporting of financial accounting information. Understanding how transactions affect the financial statements leads to a better understanding of the statements themselves.

This temporarily ends the discussion of financial accounting. The next chapter begins the treatment of managerial accounting. However, the concepts presented in Chapters 3 and 4 are used repeatedly throughout the remainder of the book. In addition, financial accounting concepts are revisited in Chapter 17, which focuses on assessing financial performance.

Questions

4.1 a. What is the difference between the income statement and balance sheet in regards to timing?

b. What is wrong with this statement: "The clinic's cash balance for 1998 was $150,000, while its net income on December 31, 1998 was $50,000."

4.2 What is the accounting identity? What is the implication of the accounting identity for the numbers on a balance sheet?

4.3 a. What are assets?

b. What are the four major categories of assets?

4.4 a. What makes an asset a current asset?

b. Provide some examples of current assets.

c. What is net working capital, and what does it measure?

4.5 a. On the balance sheet, what is the difference between long-term investments and property and equipment?

b. What is the difference between gross fixed assets and net fixed assets?

c. How does depreciation expense on the income statement relate to accumulated depreciation on the balance sheet?

4.6 a. What is the difference between liabilities and equity?

b. What makes a liability a current liability?

c. Give some examples of current liabilities.

d. What is the difference between long-term debt and current maturities of long-term debt?

4.7 a. Explain the difference between the equity section of a not-for-profit business and an investor-owned business.

b. What is the relationship between net income on the income statement and the equity section on a balance sheet?

4.8 What is fund accounting and why is it important to some healthcare providers?

4.9 a. What is the statement of cash flows and how does it differ from the income statement?

b. What are the three major sections of the statement of cash flows?

c. What is the "bottom line" of the statement of cash flows and how important is it?

Problems

4.1 Middleton Clinic had total assets of $500,000 and an equity balance of $350,000 at the end of 1997. One year later, at the end of 1998, the clinic had $575,000 in assets and $380,000 in equity. What was the clinic's dollar growth in assets during 1998 and how was this growth financed?

4.2 San Mateo Healthcare had an equity balance of $1.38 million at the beginning of the year. At the end of the year, its equity balance was $1.98 million.

a. Assume that San Mateo is a not-for-profit organization. What was its net income for the period?

b. Assume that San Mateo is an investor-owned business. Assuming zero dividends, what was San Mateo's net income?

c. Assuming $200,000 in dividends, what was its net income?

d. Assuming $200,000 in dividends and $300,000 in additional stock sales, what was San Mateo's net income?

4.3 Here is financial statement information on four not-for-profit clinics:

	Pittman	Rose	Beckman	Jaffe
December 31, 1997:				
Assets	$ 80,000	$100,000	g	$150,000
Liabilities	50,000	d	$ 75,000	j
Equity	a	60,000	45,000	90,000
December 31, 1998:				
Assets	b	130,000	180,000	k
Liabilities	55,000	62,000	h	80,000
Equity	45,000	e	110,000	145,000
During 1998:				
Total revenues	c	400,000	i	500,000
Total expenses	330,000	f	360,000	l

Fill in the missing values labeled a through l.

4.4 The following are selected entries for Warren Clinic for December 31, 1998, in alphabetical order. Create Warren Clinic's balance sheet.

Accounts payable	$ 20,000
Accounts receivable, net	60,000
Cash	30,000
Other long-term liabilities	10,000
Net property and equipment	150,000
Long-term investments	100,000
Long-term debt	120,000
Other assets	40,000
Equity	230,000

4.5 Consider the following balance sheet:

BestCare HMO
Balance Sheet
June 30, 1998
(in thousands)

Assets

Current Assets:	
Cash and cash equivalents	$2,737
Net premiums receivable	821
Supplies	387
Total current assets	$3,945
Net property and equipment	$5,924
Total assets	$9,869

Liabilities and Net Assets

Accounts payable—medical services	$2,145
Accrued expenses	929
Notes payable	141
Current portion of long-term debt	241
Total current liabilities	$3,456
Long-term debt	$4,295
Total liabilities	$7,751
Net assets—unrestricted (equity)	$2,118
Total liabilities and net assets	$9,869

a. How does this balance sheet differ from the one presented in Table 4.1 for Sunnyvale?

b. What is BestCare's net working capital for 1998?

c. What is BestCare's debt ratio? How does it compare with Sunnyvale's debt ratio?

4.6 Consider this 1998 balance sheet:

Green Valley Nursing Home, Inc.
Balance Sheet
December 31, 1998

Assets

Current Assets:

Cash and cash equivalents	$ 105,737
Investments	200,000
Net patient accounts receivable	215,600
Supplies	87,655
Total current assets	$ 608,992
Property and equipment	$2,250,000
Less accumulated depreciation	356,000
Net property and equipment	$1,894,000
Total assets	$2,502,992

Liabilities and Shareholders' Equity

Current Liabilities:

Accounts payable	$ 72,250
Accrued expenses	192,900
Notes payable	100,000
Current portion of long-term debt	80,000
Total current liabilities	$ 445,150
Long-term debt	$1,700,000

Shareholders' Equity:

Common stock, $10 par value	$ 100,000
Retained earnings	257,842
Total shareholders' equity	$ 357,842
Total liabilities and shareholders' equity	$2,502,992

a. How does this balance sheet differ from the ones presented in Table 4.1 and Problem 4.5?

      b. What is Green Valley's net working capital for 1998?

      c. What is Green Valley's debt ratio? How does it compare with the debt ratios for Sunnyvale and BestCare?

4.7 Refer to the transactions pertaining to Bayshore Radiology Center presented in the chapter. Restate the impact of the transactions on Bayshore's balance sheet using these data:

      a. Transaction 2: The $200,000 equipment purchase is made with long-term borrowings instead of cash.

      b. Transaction 3: The $20,000 in supplies are purchased with cash instead of on trade credit.

      c. Transaction 4: The $30,000 in services provided are immediately paid for by patients instead of billed to third-party payors.

Notes

1. *Treasury bills* are short-term debt instruments issued by the U.S. Government. *Commercial paper* is short-term debt issued by very large and financially strong corporations. Both types of securities are relatively safe investments because there is virtually 100 percent assurance that borrowers will repay the loans when they mature.

2. For-profit firms have to be concerned with both *book depreciation*, which is calculated according to GAAP and reported to stockholders, and *tax depreciation*, which is calculated according to IRS regulations and used to determine the firm's income for tax purposes.

3. The decision as to whether or not Sunnyvale should take the extended trade credit (pay in 30 days rather than ten) is discussed in Chapter 16. In essence, the cost of foregoing the discount to gain additional credit (financing) has to be compared to the cost of other financing alternatives.

4. The supplier would be extending $3,000 of trade credit to Sunnyvale, so its balance sheet would show $3,000 in accounts receivable attributable to its business with the clinic.

5. In general, leases that have a long life (*capital leases*) are shown directly on the balance sheet. Conversely, leases with short lives (*operating leases*) are reported only in the footnotes.

6. Conversion of a not-for-profit organization to for-profit status presents a difficult legal challenge because not-for-profit assets must be used for charitable purposes in perpetuity (forever). Thus, the monies received in conversion must be used to create a foundation that will continue to perform charitable deeds.

7. Prior to the late 1980s, a different statement—the statement of changes in financial position—was required. The statement of cash flows, which presents essentially the same information but in a much more usable format, replaced this earlier statement.

8. To be technically correct, the provision for bad debt losses amount should have been included as an inflow to the adjustments section. However, this would have created a complication best left to accountants. Also, there are two different formats prescribed for the statement of cash flows. The format used in Table 4.3, called the *indirect method*, incorporates net working capital changes into the operating flows. The *direct method* focuses attention on the operating cash flows without considering the impact

of net working capital changes. Then, adjustments for these flows are made at the bottom of the statement.

References

AICPA. 1997a. *Audit and Accounting Guide.* New York: American Institute of Certified Public Accountants.

———. 1997b. *Checklists and Illustrative Financial Statements for Health Care Organizations.* New York: American Institute of Certified Public Accountants.

Bitter, M. E. and J. Cassidy. 1992. "Perceptions of New AICPA Audit Guide." *Healthcare Financial Management* (November): 38–48.

Luecke, R. W. and D. T. Meeting. 1996. "SFAS 124, Accounting for Investments: The Rules Have Changed." *Healthcare Financial Management* (December): 58–63.

MANAGERIAL ACCOUNTING

COST BEHAVIOR AND PROFIT ANALYSIS

Learning Objectives

After studying this chapter, readers will be able to:

- Explain the two major classifications of costs.
- Conduct profit analyses to determine breakeven points and to analyze the impact of input value changes on both profitability and breakeven points.
- Explain the primary differences in profit analyses that arise when comparing fee-for-service reimbursement with capitation.

Introduction

While financial accounting focuses on organizational-level data for presentation in a business' financial statements, *managerial accounting* focuses mostly on sub-unit (say, a department) data used internally for managerial decision making.[1] For example, managerial accounting information is used for routine budgeting processes, income distribution, and pricing decisions, all of which deal with sub-units of an organization. Also, managerial accounting data can be compiled for special projects such as assessing alternative modes of delivery or projecting the profitability of a particular reimbursement contract. In short, the focus of managerial accounting is to develop information to meet the needs of managers within the organization, rather than interested parties (mainly investors) outside the organization. Thus, while financial accounting information is driven primarily by the needs of outsiders, managerial accounting information is driven by the needs of managers.

Managers are more concerned with what will happen in the future than with what has happened in the past. Unlike financial accounting, managerial accounting is for the most part forward looking. Also, because the past is much better known than the future, managerial accounting information tends to be much less certain than financial accounting data. As managers embark upon budgeting and pricing decisions, they often must make heroic assumptions regarding utilization and costs. This requirement for assumptions combined with the fact that there are no generally agreed-upon rules for managerial accounting makes it much more open to improvisation than financial accounting.

The discussion of managerial accounting spans four chapters. Cost behavior and profit analysis, which many consider the foundation of managerial accounting, are discussed in this chapter. In Chapters 6 through 8, coverage is extended to include cost allocation, pricing, planning, and budgeting.

Cost Classifications

A critical part of managerial accounting is the measurement of costs. In fact, the concept of costs is so important that it has spawned its own field of accounting—cost accounting. *Cost accounting* is generally considered to be a subset of managerial accounting, although cost-accounting systems also are used to develop the expense data reported on a business' income statement. Therefore, cost accounting bridges both managerial and financial accounting.

Unfortunately, there is no single definition of the term *cost*. Rather, there are different costs for different purposes. As a general rule for healthcare providers, cost involves a resource use associated with providing a specific service. However, the cost per service identified for pricing purposes can differ from the cost per service used for management control purposes. Also, the cost per service used for long-range planning purposes may differ from the cost per service defined for short-term purposes. Finally, as discussed in Chapters 3 and 4, costs do not necessarily reflect actual cash outflows.

Direct Versus Indirect Costs

Costs are classified in two different ways—by their relationship to the sub-unit being analyzed and by their relationship to the volume (amount) of services provided. Some costs—about 50 percent of a health services organization's cost structure—are unique to the reporting sub-unit, and hence usually can be identified with relative certainty. Such costs are called *direct costs*. To illustrate, consider the clinical laboratory at a small hospital. Certain costs are unique to the laboratory: the salaries and benefits for the six technicians who work there and the costs of the equipment and supplies used to conduct the tests. These costs, which would not occur if the laboratory were closed, are classified as the direct costs of the department.

Unfortunately for measurement purposes, direct costs constitute only a portion of the laboratory's entire cost structure. The remaining resources utilized by the laboratory are **not** unique to the laboratory; the laboratory utilizes many shared resources of the hospital as a whole. For example, the laboratory shares the organization's physical space as well as its infrastructure, which includes information systems, utilities, housekeeping, maintenance, medical records, and general administration. The costs that are not borne directly by the laboratory are called *indirect*, or *overhead*, *costs*.

Indirect costs, in contrast to direct costs, are much more difficult to measure at the sub-unit level for the precise reason that they arise from shared resources. That is, if the laboratory were closed, the indirect costs would not disappear. Perhaps some indirect costs would be reduced, but the hospital still requires a basic infrastructure to operate its remaining departments. Note that the direct/indirect classification has relevance only at the sub-unit level; if the unit of analysis is the entire hospital, all costs are direct by definition. The allocation of indirect costs is so important and complex that an entire chapter (Chapter 6) is devoted to the topic. In the remainder of Chapter 5, the concentration is on the second cost classification: the relationship of costs to volume.

Fixed Versus Variable Costs

The second classification of costs involves the relationship between costs and the amount of services provided, often referred to as *activity, utilization,* or *volume.* As stated earlier, much of managerial accounting pertains to the future. In dealing with the future, there is always volume uncertainty—the number of patient days, number of visits, number of enrollees, and so on. However, some costs, called *fixed costs,* are more or less known over some predetermined time period regardless of volume. For example, the labor costs at the clinical laboratory discussed in the previous section are fixed for some length of time, regardless of the volume of laboratory tests. A permanent increase or decrease in laboratory volume would ultimately trigger staffing changes. Thus, in the long run, no costs are fixed. But, in the short-run, changes in laboratory volume (unless extreme) would not alter the staffing level. Other examples of fixed costs include expenditures on equipment, facilities, and information systems. After an organization has purchased these items, they are locked into them for some time regardless of volume (within some reasonable range).

Conversely, other resources are more or less acquired and used as volume dictates. Costs associated with such resources are called *variable costs.* The costs of the supplies (e.g., slides, reagents, and so on) used in the laboratory would be classified as variable costs. Also, some of the equipment used in the laboratory may be leased on a per procedure basis, which would convert the cost of the equipment from a fixed cost to a variable cost.

Cost classifications play a very important role in managerial accounting. Thus, these classifications will be used again and again. Readers should keep these concepts in mind while reading the following sections and chapters.

1. Explain and provide an example of the difference between direct and indirect costs.
2. Explain and provide an example of the difference between fixed and variable costs.

Self-Test Questions

Cost Behavior

Health services managers are vitally interested in how costs are affected by changes in the organization's activity (volume). The relationship between cost and activity, called *cost behavior* or *underlying cost structure,* is used by managers in planning, control, and decision making. The primary reason for defining an organization's underlying cost structure is to provide managers with a tool for forecasting costs at different levels of activity.

To illustrate the concept of cost behavior, consider the hypothetical cost data presented in Table 5.1 for a small, single-physician, walk-in clinic. The underlying cost structure consists of both fixed and variable costs; that is, some of the costs are expected to be volume sensitive and some are not. This structure of both fixed and variable costs is typical in health services businesses as well as most other businesses.

As noted in Table 5.1, the clinic has $300,000 in fixed costs. These costs occur even if the clinic has no patients, assuming the clinic is kept open. In addition to the fixed costs, each patient visit requires $25 in variable costs on average, consisting of $20 in clinical supplies and $5 in administrative supplies. The per unit (per visit in this example) variable cost of $25 is called the *variable cost rate*. If activity at the clinic doubles, for example, from 100 visits to 200 visits, *total variable costs* double from $2,500 to $5,000. However, the variable cost rate ($25 per patient visit) remains the same whether the visit is the first, the hundredth, or the thousandth. Total variable costs, therefore, increase or decrease proportionately as activity changes, but the variable cost rate remains constant.

Fixed costs, in contrast to total variable costs, remain unchanged as the level of activity varies. When activity doubles from 100 to 200 visits, fixed costs remain at $300,000. Examples of fixed costs include depreciation of plant and equipment, salaries for permanent personnel, and overhead costs such as utilities and housekeeping.

Because all costs are either fixed or variable, *total costs* are merely the sum of the two. For example, at 50 patient visits total costs are $300,000 + (50 × $25)

TABLE 5.1
Cost Behavior
Illustration

Variable Costs Per Visit		Fixed Costs Per Year	
Clinical supplies	$20	Depreciation	$ 30,000
Administrative supplies	5	Salaries	190,000
	$25	Other fixed costs	80,000
			$300,000

Volume	Fixed Costs	Total Variable Costs	Total Costs	Average Cost
1	$300,000	$ 25	$300,025	$300,025
50	300,000	1,250	301,250	6,025
100	300,000	2,500	302,500	3,025
200	300,000	5,000	305,000	1,525
500	300,000	12,500	312,500	625
1,000	300,000	25,000	325,000	325

= $300,000 + $1,250 = $301,250. Because variable costs are tied to volume, total costs increase as activity increases.

The column to the right, in Table 5.1, contains *average cost* per unit of activity, which in this case is average cost per visit. It is calculated by dividing total costs by volume. For example, at 500 visits, with total costs of $312,500, the average cost per visit is $312,500 / 500 = $625. Because fixed costs are spread over more visits as activity increases, average cost declines as activity increases. For example, when activity doubles from 100 to 200 visits, fixed costs remain at $300,000, but fixed cost per unit declines from $300,000/100 = $3,000 to $300,000/200 = $1,500. The fact that higher volume reduces average fixed cost and average cost per visit has important implications regarding the effect of volume changes on profitability. This point will be made several times in later sections.

The cost behavior presented in Table 5.1 is graphed in Figure 5.1. Here, costs are shown on the vertical Y axis and volume (number of visits) on the horizontal X axis. Because fixed costs are independent of volume, fixed costs are shown as a horizontal dashed line at $300,000. Total variable costs appear as an upward-sloping dotted line that starts at the origin (0 visits, $0 costs) and rises at a rate of $25 for each additional visit. Thus, the slope of the total variable costs line is the variable cost rate. When fixed and total variable costs are combined to obtain total costs, the result is an upward-sloping solid line parallel to the total variable costs line, but beginning at the Y axis at a value of $300,000 (the fixed costs amount). In effect, the total costs line is nothing more than the total variable costs line shifted upward on the graph by the amount of fixed costs.

Figure 5.1 is not drawn to scale. The intent here is to emphasize the shape of the graph and not its exact position. Also, the total variable costs shown in the graph are linear—they plot as a straight line. Curvilinear total variable costs can occur in some situations. However, in all illustrations in this text, the assumption is made that the variable cost rate is constant, and hence total variable costs are linear, at least in the range of volume under consideration. Such an assumption is not unreasonable for most health services organizations in most situations.

One final point should be noted about cost behavior: fixed costs do not remain constant forever regardless of volume. At some point of increasing volume, additional fixed costs must be incurred for new property and equipment, additional staffing, and so on. Likewise, if volume shrinks enough, there could be an opportunity to shed part of an organization's fixed cost base. While this is certainly true, the predominant assumption is that within some *relevant range* of volume and time, the organization's fixed cost structure will remain constant. In general, the illustrations in this chapter will stay within such a relevant range.[2]

Self-Test Questions

1. Construct a simple table similar to the one in Table 5.1 and discuss its elements.
2. Sketch and explain a simple diagram similar to Figure 5.1 to match your table.
3. What is meant by the term *relevant range*?

FIGURE 5.1
Cost Behavior
Graph

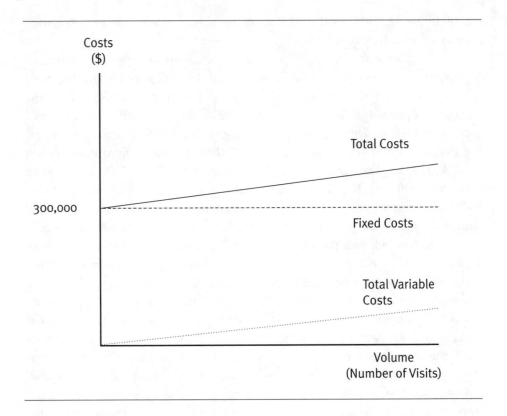

Profit (CVP) Analysis

Profit analysis is an analytical technique that typically is used to analyze the effects of volume changes on profit. The same procedures can be used to assess the effects of volume changes on costs, so this type of analysis is often called *cost-volume-profit* (*CVP*) *analysis*. CVP analysis allows managers to examine the effects of alternative assumptions regarding costs, volume, and prices. Clearly, such information is useful as managers evaluate future courses of action regarding pricing and the introduction of new services.

Basic Data

Table 5.2 presents the estimated costs for the Atlanta Clinic, a subsidiary of Atlanta Health Services, for 1999. These forecasted costs are based upon the clinic's best estimate of volume—75,000 visits. The best estimate often is called the *base case*, so the cost forecast in Table 5.2 is the clinic's base case cost analysis. Expected total costs for 1999 are $7,080,962. Because these costs support 75,000 visits, the forecasted average cost per visit is $7,080,962 / 75,000 = $94.41.

Focusing solely on total costs does not provide the clinic's managers with much information regarding potential alternative outcomes for 1999. By focusing on total costs, all costs are implicitly treated as fixed costs, which suggests that the clinic's total costs will remain constant regardless of the number of patient

	Variable Costs	Fixed Costs	Total Costs
Salaries and Benefits:			
Management and supervision	$ 0	$ 928,687	$ 928,687
Coordinators	442,617	598,063	1,040,680
Specialists	0	38,600	38,600
Technicians	681,383	552,670	1,234,053
Clerical/administrative	71,182	58,240	129,422
Social security taxes	89,622	163,188	252,810
Group health insurance	115,924	211,081	327,005
Professional fees	325,489	383,360	708,849
Supplies	313,283	231,184	544,467
Utilities	74,000	45,040	119,040
Allocated costs	0	1,757,349	1,757,349
Total	$2,113,500	$4,967,462	$7,080,962

TABLE 5.2
Atlanta Clinic:
Forecasted Cost
Data for 1999
(Based on 75,000
patient visits)

visits. Similarly, the base case cost per visit amount of $94.41 implicitly treats all costs as variable costs, which suggests that the average cost per visit would be $94.41 regardless of volume. Total cost information is necessary and useful, but the detailed breakdown in Table 5.2 gives the clinic's managers more insight into prospective financial outcomes for 1999 than is possible with a total cost focus.

As shown in Table 5.2, the clinic's total costs of $7,080,962 are broken down into two components: total variable costs of $2,113,500 and total fixed costs of $4,967,462. These cost amounts are fundamentally different, both in a quantitative sense and in a qualitative sense. The total fixed costs of $4,967,462 must be borne by the clinic no matter what volume actually occurs in 1999. However, total variable costs of $2,113,500 apply only to a volume of 75,000 patient visits. If the actual number of visits realized in 1999 is less than or greater than 75,000, total variable costs will be less than or greater than $2,133,500. (This is the primary reason why costs are classified as fixed and variable in the first place.)

The best way to show that total variable costs vary with volume is to express variable costs on a per unit (rate) basis. For Atlanta Clinic, the variable cost rate is $2,113,500 / 75,000 visits = $28.18 per visit. Thus, the clinic's total costs at any relevant volume can be calculated as follows:

Total costs = Fixed costs + Total variable costs

= $4,967,462 + ($28.18 × Number of visits).

This equation, the *cost behavior model*, explicitly shows that total costs depend on volume. To illustrate, consider three potential patient visit volumes for 1999: 70,000, 75,000, and 80,000:

Volume = 70,000:

Total costs = $4,967,462 + ($28.18 × 70,000)

= $4,967,462 + $1,972,600 = $6,940,062

Volume = 75,000:

$$\text{Total costs} = \$4,967,462 + (\$28.18 \times 75,000)$$

$$= \$4,967,462 + \$2,113,500 = \$7,080,962$$

Volume = 80,000:

$$\text{Total costs} = \$4,967,462 + (\$28.18 \times 80,000)$$

$$= \$4,967,462 + \$2,254,400 = \$7,221,862.$$

When an organization's costs are expressed in this way, it is easy to see that higher volume leads to higher total costs.

Atlanta Clinic's underlying cost structure is plotted in Figure 5.2. As first illustrated in Figure 5.1, fixed costs are shown as a horizontal dashed line, and total costs are shown as an upward-sloping solid line with a slope (rise over run) equal to the variable cost rate, $28.18 per visit. Unlike Figure 5.1, the graphical presentation has been simplified by not showing total variable costs as a separate line starting at the origin. Of course, total variable costs are represented in Figure 5.2 by the vertical distance between the total costs line and the fixed costs line.

Note that Atlanta Clinic does not literally write out a check for $28.18 for each visit, although there may be examples of variable costs in which this is the case. Rather, Atlanta's cost structure indicates that the clinic uses certain resources

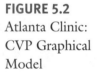

FIGURE 5.2
Atlanta Clinic:
CVP Graphical
Model

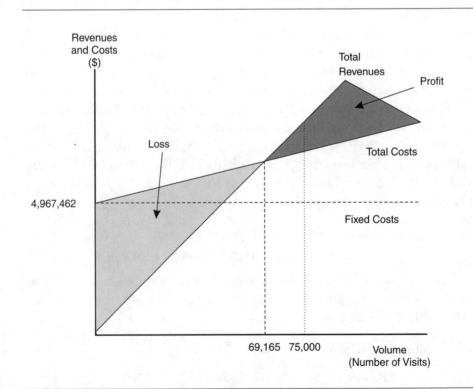

that its managers have defined as inherently variable, and the best estimate of the value of such resources is $28.18 per visit.

The cost structure shown in Figure 5.2 could be estimated in several ways. One way would be to use time-motion studies and interviews with clinic personnel. However, instead of such an intrusive approach, cost accountants could plot the total cost of the clinic at different volume levels for the past several years or months and then run a regression on these data. In this case, the beta term (slope) of the regression would be the variable cost rate, $28.18, and the alpha term (intercept) would be fixed costs, $4,967,462.

To complete the CVP model, a revenue component must be added. For 1999, Atlanta Clinic expects revenues, on average, to be $100 per patient visit. Total revenues are plotted on Figure 5.2 as an upward sloping solid line starting at the origin and having a slope of $100 per visit. If there were no visits, total revenues would be zero; at one visit, total revenues would be $100; at 10 visits, total revenues would be $1,000; and at 75,000 visits, total revenues would be $7,500,000; and so on.

The Pro-Forma P&L Statement

One of the first things that Atlanta Clinic's managers could do in terms of CVP analysis for the upcoming year is to project profit (net income), given the initial base case assumptions. Such a projection is called a *pro-forma profit and loss* (*P&L*) *statement* or *pro-forma income statement*.[3] The term *pro forma* merely means forecasted. This pro-forma income statement is different from the year-end, audited income statements that are part of Atlanta Clinic's annual report. First, the pro forma is done prior to 1999, not after year end, as part of the clinic's planning effort. Second, as with any forecast, if Atlanta's managers do not like what they see on the pro-forma income statement, they can take actions to change it, which cannot be done with historical data.

Atlanta Clinic's 1999 base case pro-forma P&L statement is shown in Table 5.3. The bottom line projects Atlanta's 1999 net income assuming that all assumptions regarding costs, volume, and prices that have been built into the base case are correct. Note that the format of a CVP pro-forma income statement distinguishes between variable and fixed costs, whereas a typical income statement does not make this distinction, which is irrelevant in financial accounting. Also, note that the pro-forma income statement contains a line labeled total contribution margin. This very important concept will be presented in the next section.

Total revenues ($100 × 75,000)	$7,500,000
Total variable costs ($28.18 × 75,000)	2,113,500
Total contribution margin ($71.82 × 75,000)	$5,386,500
Fixed costs	4,967,462
Profit (net income)	$ 419,038

TABLE 5.3 Atlanta Clinic: 1999 Base Case Pro-Forma P&L Statement (Based on 75,000 patient visits)

The pro-forma income statement used in CVP analysis is essentially a four-variable model; three of the variables are assumed and the fourth is calculated. In Table 5.3, the assumed variables are expected volume (75,000 visits), expected price ($100 per visit), and expected costs (delineated in terms of the cost structure). Profit, the fourth variable, is calculated on the basis of the three assumed variables.

The Table 5.3 base case pro-forma income statement represents only one point on the Figure 5.2 CVP model. This point is shown by the dotted, vertical line at a volume of 75,000 patient visits. Moving up along this dotted line, the distance from the X axis to the horizontal fixed costs line represents the $4,967,462 in fixed costs. The distance from the fixed costs line to the total costs line represents the $2,113,500 in total variable costs. The distance between the total costs line and the total revenues line represents the $419,038 profit. As with Figure 5.1, the graph in Figure 5.2 is not drawn to scale because it will not be used to develop numerical data. Rather, it provides the clinic's managers with a pictorial representation of Atlanta's projected financial future.

Contribution Margin

The base case pro-forma P&L statement in Table 5.3 introduces the concept of *contribution margin*, which is the difference between per unit revenue and the variable cost rate (per unit variable cost). In this illustration, the contribution margin is $100.00 − $28.18 = $71.82. What is the inherent meaning of this contribution margin value of $71.82? The contribution margin has the look and feel of profit, but because none of the fixed costs of providing service have been considered, it is **not** profit. The contribution margin is the dollar amount per visit that **first** must be used to cover Atlanta Clinic's fixed costs. Only after fixed costs are fully covered does the contribution margin contribute to profit.

With a contribution margin of $71.82 on each of the clinic's 75,000 visits, the projected base case *total contribution margin* for 1999 is $71.82 × 75,000 = $5,386,500. This amount of total contribution is sufficient to cover the clinic's fixed costs of $4,967,462 and then provide $5,386,500 − $4967,462 = $419,038 in profit. In essence, after fixed costs have been covered, any additional visits contribute to the clinic's profit at a rate of $71.82 per visit. Readers will discover that the contribution margin concept is used again and again as the discussion of CVP analysis is extended.

Self-Test Questions

1. Construct a simple P&L statement similar to the one in Table 5.3 and discuss its elements.
2. Sketch or explain a simple diagram to match your table.
3. Define and explain the contribution margin.

Breakeven Analysis

Breakeven analysis is applied in many different ways, so it is necessary to understand the context to fully understand the meaning of the term *breakeven*. Here it is used to determine the volume, called the *breakeven volume*, or *breakeven point*, at which a program or service becomes financially self-sufficient in an accounting sense. In other words, the breakeven point is that volume that generates zero accounting profit. Although the breakeven analysis discussed here is actually part of profit (CVP) analysis, the concept deserves separate consideration.

As mentioned in the previous section, the pro-forma P&L statement is a four-variable model where values for three of the four variables (costs, volume, and price) are assumed and the fourth (profit) is calculated. In breakeven analysis, the same four variables are used, but profit is assumed to be the breakeven profit, which, of course, has a value of zero. Then, volume typically is the unknown (calculated) value. However, it is also possible to assume a value for volume and price (or costs), and then calculate the breakeven value for costs (or price). The breakeven point can be obtained two ways: algebraically or graphically. To illustrate the algebraic approach, the pro-forma P&L statement presented in Table 5.3 can be expressed algebraically as follows:

$$\text{Total revenues} - \text{Total variable costs} - \text{Fixed costs} = \text{Profit}$$

$$(\$100 \times \text{Volume}) - (\$28.18 \times \text{Volume}) - \$4{,}967{,}462 = \text{Profit}.$$

By definition, at breakeven the clinic's profit equals zero, so the equation can be rewritten this way:

$$(\$100 \times \text{Volume}) - (\$28.18 \times \text{Volume}) - \$4{,}967{,}462 = \$0.$$

Rearranging the terms so that only the terms related to volume appear on the left side produces this equation:

$$(\$100 \times \text{Volume}) - (\$28.18 \times \text{Volume}) = \$4{,}967{,}462.$$

Using basic algebra, the two terms on the left side can be combined because volume appears in both. The end result is this:

$$(\$100 - \$28.18) \times \text{Volume} = \$4{,}967{,}462$$

$$\$71.82 \times \text{Volume} = \$4{,}967{,}462.$$

The left side of the breakeven equation now contains the contribution margin, $71.82, multiplied by volume. Here, the previous conclusion is reaffirmed that the clinic will break even when the total contribution margin equals fixed costs. Solving the equation for volume results in a breakeven point of $4,967,462 / $71.82 ≈ 69,165 visits. Any volume greater than 69,165 visits produces a profit for the clinic, while any volume less than 69,165 results in a loss. Note that the precise breakeven point is 69,165.4 visits. However, because partial visits are not feasible, the clinic really would not break even until 69,166 visits. One visit out of this high volume is meaningless, so 69,165 visits is used as the breakeven point.

The logic behind this breakeven point is that each patient visit brings in $100, of which $28.18 is the variable cost to treat the patient, which leaves a $71.82 contribution margin from each visit. If the clinic sets the contribution margin aside for the first 69,165 visits in 1999, it would have $4,967,430, which is enough (except for a small rounding difference) to cover its fixed costs. Once the clinic exceeds breakeven volume, each visit's contribution margin produces a profit. If the clinic achieves its 75,000 visits volume estimate, the 5,835 visits above the breakeven point result in a total profit of $5,835 \times \$71.82 = \$419,070$, which matches the profit (again, except for a rounding difference) shown on the clinic's base case pro-forma P&L statement in Table 5.3.

The second method for determining the breakeven point is by graphical analysis. At breakeven the profit is zero, so total revenues must equal total costs. On a CVP graphical model such as Figure 5.2, this condition holds at the intersection of the total revenues line and total costs line. This point is indicated by a vertical dashed line drawn at a volume of 69,165 visits. If a very large sheet of graph paper were used, the lines could be drawn perfectly to scale and the breakeven point could be read off of the graph.

The logic of the breakeven point as illustrated in Figure 5.2 goes back to the nature of the clinic's fixed and variable cost structure. Before even one patient walks in the door, the clinic has already committed to $4,967,462 in fixed costs. Because the total revenues line is steeper than the total variable costs line, and hence the total costs line, total revenue eventually catches up to the clinic's cost structure. Any utilization to the right of the breakeven point, which is shown as a dark-shaded area, produces a profit; any utilization to the left, which is shown as a light-shaded area, results in a loss.

The relationship between breakeven analysis and the pro-forma P&L statement is important to understand. To an extent, breakeven analysis is a neurotic pro forma. That is, based on the clinic's base case marketing projection of 75,000 visits, it can anticipate a profit of $419,038. However, management may worry that the clinic will not achieve this projected volume and ask the following question: What is the minimum number of visits that are needed to at least break even?

To verify the breakeven point, Table 5.4 contains a pro-forma P&L statement for 69,165 visits. Except for a small rounding difference, the net income at the breakeven point is $0. (Remember that the breakeven point was actually 69,165.4 visits.) As mentioned previously, at breakeven the total contribution margin just covers fixed costs, resulting in zero profit.

This breakeven analysis contains important assumptions. The first assumption is that the price or set of prices for different types of patients and different payors is independent of volume. In other words, volume increases are not attained by lowering prices, and price increases are not met with volume declines. The second assumption is that costs can be reasonably subdivided into fixed and variable components. The third assumption is that both fixed costs and the variable cost rate are independent of volume over the relevant range, which makes both the total costs and total revenues lines linear.

Total revenues ($100 × 69,165)	$6,916,500	
Total variable costs ($28.18 × 69,165)	1,949,070	
Total contribution margin	$4,967,430	
Fixed costs	4,967,462	
Profit (net income)	($ 32)	

TABLE 5.4

Atlanta Clinic: 1999 Pro-Forma P&L Statement (Based on 69,165 patient visits)

Breakeven analysis is often performed in an iterative manner. After the breakeven volume is calculated, managers must determine whether or not the resulting volume can realistically be achieved at the price assumed in the analysis. If the price appears to be unreasonable for the breakeven volume, a new price has to be estimated and the breakeven analysis repeated. Likewise, if the cost structure used for the calculation appears to be unrealistic at the breakeven volume, operational assumptions, and hence cost assumptions, should be changed and the analysis should be repeated again.

Both concepts—the pro-forma P&L statement and breakeven analysis—are consistent with the broader intent of CVP analysis; that is, to model relationships between cost, volume, price, and profit. To take this logic a step further, the base case pro-forma P&L statement and the breakeven point are only two points on a continuum of possibilities. Instead of asking the number of visits needed to break even, Atlanta's managers may ask the number of visits needed to achieve a $100,000 profit, or any other profit for that matter. They know that the clinic will have a $419,038 profit if it has 75,000 visits, and that it will have no profit if it has 69,165 visits. Thus, the number of visits required to achieve a $100,000 profit is somewhere in between 69,165 and 75,000. In fact, the number of visits required is 70,558:

$$\text{Total revenues} - \text{Total variable costs} - \text{Fixed costs} = \text{Profit}$$
$$(\$100 \times \text{Volume}) - (\$28.18 \times \text{Volume}) - \$4,967,462 = \$100,000$$
$$(\$71.82 \times \text{Volume}) - \$4,967,462 = \$100,000$$
$$\$71.82 \times \text{Volume} = \$5,067,462$$
$$\text{Volume} = 70,558.$$

Self-Test Questions

1. What is the purpose of breakeven analysis?
2. What is the equation for volume breakeven?
3. Why is breakeven analysis often conducted in an iterative manner?
4. Can breakeven concepts be applied to a profit value other than zero?

Operating Leverage

The movement from a pro-forma analysis at 75,000 visits to one at 69,165 visits is quite easy. In fact, the pro-forma analysis could be entered on a spreadsheet and the results could be quickly examined at any given volume. This way, "what if" questions could be answered about the impact of changing volume, costs, or prices. With that in mind, assume that marketplace changes have occurred, forcing Atlanta Clinic's managers to estimate a new volume of 82,500 visits—an increase of 7,500 visits over the original 75,000 visit base case estimate. Table 5.5 contains the clinic's pro-forma P&L statements at 69,175 (breakeven), 75,000 (base case), and 82,500 visits. The first two columns are the same as previously constructed. The third column, which represents the 82,500 visit estimate, is new.

Now that P&L statements exist at three different volume levels, the consequences of volume changes can be better understood. As the clinic's forecasted volume moves from 75,000 visits to 82,500 visits, its profit increases by $957,688 − $419,038 = $538,650. This increase is equal to the additional 7,500 visits multiplied by the $71.82 contribution margin. When the volume is beyond the breakeven point, any additional visits are "gravy." That is, the clinic's fixed costs are now covered, so all additional contribution margin flows directly to profit. Similarly, the outcome is known if the clinic's projected volume dropped from 75,000 to 69,165 visits. In this case, the decrease of 5,835 visits multiplied by the $71.82 contribution margin equals $419,670, which is the loss of profit, except for a rounding difference, that results from the volume decrease.

The movement from 75,000 to 82,500 visits resulted in a (82,500 − 75,000) / 75,000 = 7,250 / 72,500 = 0.10 = 10% increase in volume, and thus total revenues. While the top line of the P&L statement—total revenues—increased by 10 percent, the bottom line of the P&L statement—net income—increased by 128.5 percent ($538,650 / $419,038 = 1.285 = 128.5%). This incredible increase in profit occurs because the clinic is reaping the benefit of the fixed cost structure, which does not change with volume.

If a high proportion of a business' total costs are fixed, the business is said to have high *operating leverage*. In physics, leverage implies the use of a lever to raise a heavy object with a small amount of force. In politics, individuals who have leverage can accomplish much with the smallest word or action. In finance, high

TABLE 5.5

Atlanta Clinic: 1999 Pro-Forma P&L Statements (Based on 69,165, 75,000 and 82,500 patient visits)

	Number of Visits		
	69,165	75,000	82,500
Total revenues ($100 × volume)	$6,916,500	$7,500,000	$8,250,000
Total variable costs ($28.18 × volume)	1,949,070	2,113,500	2,324,850
Total contribution margin ($71.82 × volume)	$4,967,430	$5,386,500	$5,925,150
Fixed costs	4,967,462	4,967,462	4,967,462
Profit (net income)	($ 32)	$ 419,038	$ 957,688

operating leverage means that a relatively small change in volume results in a large change in profit (net income).

Operating leverage is measured by the *degree of operating leverage* (*DOL*), which at any volume is calculated by dividing the total contribution margin by **pre-tax income**, which for not-for-profit businesses is net income. At a volume of 75,000 visits, Atlanta Clinic's degree of operating leverage is $5,386,500 / $419,038 = 12.85. The DOL indicates how much income will change for each 1 percent change in volume. In this example, each 1 percent change in volume produces a 12.85 percent change in net income. Therefore, a 10 percent increase in volume results in a $10\% \times 12.85 = 128.5\%$ increase in profit. The DOL changes with volume, so the 12.85 DOL only is applicable to a starting volume of 75,000 visits.

Cost structures differ widely among industries and among organizations within a given industry. The DOL is greatest in health services organizations with a large proportion of fixed costs, and consequently a low proportion of variable costs. The end result is a high contribution margin, which contributes to a high DOL. In economics terminology, high-DOL businesses are said to have *economies of scale* because higher volumes lead to lower per unit total costs. In such businesses, a small increase in revenue produces a relatively large increase in income. However, high-DOL businesses have relatively high breakeven points, which increase the risk of losses. Also, operating leverage is a double-edged sword: high-DOL businesses suffer large profit declines, and potentially large losses, if volume falls.

To illustrate the negative effect of a high DOL, consider this question: What would happen to Atlanta Clinic's profit if volume falls by 7.8 percent from the base case level of 75,000 visits? To answer this question, recognize that profit would decline by $7.8\% \times 12.85 \approx 100\%$, so the clinic's profit would fall to zero. The data in Table 5.5 confirm this answer. At a projected volume of 69,165 visits (a decrease of 7.8 percent from 75,000 visits), the clinic's profit is zero. Of course, this volume was previously identified as the breakeven point.

To what extent can managers influence a business' operating leverage? In many respects, operating leverage is determined by the inherent nature of the business. In general, hospitals must make large investments in fixed assets, and hence they have a high proportion of fixed costs and high operating leverage. Conversely, home health care businesses need few fixed assets, so they tend to have relatively low operating leverage. Still, managers can somewhat influence operating leverage. For example, organizations can make use of temporary rather than permanent employees to handle peak patient loads. Assets also can be leased, especially on a per use basis, rather than purchased. Actions such as these tend to reduce the proportion of fixed costs in an organization's cost structure.

1. What is operating leverage and how is it measured?
2. Why is the operating leverage concept important to managers?
3. Can managers influence their firms' operating leverage?

Self-Test Questions

4. How does an organization's cost structure affect its exposure to economies of scale?

CVP Analysis in a Discounted Fee-for-Service Environment

As noted in the previous discussion, CVP analysis is quite valuable to managers in that it provides information about expected costs and profitability given an estimate of volume. To learn more about its usefulness, suppose that one third (25,000) of Atlanta Clinic's expected 75,000 visits would come from Peachtree HMO, which has proposed that their new contract with the clinic contain a 40 percent discount from charges. Thus, the net price for their patients would be $60 instead of the undiscounted $100. If the clinic refuses, Peachtree has threatened to take its patients elsewhere.

At first blush, Peachtree's proposal appears to be unacceptable. Among other reasons, $60 is less than the full cost of providing service, which was determined earlier to be $94.41 per visit at a volume of 75,000. Thus, on a full-cost basis, Atlanta would lose $94.41 − $60 = $34.41 per visit on Peachtree's patients. With an estimated 25,000 visits, the discounted contract would result in a loss of 25,000 × $34.41 = $860,250. Before Atlanta's managers reject Peachtree's proposal, however, it must be examined more closely.

The Impact of Rejecting the Proposal

If Atlanta's managers reject the proposal, the clinic would lose market share—an estimated 25,000 visits. The pro-forma P&L statement that would result, which is based on 50,000 undiscounted visits, is shown in Table 5.6. At the lower volume, the clinic's total revenues, total variable costs, and total contribution margin decrease proportionately (i.e., by one third). However, fixed costs are not reduced, so Atlanta would not cover its fixed costs, and hence a loss of $3,591,000 − $4,967,462 = −$1,376,462 would occur. To view the situation another way, the expected volume of 50,000 visits is 19,165 short of the breakeven point, so the clinic would be operating to the left of the breakeven point in Figure 5.2. This shortfall from breakeven of 19,165 visits when multiplied by the contribution margin of $71.82 produces a loss of $1,376,430, which is the same as shown in Table 5.6 (except for a rounding difference).

Clearly, the major factor behind the projected loss is the clinic's fixed cost structure of $4,967,462. With a projected decrease in volume of 33 percent,

TABLE 5.6

Atlanta Clinic: 1999 Pro-Forma P&L Statement (Based on 50,000 undiscounted patient visits)

Total revenues ($100 × 50,000)	$5,000,000
Total variable costs ($28.18 × 50,000)	1,409,000
Total contribution margin ($71.82 × 50,000)	$3,591,000
Fixed costs	4,967,462
Profit (net income)	($1,376,462)

perhaps the clinic could reduce its fixed costs. If Atlanta's managers perceive the volume reduction to be permanent, they would begin to reduce the fixed costs currently in place to meet an anticipated volume of 75,000 visits. However, if the clinic's managers believe that the loss of volume is merely a temporary occurrence, they may choose to maintain the current fixed cost structure and absorb the loss expected for next year. It would not make sense for them to start selling off equipment and facilities and firing workers, only to reverse these actions one year later. The critical point, though, is that the loss of market share caused by rejecting Peachtree's proposal can have a significant negative impact on the clinic's profit, which indicates that the clinic's fixed cost structure should be reexamined.

The Impact of Accepting the Proposal

An alternative strategy for the clinic's managers would be to accept Peachtree's proposal. The resulting pro-forma P&L statement is contained in Table 5.7. The average per visit revenue of serving these two different payor groups is $(2/3 \times \$100) + (1/3 \times \$60) = \$86.67$. Total revenues based on this average revenue per visit would be $75,000 \times \$86.67 = \$6,500,250$, which equals the value for total revenues shown in the table (except for a rounding difference). With a lower average revenue per visit, the contribution margin falls to $\$86.67 - \$28.18 = \$58.49$, which leads to a lower total contribution margin.

The critical point here is that the clinic's total revenues have decreased significantly from the previous situation in which all visits bring in $100 in revenue (see Table 5.3). The clinic's cost structure remains the same, however, because it is handling same number of visits—75,000. The impact of the discount is strictly on revenues, and the end result of accepting Peachtree's proposal is a projected loss of $580,962.

Another way of confirming the expected loss at 75,000 visits is to calculate the clinic's breakeven point at the new average per visit revenue of $86.67. The new higher breakeven point is 84,928 visits, so the breakeven analysis confirms that the clinic will lose money at 75,000 visits because of the lower revenue function ($86.67 volume). Because the clinic is projected to be $84,928 - 75,000 = 9,928$ visits below breakeven and the contribution margin is now $58.49, the projected loss is $9,928 \times \$58.49 = \$580,689$, which is the amount shown in Table 5.7 (except for a rounding difference).

Undiscounted revenue ($100 × 50,000)	$5,000,000
Discounted revenue ($60 × 25,000)	1,500,000
Total revenues ($86.67 × 75,000)	$6,500,000
Total variable costs ($28.18 × 75,000)	2,113,500
Total contribution margin ($58.49 × 75,000)	$4,386,500
Fixed costs	4,967,462
Profit (net income)	($ 580,962)

TABLE 5.7 Altanta Clinic: 1999 Pro-Forma P&L Statement (Based on 50,000 visits at $100 and 25,000 visits at $60)

The change in breakeven point that results from accepting Peachtree's proposal is graphed in Figure 5.3, along with the original breakeven point. The new total revenues line (the dot-dashed line), is flatter than the original line. The new total revenues line, combined with the existing cost structure results in the breakeven point being pushed to the right to 84,928 visits. However, any cost-control actions taken by Atlanta's managers would either flatten, if variable costs are lowered, or lower, if fixed costs are reduced, the total costs line, and hence push the breakeven point back to the left.

Nothing much has changed in terms of core economic underpinnings because of the new discounted-charge environment. The clinic is worse off economically, but the clinic's cost structure, managerial incentives, and solutions to financial problems are essentially the same. To increase profit, more services must be provided. In short, the movement from charges to discounted charges does not make a radical impact on managerial decision making. The major difference is that the clinic is now under greater financial pressure. As discussed in the next major section, the clinic's entire incentive structure will change if it moves to a capitated environment.

Evaluating the Alternative Strategies

What should Atlanta's managers do? If Peachtree's proposal is accepted, the clinic is expected to lose $580,962 rather than make a profit of $419,038 when no

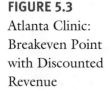

FIGURE 5.3
Atlanta Clinic: Breakeven Point with Discounted Revenue

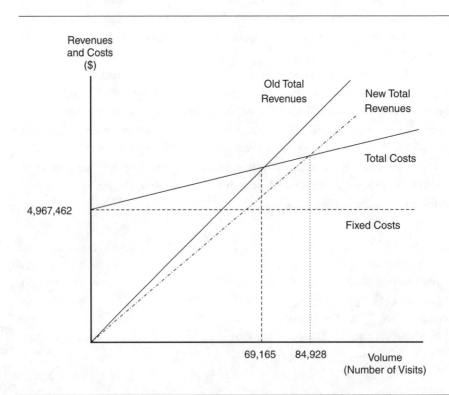

discount was demanded. The difference is a swing of $1 million in profit in the wrong direction, hardly an enticing prospect. What happened to the "missing" $1 million? It is now in the hands of Peachtree HMO, which is paying $1 million less to one of its providers (25,000 visits × $40 savings = $1,000,000). This will be reflected as a cost savings on Peachtree's income statement and, if the savings is not passed on to the ultimate payors, will result in a profit increase.

If market forces in Atlanta Clinic's service area suggest that making a counter offer to Peachtree is not feasible—perhaps because the clinic is being pitted against another provider—the comparison of a loss of $580,792 to a profit of $419,038 is irrelevant. The only relevant issue at hand for the short term is the comparison of the $580,792 loss if the clinic accepts the proposal versus the $1,376,462 loss if the proposal is rejected and Peachtree's patients are lost to the clinic. Although neither outcome is very appealing, the acceptance of the discount is the lesser of two evils. In fact, the acceptance of the discount is better by $1,376,462 − $580,792 = $795,670. Accepting the discount proposal is Atlanta's best short-term strategy because Peachtree's patients still produce a positive contribution margin of $60 − $28.18 = $31.82 per visit, which would be foregone if the clinic rebuffs Peachtree's offer. That $31.82 per visit contribution margin, when multiplied by the expected 25,000 visits on the contract, puts $795,500 on the total contribution margin table that would otherwise be lost.

Marginal Analysis: Short-Term Versus Long-Term Implications

The Atlanta/Peachtree illustration points out how the contribution margin can be used in managerial decision making. To help see this, the analysis needs to be viewed from a different perspective. Suppose the clinic is forecasting a volume of 50,000 visits for 1999, and Peachtree HMO offers to provide the clinic 25,000 additional visits at $60 revenue per visit. These 25,000 visits are called *marginal*, or *incremental, visits* because they add to the exiting base of visits. Should the clinic's managers accept this offer?

Although each marginal visit from the contract brings in only $60 compared with $100 on the clinic's other contracts, the *marginal cost*, which is the cost associated with each additional visit, is the variable cost rate of $28.18. The clinic's $4,967,462 in fixed costs will be incurred whether the offer is accepted or rejected, so these costs are not relevant to the decision. In finance parlance, the clinic's fixed costs are *nonincremental* to the decision. Because the contribution margin of each visit at the margin (the *marginal contribution margin*) is a positive $31.82, each visit contributes positively to Atlanta's recovery of fixed costs and ultimately to net income. The offer should be accepted, or at least seriously considered.

However, Atlanta's managers cannot ignore the long-term implications associated with accepting the proposal. These are not addressed in detail here, but clearly the clinic cannot survive this scenario in the long run because the clinic's revenues are not covering the full costs of providing services. In the meantime, bleeding $580,962 of losses in 1999 may be better than bleeding $1,376,462 until the clinic can adjust to market forces in its service area. This adjustment may be as simple as merely absorbing the losses while the clinic's competitors, perhaps in poorer financial condition, exit the market as they too face the same difficult economic choices. Should this happen, a new equilibrium would be established in the market that would allow the clinic to raise its prices. If the long-term solution is not that simple, Atlanta must reduce its cost structure or perish.

Another problem associated with accepting the discount offer is that the clinic's other payors will undoubtedly learn about the reduced payments and want to renegotiate their contracts with the same, or even greater, discount. Such a reaction would clearly place the clinic under even more financial pressure, and a draconian change in either volume or operating costs would be required for survival.

Self-Test Questions

1. What is the impact of a discount contract on fixed costs, total variable costs, and the breakeven point?
2. What is meant by marginal analysis?
3. What is meant by the following statement: "Marginal analysis is made more complicated by long-run considerations."?

CVP Analysis in a Capitated Environment

As a review of CVP analysis, consider how the analysis is changed when a provider operates in a capital environment. In addition to solidifying CVP concepts, this section provides insight into the basic differences between fee-for-service reimbursement and capitation.

To begin, assume that the purchaser of services from Atlanta Clinic is the Alliance, a local business coalition. As in previous illustrations, assume the Alliance is paying the clinic $7,500,000 to provide services for an expected 75,000 visits, but now the amount is capitated. Although projected total revenues remain the same under the Alliance as the previous base case (see Table 5.3), they are qualitatively quite different. The $7,500,000 that the Alliance is paying is not explicitly related to the amount of services (visits) provided, but rather to the size of the covered employee group. In essence, the clinic is no longer merely selling healthcare services as it had in the fee-for-service or discounted fee-for-service environment. Now, the clinic is taking on the insurance function, in that it is responsible for the health (utilization) of the covered population and must bear the attendant risks. If the total costs of services delivered by the clinic exceed the insurance revenue (paid up-front on a per member basis), the clinic will suffer the financial consequences. However, if the clinic can efficiently manage the healthcare of the served population, it will be the economic beneficiary.

How might Atlanta's managers evaluate whether or not the $7,500,000 revenue attached to the contract is financially attractive? To do the analysis, they need two critical pieces of information: cost information and actuarial information. The clinic already has the cost-accounting information; the full cost per visit is expected to be $94.41 (at a volume of 75,000 visits), with an underlying cost structure of $28.18 per visit in variable costs and $4,967,462 in fixed costs. For its actuarial information, Atlanta's managers estimate that the Alliance will have a covered population of 18,750 members with an expected utilization of four visits per year. Thus, the total number of visits expected is $18,750 \times 4 = 75,000$. Although this appears to be the same 75,000 visits as in the fee-for-service environment, significant difference exists in the implications of this volume. Because there is no direct tie between total revenues and volume, utilization above that expected will bring increased costs with **no corresponding** increase in revenues.

The revenues expected from this contract, $7,500,000, exceed the expected costs of serving this population, which are 75,000 visits multiplied by $94.41 per visit, or $7,080,750. Thus, this contract is expected to generate a profit of $419,250, which, not unexpectedly, is the same as the original base case fee-for-service result (except for a rounding difference) (see Table 5.3).

A Graphical View in Terms of Utilization

Figure 5.4 contains the graphical CVP analysis for the capitation contract. To begin the graphical analysis, note that Figure 5.4 is constructed similar to the fee-for-service graphs shown in Figures 5.2 and 5.3. The horizontal axis shows the number of visits, while the vertical axis shows dollars of revenues and costs. Also shown is the same underlying cost structure of $4,967,463 in fixed costs coupled with a variable cost rate of $28.18. One very significant difference exists, however. Instead of being upward sloping, the total revenues line is horizontal, which shows that total revenue is $7,500,000 regardless of volume as measured by the number of visits.

Several subtle messages are inherent in this flat revenue line. First, it tells managers that revenue is being driven by something other than the volume of services provided. Under capitation, revenue is being driven by the insurance contract (i.e., by the monthly or annual premium based on the number of covered lives, or *enrollees*). This change in the revenue source is the core of the logic switch from fee-for-service to capitation; the clinic is being rewarded to manage the healthcare of the population served rather than to provide services. However, the clinic's costs are still driven by the amount of services provided (in this case, the number of visits).

A second critical point about Figure 5.4 is the difference between the flat revenue and the flat fixed cost base. Atlanta has a spread of $7,500,000 − $4,967,462 = $2,532,538 to work with in the management of the healthcare of this population for the period of the contract. If total variable costs equal $2,532,538, the clinic breaks even; if total variable costs exceed $2,532,538, the clinic loses. If everyone in the organization, especially the managers and clinicians, does not understand this inherent risk of capitation, the clinic could find itself in serious financial trouble. On the other hand, if Atlanta's managers and clinicians at all levels understand and manage this risk, a handsome reward may be gained.

FIGURE 5.4

Atlanta Clinic:
Breakeven Point
Under Capitation

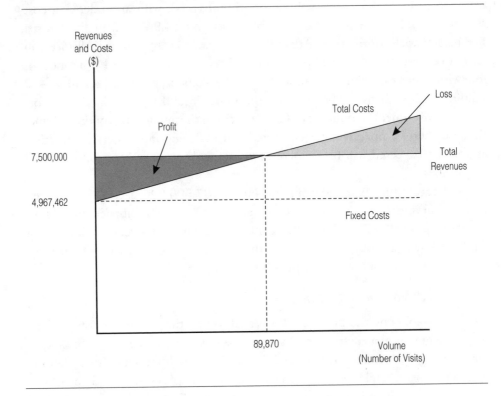

A key feature of capitation is the reversal of the profit and loss portions of the graph. To see this, compare Figure 5.4 with Figure 5.2. The idea that profits occur at lower volumes under capitation is contrary to the fee-for-service environment. In fact, the optimal short-term response to capitation from a purely financial perspective is to take the money and run (provide no services) because zero visits allow the clinic to capture the full spread between total revenues and fixed costs. The clinic may have trouble renewing the contract in subsequent years, but it will have maximized short-term profit. Obviously, this course of action is neither appropriate nor feasible. Still, its implications are at the heart of concerns expressed by critics of managed care about the incentives to withhold patient care inherent in a capitated environment.

A Graphical View in Terms of Membership

Figure 5.5 recasts the situation shown in Figure 5.4 to reflect a different definition of volume. Figure 5.4 is like Alice of *Alice in Wonderland*, peering through the looking glass and finding that everything is backwards. The key to this problem is that the horizontal axis does not measure the volume to which revenues are related. That is, the horizontal axis in Figure 5.4 has number of visits, just as if Atlanta Clinic were selling healthcare services. It is not; it is now selling insurance, so the appropriate horizontal axis value is the number of members (enrollees).

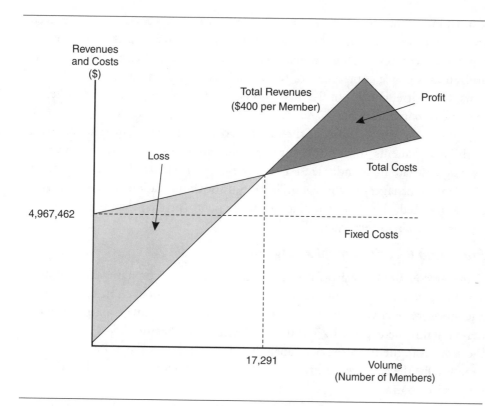

FIGURE 5.5

Atlanta Clinic: Breakeven Point Under Capitation in Insurance Terms

Figure 5.5 recognizes that membership, rather than the amount of services provided, drives revenues. With the number of members on the horizontal axis, the total revenues line is no longer flat; revenues only look flat when they are considered relative to the number of visits. The revenue earned by the clinic is actually $400 per member, which could be broken down to a monthly premium. The expected $7,500,000 revenue shown on Figure 5.4 results from an expected enrollee population of 18,750 members. The cost structure can easily be expressed on a membership basis as well. Fixed costs are no problem within the relevant range; they are inherently volume insensitive, whether volume is measured by number of visits or members. Thus, Figure 5.5 shows fixed costs as the same flat, dashed line as before. However, the variable cost rate based on number of enrollees is not the same as the variable cost rate based on number of visits. Per member variable cost must be estimated from two other factors: the variable cost of $28.18 per visit and the expected utilization of four visits per year. The combination of the two is 4 × $28.18 = $112.72, which is the clinic's expected variable cost per member.

There are two elements to controlling total variable costs under capitation: the underlying variable cost of the service ($28.18 per visit) and the number of visits per member (four). The two-variable nature of the variable cost rate makes cost control more difficult under capitation. In a fee-for-service environment, cost control entails only minimizing per visit expenses. Utilization is not an issue.

If anything, utilization is good because per visit revenue almost always exceeds the variable cost rate. (In other words, there is a positive contribution margin.) Capitation requires a change in management thinking about cost control because utilization is now a component of the variable cost rate, and hence total variable costs. Of course, control of fixed costs is always financially prudent regardless of the type of reimbursement.

Also, a positive feature of the variable cost structure under capitation exists. With two elements to control, the clinic has more opportunity to lower the variable cost rate than under fee-for-service reimbursement. The key is the ability of Atlanta's managers to control utilization. If **both** utilization and per visit costs can be reduced, the clinic can reap greater benefits (profits) than possible under fee-for-service reimbursement.

Pro-Forma P&L Statement Analysis

Table 5.8 contains three pro-forma P&L statements in this capitated environment. The three volume levels shown are the same as those contained in Table 5.5 for a fee-for-service environment. To begin, start with the middle column—the one that contains the expected 75,000 patient visits. The bottom line ($419,038) is the same as in the fee-for-service analysis, which reinforces the point that at least superficially, the capitated contract is not inherently better or worse than the fee-for-service contract.

Although the profit at 75,000 visits is the same, some of the values in the pro-forma analyses and their economic meanings differ. For example, although total revenues are $7,500,000, it is a flat amount in Table 5.8, while it varies with volume in Table 5.5. The variable cost rate is the same in both tables, $28.18 per visit. However, because each visit does not result in additional revenue, the revenue per visit is zero in Table 5.8. The end result is a strange-looking contribution margin of $0 − $28.18 = −$28.18. In essence, each visit contributes nothing in revenues to the clinic, but it costs the clinic $28.18 in variable costs. This feature of capitation explains why the clinic's profits decline as volume moves to the right on a CVP graph such as Figure 5.4.

What would happen if the clinic experienced more visits than predicted? If the number of visits increases by 10 percent or by 7,500 to 82,500, the right

TABLE 5.8

Atlanta Clinic: 1999 Pro-Forma P&L Statement (Based on 69,165, 75,000 and 82,500 patient visits)

	Number of Visits		
	69,165	75,000	82,500
Total revenues	$7,500,000	$7,500,000	$7,500,000
Total variable costs ($28.18 × volume)	1,949,070	2,113,500	2,324,850
Total contribution margin	$5,550,930	$5,386,500	$5,175,150
Fixed costs	4,967,462	4,967,462	4,967,462
Profit (net income)	$ 583,468	$ 419,038	$ 207,688

column in Table 5.8 shows that profit would decrease by $419,038 − $207,688 = $211,350. This occurs because total revenues stay constant while costs are increasing at a rate of $28.18 for each additional visit. With 7,500 additional visits, the clinic's costs increase by 7,500 × $28.18 = $211,350. Obviously, this is quite in contrast to the significant increase in profit at this volume level that occurs in a fee-for-service environment (see Table 5.5).

Under capitation, a decrease in visits will improve the profitability of the clinic. When the number of visits decreases to 69,165, which is the breakeven point in a fee-for-service environment, profit in a capitated environment increases by $164,430, to $583,468. This increase is explained by the decrease in visits (5,835) multiplied by the contribution margin (−$28.18), which results in a $164,430 decrease in costs while revenues remain constant.

Finally, what is Atlanta Clinic's breakeven point under capitation? The three pro-forma income statements in Table 5.8 show that profit gets smaller as the number of visits increase. Because the clinic is projected to operate at a profit, it must be to the left of breakeven, so the breakeven point must be greater than 82,500 visits. Actually, the breakeven point is 89,870 visits, calculated as follows:

$$\text{Total revenues} - \text{Total variable costs} - \text{Fixed costs} = \text{Profit}$$

$$\$7,500,000 - (\$28.18 \times \text{Volume}) - \$4,967,462 = \$0$$

$$\$28.18 \times \text{Volume} = \$2,532,538$$

$$\text{Volume} = 89,870.$$

Any volume less than 89,870 visits results in a profit, while any volume greater than this amount results in a loss.

The Importance of Controlling Utilization

To determine the impact of utilization changes on profitability, refer to Table 5.8. The center column, the base case, is once again our starting point. With an assumed utilization of four visits for each of Peachtree's 18,750 members, 75,000 visits result in a projected profit of $419,038.

However, if Atlanta's managers are not able to attain the utilization forecasted, the clinic's profit would fall. Assume that realized utilization is actually 4.4 visits per member, rather than the 4.0 forecasted. This higher utilization would result in 4.4 × 18,750 = 82,500 visits, which produces the results shown in the right column in Table 5.8. Because revenues are fixed and costs are tied to volume, higher utilization leads to higher costs and lower profit. With the same 82,500 visits but total variable costs of $2,324,850 at the higher utilization rate, the variable cost per member increases to $2,324,850 / 18,750 = $124.99, which could also be found by multiplying 4.4 visits per member times the variable cost rate of $28.18.

The left column of Table 5.8 shows what the clinic's profitability would be if utilization was reduced to 3.69 visits per member, producing about 69,165 total visits. With lower utilization, total variable costs are reduced and profit increases. The key point is that the ability of a provider to control utilization is the key to profitability in a capitated environment. Less utilization means lower total costs, and lower total costs mean greater profit.

In the discussion of fee-for-service CVP analysis, operating leverage is related to the cost structure of the organization—the higher the proportion of fixed costs, the greater the operating leverage. In a fee-for-service environment, high operating leverage means a low variable cost rate, a high per visit contribution margin, and hence high risk in that small volume decreases lead to large cuts in profitability. On the other hand, small volume increases can have a significant positive impact on the bottom line.

Under capitation, the situation is reversed because the per visit contribution margin is negative. Whereas a higher proportion of fixed costs drives the positive per visit contribution margin even higher under fee-for-service reimbursement, it drives the negative per visit contribution margin toward zero under capitation. In fact, if all of Atlanta Clinic's costs were fixed, its contribution margin would be zero and the clinic's profit would be assured regardless of the number of visits.[4] Thus, a higher fixed cost structure leads to lower risk in a capitated environment, while a higher variable cost (lower fixed cost) structure leads to lower risk in a fee-for-service environment. Of course, reduced risk also reduces the rewards that an organization can attain from utilization management.

The Importance of the Number of Members

Table 5.9 contains the pro-forma P&L statements under capitation, recast to focus on the number of members. Assuming a per member utilization of four visits per year, a 10 percent membership increase to 20,625 members increases the projected profit by about 128 percent. However, if membership declines to 17,291, the clinic just about breaks even. To verify the breakeven point, use the breakeven equation:

$$\text{Total revenues} - \text{Total variable costs} - \text{Fixed costs} = \text{Profit}$$

$$(\$400 \times \text{Members}) - (\$112.72 \times \text{Members}) - \$4,967,462 = \$0$$

$$\$287.28 \times \text{Members} = \$4,967,462$$

$$\text{Members} = 17,291.$$

Thus, breakeven analysis reaffirms that the clinic needs 17,291 members in its contract with Peachtree HMO to break even, given the assumed cost structure, which in turn assumes utilization of four visits per member and a variable cost rate of $28.18 per visit.

What happens to breakeven when utilization changes? In Table 5.9, the utilization is held constant at four visits per member per year. If utilization increases to 4.4 visits per member, the variable cost per member increases to 4.4 × $28.18

	Number of Members			TABLE 5.9
	17,291	18,750	20,625	
Total revenues ($400 × Number of members)	$6,916,400	$7,500,000	$8,250,000	
Total variable costs ($112.72 × Members)	1,949,042	2,113,500	2,324,850	
Total contribution margin	$4,967,359	$5,386,500	$5,025,150	
Fixed costs	4,967,462	4,967,462	4,967,462	
Profit (net income)	($ 104)	$ 419,038	$ 957,688	

TABLE 5.9
Atlanta Clinic:
1999 Pro-Forma
P&L Statement
(Based on 17,291,
18,750, and 20,625
members)

= $123.99. This higher variable cost rate increases total variable costs for any number of members, which pushes the breakeven point to the right:

$$\text{Total revenues} - \text{Total variable costs} - \text{Fixed costs} = \text{Profit}$$

$$(\$400 \times \text{Members}) - (\$123.99 \times \text{Members}) - \$4{,}967{,}462 = \$0$$

$$\$276.01 \times \text{Members} = \$4{,}967{,}462$$

$$\text{Members} = 17{,}997.$$

Alternatively, if the clinic's utilization falls to 3.69 visits per member, the variable cost rate falls to $3.69 \times \$28.18 = \$103.98$, resulting in a lower breakeven point of 16,781 members:

$$\text{Total revenues} - \text{Total variable costs} - \text{Fixed costs} = \text{Profit}$$

$$(\$400 \times \text{Members}) - (\$103.98 \times \text{Members}) - \$4{,}967{,}462 = \$0$$

$$\$296.02 \times \text{Members} = \$4{,}967{,}462$$

$$\text{Members} = 16{,}781.$$

To close this chapter, consider some of the important points brought out by the fee-for-service and capitation analyses. First, the financial incentives for providers under capitation are opposite of the incentives created in a fee-for-service environment. Less utilization rather than more utilization enhances profitability because under capitation each additional visit creates costs without a corresponding increase in revenues.

Second, assuming constant per member utilization, more members increases profitability because additional members create additional revenues that hopefully exceed their incremental (variable) costs. Indeed, the degree of operating leverage concept can be applied here. Consider Table 5.9 again. With base case membership of 18,750, a 10 percent increase to 20,625 members results in a (roughly) 128.5 percent increase in profit (from $419,038 to $957,688, or by $538,650). Thus, each 1 percent increase in membership increases profitability by 12.85 percent. Similarly, if membership decreases to the breakeven point of

17,291, a decrease of 7.8 percent, profitability falls by $7.8\% \times 12.85 \approx 100\%$, which leads to a profit of zero.

Many people believe capitation is going to become more widely used than it is today. If that is the case, health services managers will have to fully understand its implications for profitability and provider behavior. Without such an understanding, providers face a future that is fraught with difficulties.

Self-Test Questions

1. Under capitation, what is the difference between a CVP graph with the number of visits on the X axis and one with the number of members on the X axis?
2. What is unique about the contribution margin under capitation?
3. Why is utilization management so important in a capitated environment?

Key Concepts

Managers rely on managerial accounting information to plan and control a health services organization's operations. A critical part of managerial accounting information is the measurement of costs and the use of this information in profit analysis. The key concepts of this chapter are:

- Costs are classified along two dimensions: by their relationship to the *unit of analysis* (direct versus indirect) and by their relationship to the *amount of services provided* (fixed versus variable).
- *Direct costs* are unique to the reporting sub-unit, while *indirect costs* represent the use of shared resources not unique to the reporting sub-unit.
- *Variable costs* are those costs that are expected to increase and decrease with volume (patient days, number of visits, and so on), while *fixed costs* are the costs that are expected to remain constant regardless of volume (within some relevant range).
- The relationship between cost and activity (volume) is called *cost behavior* or *underlying cost structure.*
- *Profit analysis,* often called *cost-volume-profit (CVP) analysis,* is an analytical technique that typically is used to analyze the effects of volume changes on revenues, costs, and profit.
- A *pro-forma (P&L) profit and loss statement* is a projected income statement that uses assumed values for volume, price, and costs to forecast profit.
- *Breakeven analysis* is used to estimate the volume needed (or the value of some other variable) for the organization to break even in profitability.
- *Contribution margin* is the difference between unit price and the variable cost rate. Hence, it is the per unit dollar amount available to first cover an organization's fixed cost structure and then to contribute to profits.
- *Operating leverage* reflects the extent to which an organization's costs are fixed. It is measured by the *degree of operating leverage (DOL).* Assuming fee-for-service reimbursement, a business with a high DOL has more risk than

a business with a low DOL because DOL measures the impact of utilization changes on profits. Conversely, high-DOL businesses benefit most from increases in utilization when operating in a fee-for-service environment.

- In *marginal analysis*, the focus is on the incremental (marginal) profitability associated with increasing or decreasing volume.
- A *capitated environment* dramatically changes the situation for providers vis-à-vis a fee-for-service environment. In essence, a capitated provider takes on the insurance function, so the key to profitability is higher membership and lower per member utilization.

In chapter 6, the discussion of managerial accounting continues with a examination of cost allocation (direct versus indirect costs).

Questions

5.1 What are the two major cost classifications?

5.2 Total costs are made up of what two components?

5.3 a. What is cost-volume-profit (CVP) analysis?
   b. Why is it so useful to health services managers?

5.4 a. Define contribution margin.
   b. What is its economic meaning?

5.5 a. Write out and explain the equation for volume breakeven.
   b. What role does contribution margin play in this equation?

5.6 a. What is operating leverage?
   b. How is it measured?

5.7 What elements of CVP analysis change when a provider moves from a fee-for-service to a discounted fee-for-service environment?

5.8 What are the critical differences in CVP analysis when conducted in a capitated environment versus a fee-for-service environment?

5.9 How do provider incentives differ when it moves from a fee-for-service to a capitated environment?

Problems

5.1 Consider the CVP graphs (shown on the next page) for two providers operating in a fee-for-service environment to answer the following questions:
   a. Assuming the graphs are drawn to the same scale, which provider has the greater fixed costs? The greater variable cost rate? The greater per unit revenue?
   b. Which provider has the greater contribution margin?
   c. Which provider needs the higher volume to break even?
   d. How would the graphs above change if the providers were operating in a discounted fee-for-service environment? In a capitated environment?

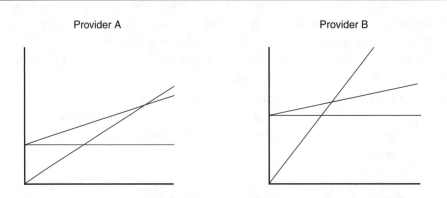

5.2 Consider the data in the table below for three independent health services organizations:

	Sales	Total Variable Costs	Fixed Costs	Total Costs	Profit
a.	$2,000	$1,400	?	$2,000	?
b.	?	1,000	?	1,600	$2,400
c.	4,000	?	$600	?	400

Fill in the missing data indicated by question marks.

5.3 Assume that a radiologist group practice has the following cost structure:

Fixed costs	$500,000
Variable cost per procedure	$25
Charge (revenue) per procedure	$100

Furthermore, assume that the group expects to perform 7,500 procedures in the coming year.

a. Construct the group's base case pro-forma profit and loss statement.

b. What is the group's contribution margin? What is its breakeven point?

c. What volume is required to provide a pre-tax profit of $100,000? A pre-tax profit of $200,000?

d. Sketch out a CVP analysis graph depicting the base case situation.

e. Now, assume that the practice contracts with one HMO, and the plan proposes a 20 percent discount from charges. Redo questions a, b, c, and d under these conditions.

5.4 General Hospital, a not-for-profit acute care facility, has the following cost structure for its inpatient services:

Fixed costs	$10,000,000
Variable cost per inpatient day	$200
Charge (revenue) per inpatient day	$1,000

The hospital expects to have a patient load of 15,000 inpatient days next year.

a. Construct the hospital's base case pro-forma P&L statement.

b. What is the hospital's breakeven point?

c. What volume is required to provide a profit of $1,000,000? A profit of $500,000?

d. Now, assume that 20 percent of the hospital's inpatients come from a managed care plan that wants a 25 percent discount from charges. Should the hospital agree to the discount proposal?

5.5 You are considering starting a walk-in clinic. Your financial projections for the first year of operations are as follows:

Revenues (10,000 visits)	$400,000
Wages and benefits	220,000
Rent	5,000
Depreciation	30,000
Utilities	2,500
Medical supplies	50,000
Administrative supplies	10,000

Assume that all costs are fixed except supply costs, which are variable. Furthermore, assume that the clinic must pay taxes at a 30 percent rate.

a. Construct the clinic's pro-forma P&L statement.

b. What number of visits is required to break even?

c. What number of visits is required to provide you with an after-tax profit of $100,000?

5.6 Review the walk-in clinic data presented in Problem 5.5.

a. Construct pro-forma profit and loss statements at volume levels of 8,000, 9,000, 10,000, 11,000, and 12,000 visits.

b. Assume that the base case forecast is 10,000 visits. What is the clinic's degree of operating leverage (DOL) at this volume level? Confirm the net incomes at the other volume levels using the DOL combined with the percent changes in volume.

c. Now, assume that the base case volume is 9,000 visits. What is the DOL at this volume?

5.7 Grandview Clinic has fixed costs of $2 million and an average variable cost rate of $15 per visit. Its sole payor, an HMO, has proposed an annual capitation payment of $150 for each of its 20,000 members. Past experience indicates the population served will average 2 visits per year.

a. Construct the base case pro-forma profit and loss statement on the contract.

b. Sketch two CVP analysis graphs for the clinic—one with number of visits on the X axis, and one with number of members on the X axis. Compare and contrast these graphs with the one in Problem 5.3.d.

c. What is the clinic's contribution margin on the contract? How does this value compare with the value in Problem 5.3.b?

d. What profit gain can be realized if the clinic can lower per member utilization to 1.8 visits?

Notes

1. The term *management accounting* is sometimes used in place of managerial accounting. Although some accountants differentiate between managerial and management accounting, the differences are small and beyond the scope of this book. Thus, for purposes here, managerial and management accounting are the same.

2. Some costs are classified as *semi-fixed*. These costs are fixed over a range of activity that is less than the relevant range of analysis. For example, a clinic may have to add an additional nurse if the number of patient visits exceeds 50 per day. If the anticipated utilization ranges from 40 to 60 visits per day, then nursing salaries and benefits would be fixed from 40 to 50 visits and then again from 51 to 60 visits. However, these costs are not fixed throughout the entire relevant range of analysis (40 to 60 visits). Because this is an introductory text, semi-fixed costs are not included in the illustrations.

3. To be technically correct, an income statement should be prepared according to the GAAP, while a profit and loss statement can be based on internal guidelines. However, both statements are intended to show an organization's profitability, so the terms will be used interchangeably for managerial accounting purposes.

4. The assumption here is that the number of visits will fall within the relevant range. That is, estimated fixed costs provide the appropriate resources needed to accommodate any number of visits within some predetermined range.

References

For a more in-depth treatment of cost measurement in healthcare organizations, see

Herkimer, A. G., Jr. 1989. *Understanding Health Care Accounting.* Rockville, MD: Aspen Publishers.

Prince, T. R. 1992. *Financial Reporting and Cost Control for Health Care Entities.* Chicago: AUPHA/Health Administration Press.

Suver, J. D., B. R. Neumann, and K. E. Boles. 1992. *Management Accounting for Health-care Organizations.* Chicago: Healthcare Financial Management Association and Pluribus Press.

For an interesting view on breakeven under capitation, see

Boles, K. E. and S. T. Fleming. 1996. "Breakeven Under Capitation." *Health Care Management Review* (Winter): 38–47.

COST ALLOCATION

Learning Objectives

After studying this chapter, readers will be able to:

- Explain why proper cost allocation is important to health services organizations.
- Define a cost driver and explain the characteristics of a good driver, as opposed to a poor one.
- Describe the three primary methods used to allocate overhead costs among revenue producing departments.
- Apply cost-allocation principles across a wide range of situations within health services organizations.

Introduction

In the introduction to profit analysis presented in Chapter 5, the concept of classifying costs according to their relationship to the unit of analysis was introduced (e.g., a department, service, or third-party payor contract). *Direct costs* are those costs that are unique and exclusive to the unit and, as such, often are relatively easy to measure. For example, the direct costs of a clinical department would include the labor costs for department personnel, the costs of equipment and supplies used by the department, and so on. In contrast, *indirect,* or *overhead, costs* are inherently difficult to measure because these costs result from the sharing of resources by two or more units. To illustrate, a clinical department shares the physical space of the entire organization, as well as infrastructure services, so the department must share in the costs of physical plant, utilities, information systems, housekeeping, maintenance, medical records, general administration, and so on.

A critical part of the cost-measurement process is the assignment or allocation of indirect costs, which is the topic of this chapter. *Cost allocation* is essentially a pricing process within the organization whereby managers allocate the costs of one department to other departments. Because this pricing process does not occur in a market setting, no objective supply-and-demand process exists that establishes the price for the transferred services. Thus, the cost-allocation process must, to the extent possible, establish prices that proxy those that would be set under market conditions.

What costs within a health services organization must be allocated? In general, the costs of support functions, such as those provided by administrators, facilities management personnel, financial staffs, and housekeeping and maintenance personnel, must be allocated to those departments that generate revenues for the organization (generally patient services departments). The allocation of support costs to patient services departments is necessary because there would be no need for support costs if there were no patient services departments. Thus, decisions regarding pricing and service offerings by the patient services departments must be based on the full costs associated with each service, including both direct and overhead (indirect) costs. Clearly, the proper allocation of overhead costs is essential to good decision making within health services organizations.

In general, the goal of cost allocation is to assign as many costs of the organization as possible directly to the activities that cause them to be incurred. Ideally, managers of healthcare providers would like to track and assign costs by individual patient, physician, diagnosis, reimbursement contract, and so on. With complete cost data at hand in the organization's managerial accounting system, managers can make better decisions regarding cost control, what services should be offered, and how these services should be priced. Of course, the more complex the managerial accounting system, the higher the costs of developing, implementing, and operating the system. As in all situations, the benefits associated with more accurate cost data must be weighed against the costs required to develop the data.

Interestingly, much of the motivation for more accurate cost-allocation systems comes from the "customer" or recipient of overhead services. Managers at all levels within health services organizations are coming under increased pressure to optimize economic performance, which translates into reducing costs. Indeed, many department heads are being evaluated, and hence compensated and promoted, primarily on the basis of economic results—assuming that performance along other dimensions is satisfactory. For such a performance-evaluation system to work, all parties must perceive the cost-allocation process to be accurate and fair because managers are being held accountable for both direct and indirect costs.

Self-Test Questions

1. What is meant by the term *cost allocation*?
2. What is the goal of cost allocation?
3. Why is cost allocation important to health services managers?

A Historical Perspective on Cost Allocation

Before the inception of Medicare and Medicaid programs, accurate information regarding the full (direct plus indirect) cost of providing services was not the predominant basis for pricing decisions, and therefore not important. Prices for healthcare services were based mostly on informal factors including historical precedent, and *cross subsidization* (*price shifting*) was common. (Under cross subsidization, profit shortages on some services are covered by setting inflated prices on other services.) Furthermore, contributions and government grants often covered shortfalls that resulted from improper pricing, so a close link between the cost of providing services and the prices set on those services was not necessary.

With the introduction of Medicare in the mid-1960s, healthcare providers' costing practices began to revolve around the Medicare cost report. To some extent, the arrival of Medicare and Medicaid on the scene contributed to even less concern by health services managers over the true cost of providing services. In essence, reimbursement systems were designed to ensure that the government paid for all costs of providing healthcare services to Medicare patients. As a result, providers developed managerial accounting systems that focused on maximizing Medicare reimbursement. This meant that cost-allocation systems were purposely distorted to allocate the highest amount of costs possible to government-sponsored patients, regardless of the true source of the costs. In short, managerial accounting systems and their underlying cost-allocation systems were designed to maximize revenues rather than to properly identify and allocate costs.

Unfortunately, during the early years of Medicare and Medicaid, healthcare providers lost ground in the quest for good cost-accounting systems, moving from systems that had at least some ability to identify true costs to systems that stressed revenue maximization. However, this movement away from legitimate cost-accounting efforts was stopped when Medicare introduced fixed-rate payments in 1983. Under Medicare's new diagnosis related group (DRG) system, healthcare providers, particularly hospitals, received a rude awakening. Providers now received fixed amounts to treat patients having a single diagnosis, yet most providers had no idea how much it actually cost to treat different diagnoses. As time passed, more third-party payors changed to fixed-payment reimbursement systems such as DRG, per diem, or capitation; therefore, providers were forced to ensure that total costs did not exceed fixed payment amounts. What is somewhat paradoxical is that the movement to various forms of fixed-payment reimbursement, with no explicit relationship to costs, has made cost measurement more important for providers than ever before.

1. Briefly trace the evolution of cost-accounting systems among healthcare providers.
2. Are good cost-accounting systems more or less important to healthcare providers today than they were in the past?

Self-Test Questions

Cost Allocation Basics

To assign costs from one area to another, two important elements of cost accounting must be identified: a cost pool and a cost driver. A *cost pool* is any grouping of costs that must be allocated, while a *cost driver* is the criterion upon which the allocation is made. To illustrate, a hospital may allocate housekeeping costs to its other departments on the basis of the size of each department's physical space. In this situation, total housekeeping costs would be the cost pool and the number of square feet of occupied space would be the cost driver.

When the cost pool is divided by the cost driver, the result is the overhead *allocation rate*. Thus, in the housekeeping illustration, the allocation rate is total housekeeping costs divided by the total space (square footage) occupied by the departments receiving the allocation. This procedure results in an allocation rate measured in dollar cost per square foot of space utilized. In the patient services departments, total costs would include not only the direct costs of each department, but also an allocation for the cost of providing housekeeping services made on the basis of the amount of occupied space. Clearly, the development of meaningful allocation rates enhances the ability of managers to make judgments concerning price negotiations, service profitability, and cost reduction.

Cost Drivers

Perhaps the most important step in the cost-allocation process is the identification of proper cost drivers. Traditionally, overhead costs (e.g., for a hospital) were accumulated and then divided by a rough measure of output (e.g., patient days), which resulted in a cost driver of a dollar amount per patient day (called the *per diem overhead rate*). For example, if a hospital had 72,000 patient days in 1998 and total overhead costs for the hospital were $36 million, the overhead allocation rate would be $36,000,000 / 72,000 = $500 per patient day (per diem). Regardless of the type of patients treated within a department (adult versus child, trauma versus illness, acute versus critical care, and so on), the $500 per diem allocation rate would be applied to determine indirect costs for that department.

However, not all overhead costs are tied to the number of patient days. For example, overhead costs associated with admission, discharge, and billing are typically not related to the number of patient days, but to the number of admissions. Tying all overhead costs to a single cost driver improperly allocates such costs, which distorts reported costs for patient services, and hence raises concerns about the effectiveness of decisions based on such costs.

In most organizations, different types of overhead costs respond to widely different cost drivers. As illustrated previously, it is inappropriate to lump all clinical overhead costs together and conclude that they are driven by the number of patient days, the number of patient visits, or the amount of revenue dollars generated. In state-of-the-art cost-management systems, the various types of overhead costs are separated into different cost pools and the most appropriate cost driver for each pool is identified.

The key to identifying effective cost drivers is the extent to which costs from a pool actually vary as the value of the driver changes. The better the relationship (correlation) between actual costs and the cost driver, the better the cost driver, and hence the better the resulting cost allocations. The remainder of this chapter emphasizes the importance of good cost drivers, including several illustrations that distinguish good drivers from poor ones.

The Allocation Process

The steps involved in allocating overhead costs are summarized in Table 6.1, which illustrates how Prairie View Clinic allocated its housekeeping costs for 1999.[1] First, the cost pool must be established. In this case, the clinic is allocating housekeeping costs, so the cost pool is the projected total costs of the Housekeeping Department, $100,000.

Next, a meaningful cost driver must be identified. After considerable investigation, Prairie View's managers concluded that the best cost driver for housekeeping costs is labor hours. That is, the number of hours of housekeeping services required by the clinic is the variable most closely related to total housekeeping costs. The intent here, of course, is to pick the cost driver that provides the most accurate cause-and-effect relationship between the use of housekeeping services and the costs of the Housekeeping Department. For 1999, Prairie View's managers estimate that the Housekeeping Department will provide 10,000 hours of service to the departments that will receive the allocation.

Now that the cost pool and cost driver have been defined and measured, the allocation rate is established by dividing the expected total overhead cost (the cost pool) by the expected total volume of the cost driver: $100,000 / 10,000 hours = $10 per hour of services provided. The final step in the process is to make the allocation to the clinical departments.

To illustrate the allocation, consider Physical Therapy (PT), one of Prairie View's patient services departments. For 1999, PT is expected to utilize 3,000 hours of housekeeping services, so the dollar amount of housekeeping overhead allocated to PT is $10 × 3,000 = $30,000. Other departments within the clinic will also utilize housekeeping services, and their allocations would be made in a similar manner. To obtain the dollar allocation, the $10 allocation rate per hour of services utilized is multiplied by the amount of each department's utilization of housekeeping services. When all departments are considered, the entire clinic is projected to use 10,000 hours of housekeeping services, so the total amount allocated across the entire clinic must be $10 × 10,000 = $100,000. For any department, the amount allocated depends on both the allocation rate and the amount of the cost driver utilized.

TABLE 6.1

Prairie View Clinic: Allocation of Housekeeping Overhead to the Physical Therapy Department

Step One: Determine the Cost Pool
  The departmental costs to be allocated are for the Housekeeping Department, which has total budgeted costs for 1999 of $100,000.

Step Two: Determine the Cost Driver
  The best cost driver was judged to be the number of hours of housekeeping services provided. An expected total of 10,000 hours of such services will be provided in 1999 to those departments that will receive the allocation.

Step Three: Calculate the Allocation Rate
  $100,000 / 10,000 hours = $10 per hour of housekeeping services provided.

Step Four: Determine the Allocation Amount
  Physical Therapy utilizes 3,000 hours of housekeeping services, so its allocation of Housekeeping Department overhead is $10 × 3,000 = $30,000.

Allocation Methods

Cost allocation can be accomplished a variety of ways, and the method to use is somewhat discretionary. No matter what method is chosen, all support department costs eventually must be allocated to the departments that create the need for overhead costs, primarily patient services departments.

The key differences among the methods are how support services provided by one department are allocated to other support departments. The direct method totally ignores services provided by one support department to another; the reciprocal method recognizes all of the intrasupport department services; and the step-down method represents a compromise that recognizes some, but not all, of the intrasupport department services. Regardless of the method, all of the support costs within an organization ultimately are allocated from support departments to the departments that generate revenues for the organization, and hence creates the need for the support services.

Figure 6.1 summarizes the three allocation methods. Prairie View Clinic, which is used in the illustration, has three support departments (Human Resources, Housekeeping, and Administration) and two patient services departments (Physical Therapy and Internal Medicine). The direct method shown in the top section of Figure 6.1 is simple and straightforward. In this method, costs are allocated directly from each support department to the patient services departments and no allocation is made to other support services departments. Unfortunately, in creating a method that is easy to use, the direct method fails to capture the fact that support departments provide services to other support departments in addition to those provided to patient services departments.

Under the *direct method*, each support department's costs are allocated directly to the patient services departments that utilize the services. In the illustration, both Physical Therapy and Internal Medicine use the services of all three support departments, so the costs of each support department are allocated to both patient services departments. The key feature of the direct method, and the feature that makes it relatively simple to apply, is that none of the costs of providing support services is allocated to other support departments. In effect, under the direct method, only the direct costs of the support departments are allocated to the patient services departments because no indirect costs have been created by intrasupport department allocations.

The *reciprocal method* generally is considered to be more accurate and objective than the direct method because it recognizes support department interdependencies. The reciprocal method derives its name from the fact that it recognizes all services that departments provide to and receive from other departments. The good news is that this method captures all of the intrasupport department relationships, so no information is ignored and no biases are introduced into the cost-allocation process. As shown in the center section of Figure 6.1, the support department interdependencies between Human Resources, Housekeeping, and Administration are recognized through cost allocation. This

FIGURE 6.1
Prairie View Clinic:
Alternative Cost
Allocation Methods

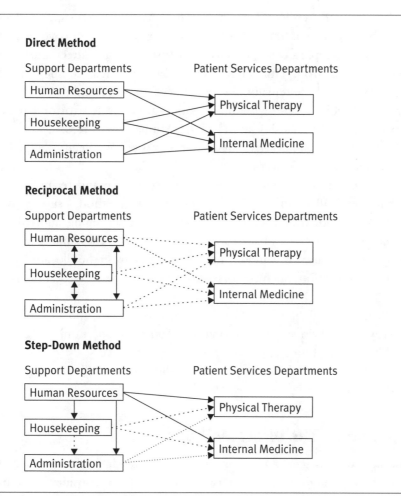

intrasupport department allocation is made prior to any allocation to the patient services departments. After the intrasupport department allocation is completed, the total costs (both direct and indirect) of these departments are allocated to Physical Therapy and Internal Medicine. Unfortunately, the reciprocal method relies on the simultaneous solution of a series of equations that represent the utilization of intrasupport department services, and hence this method is complex and difficult to implement in practice.

The *step-down method* represents a compromise between the simplicity of the direct method and the complexity of the reciprocal method. The step-down method recognizes some of the intrasupport department effects that the direct method ignores, but it does **not** recognize the full range of interdependencies. Therefore, the step-down method does not require the complexity of mathematics needed for the reciprocal method. The step-down method derives its name from the sequential, stair-step pattern of the allocation process. The lower section in Figure 6.1 illustrates the step-down method. The allocation takes place in a specific sequence. First, all the direct costs of Human Resources are allocated to both the patient services departments and the other two support departments. Human Resources is then *closed out* because all its costs have been allocated. Next, Housekeeping costs, which now consist of both direct and indirect costs (the allocation from Human Resources), are allocated to the patient services departments and the remaining support department, Administration. Finally, the direct and indirect costs of Administration are allocated to the patient services departments. The final allocation includes Human Resources, Housekeeping, and Administration costs because these support costs have been "stepped down" to the Administration Department.

The critical difference between the step-down and reciprocal methods is that after each allocation is made in the step-down method, a support department is removed from the process. Even though Housekeeping and Administration provide support services back to Human Resources, these indirect costs are not recognized because Human Resources is removed from the allocation process after the initial allocation. Such costs are recognized in the reciprocal method.

Self-Test Questions

1. What are the definitions of a cost pool, a cost driver, and an allocation rate?
2. Why are cost drivers so important to good cost allocation?
3. What are the four steps in the cost-allocation process?
4. Briefly, what are the three primary methods of cost allocation and their key differences?

Cost Allocation Illustration I: The Direct Method

The best way to gain a more in-depth understanding of cost allocation basics is to work through allocation illustrations. To begin, consider Table 6.2, which contains revenue and cost data for Kensington Hospital. The hospital has three revenue producing patient services departments or *revenue centers*: Routine Care, Laboratory, and Radiology. Hospital costs are broken into those attributable to the revenue centers (direct costs) and those attributable to the support departments (overhead costs). Of course, the overhead costs are direct costs to the support departments, but when allocated, become indirect costs to the revenue centers (patient services departments).

The data show that the revenues for each of the patient services departments are much greater than their direct costs. Furthermore, Kensington's projected total revenues of $27,000,000 exceed the hospital's projected total costs of $25,450,000. However, the aggregate cost amounts provide no information to Kensington's managers concerning the profitability of each revenue center (i.e., each patient services department). To determine profitability by revenue center, the full costs of providing patient services, including both direct and indirect costs, must be measured. Only then will the hospital's managers develop rational pricing and cost-control strategies for each patient services department.

As previously discussed, there are two primary issues in cost allocation: choosing the cost driver and the method of allocation. This illustration sticks to

TABLE 6.2
Kensington
Hospital:
1999 Revenue and
Cost Projections

Projected Revenues by Patient Services Department:	
Routine Care	$16,000,000
Laboratory	5,000,000
Radiology	6,000,000
Total revenues	$27,000,000
Projected Costs for All Departments:	
Patient Services Departments (Direct Costs):	
Routine Care	$ 5,500,000
Laboratory	3,300,000
Radiology	2,800,000
Total costs	$ 11,600,000
Support Services Departments (Overhead Costs):	
Food Services	$ 1,500,000
Facilities	3,800,000
Housekeeping	1,600,000
Administration	4,400,000
Personnel	2,550,000
Total costs	$13,850,000
Total costs of both patient and support services	$25,450,000
Projected profit	$ 1,550,000

the basics, so the assumption is that Kensington Hospital uses the direct method of cost allocation. The step-down method is discussed in a later illustration.

The cost pools (total costs) for the support services departments are given in the lower section of Table 6.2. Food Services costs are $1,500,000; Facilities costs equal $3,800,000; Housekeeping costs are $1,600,000; Administration costs total $4,400,000; and Personnel costs equal $2,550,000. Thus, total overhead costs equal $13,850,000. The allocation process must allocate these costs to the hospital's three patient services departments.

The next and most important step in the process is to identity the best cost drivers for each category of overhead costs. Table 6.3 provides a summary of the support departments and their assigned cost drivers. Unfortunately, the selection of cost drivers is not an easy process and, to a large extent, the usefulness of the entire cost allocation process depends on choosing the most appropriate drivers. As discussed later in this chapter, Kensington's selection of cost drivers, like most real-world situations, has its problems.

The cost driver for Financial Services is patient services revenue. Financial Services provides a full range of financial support to the hospital. The bulk of its efforts are devoted to patient accounts, but it is also involved in financial and managerial accounting, report preparation, and a host of other financial tasks.

TABLE 6.3
Kensington
Hospital: Assigned
Cost Drivers

Support Services Department	Cost Driver
Financial Services	Patient services revenue
Facilities	Space utilization (square footage)
Housekeeping	Labor hours
Administration	Salary dollars
Personnel	Salary dollars

Tying the allocation of this support department to the amount of patient services revenues assumes a strong positive relationship between the amount of financial services provided to each patient services department and revenues generated by that department. Clearly, patient services revenue is a relatively rough cost driver, and hence the resulting cost allocation has limited economic meaning. The next illustration includes a discussion of the benefits gained by moving from a rough cost driver to a more precise one.

The amount of space utilized (square footage) is the basis for allocating the costs of Facilities. This cost driver is often used by health services organizations to allocate facilities services. The logic applied here is that the patient services departments with the most space require the most facilities support. Of course, this assumption does not always hold. For example, in any year, Facilities may be required to support a special, large project for one of the patient services departments that results in costs that far exceed that department's proportional space utilization. Nevertheless, over the long run at Kensington Hospital, the relative costs of facilities utilization by the patient services departments track closely with the space occupied by those departments.

Two of the support departments, Administration and Personnel, also use a fairly rough cost driver instead of a more precise one: salary dollars. For example, if Radiology has payroll costs that are five times larger than those of Laboratory, Radiology will be charged (allocated) five times as much of the costs incurred by Administration and Personnel. This cost driver is often used, but in reality, it is not very precise or meaningful. Thus, the allocated costs do not truly represent the relative amounts of utilization of these overhead services.

Housekeeping has pushed the selection of a cost driver further than the other support departments in terms of choosing a meaningful cost driver, namely, the number of labor hours of housekeeping services consumed. In many organizations, housekeeping costs are allocated on the basis of square footage, which uses the logic that the spatial size of a department accurately reflects housekeeping efforts, and hence costs. This assumption may or may not be valid, however. In effect, large-space departments may be subsidizing small-space departments such as emergency services where space may be limited, but the intensity of work requires a significant amount of housekeeping services. To account for such situations at Kensington Hospital, Housekeeping is using a more meaningful cost driver—one that is more closely aligned with the actual relative costs of providing services to the patient services departments.

Note three important points about the cost driver selected for Housekeeping. First, the motivation to use labor hours instead of square footage as the cost driver probably came from one of the patient services departments rather than from Housekeeping. More often than not, it is the recipients of the allocation (i.e., the department heads of the patient services departments) who feel that a particular cost driver is unfair, and who demand the development of more meaningful cost drivers.

Second, similar to most situations, the development and use of a more meaningful cost driver is a cost-benefit issue. Housekeeping must now devote resources to track where their workers spend their time, an effort that would not be required if the cost driver were square footage. The benefit is that the resource expenditure required to monitor housekeeping hours results in a more meaningful cost driver, which makes it easier for Kensington's senior managers to hold department heads responsible for both direct and indirect costs. Now, if the head of Radiology does not like the amount of housekeeping costs that are being charged to the department, he or she can do something about it: use less housekeeping services. Under a less meaningful cost driver such as square footage, patient services department heads can do little if they do not like the Housekeeping allocation. In most cases, reduction of square footage is not very practical. With labor hours consumed as the cost driver, however, the cost control solution is to reduce the amount of housekeeping services utilized, which is a response that—if it can be accomplished—has positive implications both for the allocated costs and for the cost structure of the organization.

This discussion leads to an important point about cost drivers. Often, cost driver selection is not so much a fairness issue regarding the relative allocation of overhead costs to departments, but rather an organizational cost-control issue. By moving from a less meaningful cost driver, such as space utilization, to a more meaningful one, such as housekeeping hours, Kensington's senior management can now legitimately hold patient services department heads accountable for the indirect costs allocated to their departments. This accountability, in turn, creates an incentive for these department heads to reduce overhead costs. With a good cost driver in place, department heads will not treat housekeeping services as if it is a free resource and will examine ways to reduce usage.

If all patient services department heads are made to think this way by having the right incentive system in place, ultimately, the hospital will discover it is as efficient as possible in utilizing housekeeping services. In the long run or even mid-range, the direct costs of the Housekeeping Department, currently $1,600,000, will fall as these services are more efficiently utilized. In reality, the secondary benefit of moving from a rough cost driver, such as square footage, to a more precise cost driver, such as labor hours, is a more equitable allocation. The primary benefit is that a more meaningful cost driver creates an incentive to use less of a support service, which ultimately leads to lower overall costs for the organization.

Table 6.4 contains the initial data necessary for Kensington's managers to allocate overhead costs to the revenue producing (patient services) departments. The first column of Table 6.4 lists the patient services departments. The amounts of the chosen cost drivers consumed by each patient services department are listed after that. These amounts include: patient services revenue used for allocating Financial Services costs; square footage used for Facilities allocations; housekeeping labor hours used for Housekeeping allocations; and departmental salary dollars used both for Administration and Personnel allocations.

If Kensington were using the step-down or reciprocal allocation methods, the information shown in Table 6.4 would have included the support departments because it would be needed for intrasupport department allocations. By using the direct method, the hospital ignores the realities of intrasupport department utilization, so the totals indicated at the bottom of each column reflect only the utilization of the patient services departments, which are allocated all of the support costs.

Table 6.5 combines the cost pools (total costs) of each support department with the total cost-driver utilization of the patient services departments to derive the allocation rates. For example, the direct costs of Financial Services are $1,500,000. These direct costs will be allocated as indirect costs to the patient services departments that have a total of $27,000,000 in patient services revenues. The allocation rate for Financial Services, therefore, is $1,500,000 / $27,000,000 = $0.05556 per dollar of patient services revenue.

As previously mentioned, the allocation of indirect costs can be viewed as an internal pricing mechanism. Thus, the revenue producing department heads can look at Table 6.5 and see the rate that they are being charged for support services. The patient services departments are being charged:

- $0.05556 for each dollar of patient services revenue generated for Financial Services support;
- $12.64 per square foot of space utilized for Facilities support;
- $17.58 per labor hour consumed for Housekeeping support;

TABLE 6.4
Kensington Hospital: Patient Services Departmental Summary Data

Department	Patient Services Revenues	Square Feet	Housekeeping Labor Hours	Salary Dollars
Routine Care	$16,000,000	199,800	76,000	$ 5,709,000
Laboratory	5,000,000	39,600	6,000	2,035,000
Radiology	6,000,000	61,200	9,000	2,439,000
Total	$27,000,000	300,600	91,000	$10,183,000

- $0.432 per salary dollar paid to department employees for Administrative overhead; and
- $0.250 per salary dollar for Personnel support.

If Radiology pays a technician $10.00 an hour in direct labor costs for each hour the technician works, the department will also be charged $0.432 \times $10.00 = $4.32 for Administrative overhead and $0.250 \times $10.00 = $2.50 for Personnel overhead, plus additional allocations for Financial Services, Facilities, and House-keeping support.

Having two support services, in this case Administration and Personnel, that utilize the same cost driver, salary dollars, is not unusual. The allocation rate is different for the two support departments because they have different cost pools (total costs).

The final step in the allocation process is to determine the actual dollar allocation to each of the patient services departments, which is shown in Table 6.6. The support departments are listed in the first column along with the applicable allocation rate, while the patient services departments are listed across the top. To illustrate the calculations, consider Routine Care. It produces $16,000,000 in patient services revenue and the overhead allocation rate for Financial Services is $0.05556 per dollar of patient services revenue, so the allocation for such support is 0.05556 \times $16,000,000 = $888,960. Routine Care has 199,800 square feet of space; with a Facilities rate of $12.64 per square foot, its allocation for Facilities support is $12.64 \times 199,800 = $2,525,472.

The allocations to Routine Care for Housekeeping, Administration, and Personnel services support shown in Table 6.6 were calculated similarly. The end result is that $8,644,050 out of a total of $13,850,000 of the indirect (overhead) costs of Kensington Hospital are allocated to Routine Care. Routine Care also has direct costs of $5,500,000, so the total costs of the department, including both direct and indirect, are $8,644,050 + $5,500,000 = $14,144,050. The cost allocations and total cost calculations for Laboratory and Radiology shown in Table 6.6 were done in a similar manner.

For general management, as opposed to accounting purposes, understanding the mechanics of the allocation is less important than recognizing the value of

Department	Cost Pool (Total Costs)	Cost Driver	Total Utilization	Allocation Rate	
Financial Services	$1,500,000	Patient revenue	$27,000,000	$0.05556	**TABLE 6.5** Kensington Hospital: Overhead Allocation Rates
Facilities	3,800,000	Square feet	300,600	12.64	
Housekeeping	1,600,000	Labor hours	91,000	17.58	
Administration	4,400,000	Salary dollars	$10,183,000	0.432	
Personnel	2,550,000	Salary dollars	$10,183,000	0.250	

TABLE 6.6
Kensington Hospital: Final Allocations

		Patient Services Department	
Support Department	Routine Care	Laboratory	Radiology
Financial Services ($0.05556)	× $16,000,000 = $ 888,960	× $5,000,000 = $ 277,800	× $6,000,000 = $ 333,360
Facilities ($12.64)	× 199,800 = 2,525,472	× 39,600 = 500,544	× 61,200 = 773,568
Housekeeping ($17.58)	× 76,000 = 1,336,080	× 6,000 = 105,480	× 9,000 = 158,220
Administration ($0.432)	× 5,709,000 = 2,466,288	× 2,035,000 = 879,120	× 1,439,000 = 1,053,648
Personnel ($0.250)	× 5,709,000 = 1,427,250	× 2,035,000 = 508,750	× 1,439,000 = 609,750
Total indirect costs	$ 8,644,050	$ 2,271,694	$ 2,928,546
Direct cost	$ 5,500,000	$ 3,300,000	$ 2,800,000
Total costs	$ 14,144,050	$ 5,571,694	$ 5,728,546

Total indirect costs = $8,644,050 + $2,271,694 + $2,928,546 = $13,844,290

Total costs = $14,144,050 + $5,571,694 + $5,728,546 = $25,444,290

Note: Because of rounding in the allocation process, the totals here are slightly different from the values contained in Table 6.2.

choosing good cost drivers. The cost driver for Housekeeping (i.e., the number of service hours provided) is good in the sense that it reflects the true level of effort expended by this department in support of the patient services departments. The patient services department heads are being charged fairly for Housekeeping services and, more importantly, patient services managers can take actions to lower the allocated amounts by reducing the amount of these services utilized.

The costs of the other four support departments (Financial Services, Facilities, Administration, and Personnel) are allocated on a basis that depends more on assumed correlations than on actual economic linkages. For example, the head of Routine Care has little control over the $2,525,472 of Facilities costs allocated to the department because the allocation basis is space utilization. In reality, the amount of resources that Facilities expends in supporting Routine Care is not truly captured by the cost driver assigned, as was the case with Housekeeping. Because Routine Care has approximately 66 percent of the total square footage of the patient services departments (i.e., 199,800 out of a total of 300,600 square feet), this same proportion of Facilities costs are allocated to the department.

As discussed previously, but worth another mention, Kensington's managers face two important issues in choosing cost drivers. First, and perhaps the less important of the two, is the issue of fairness. That is, do the cost driver's chosen result in an allocation fair to the patient services departments? Routine Services may occupy a significant portion of the space utilized by Kensington's patient services departments, but it may not require a significant amount of Facilities support. Perhaps another department with less square footage utilizes more technology, has special needs, and requires a great deal of Facilities support. In this situation, the allocation of Facilities overhead would not be perceived as being fair, especially by the head of any department that has an allocation that is too high compared to true costs.

The second, and perhaps more important, issue is cost control. The patient services department managers can do little to lower their Facilities cost allocations. This inability to lower allocated costs occurs because the allocation basis is based on an assumed correlation, as opposed to a meaningful cost driver. Unlike Housekeeping, in which the allocation provides an incentive for patient services managers to use the support services more efficiently (which ultimately can lower Housekeeping costs), no such direct linkage exists with Facilities. The same logic applies to the allocation of Administration and Personnel costs. Basing allocations on assumed correlations does have the advantage of simplicity, but simplicity brings fairness and cost-control limitations.

In closing this illustration, note how Table 6.6, after the allocation process, reconciles with Table 6.2, before the allocation process. First, as shown in Table 6.2, total support services (overhead) costs are $13,850,000. This is the same amount shown in Table 6.6, except for a rounding difference, as the total overhead allocated to the patient services departments: $8,644,050 (to Routine Care) + $2,271,694 (to Laboratory) + $2,928,546 (to Radiology) = $13,844,290. The total after-allocation costs of $25,444,290 shown in Table 6.6 also equal the original forecast for total costs in Table 6.2 of $25,450,00, except for a rounding difference.

Finally, the patient services department revenues shown in Table 6.2 appear to be more reasonably related to costs after the allocation of overhead costs. For example, the $16,000,000 revenue generated by Routine Care, which seemed unreasonably high relative to the department's direct costs of $5,500,000, now makes more sense when viewed relative to the department's full costs (direct plus indirect) of $14,144,050.

Self-Test Questions
1. Briefly outline the allocation procedures used by Kensington Hospital.
2. What underlying characteristic makes a good cost driver?
3. What are the two primary issues that must be considered when choosing a cost driver?

Cost Allocation Illustration II: Direct Method with Changing Cost Drivers

The Kensington Hospital illustration presents the big picture—the overall application of the direct method of cost allocation. The second cost-allocation illustration provides closer details of the benefits of moving from a cost driver based on an assumed correlation to one that better measures true cost relationships.

The illustration examines one part of the overhead allocation process at Fargo Medical Center, a multi-specialty outpatient services facility. As shown in Table 6.7, the issue at hand is the choice of a cost driver for the Financial Services Department, which has total costs of $665,031. Of course, these support costs must be allocated on some basis to the center's various revenue producing patient services departments including Home Care, Learning and Behavior (L and B), Developmental Medicine (DM), Family Intervention (FI), Children's Clinic, and Diagnostic Services. Additionally, the center has four other patient services departments that, for purposes of this illustration, have been lumped into a single category called Other.

Like Kensington Hospital, Fargo Medical Center historically has allocated the $665,031 in Financial Services costs to the patient services departments on the basis of an assumed correlation between the volume of patient services provided and the utilization of Financial Services resources. Specifically, the revenue producing departments were allocated Financial Services costs on the basis of the amount of patient services revenues generated. As shown in Table 6.7, the amount to be allocated, $665,031, was spread across total patient services revenues of $28,150,418, which results in an allocation rate of $665,031 / $28,150,418 = $0.023624 per dollar of revenue.

Home Care generates $4,112,776 of patient services revenue, so application of the allocation rate produces an allocation of 0.023624 × $4,112,776 = $97,160. L and B generates much less revenue than Home Care—$647,705 versus $4,112,776—so its allocation of Financial Services costs is only 0.023624 × $647,705 = $15,301. In other words, Home Care generates 14.6 percent

TABLE 6.7
Fargo Medical Center: Direct Allocation of Financial Services Costs Under Different Costs Drivers

Allocation on the Basis of Patient Services Revenues:
Financial Services Department costs = $665,031
Allocation rate = $665,031/$28,150,418 = $0.023624 per dollar of revenue

	Home Care	L and B	DM	FI	Children's Clinic	Diagnostic Services	Other	Total
Patient revenue	$ 4,112,776	$ 647,705	$ 630,294	$2,971,533	$1,626,441	$ 1,339,716	$ 16,821,953	$ 28,150,418
Percent of total	14.6%	2.3%	2.2%	10.6%	5.8%	4.8%	59.8%	100.0%
Allocation	$ 97,160	$ 15,301	$ 14,890	$ 70,200	$ 38,423	$ 31,650	$ 397,405	$ 665,031

Allocation on the Basis of Number of Bills Generated:
Allocation rate = $665,031/100,915 = $6.59 per bill

	Home Care	L and B	DM	FI	Children's Clinic	Diagnostic Services	Other	Total
Number of bills	2,508	1,948	3,379	12,660	7,048	1,620	71,752	100,915
Percent of total	2.5%	1.9%	3.3%	12.5%	7.0%	1.6%	71.1%	100.0%
Allocation	$ 16,528	$ 12,837	$ 22,268	$ 83,429	$ 46,446	$ 10,676	$ 472,832	$ 665,031

Allocation Difference Between Cost Drivers:

	Home Care	L and B	DM	FI	Children's Clinic	Diagnostic Services	Other	Total
In dollars	($ 80,632)	($ 2,464)	$ 7,378	$ 13,229	$ 8,023	($ 20,974)	$ 75,427	$ 0
In percent	−83.0%	−16.1%	+49.6%	+18.8%	+20.9%	−66.3%	+19.0%	0%

of Fargo's total patient services revenue, so it is allocated 14.6 percent of Financial Services costs, while L and B's allocation is only 2.3 percent.

The major advantage of basing the allocation of Financial Services costs on patient services revenues is the ease of calculation. All the information required for the allocation process is readily available in Fargo's managerial accounting system, so the allocation is a simple matter. The key variable used in the allocation, patient services revenue, is already in the center's database, along with other relevant statistics such as number of visits, number of full-time equivalents (FTEs), payroll dollars, square footage, and so on.

To take advantage of the data availability, Fargo's managers had to assume that the utilization of Financial Services by the patient services departments is highly correlated with patient services revenue. That is, if one department generates twice as much patient services revenue as another, it will, by assumption, use twice as much Financial Services support. While the strength of such a traditional volume-based approach is ease of calculation, the weaknesses, discussed in the previous illustration, are fairness inequities and the lack of incentive for patient services departments to control Financial Services costs.

A shift to a cost driver that better reflects the actual work done by Financial Services requires that Fargo's managers develop at least a rough definition and measurement of the output of this department. The critical issue is what factor drives the costs of the department, which depends on the primary work output of the department. Such information may be answered through time/motion studies or by interviewing department personnel. In Fargo's case, an analysis revealed that the primary work done in Financial Services was sending bills to third-party payors. Thus, this action was chosen as the new cost driver. Given that the generation of bills best reflects the output of the department, Fargo's managers must estimate the expected output (number of bills) for Financial Services for the coming year. After analyzing historical data, an estimate of 100,915 bills was made.

With number of bills as the cost driver, the allocation rate is \$665,031 / 100,915 = \$6.59 per bill, compared to the previous rate of \$0.023624 per revenue dollar. The move to a different cost driver represents more than just change for the sake of change. It represents an attempt by Fargo's managers to base the allocation on the actual work performed by Financial Services, and thus to create an allocation that has economic meaning that is perceived to be fair and that will encourage department heads to reduce their utilization of Financial Services.

In spite of the improvement that results from the change, the new cost driver is not perfect. Other changes could be made to improve the allocation even more. For example, the Financial Services department performs tasks other than billing such as generating numerous reports for the organization, including both financial statements and managerial accounting reports. Indeed, the department has one analyst whose full-time job is creating and helping to interpret managerial accounting reports. (Managerial accounting reports are discussed in Chapter 8.) A better allocation of Financial Services costs, therefore, may be based on multiple cost drivers. If this were done, some proportion of the department's total costs of $665,031 would be assigned to report preparation, and a separate cost driver would be identified to allocate these costs to the other departments.

Even though a better cost driver may be developed, the change that has taken place is still meaningful. Cost accounting studies have discovered that a presumed strong correlation between overhead cost usage and volume, as measured by revenues or units produced, is incorrect and results in systematic, as opposed to random, errors. Volume-based allocation schemes create a bias against larger revenue producing departments or product lines by over-allocating costs, and in favor of smaller revenue producing departments or product lines by under-allocating costs. This bias occurs largely because a volume-based allocation rate fails to recognize the economies of scale inherent with larger departments in the utilization of overhead services. For example, it probably costs no more to bill a third-party payor for $5,000 than it does to bill for $500, in terms of the resources required to produce and transmit the bill and to monitor payment. Yet, a volume-based allocation scheme would tend to allocate more financial services costs to a patient services department with relatively high charges than to a department with relatively low charges that had exactly the same patient load, and hence the same number of bills.

As shown in Table 6.7, now that Fargo has established an allocation rate of $6.59 per bill, the Financial Services Department must track the number of bills produced for each revenue producing department. This is the downside of the change in cost drivers. However, computerized management information systems are making the development of such data relatively easy. For example, Home Care is expected to generate 2,508 bills for the year, and hence is allocated $16,528 in Financial Services costs.

The new amount allocated to Home Care is $80,632 less than the amount allocated under the old volume-based system, which represents an 83 percent decrease in allocated costs. This large change in allocation makes a very strong statement about the inadequacies of volume-based allocation based on patient services revenue. In effect, the assumed correlation between Financial Services costs and patient services revenue was incorrect—the correlation was not very strong at all. Likewise, Developmental Medicine (DM) is expected to generate 3,379 bills, and hence is allocated $22,268 of Financial Services costs, which is an increase of almost 50 percent over the volume-based system. The large percentage changes listed across the bottom of Table 6.7 are strong evidence that the old allocation system was not doing a good job.

What is the final result of Fargo's transition to a better cost driver? Again, think in terms of the two primary allocation issues: equity and cost control. Regarding equity, the critical point in this illustration is that the total costs of Financial Services support ($665,031) are now more fairly assigned to the departments that utilize those services. There is no question that the more equitable distribution was good news to the department head of Home Care, which was allocated a lower amount of Patient Services costs. Of course, the change in cost driver was not well-received by the department head of DM, but even she had to admit that the new allocation was more fair.

Although the allocation change appears to be a zero-sum game (i.e., one patient services department gains while another loses), the decision to make the change was not really difficult for Fargo's top managers. The original volume-based allocation was adopted solely because of its ease of calculation, and not because of any inherent rationale for fairness. With a better cost driver, Fargo has moved to a more equitable allocation of Financial Services costs, even though it may not seem that way to the department heads who saw their allocated amounts increase. However, those departments with allocation increases for Financial Services, such as DM and Family Intervention (FI), are now being allocated the appropriate amounts. They were formerly being subsidized by other departments, such as Home Care and Diagnostic Services, whose allocations were too high.

In spite of the equity appeal of the change, the greatest potential benefit for Fargo is in terms of cost control. How to allocate the $665,031 of Financial Services costs fairly to the various revenue departments is not as important to the financial well-being of Fargo Medical Center as how to control and potentially decrease these costs. Put simply, the goal of cost allocation is not merely how to divide the pie (equity), but also how the organization can shrink the pie (cost control). The movement from an allocation based on an assumed correlation with volume to an allocation based on an actual cost driver provides the potential for better cost control.

To reinforce this point, consider the old system of allocation on a per-dollar-of-revenue basis. How can a revenue producing department head decrease the amount of Financial Services costs being allocated to the department? The answer is to decrease the amount of patient services revenue. Such an action makes no sense at all, which is exactly the point. Because there was no direct connection between the amount allocated and the work done by Financial Services under the initial cost driver, the result is a cost-control conclusion that is nonsensical. No department head is going to sacrifice $1 worth of revenue to eliminate $0.023624 of Financial Services costs, so none of the revenue producing department heads will make any effort to create a more efficient financial support system. Even if Home Care were to change its billing procedures such that they utilized significantly less Financial Services support, it would not reap the benefits of such efforts. Home Care would continue to be allocated $97,160 in Financial Services costs because its revenue would remain at $4,112,776.

Now that Fargo is allocating Financial Services costs on the basis of the number of bills, revenue producing department heads can reap the benefits of their efforts to make the billing process more efficient. If the head of the Children's Clinic does not like the new higher allocation, he or she can do something about it—generate fewer bills. The task must be done without lowering the total billing amount, which may not be easy. In fact, the effort will probably have to be done jointly with Financial Services, and perhaps with third-party payors.

The critical point is that the head of the Children's Clinic is now motivated to participate in making the billing process more efficient. If the Children's Clinic can cut the number of bills in half, it can cut its allocation in half. If enough patient services departments do this, Fargo will eventually discover that it can get along with fewer resources devoted to Financial Services, and thus reduce total overhead costs. A reduction in overhead costs is the ultimate benefit of utilizing a meaningful cost driver. A well-chosen cost driver makes department heads accountable for the use of support department resources, which is the starting point in gaining control of overhead costs within any organization.

Despite honest efforts, what if the head of the Children's Clinic cannot reduce the number of bills generated? For example, maybe Home Care has an inherent advantage over the other patient services departments because it has only a few major payors, and hence more opportunity to consolidate bills. Or perhaps each bill is significantly larger. This difference in payor mix or average billing amount allows Home Care to generate $4,112,776 in revenue with 2,508 bills, while Children's Clinic requires 7,048 bills to generate only $1,626,441 in revenue. Perhaps these differences are such that managerial actions at Fargo cannot change the situation. One response may be that this is fine—this is exactly the type of information that Fargo's managers need to know. If the Children's Clinic is inherently less efficient in billing, and therefore the use of Financial Services support, it should be recognized in the cost-allocation process. Thus, Children's Clinic is charged $46,446 in Financial Services costs instead of $38,423 under the old cost driver, and the inherent inefficiency is not disguised by cross subsidization from other departments.

The same logic applies to Home Care. If they have inherent efficiencies in the billing process, why should they not be the beneficiaries of such efficiencies, and hence charged less? The correct information regarding the allocation of Financial Services costs is important to Fargo's managers when they make pricing and service decisions. Maybe Fargo has been under-pricing Children's Clinic services because the department's overhead costs have been understated. Fargo's costing system should reflect the true total cost of operating the Children's Clinic, including $46,446 versus $38,423 of Financial Services costs, and the clinic should seek to recover the true costs of providing these services in its pricing.

If the true cost of Financial Services support cannot be recovered, Fargo's managers have a bigger issue to consider—what actions can be taken to produce healthcare services at a total cost that is less than the revenues generated. In any event, the Children's Clinic should not be made to look artificially profitable by understating its overhead costs. What is important to the efficient management of Fargo Medical Center is that overhead costs are allocated as accurately as possible. Perhaps Home Care is not as unprofitable as it had looked in the past, now that Fargo's managers recognize the efficiencies inherent in its use of Financial Services support. Again, such information will make an impact on operational decisions, such as pricing strategies, and also on long-term decisions, such as which service lines to operate and which ones to close.

1. What are the advantages of changing from a poor cost driver to a better one?
2. What are the costs involved in the change?
3. Why is a good cost allocation critical to good decision making?

Cost Allocation Illustration III: The Step-Down Method

This series of three cost-allocation illustrations closes with a simple illustration of the step-down method. Fargo Medical Center will again be used for this illustration, but in addition to Financial Services, Administration, a second overhead department, is added, which has total direct costs of $312,425. In the previous illustration, the direct method of allocation was assumed; therefore, Financial Services costs were allocated directly to the patient services departments without any intrasupport department allocation. In this illustration, which is highlighted in Table 6.8, the complexities of allocating overhead costs from one support department to another is added.

To simplify the illustration, assume that Fargo Medical Center has only two support departments: Administration and Financial Services. The first decision that must be made under the step-down method is which of the two support departments is the most primary (i.e., which department provides the most services to the other). In this illustration, assume that Administration provides more support to Financial Services than Financial Services provides to Administration. Thus, in the step-down process, the first support department to be allocated is Administration.[2]

In the step-down method, Administration costs are allocated to the revenue producing departments and also to the other support departments. The process has been simplified somewhat by lumping together most of Fargo's patient services departments in the category called Other. Thus, the initial allocation in the top section of Table 6.8 shows that Administration costs are allocated to Financial Services, Home Care, L and B, DM, and the remaining patient services departments aggregated and shown as Other.

The allocation of Administration costs is made using payroll costs of the receiving departments as the cost driver. The total payroll for Fargo, less the Administration Department, is $10,625,400, so the $312,425 in Administration costs are allocated at a rate of $312,425 / $10,625,400 = $0.029404 per dollar of payroll. For example, the allocation of Administration costs to Financial Services is $0.029404 \times \$505,321 = \$14,858$, while the allocation to Home Care is $0.029404 \times \$1,376,845 = \$40,485$. The key point is that under the step-down method, overhead costs are allocated to support departments and to patient services departments. Table 6.8 places Financial Services in the allocation scheme, while Table 6.7 listed only patient services departments.

Now that Administration costs have been allocated across support and patient services departments, the role of Administration in the allocation process is closed out. The next step is to allocate Financial Services costs, which now include both direct costs plus the indirect costs from the allocation for Administration overhead. This allocation is shown in the bottom section of Table 6.8. In

TABLE 6.8
Fargo Medical Center: Step-Down Allocation of Administration and Financial Services Costs

Initial Allocation of Administration Department Costs:

Administration costs = $312,425

Allocation rate = $312,425/$10,625,400 = $0.029404 per dollar of payroll

	Financial Services	Home Care	L and B	DM	Other	Total
Payroll costs	$505,321	$1,376,845	$425,115	$257,316	$8,060,803	$10,625,400
Percent of total	4.8%	13.0%	4.0%	2.4%	75.9%	100.0%
Allocation	$ 14,858	$ 40,485	$ 12,500	$ 7,566	$ 237,017	$ 312,425

Subsequent Allocation of Financial Services Department Costs:

Financial Services costs = $665,031 + $14,858 = $679,889

Allocation rate = $679,889/100,915 = $6.737 per bill

	Financial Services	Home Care	L and B	DM	Other	Total
Number of bills		2,508	1,948	3,379	93,080	100,915
Percent of total		2.5%	1.9%	3.3%	92.2%	100.0%
Allocation	$ 0	$ 16,896	$ 13,124	$ 22,764	$ 627,080	$ 679,864

Table 6.7, Financial Services had $665,031 in direct costs to be allocated. However, in Table 6.8, Financial Services has $679,889 in total costs (direct plus indirect) to be allocated because the department has been allocated $14,858 of Administration overhead. The allocation of Financial Services costs proceeds as before except that the allocation rate is now $6.737 per patient services bill, as opposed to $6.59 per bill in Table 6.7. Because some of the costs of Administration now flow through Financial Services, the allocation of Financial Services costs to the patient services departments is somewhat greater than before. However, the allocation of Administration costs to the patient services departments is less under the step-down method than under the direct method because some costs that had been allocated directly to patient services departments are now allocated to another support department, Financial Services.

The step-down method of allocation is more complex than the direct method, and therefore more costly. Whether the added cost is worth it depends on the situation. For the reasons discussed previously (equity and cost control), managers want the best possible allocation system. However, the marginal costs associated with a more sophisticated allocation system are only worth incurring if the benefits (primarily cost control) associated with improved decision making exceed such costs.

Self-Test Questions

1. What is the primary difference between the direct and step-down methods of cost allocation?
2. Why would organizations adopt a more costly allocation system?

Activity-Based Costing

The discussion thus far has focused on traditional cost-allocation methods. In essence, the traditional methods begin with aggregate costs, typically at the department level. Overhead costs are then allocated downstream to the patient services departments. Thus, traditional methods can be thought of as a top-down allocation.

Activity-based costing (ABC) is a relatively new allocation system that is gaining popularity in the health services industry. ABC uses an upstream approach to cost allocation. Its premise is that the foundation of all costs within an organization stems from *activities*, hence its name. In fact, the term *cost driver*, which has been used throughout the chapter, originated with ABC; a cost driver is the basic activity that causes costs to be incurred in the first place. In ABC, because activities are the focus of the cost-accounting system, costs can be more easily assigned to individual patients, individual physicians, particular diagnoses, a reimbursement contract, a managed care population, and so on. The key to cost allocation under ABC is to identify the activities that are performed and then aggregate the costs of the activities.

Clearly, ABC holds great promise for healthcare providers. The ability to assess costs at multiple levels provides managers with much better information regarding the true costs of providing services. However, the information and resource requirements to establish an ABC system far exceed those required for a traditional cost-allocation system. For this reason, traditional cost allocation still dominates the scene, but ABC will probably become more prevalent as providers invest in newer and more powerful managerial accounting information systems.

1. What are the key differences between traditional and activity-based costing?
2. Why does ABC hold so much promise for healthcare providers?

Self-Test Questions

Final Thoughts on Cost Allocation

This chapter has been more mechanical than conceptual, but readers should not lose sight of the basic principles of cost allocation. The primary goal of cost allocation is to allocate as many costs as possible to those activities that create the need for the costs. In addition, the cost drivers used in the allocation must create a system that meets two tests. First, a good cost-allocation system must be fair; managers must believe that the overhead allocations to their departments truly reflect the amount of overhead services consumed. Second, the allocation process should foster cost reduction within the organization. To ensure fairness and cost-control incentives, cost drivers must reflect those factors that truly influence the total costs to be allocated.

For any organization, the better its cost-allocation process meets these two tests, the better the managerial decisions. After all, costs play a major role in provider decisions, such as what prices to charge and what services to offer. If the cost-allocation system is faulty, those decisions may be flawed and the financial condition of the business will be degraded. Although the allocation process may seem painful, the more confidence that all managers have in its validity, the better the organization will function.

1. What is the goal of cost allocation?
2. What are the two primary tests that good cost-allocation processes pass?
3. Why is the cost-allocation process important to health services managers?

Self-Test Questions

Key Concepts

This chapter focused on cost allocation. The key concepts of this chapter are:

- *Direct costs* are the unique and exclusive resources utilized only by one unit of an organization, such as a department, and therefore are fairly easy to measure.
- *Indirect costs*, in contrast, are inherently difficult to measure because these costs constitute a shared resource of the organization as a whole, such as administrative costs.
- The *goal* of cost allocation is to assign as many costs of an organization as possible directly to the activities that cause them to be incurred.

- *Cost allocation* is a critical part of the costing process because it addresses the issue of how to assign the costs of support activities to the revenue producing (patient services) departments.
- The motivation to improve cost-allocation systems comes largely from the increasing pressure to optimize economic performance within health services organizations, and the resultant managerial incentive systems that focus on financial parameters.
- The identification of meaningful *cost drivers* is an important step in developing a sound cost-allocation system.
- The best cost drivers are based on the *critical activities* that cause the overhead costs to be incurred.
- There are three primary *methods for cost allocation*: direct, reciprocal, and step down.
- The *direct method* recognizes no intrasupport department services. Thus, support department costs are allocated exclusively to patient services departments.
- The *reciprocal method* recognizes all intrasupport department services. Unfortunately, the reciprocal method is difficult to implement because it requires the simultaneous solution of a series of equations.
- The *step-down method* represents a compromise that recognizes some of the intrasupport department services.
- Regardless of the allocation method, all costs eventually end up in the patient services departments.
- A good cost driver will be perceived by department heads as being *fair* and will promote *cost control measures* within the organization.
- *Activity-based costing (ABC)* allocates costs on the basis of activities, and hence aggregates costs from the basic components that create costs in the first place. ABC can provide a much more meaningful allocation of costs because costs can be assigned to individual patients, diagnoses, patient populations, and so on. The problem with ABC is that it requires a very sophisticated and costly managerial accounting information system.

Although this chapter has been mostly mechanical in nature, the most important point to remember is that a sound cost-allocation system is required for making good pricing and service decisions, which are discussed in the next chapter.

Questions

6.1 What are the primary differences between direct and indirect costs?

6.2 What is the goal of cost allocation?

6.3 a. What are the three primary methods of cost allocation?

     b. What are the differences among them?

6.4 a. What is a cost pool?

b. What is a cost driver?

c. How is the cost-allocation rate determined?

6.5 Effective cost drivers, and hence the resulting allocation system, must have what two important attributes?

6.6 Briefly describe (illustrate) the cost-allocation process. (To keep things simple, use the direct method for your illustration.)

6.7 Which is the better cost driver for the costs of a hospital's Financial Services Department: patient services department revenues or number of bills generated? Explain your rationale.

6.8 How does activity-based costing (ABC) differ from traditional costing approaches?

Problems

6.1 The Housekeeping Services department of the Ruger Clinic, a large multi-specialty clinic in Toledo, Ohio, had $100,000 in direct costs during 1998. These costs must be allocated to Ruger's three revenue producing patient services departments using the direct method. Two cost drivers are under consideration: patient services revenue and hours of housekeeping services utilized. The patient services departments generated $5 million in total revenues during 1998, and to support these clinical activities, used 5,000 hours of housekeeping services.

a. What is the value of the cost pool?

b. What is the allocation rate if:

(1) patient services revenue is used as the cost driver?

(2) hours of housekeeping services is used as the cost driver?

6.2 Refer to Problem 6.1. Assume that the three patient services departments are Adult Services, Pediatric Services, and Other Services. The patient services revenue and hours of housekeeping services for each department are:

Department	Revenue	Housekeeping Hours
Adult Services	$3,000,000	1,500
Pediatric Services	1,500,000	3,000
Other Services	500,000	500
Total	$5,000,000	5,000

a. What is the dollar allocation to each patient services department if patient services revenue is used as the cost driver?

b. What is the dollar allocation to each patient services department if hours of housekeeping support is used as the cost driver?

c. What is the difference in the allocation to each department between the two drivers?

d. Which of the two drivers is better? Why?

The following data pertain to the remaining problems:

St. Benedict's Hospital has three support departments and four patient services departments. The direct costs to each of the support departments are:

General Administration	$2,000,000
Facilities	5,000,000
Financial Services	3,000,000

Selected data for the three support and four patient services departments are:

Department	Patient Services Revenue	Space (Square Feet)	Housekeeping Labor Hours	Salary Dollars
Support:				
General Administration		10,000	2,000	$1,500,000
Facilities		20,000	5,000	3,000,000
Financial Services		15,000	3,000	2,000,000
Total		45,000	10,000	$6,500,000
Patient Services:				
Routine Care	$30,000,000	400,000	150,000	$12,000,000
Intensive Care	4,000,000	40,000	30,000	5,000,000
Diagnostic Services	6,000,000	60,000	15,000	6,000,000
Other Services	10,000,000	100,000	25,000	7,000,000
Total	$50,000,000	600,000	220,000	$30,000,000
Grand total	$50,000,000	645,000	230,000	$36,500,000

6.3 Assume that the hospital uses the direct method for cost allocation. Furthermore, the cost driver for General Administration and Financial Services is patient services revenue while the cost driver for Facilities is space utilization.

a. What are the appropriate allocation rates?

b. Use an allocation table similar to Table 6.6 to allocate the hospital's overhead costs to the patient services departments.

6.4 Assume that the hospital uses salary dollars as the cost driver for General Administration, housekeeping labor hours as the cost driver for Facilities, and patient services revenue as the cost driver for Financial Services. (The majority of the costs of the Facilities department are devoted to housekeeping services.)

a. What are the appropriate allocation rates?

b. Use an allocation table similar to the one used for Problem 6.3 to allocate the hospital's overhead costs to the patient services departments.

    c. Compare the dollar allocations with those obtained in Problem 6.3. Explain the differences.

    d. Which of the two cost driver schemes is better? Explain your answer.

6.5 Now, assume that the hospital uses the step-down method for cost allocation, with salary dollars as the cost driver for General Administration, housekeeping labor hours as the cost driver for Facilities, and patient services revenue as the cost driver for Financial Services. Assume also that General Administration provides the most services to other support departments, followed closely by Facilities. Financial Services provides the least services to the other support departments.

    a. Use an allocation table to allocate the hospital's overhead costs to the patient services departments.

    b. Compare the dollar allocations with those obtained in Problem 6.4. Explain the differences.

    c. Is the direct method or the step-down method better for cost allocation within St. Benedict's? Explain your answer.

6.6 Return to the direct method of cost allocation and use the same cost drivers as specified in Problem 6.4 for General Administration and Facilities. However, assume that $2,000,000 of Financial Services costs are related to billing and managerial reporting, and $1,000,000 are related to payroll and personnel management.

    a. Devise and implement a cost-allocation scheme that recognizes that Financial Services has two widely different functions.

    b. Is there any additional information that would be useful in completing Part a?

    c. What are the costs and benefits to St. Benedict's of creating two cost pools for Financial Services?

Notes

1. Cost allocation takes place both for historical purposes, in which realized costs over the past year are allocated, and for planning purposes, in which estimated future costs are allocated to aid in pricing and other decisions. The examples in this chapter generally assume that the purpose of the allocation is for pricing, so the data presented is estimated for the coming year, 1999, rather than historical.

2. If the two support departments were Human Resources and Housekeeping, the decision on which department to allocate first may be more difficult because each of these departments provides significant support to the other. In such a situation, the best allocation method may be the reciprocal method. (See Figure 6.1.)

References

Baker, J. J. and G. F. Boyd. 1997. "Activity-Based Costing in the Operating Room at Valley View Hospital." *Journal of Health Care Finance* (Fall): 1–9.

Baker, J. J. 1995. "Activity-Based Costing for Integrated Delivery Systems." *Journal of Health Care Finance* (Winter): 57–61.

Hill, N. T. and E. L. Johns. 1994. "Adoption of Costing Systems by U.S. Hospitals." *Hospital & Health Services Administration* (Winter) 521–537.

Hoyt, R. E. and C. M. Lay. 1995. "Linking Cost Control Measures to Health Care Services by Using Activity-Based Information." *Health Services Management Research* (November): 221–233.

Ramsey, R. H., IV. 1994. "Activity-Based Costing for Hospitals." *Hospital & Health Services Administration* (Fall): 385–396.

Stiles, R. A. and S. S. Mick. 1997. "What is the Cost of Controlling Quality." *Hospital & Health Services Administration* (Summer): 193–204.

Upda, S. 1996. "Activity-Based Costing for Hospitals." *Health Care Management Review* (Summer): 83–96.

PRICING AND SERVICE DECISIONS

Learning Objectives

After studying this chapter, readers will be able to:

- Describe the difference between providers as price setters and providers as price takers, and how this difference affects pricing and service decisions.
- Explain the difference between full-cost, marginal-cost, direct-cost, and competitive pricing.
- Explain how accounting and actuarial information are used to make pricing and service decisions.
- Conduct basic analyses both to set prices and determine service offerings, particularly under capitated reimbursement.

Introduction

One of the most important uses of accounting data involves either establishing a price for a particular service or, given a price, deciding whether or not the service should be offered. For example, in a charge-based environment, managers of healthcare providers must set prices on the services that their organizations offer. Managers also must determine whether or not to offer volume discounts to valued payor groups such as managed care plans or business coalitions, and how large these discounts should be. Such decisions are called *pricing decisions.*

In many situations, insurers, especially governmental and managed care plans, dictate the reimbursement amount. Therefore, health services managers must decide whether or not the payment is sufficient to assume the risks associated with providing services to the covered populations. These decisions are called *service decisions.* Because service decision analyses are similar to pricing decision analyses, the two types of analyses are discussed jointly.

Pricing and service decisions affect a business' revenues and costs, and hence its financial condition, which ultimately determines its long-term viability. The importance of such decisions is easy to understand. In essence, pricing and service decisions determine both the strategic direction of the business and the ability of the organization to survive and prosper. In this chapter, the focus is on the analyses behind such decisions, with particular emphasis on doing so in a capitated environment.

Healthcare Providers and the Power to Set Prices

Two extremes exist regarding the power of healthcare providers to set prices. At one extreme, providers have no power whatsoever and must accept the reimbursement levels set by payors. At the other extreme, providers can set any prices (within reason) desired and payors must accept those prices. Clearly, few real-world markets support such extreme positions. Nevertheless, thinking in such terms can help managers better understand the pricing and service decisions that providers face.

Providers as Price Takers

As indicated throughout this text, healthcare services are provided in an increasingly competitive marketplace. As providers respond to market competition, managers must assess the ability of their organizations to influence the prices paid for the services offered. If the organization is one of a large number of providers in a service area with a large number of commercial fee-for-service purchasers and if little distinguishes the services offered by different providers, economic theory suggests that prices will be set by local supply and demand conditions. Thus, the actions of a single participant, whether a purchaser or provider, cannot influence the prices set in the marketplace. In this competitive market situation, healthcare providers are said to be *price takers* because they are constrained by the prices set in the marketplace.

Some purchasers of healthcare services, notably government payors as well as managed care plans and employer purchasing groups with market power, can set reimbursement levels on a "take it or leave it" basis. In this situation, providers also are price takers because they cannot influence market rates. Because many markets either are reasonably competitive or are dominated by large payor groups, and because governmental payors cover a significant proportion of the population, most providers probably qualify as price takers for the majority of services offered.

As a general rule, providers that are price takers for services must take price as a given and concentrate managerial efforts on cost structure and utilization to ensure that their services are profitable. From a pure financial perspective, such a price taking provider should offer all services with costs that are less than the given price, even if that price falls because of discounting or other market actions.

Although the pure financial approach to service decisions is obviously simplistic, it does raise two important managerial accounting issues. First, managers must determine what costs are relevant to the decision at hand. As discussed in previous chapters, direct costs usually are easy to identify, but how are overhead costs affected by the decision to offer a particular service at some expected volume level? Often, this question is not easy to answer. Second, managers must recognize that costs can be covered in either the short run or the long run. To ensure long-term sustainability, prices must cover full costs. Such matters are discussed in the next major section.

Providers as Price Setters

In contrast to the previous discussion, healthcare providers with market dominance enjoy large market shares, and hence exercise pricing power. Within limits, managers of such providers can decide what prices to set on the services offered. Furthermore, if a provider's services can be differentiated from others on the basis of quality, convenience, or some other characteristic, the provider also has the ability, again within limits, to set prices on the differentiated services. Healthcare providers that have such pricing power are called *price setters*.

The situation would be much easier for managers if a provider's status as a price taker or price setter were fixed for all services for long periods of time. Unfortunately, the market for healthcare services is ever changing, and hence providers can quickly move from one status to the other. For example, the merger of two healthcare providers may create sufficient market power to change two price takers, as separate entities, into one price setter, as a combined entity. Furthermore, providers can be price takers for some services and price setters for others. To make matters even more complicated, a large provider that serves separate market areas may be a price taker for a particular service in one geographical market, and yet be a price setter in another geographical market.

1. What is the difference between a price taker and a price setter?
2. Are healthcare providers generally either price takers or price setters exclusively? Explain your answer.

Self-Test Questions

Pricing Strategies

Numerous strategies are used to price healthcare services. Unfortunately, no single strategy is most appropriate in all situations. In this section, a few of the pricing strategies most frequently used by health services organizations are discussed.

Full-Cost Pricing

Full-cost pricing recognizes that to remain viable in the long run, health services organizations must set prices that recover all costs associated with operating the business. Thus, the full cost of a service, whether a patient day in a hospital, a visit to a clinic, a laboratory test, or the treatment of a particular diagnosis, must include the following: (1) the direct variable costs of providing the service; (2) the direct fixed costs; and (3) the appropriate share of the overhead expenses of the organization.

Because of the difficulties inherent in allocating overhead costs discussed in Chapter 6, the full costs of an individual service are difficult to measure with precision, and hence have to be viewed with some skepticism, especially by payors. Nevertheless, in the aggregate, revenues must cover both direct and overhead costs, and hence prices in total must cover all costs of an organization. Furthermore, all businesses need profits to survive in the long run. In not-for-profit businesses, prices must be set high enough to provide the profits needed to support asset replacement and to meet expansion plans. In addition, for-profit providers must provide equity investors with a return on their investment.

Marginal-Cost Pricing

In economics, the *marginal cost* of an item is the cost of providing one additional unit of output, whether that output is a product or service. For example, suppose that a hospital currently provides 40,000 patient days of care. Its marginal cost, based on inpatient day as the unit of output, is the cost of providing the 40,001th day of care. In this situation, fixed costs, both direct and overhead, have already been covered, at least in theory, by the existing patient base (the 40,000 patient days), so the marginal cost consists solely of the variable costs associated with an additional one-day stay. In most situations, no additional labor costs would be involved; additional personnel would not be hired nor overtime required. The marginal cost, therefore, consists of expenses such as laundry costs, costs of expendable supplies, and costs of utility services consumed during that day. Obviously, the marginal cost associated with one additional patient day is far less than the full cost.

Many proponents of government programs, such as Medicare and Medicaid, argue that payments to providers should be made on the basis of marginal rather than full costs. The argument here is that some price above marginal cost is all that is required for the provider to "make money" on government-sponsored patients. However, what would happen if all payors for a particular provider set reimbursement rates based on marginal costs? If such a situation were allowed to occur, the organization would not recover its fixed costs, including both direct and overhead, and hence would ultimately fail.

Should any prices be set on the basis of marginal costs? **In theory**, the answer is no. For prices to be equitable, all payors should pay their fair shares in covering providers' total costs. Furthermore, if *marginal-cost pricing* should be adopted, which payor(s) should receive its benefits by being charged lower prices? Should it be the government because it is taxpayer funded, or should it be the latest payor to contract with the provider? There are no good answers to these questions, so the easy way out, at least conceptually, is to require all payors to pay full costs, and hence equitably share the burden of the organization's fixed costs.

However, as a practical matter, what may make sense for health services providers is to occasionally use marginal-cost pricing to attract a new patient clientele or to retain an existing clientele (i.e., gain or retain market share). To survive in the long run, however, businesses must earn revenues that cover their full costs. Thus, marginal-cost pricing either must be a temporary measure or the organization must employ *cross subsidization*, or *price shifting*. In such situations, some patients or covered populations are overcharged for services, as compared to full costs, while others are undercharged.

Historically, price shifting was used by providers to support services, such as emergency care, teaching and research, and indigent care, that were not self-supporting. Without such price-shifting strategies, many providers would not have been able to offer a full range of services. Payors were willing to accept price shifting because the additional burden was not excessive. Today, however, overall healthcare costs have risen to the point where the major purchasers of healthcare services are not willing to support the costs associated with providing services to others, and hence purchasers are demanding prices that cover only true costs, without cross subsidies. Payors perhaps rightly believe that they do not have the moral responsibility to fund healthcare services for those outside of their covered populations.

Direct-Cost Pricing

Direct-cost pricing falls between full-cost pricing and marginal-cost pricing. In direct-cost pricing, prices are set to cover the direct costs of providing services, including both variable and fixed costs. Thus, fixed direct costs are covered in this strategy, whereas such costs are not covered in marginal-cost pricing. Indirect (overhead) costs are not covered, however, so this strategy does not provide revenues that cover the full costs of providing services. The ramifications of direct-cost pricing are similar to those of marginal-cost pricing, except the former are less severe. Because of the recognition of additional costs, direct-cost pricing produces higher prices than does marginal-cost pricing.

Competitive Pricing

In certain situations, health services organizations may be required to price in accordance with market conditions out of necessity. Here, cost structure is not relevant to the pricing decision. All that counts is what it takes to be competitive in the marketplace. Thus, such a pricing strategy is called *competitive pricing*. Under moderate competition, some prices may be set lower than those under full-cost pricing, but higher than under marginal- or direct-cost pricing—a condition that could endure for a relatively long period. Under severe competition, however, competitive pricing leads to prices that are based on marginal costs, and hence that are unsustainable in the long run. In such situations, weaker competitors often drop out of the marketplace either through acquisition or closure, and the end result is less competition and a return to sustainable full-cost pricing.

Self-Test Questions

1. Describe four common pricing strategies and their implications for financial survivability.
2. What is cross subsidization (price shifting)?
3. Is cross subsidization used by providers as frequently today as it was in the past? If not, why?

Target Costing

Target costing is a management strategy often used in competitive markets. Target costing assumes the price for a service is a given, and then subtracts the desired profit on that service to obtain the target cost level. If possible, management then will reduce the full cost of the service to the target level, with a goal of continuous cost reduction that will eventually push costs below the target. Essentially, target costing backs into the cost at which a healthcare service must be provided in the long run to attain a given profitability target.

Perhaps the greatest value of target costing lies in the fact that it forces managers to take market prices seriously. That is, it recognizes that purchasers do not really care whether or not prices are based on the underlying costs of the services provided. Rather, purchasers are concerned only with their own costs, which are the selling prices of insurers and providers.

Self-Test Questions

1. What is target costing?
2. What is its greatest value?

Illustration I: Setting Prices on Individual Services

The best way to understand the mechanics of pricing and service decisions is to work through several illustrations. The first illustration examines how prices can be set on individual services.

Assume that the managers of Windsor Clinic, a not-for-profit provider, are planning to offer a new outpatient service. The clinic's managerial accountants have estimated the following cost data for the service:

Variable cost per visit	$10
Annual direct fixed costs	$100,000
Annual overhead allocation	$25,000.

Furthermore, the clinic's marketing staff believes that demand for the new service will be 5,000 visits during its first year of operation.

To begin, Windsor's managers want to know what price must be set on each visit for the service to break even during the first year. To break even, the net income of the service must be zero, so revenues less costs must equal zero. One way to calculate the breakeven price is to express the relationship between revenues, costs, and profit in equation form:

$$\text{Total revenues} - \text{Total costs} = \$0$$

$$\text{Total revenues} - \text{Total variable costs} - \text{Direct fixed costs} - \text{Overhead} = \$0$$

$$(5,000 \times \text{Price}) - (5,000 \times \$10) - \$100,000 - \$25,000 = \$0$$

$$(5,000 \times \text{Price}) - \$175,000 = \$0$$

$$5,000 \times \text{Price} = \$175,000$$

$$\text{Price} = \$175,000 \, / \, 5,000 = \$35.$$

Thus, under the utilization and cost assumptions developed by Windsor's managers, a price of $35 per visit must be set on the new service to break even.

Of course, Windsor's managers want the service to do better than just break even. Suppose the goal is to make a profit of $100,000. Examining the calculations above show that costs at 5,000 visits are expected to total $175,000. Thus, to make a profit of $100,000, service revenues must total $175,000 + $100,000 = $275,000. With 5,000 visits, the price must be set at $275,000 / 5,000 = $55 per visit.

To this point, the analysis has focused on full-cost pricing. Suppose that Windsor's managers wanted to price the service aggressively to quickly build market share. What price would be set under marginal-cost pricing? Now, the service must only cover the variable (marginal) cost of $10 per visit, so a price of $10 is all that is required. This price, which is well below the full costs breakeven of $35, would result in a loss of $125,000 ($100,000 in direct fixed costs and $25,000 in overhead) during the first year the service is offered, assuming that the aggressive pricing does not affect the 5,000 visit utilization estimate.

What price must be set under direct-cost pricing, whereby the clinic would recover all of the service's direct costs (both variable and fixed), but none of its overhead costs? With $25,000 less in total costs to cover, the 5,000 visits must generate only $150,000 in revenues, so the price under direct costing is $150,000 / 5,000 = $30 per visit.

What price should Windsor's managers actually set on the new service? It should be obvious to readers that a great deal of judgment is required to make this decision. The key is the relationship between price and utilization, which the analysis has ignored by assuming that the service would produce 5,000 visits regardless of price. A more complete analysis would examine the effect of different prices and utilization levels on profits. However, rather than extend this illustration, it is best to defer this discussion until later.

1. Briefly explain the process for pricing individual services.
2. What do you think the price should be on Windsor's new service? Justify your answer.

Self-Test Questions

Illustration II: Hospital Price Setting Under Capitation

The second illustration focuses on how one hospital priced a new capitated product.

Base Case Analysis

Table 7.1 contains the 1999 forecasted, pro-forma payor worksheet and profit and loss (P&L) statement for Montana Medical Center (MMC), a 350-bed, not-for-profit hospital. According to its managers' best estimates, MMC is expecting to earn a profit of $1,662,312 in 1999. The data consist first of a worksheet, which breaks down the cost data by product line, in this case, by payor. Here, the assumption is that all payors pay on a fee-for-service basis, including discounted fee-for-service. Table 7.1 cost data also include the hospital's cost structure, broken down by variable costs, fixed costs including both direct and overhead (the $71,746,561 given in the P&L statement), and contribution margin.

To illustrate the data, consider MMC's Medicare patients. Medicare is expected to provide the hospital with 4,268 admissions at an average revenue of $7,327 per admission, for total revenues of 4,268 × $7,327 = $31,271,636. Expected variable cost per admission for a Medicare patient is $2,529, which results in expected total variable costs of 4,268 × $2,529 = $10,793,772. The difference between expected total revenues and the expected total variable costs produces a forecasted total contribution margin of $31,271,636 − $10,793,772 = $20,477,864 for the Medicare patient group. This total contribution margin is combined with the total contribution margins of the other payor groups to produce an expected total contribution margin for the hospital of $73,408,873. As shown in the P&L statement portion of Table 7.1, the total contribution margin both covers MMC's forecasted fixed costs of $71,746,561 and produces an expected profit (net income) of $1,662,312.

MMC's managers are considering taking a bold strategic action—offering a capitated plan for inpatient services. One of the first tasks that must be performed is setting the price for the new plan. Table 7.2 contains the key assumptions inherent in the pricing decision. The hospital's managers believe that about 13 percent of the current patient base would be converted to the capitated plan. To be conservative, the assumption was made that no additional patients would be generated. Thus, at least initially, patients in the capitated plan would come from MMC's current patient base. In effect, MMC would have to cannibalize from its

TABLE 7.1

Montana Medical Center (MMC): Pro-Forma Payor Worksheet and P&L Statement for 1999

Payor	Number of Admissions	Average Revenue per Admission	Revenues by Payor	Variable Cost per Admission	Total Variable Costs	Contribution Margin
Payor Worksheet:						
Medicare	4,268	$7,327	$ 31,271,636	$2,529	$10,793,772	$20,477,864
Medicaid	5,895	5,448	32,115,960	1,575	9,284,625	22,831,335
Montana Care	828	4,305	3,564,540	1,907	1,578,996	1,985,544
Managed Care	1,885	3,842	7,242,170	1,638	3,087,630	4,154,540
Blue Cross	332	5,761	1,912,652	2,366	785,512	1,127,140
Commercial	1,408	11,770	16,572,160	2,969	4,180,352	12,391,808
Self-Pay	1,289	2,053	2,646,317	1,489	1,919,321	726,996
Other	1,149	11,539	13,258,311	3,085	3,544,665	9,713,646
Total	17,054		$108,583,746		$35,174,873	$73,408,873
Weighted average		$6,367		$2,063		
P&L Statement:						
Total revenues	$108,583,746					
Variable costs	35,174,873					
Contribution margin	$ 73,408,873					
Fixed costs	71,746,561					
Net income	$ 1,662,312					

own business with the expectation of protecting current market share and using the capitated plan as a marketing tool to expand market share in the future.

Assumptions also have been made regarding where the cannibalization would occur and the number of admissions under the capitated plan. These data are provided in Points 2 and 3 of Table 7.2. The patient mix assumptions will be important when costs are estimated for the new plan. Note that the new plan's 25,000 enrollees are expected to produce 2,258 admissions.

MMC's managers believe, at least initially, that hospital utilization will be unaffected by the transfer of some patients from current contracts to capitation. Another expectation is that variable costs for the new plan would be the same as experienced in the past with each payor group. Here, MMC's managers are making a very important assumption: the delivery of healthcare services to the capitated population will be exactly the same as provided to the fee-for-service population. Because the capitated population initially will come from existing Medicaid, commercial, and self-pay groups, the expected utilization and cost behavior is assumed to be the same as when these patients were treated in a fee-for-service environment. This is probably a reasonable starting assumption given that the capitated population will represent only a small portion of MMC's overall business. However, as managed care penetration increases in MMC's service area, and hence MMC's proportion of capitated patients increases, both utilization patterns and the underlying cost structure are likely to change as the hospital responds to the incentives created by fixed payment-per-enrollee reimbursement.

Finally, and perhaps most importantly in terms of pricing strategy, the capitated price that MMC plans to offer to the market must result in at least the same net income as expected if the hospital were to remain totally fee-for-service. This amount is the pro-forma net income of $1,662,312 developed in Table 7.1. The underlying logic here is that MMC's managers want to experiment

---

TABLE 7.2

Montana Medical Center (MMC): Initial Assumptions for a Capitated Plan

1. The capitated plan will initially enroll the following percentages of the hospital's current patients:
   a. Medicaid: 20 percent
   b. Commercial: 40 percent
   c. Self-pay: 40 percent
2. Assuming that utilization rates are not affected by the change to a capitated plan, admissions from the capitated group are expected to total $(0.20 \times 5,895) + (0.40 \times 1,408) + (0.40 \times 1,289) = 2,258$.
3. Based on current coverage information, the patient population under capitation (number of enrollees) would be 25,000.
4. Variable costs for capitated patients will remain the same as currently estimated for each payor group.
5. Total fixed costs will remain the same.
6. All other assumptions inherent in the Table 7.1 forecast hold for the capitated plan.
7. The goal for the price set for capitated enrollees will be to generate, at a minimum, the net income forecasted in Table 7.1 under fee-for-service reimbursement.

with capitation, but they are unwilling to do so at the expense of the bottom line. This pricing goal and the expected cost structure of serving the capitated population, therefore, will drive the monthly premium established for the capitated product. If the goal of preserving the bottom line while adding the new product proves to be unattainable, MMC's managers would have to reevaluate their initial pricing strategy.

Table 7.3 contains an analysis similar to the one shown in Table 7.1, except that Table 7.3 includes the proposed capitated plan. Changes from the Table 7.1 values are shown in boldface. For example, the entire first line of the worksheet, labeled "Capitated", is in boldface because this is MMC's new product line, which does not appear in Table 7.1. Also in boldface are selected values on the Medicaid, commercial, and self-pay lines because these values will change because of the shift of some of these payor groups' patients to the capitated plan.

Notice the volume levels in each of the payor groups. The Medicaid group, for example, reflects the 20 percent decrease that results from patients' shift to the capitated plan: $0.80 \times 5,895 = 4,716$. The commercial and self-pay payor groups also reflect their 40 percent losses in admissions to the new plan. In total, the capitated plan is expected to siphon off $0.20 \times 5,895 = 1,179$ Medicaid admissions, $0.40 \times 1,408 = 563$ commercial admissions, and $0.40 \times 1,289 = 516$ self-pay admissions, for a total of 2,258 admissions.

TABLE 7.3

Montana Medical Center (MMC): Pro-Forma Analysis Assuming 25,000 Enrollees and Constant Net Income

Payor	Number of Admissions	Average Revenue per Admission	Revenues by Payor	Variable Cost per Admission	Total Variable Costs	Contribution Margin
Payor Worksheet:						
Capitated	**2,258**	**$ 6,250**	**$ 14,110,583**	**$1,903**	**$ 4,296,794**	**$ 9,813,789**
Medicare	4,268	7,327	31,271,636	2,529	10,793,772	20,477,864
Medicaid	**4,716**	5,448	**25,692,768**	1,575	**7,427,700**	**18,265,068**
Montana Care	828	4,305	3,564,540	1,907	1,578,996	1,985,544
Managed Care	1,885	3,842	7,242,170	1,638	3,087,630	4,154,540
Blue Cross	332	5,761	1,912,652	2,366	785,512	1,127,140
Commercial	**845**	11,770	**9,943,296**	2,969	**2,508,211**	**7,435,085**
Self-Pay	**773**	2,053	**1,587,790**	1,489	**1,151,593**	**436,198**
Other	1,149	11,539	13,258,331	3,085	3,544,665	9,713,646
Total	17,054		$108,583,746		$35,174,873	$73,408,873
Weighted average		$ 6,367		$2,063		

Annual capitated revenue requirements = $14,110,583/25,000 = $564.42 per member
Monthly capitated revenue requirements = $564.42/12 = $47.04 per member per month (PMPM)

P&L Statement:

Total revenues	$108,583,746
Variable costs	35,174,873
Contribution margin	$ 73,408,873
Fixed costs	71,746,561
Net income	$ 1,662,312

Note: Some rounding differences occur in the table.

For now, pass by the revenue columns in Table 7.3 and focus on the variable cost columns for the capitated patients. Because each capitated patient is expected to have the same variable cost as the previous plans, variable costs for the capitated plan are expected to total $(1,179 \times \$1,575) + (563 \times \$2,969) + (516 \times \$1,489)$ = $4,296,794.[1] With an expected number of admissions of 2,258, the average variable cost per capitated admission is $4,296,794 / 2,258 = $1,903.

Now consider the revenue columns. To keep the net income the same as in Table 7.1, revenues must total $108,583,746. Furthermore, expected total revenues from all payor groups, except the new plan, amount to $94,473,163. Thus, the capitated plan must bring in revenue of $108,583,746 − $94,473,163 = $14,110,583 to achieve MMC's target profit. This calculation can be thought of as working backwards on (or up) the pro-forma P&L statement shown on the bottom of Table 7.3.

With expected admissions at 2,258, the average revenue per admission can be calculated as $14,110,583/2,258 = $6,250. However, this implied average revenue per admission has no real meaning in a capitated plan because MMC will not be charging these patients on a per admission basis. The calculated per admission revenue value of $6,250 is really a *fee-for-service equivalent revenue*, and every worker at MMC must recognize that the hospital will not actually receive $6,250 per admission under the new plan. As MMC's patients move from fee-for-service to capitation, revenue will be based on enrollment rather than admissions.

With all this information at hand, MMC's managers now can price the new plan. Total revenues of $14,110,583 are required from 25,000 enrollees, so the annual revenue per enrollee is $14,110,583 / 25,000 = $564.42. Because premiums are normally expressed on a *per member per month (PMPM)* basis, the annual revenue requirement must be divided by 12 to obtain $47.04 PMPM. This PMPM charge is what MMC's managers would set as the initial price when marketing the new plan.

Sensitivity Analysis

The previous section illustrated how MMC's managers could establish a price for a new capitated plan. However, a good pricing analysis goes well beyond the base case analysis (or *base case scenario*), which uses a single (point) estimate for all input variables—number of enrollees, variable costs, and so on. The second part of a complete pricing analysis involves *sensitivity analysis*, whereby MMC's managers assess the impact of assumptional changes in key variable values from the base case scenario.[2] For example, the $47.04 PMPM may not work in the marketplace. Perhaps that premium is too high to be competitive, so the volume of enrollees in the new plan falls far short of the 25,000 estimate. In this case, what would be the financial results?

To begin the sensitivity analysis, assume that the premium was set and held at $47.04 PMPM, but only 15,000 enrollees—60 percent of the original estimate of 25,000—resulted. Also, assume that the proportional mix remains the same as in the base case. That is, assume that the enrollees in the capitated product consist of $0.60 \times 20\% = 12\%$ of the original Medicaid payor group, 24 percent of the commercial payor group, and 12 percent of the self-pay payor group. To assess the results under this reduced enrollee scenario, the analysis must be repeated, but with a smaller proportion of existing patients moving to the capitated plan. Now, a premium amount is not being solved for, as in the previous example, but rather net income is being calculated in the normal way, given the pricing and new volume assumptions. The results of the analysis are presented in Table 7.4.

Changes from the previous table (Table 7.3) have been indicated in bold-face. The reduction in capitated plan enrollees results in a greater number of admissions and revenues from Medicaid, commercial, and self-pay payor groups and a lower patient population and revenues from the capitated plan. The end result is no change in expected net income. This occurs because the analysis assumes that all patients incur the same costs whether admitted from their original payor groups or under the capitated plan, and the premium used for capitated enrollees was initially calculated to force revenue and profit neutrality. Thus, shifting patients from a payor group to the capitated plan, or vice versa, does not have an impact on MMC's bottom line. The goal of MMC's managers is **not** to increase total revenue by shifting current patients from one plan to another, but to increase revenues by attracting new enrollees into the capitated plan, and thus increasing market share.

What would be the impact of additional enrollees? Table 7.5 repeats the analysis, but now the assumption is that 10,000 new enrollees are added to the

TABLE 7.4
Montana Medical Center (MMC): Pro-Forma Analysis Assuming 15,000 Enrollees at $47.04 PMPM

Payor	Number of Admissions	Average Revenue per Admission	Revenues by Payor	Variable Cost per Admission	Total Variable Costs	Contribution Margin
Payor Worksheet:						
Capitated	**1,355**	$ 6,250	$ **8,466,350**	$1,903	$ 2,578,077	$ 5,888,273
Medicare	4,268	7,327	31,271,636	2,529	10,793,772	20,477,864
Medicaid	**5,188**	5,448	**28,262,045**	1,575	**8,170,470**	**20,091,575**
Montana Care	828	4,305	3,564,540	1,907	1,578,996	1,985,544
Managed Care	1,885	3,842	7,242,170	1,638	3,087,630	4,154,540
Blue Cross	332	5,761	1,912,652	2,366	785,512	1,127,140
Commercial	**1,070**	11,770	**12,594,842**	2,969	**3,177,068**	9,417,774
Self-Pay	**980**	2,053	**2,011,201**	1,489	**1,458,684**	552,517
Other	1,149	11,539	13,258,331	3,085	3,544,665	9,713,646
Total	17,054		$108,583,746		$35,174,873	$73,408,873
Weighted average		$ 6,367		$2,063		

P&L Statement:

Total revenues	$108,583,746
Variable costs	35,174,873
Contribution margin	$ 73,408,873
Fixed costs	71,746,561
Net income	$ 1,662,312

Note: Some rounding differences occur in the table.

capitated plan. Coupled with the base case estimate of 25,000 enrollees from MMC's other payor groups, total enrollment in the capitated plan is increased to 35,000. The assumptions are that the new enrollees would utilize hospital services at the same rate as current plan members, and the variable cost per admission would be the same for the new enrollees as for the existing 25,000 enrollees.

Again, those entries that differ from Table 7.3 are boldfaced. The addition of new capitated enrollees does not affect any of the other payor groups, so the changes in Table 7.5 are limited to the first line of the payor worksheet, the totals and averages, and the P&L statement. Adding 10,000 enrollees increases MMC's total revenues by $114,227,979 − $108,583,746 = $5,644,233, but only increases total variable costs by $36,893,591 − $35,174,873 = $1,718,718, thus resulting in a total contribution margin gain of $5,644,233 − $1,718,718 = $3,925,515. Assuming that fixed costs remain at $71,746,561, the entire amount of the contribution margin increase will flow to the bottom line, so net income increases by a similar amount.

An alternative way to consider the effect of additional enrollees on the bottom line is to examine the contribution margin on capitated patients. Each additional enrollee brings in $47.04 × 12 = $564.48 per year. What about the cost side? The 35,000 enrollees are expected to have 3,161 admissions, for an average rate of 3,161 / 35,000 = 0.0903 admissions per enrollee, so the expected cost per enrollee is 0.0903 × $1,903 = $171.84. Thus, the contribution margin

TABLE 7.5
Montana Medical Center (MMC): Pro-Forma Analysis Assuming 35,000 Enrollees at $47.04 PMPM

Payor	Number of Admissions	Average Revenue per Admission	Revenues by Payor	Variable Cost per Admission	Total Variable Costs	Contribution Margin
Payor Worksheet:						
Capitated	**3,161**	$6,250	**$ 19,754,816**	$1,903	**$ 6,015,512**	**$ 13,739,304**
Medicare	4,268	7,327	31,271,636	2,529	10,793,772	20,477,864
Medicaid	4,716	5,448	25,692,768	1,575	7,427,700	18,265,068
Montana Care	828	4,305	3,564,540	1,907	1,578,996	1,985,544
Managed Care	1,885	3,842	7,242,170	1,638	3,087,630	4,154,540
Blue Cross	332	5,761	1,912,652	2,366	785,512	1,127,140
Commercial	845	11,770	9,943,296	2,969	2,508,211	7,435,085
Self Pay	773	2,053	1,587,790	1,489	1,151,593	436,198
Other	1,149	11,539	13,258,331	3,085	3,544,665	9,713,646
Total	**17,957**		**$ 114,227,979**		**$36,893,591**	**$77,334,388**
Weighted average		**$6,361**		**$2,055**		

P&L Statement:

Total revenues	**$ 114,227,979**
Variable costs	**36,893,591**
Contribution margin	**$ 71,334,388**
Fixed costs	71,746,561
Net income	**$ 5,587,827**

Note: Some rounding differences occur in the table.

per enrollee is $564.48 − $171.84 = $392.64, and 10,000 new enrollees would add $3,926,400 to the bottom line, which is the same as calculated previously, except for a rounding difference.

   This analysis confirms the benefit that would accrue to MMC if the capitated plan does indeed increase the hospital's market share. Note, however, that the increased market share analysis has several key assumptions, notably that the premium remains at $47.04 PMPM and utilization and costs associated with new enrollees are the same as the initial cannibalized enrollees.

   What would happen if the initial premium of $47.04 PMPM is too high and MMC has to lower it to $40 to be attractive in the marketplace? To examine the effects of a lower premium, consider the analysis presented in Table 7.6. In this case, the assumption is that a premium of $40 results in the same 35,000 enrollees as analyzed in the last scenario. The only changes from Table 7.5 stem from the reduced revenues associated with lowering the premium from $47.04 PMPM to $40 PMPM, or by $7.04 PMPM. The loss of annual revenue of 35,000 × $7.04 × 12 = $2,956,800 with no offsetting reduction in costs flows directly to the bottom line. The end result is a corresponding reduction in net income, except for a rounding difference.

   It would be useful for MMC's managers to know what premium would be required to obtain the original forecasted net income of $1,662,312 (see Tables 7.1 and 7.3), assuming a capitated plan enrollment of 35,000. By using

TABLE 7.6
Montana Medical
Center (MMC):
Pro-Forma Analysis
Assuming 35,000
Enrollees at $40
PMPM

Payor	Number of Admissions	Average Revenue per Admission	Revenues by Payor	Variable Cost per Admission	Total Variable Costs	Contribution Margin
Payor Worksheet:						
Capitated	3,161	**$5,315**	$ 16,800,000	$1,903	$ 6,015,512	**$10,784,488**
Medicare	4,268	7,327	31,271,636	2,529	10,793,772	20,477,864
Medicaid	4,716	5,448	25,692,768	1,575	7,427,700	18,265,068
Montana Care	828	4,305	3,564,540	1,907	1,578,996	1,985,544
Managed Care	1,885	3,842	7,242,170	1,638	3,087,630	4,154,540
Blue Cross	332	5,761	1,912,652	2,366	785,512	1,127,140
Commercial	845	11,770	9,943,296	2,969	2,508,211	7,435,085
Self-Pay	773	2,053	1,587,790	1,489	1,151,593	436,198
Other	1,149	11,539	13,258,331	3,085	3,544,665	9,713,646
Total	17,957		$ 111,273,163		$36,893,591	$ 74,379,573
Weighted average		**$6,197**		**$2,055**		

P&L Statement:

Total revenues	$ 111,273,163
Variable costs	36,893,591
Contribution margin	$ 74,379,573
Fixed costs	71,746,561
Net income	$ 2,633,012

Note: Some rounding differences occur in the table.

a spreadsheet model, MMC's managers found that a PMPM premium of about $37.69 would produce a net income of $1,662,312. Therefore, MMC could lower the premium to that amount, if necessary, to obtain 35,000 enrollees without reducing its net income below the initial forecast. Furthermore, MMC could set the premium as low as $33.73 and still break even overall (i.e., have a forecasted net income of zero), assuming 35,000 enrollees.

Finally, consider the value inherent in utilization and cost reduction efforts. Suppose that MMC actually obtained 25,000 enrollees at a premium of $47.04. The expected net income in this scenario is $1,662,312 (see Table 7.3). However, assume that MMC instituted a utilization review process that lowered annual utilization rates for capitated enrollees from the current 0.0903 admissions per enrollee to 0.08 admissions per enrollee for a reduction of about 11 percent. Furthermore, assume that MMC conducted a review of its clinical guidelines for capitated patients, which results in a variable cost-per-admission reduction from $1,903 per admission to $1,800 per admission, or by about 5 percent. The results of such utilization and cost control efforts are shown in Table 7.7.

Again, the changes from Table 7.3 occur on the first line of the payor worksheet, except for aggregate and average values. The overall result is that variable costs, both for capitated patients and in total, are lowered by $35,174,873 − $34,478,079 = $696,794, so net income increases to $1,662,312 + $696,794 = $2,359,106. A reduction in utilization alone produces a cost savings of $490,616,

TABLE 7.7 Montana Medical Center (MMC): Pro-Forma Analysis Assuming 25,000 Enrollees at $47.04 PMPM plus Utilization and Cost Improvements

Payor	Number of Admissions	Average Revenue per Admission	Revenues by Payor	Variable Cost per Admission	Total Variable Costs	Contribution Margin
Payor Worksheet:						
Capitated	**2,000**	**$7,055**	$ 14,110,583	**$1,800**	$ 3,600,000	**$10,510,583**
Medicare	4,268	7,327	31,271,636	2,529	10,793,772	20,477,864
Medicaid	4,716	5,448	25,692,768	1,575	7,427,700	18,265,068
Montana Care	828	4,305	3,564,540	1,907	1,578,996	1,985,544
Managed Care	1,885	3,842	7,242,170	1,638	3,087,630	4,154,540
Blue Cross	332	5,761	1,912,652	2,366	785,512	1,127,140
Commercial	845	11,770	9,943,296	2,969	2,508,211	7,435,085
Self-Pay	773	2,053	1,587,790	1,489	1,151,593	436,198
Other	1,149	11,539	13,258,331	3,085	3,544,665	9,713,646
Total	16,796		$108,583,746		$34,478,079	$ 74,105,667
Weighted average		**$6,465**		**$2,053**		

P&L Statement:

Total revenues	$108,583,746
Variable costs	34,478,079
Contribution margin	$ 74,105,667
Fixed costs	71,746,561
Net income	$ 2,359,106

Note: Some rounding differences occur in the table.

and a reduction in variable cost per admission alone produces a cost savings of $232,754. Each effort, therefore, contributes to the projected increase in MMC's profitability.[3] The utilization and cost cutting benefits would be even greater if they could be applied to payor groups other than capitated enrollees.

Self-Test Questions

1. Briefly explain why the base case analysis required the calculation to move up the income statement rather than down (the normal direction).
2. How are capitated revenue requirements typically expressed?
3. What is sensitivity analysis and why is it so critical to good pricing decisions?
4. What is the most uncertain variable in MMC's capitated plan pricing analysis?

Illustration III: Managed Care Plan Premium Rate

A primary finance task within managed care plans and integrated delivery systems (IDSs) is the development of premium rates. In this section, several methods that an HMO or an IDS can use to estimate the payments it must make to its providers to cover a defined population are illustrated, which it can then aggregate and combine with its own costs to estimate a premium rate. Rates typically are developed as if all providers in the system were capitated because the final premium rate will be quoted on a PMPM basis. However, actual reimbursement to the providers in the plan (or system) could be by capitation, discounted fee-for-service, or another method.

Assume that BetterCare, Inc., an aggressively managed HMO, must develop a premium bid to submit to Big Business, a major employer in the BetterCare service area. To keep the illustration manageable, assume that all medically necessary in-area services can be provided by a single hospital that offers both inpatient and outpatient services including emergency room services, a single nursing home, a panel of primary care physicians, and a panel of specialist physicians. In addition, BetterCare must budget for covered care to be delivered out of area when its members are traveling. Thus, to develop its bid, BetterCare has to estimate the amount of payments to this set of providers for the covered population, plus allow for administrative expenses and profits.

Institutional Rates

The *fee-for-service equivalent method* is often used to set the within-system hospital inpatient capitation rate. This method is based on expected utilization and negotiated charges rather than underlying costs, although there clearly should be a link between charges and costs. To illustrate, assume that BetterCare targets 350 inpatient days for each 1,000 members, or 0.350 inpatient days per member. Furthermore, BetterCare believes that a fair fee-for-service charge in a competitive environment would be $938 per inpatient day. The number of inpatient days reflects a highly managed working-age population, and the fee-for-service charge is designed to cover all hospital costs, including profits, in an efficiently run hospital that operates in a highly competitive environment. The inpatient cost PMPM is found this way:

$$\text{Inpatient cost PMPM} = \frac{\text{Per member utilization rate} \times \text{Fee-for-service rate}}{12}$$

$$= \frac{0.350 \times \$938}{12} = \$27.35 \text{ PMPM}.$$

Thus, using the fee-for-service equivalent method, BetterCare estimates that inpatient costs for Big Business' HMO enrollees is $27.35 PMPM.

The rates for out-of-area hospital usage, hospital outpatient visits, and skilled nursing home stays also were developed using the fee-for-service equivalent method. Here is a summary of BetterCare's estimates for these services:

Service	Annual Usage per 1,000 Members	Fee-For-Service Rate	Capitation Rate PMPM
Out-of-area inpatient days	25	$1,495	$3.11
Outpatient surgeries	50	1,082	4.51
Emergency room visits	125	138	1.44
Skilled nursing home days	5	150	0.06
			$9.12

Here, each PMPM capitation rate was calculated by multiplying annual usage by the fee-for-service rate and dividing the resulting product first by 1,000 to obtain a per member amount, and then by 12 to get the PMPM rate. The end result is a capitation estimate of $9.12 PMPM for the services listed. Actual payments to these providers typically would be made on a fee-for-service basis.

Physician Rates

The *budgetary*, or *cost*, *approach* will be used to estimate physicians' costs for Big Business' enrollees. This method, which is the most common for setting physicians' payments, is based on usage and underlying costs as opposed to charges. The starting point is expected patient demand, by specialty, for physicians' services. This demand is then translated into the number of full-time equivalent (FTE) physicians required per 1,000 enrollees, which depends on physician productivity. Finally, the cost for physician services is estimated by multiplying physician staffing requirements by the average cost per FTE, including base compensation, fringe benefits, and malpractice premiums. In addition, an amount is added for clinical and administrative support for physicians, usually some dollar amount per 1,000 members.

In developing its rate for primary care physicians, BetterCare made the following assumptions:

- On average, each enrollee makes 3.0 visits to a primary care physician per year, so each 1,000 enrollees make 3,000 visits per year.

- Each primary care physician can handle 4,000 patient visits per year.
- Total compensation per primary care physician is $175,000 per year.

Under these assumptions, each 1,000 enrollees will require 3,000 / 4,000 = 0.75 primary care physicians, and hence each 1,000 enrollees will require 0.75 × $175,000 = $131,250 in primary care physicians' services. Finally, the annual cost per member is $131,250 / 1,000 = $131.25 and the cost PMPM = $131.25/12 = $10.94. Thus, the rate that BetterCare will propose to Big Business will include a payment of $10.94 PMPM for primary care physician compensation.

The rate for specialists' care is developed in a similar way. Here are Better-Care's assumptions:

- On average, each enrollee is referred for 1.2 visits to specialty care physicians per year, so each 1,000 enrollees make 1,200 visits per year.
- Each physician specialist can handle 2,000 patient visits per year.
- Total compensation per specialist is $284,000 per year.

Under these assumptions, each 1,000 enrollees will require 1,200 / 2,000 = 0.60 specialists. Thus, each 1,000 enrollees will require 0.60 × $284,000 = $170,400 in specialists' services. Finally, the annual cost per member is $170,400 / 1,000 = $170.40, so the cost PMPM = $170.40 / 12 = $14.20. The rate that BetterCare will propose to Big Business will therefore include a payment of $14.20 PMPM for physician specialist compensation.

Thus far, the capitation rate for physicians' compensation has been estimated, but BetterCare's analysis has not accounted for the other costs associated with physicians' practices. First, on average, physicians require 1.7 FTEs for clinical and administrative support, and each supporting staff member receives an average of $35,000 per year in total compensation. Because the physician requirement to support 1,000 members is 0.75 primary care plus 0.60 specialists, for a total of 1.35 physicians, each 1,000 members will require 1.35 × 1.7 × $35,000 ≈ $80,000 of physician's support, or $80,000 / 1,000 / 12 = $6.67 PMPM.

Next, expenditures on supplies, including administrative, medical, and diagnostic supplies, average $10 per visit and members are expected to make 4.2 visits per year to both primary and specialty care physicians. Thus, the annual cost per member is $42 and the cost PMPM is estimated to be $42 / 12 = $3.50 PMPM. Finally, overhead expenses including depreciation, rent, utilities, and so on are estimated at $6.00 PMPM.

BetterCare has estimated numerous categories of costs attributable solely to physicians. For ease, assume that BetterCare plans to contract with a single medical group practice to provide all physicians' services and to pay the group a capitated rate. The total capitation rate for the medical group would be as follows:

Primary care	$10.94	PMPM
Specialist care	14.20	
Support staff	6.67	
Supplies	3.50	
Overhead	6.00	
Subtotal	$41.31	PMPM
Profit (10%)	4.13	
In-area total	$45.44	PMPM
Outside referrals	3.40	
Total	$48.84	PMPM

The $48.84 PMPM total capitation rate for the medical group is the aggregate of the rates previously developed for physicians' services, plus two additional elements. First, BetterCare believes that a fair profit margin on medical services is 10 percent, so $4.13 PMPM is allowed for profit on the in-area physician subtotal of $41.31 PMPM. Second, $3.40 PMPM is allocated to cover referrals outside the group practice when needed either because a particular specialty is not available within the group or the covered member is outside the service area. Finally, note that the medical group may not capitate all its physicians, even though it receives a capitated rate from BetterCare.

In general, the rates obtained from the first two methods would include adjustments for age and sex. An alternative method would be to start with utilization data broken down by age and sex. The *demographic based approach* focuses on the age/sex distribution of the population being served, which is then coupled with cost or fee-for-service data to estimate the capitation rate. Table 7.8 illustrates the demographic based approach by applying it to the population that would be served if BetterCare wins the contract to provide a HMO plan for Big Business. The male/female costs were calculated by multiplying the population percentages for each sex by the applicable costs PMPM. The total cost for each service is the sum of the male and female costs.

The total cost for physicians, $16.17 + $29.27 = $45.44 PMPM, is the same as BetterCare estimated using the budgetary approach. If the data are consistent, both methods should lead to the same capitation rate. Also, the hospital/other institutional capitation rate of $36.47 PMPM is the same as the rate obtained earlier for these services: $27.35 + $9.12 = $36.47. Clearly, the data were fudged so the results would be consistent. In most cases, capitation rates that are developed using different methodologies will be different, and hence a great deal of judgment must be applied in the rate-setting process.

Setting the Final Rate

The goal in this illustration is to set a premium rate that BetterCare can use to make a bid to cover Big Business' employees. Thus far, the capitation rates required to pay all the providers needed to serve the population have been estimated for both in-area and out-of-area services. The assumption is that pharmacy and durable medical equipment (DME) benefits will be handled separately, or *carved out*, and

TABLE 7.8
Demographic
Based Rates

| | Demographics | | Cost Per Member Per Month | | | | | |
| | | | Primary Care | | Specialist/Referral | | Hospital/Other | |
Age Band	Male	Female	Male	Female	Male	Female	Male	Female
0–1	1.9%	1.9%	$47.00	$47.00	$31.42	$31.42	$ 29.93	$29.93
2–4	2.8	2.8	20.25	20.25	11.19	11.19	16.29	16.29
5–19	12.4	12.4	11.04	11.04	11.19	11.19	15.35	15.35
20–29	11.4	15.4	10.53	15.92	18.44	49.30	11.58	55.65
30–39	9.6	10.0	13.04	17.56	23.26	44.51	24.95	58.97
40–49	5.3	5.7	16.40	19.56	32.64	41.05	53.74	52.31
50–59	3.6	3.6	20.74	22.74	47.13	47.74	80.60	66.91
60+	0.7	0.5	24.93	25.60	73.43	58.91	121.54	87.60
Total	47.7%	52.3%						
Male/female cost			$ 7.07	$ 9.10	$10.58	$18.69	$ 13.24	$23.23
Total service cost			$16.17		$29.27		$36.47	

that the cost of these benefits would be $7.00 PMPM. After all costs have been considered, BetterCare's managers conclude that they should submit a bid of $108.21 PMPM.

Hospital inpatient	$ 27.35	PMPM
Other institutional	9.12	
Pharmacy and DME benefits	7.00	
Physician care	48.84	
Total medical care costs	$ 92.31	PMPM
HMO costs:		
Administration	$ 13.85	PMPM
Contribution to reserves/profits	2.05	
Total HMO costs	$ 15.90	PMPM
Total premium	$108.21	PMPM

If BetterCare wins the contract from Big Business, the monthly revenue to providers usually will be about 5 percent higher than the embedded capitated rates because enrollees will be required to make copayments for selected services.

BetterCare's bid most likely will be subject to market forces. That is, there will be multiple bidders for Big Business' health contract. If BetterCare's bid is to be accepted, it must offer the right combination of price and quality. If BetterCare's costs, and therefore bid, is too high, or its quality is too low, it will not get the contract. In that case, it must reassess its cost and quality structure to ensure that it is competitive on future bids.

Self-Test Questions

1. Briefly describe the following three methods for developing premium rates:
   a. Fee-for-service equivalent method
   b. Budgetary, or cost, approach
   c. Demographic based approach

2. Of the three approaches, which one would be the most accurate? Which approach is the easiest to apply in practice?

3. It is common to express premium rates as PMPM. Does this mean that all providers will be capitated?

Illustration IV: Hospital Service Decision

The primary focus of the Montana Medical Center (MMC) and BetterCare HMO illustrations was price setting. This illustration moves to a related decision—the service decision.

Base Case Analysis

County Health Plan (CHP), an HMO with 40,000 members, has proposed a new contract that would capitate Baptist Memorial Hospital for all inpatient services provided to CHP's commercial enrollees whose primary care physicians are affiliated with the hospital. The proposal calls for a capitation payment of $35 PMPM for the first year of the contract. Baptist's managers must make the decision whether or not to accept the proposal.

To begin the analysis, Baptist's managed care analysts developed the inpatient actuarial data contained in Table 7.9. The data are presented under two levels of utilization management. The data in the top section, Loosely Managed (Suboptimal) Utilization, are based on a loosely managed delivery system in Baptist's service area. These data represent a bare minimum of utilization management effort, and hence reflect relatively poor utilization management practices. The bottom section, Tightly Managed (Optimal) Utilization, contains data that represent the best-observed practices throughout the United States. These data are based on hospitals located in service areas that have extremely high managed care penetration. The differences between the two data sets illustrate the potential for improved financial performance that comes with more sophisticated utilization management systems. Both sets of data reflect populations with characteristics similar to CHP's commercial enrollees.

To illustrate the calculations, consider the top line in the top section (General). Under loosely managed utilization, the covered population is expected to utilize 157 days of general medical services for each 1,000 enrollees. Furthermore, the costs associated with one day of such services total $1,500. Thus, the general services costs for each 1,000 enrollees are expected to be $157 \times \$1,500 = \$235,500$, or $19.62 PMPM. Calculations for other inpatient services were performed similarly, and added to obtain total medical costs of $50.39 PMPM.

There are two additional categories of costs besides medical costs. Each section of the table has lines for administrative costs and risk margin. Administrative costs include costs incurred in managing the contract, such as those associated with

TABLE 7.9

CHP/Baptist
Memorial Hospital:
Contract Analysis
Under Two
Utilization
Management
Scenarios

Loosely Managed (Sub-optimal) Utilization:

Service Category	Inpatient Days per 1,000 Enrollees	Average Cost per Day	Average Cost Per Member Per Month*
General	157	$1,500	$19.62
Surgical	132	1,800	19.80
Psychiatric	71	700	4.14
Alcohol/Drug abuse	38	500	1.58
Maternity	42	1,500	5.25
Total medical costs	440	$1,374	$50.39
Administrative costs			2.80
Risk (profit) margin			2.80
Total			$55.99

Tightly Managed (Optimal) Utilization:

Service Category	Inpatient Days per 1,000 Enrollees	Average Cost per Day	Average Cost Per Member Per Month*
General	79	$1,600	$10.53
Surgical	58	1,900	9.18
Psychiatric	13	800	0.87
Alcohol/Drug abuse	4	600	0.20
Maternity	26	1,600	3.47
Total medical costs	180	$1,617	$24.25
Administrative costs			1.35
Risk (profit) margin			1.35
Total			$26.95

*Based on 40,000 members (enrollees).
Note: Some rounding differences occur in the table.

patient verification, utilization management, quality assurance, and member services. The second category of nonmedical costs is the *risk (profit) margin*. Because Baptist would be bearing inpatient utilization risk for the covered population, it builds in a margin both to provide a profit on the contract commensurate with the risk assumed and to create a reserve that could be tapped if utilization, and hence costs, exceeds the amount estimated. It is Baptist's practice to allow 10 percent of the total premium for these two nonmedical costs, so medical costs represent 90 percent of the total premium. For example, in the upper section of Table 7.9, 0.9 × Total Premium = $50.39, so Total Premium = $50.39 / 0.9 = $55.99. Furthermore, it is Baptist's policy to evenly split the $55.99 − $50.39 = $5.60 in nonmedical costs evenly between the two categories, so administrative costs and risk margin are allocated $2.80 each.[4]

Table 7.9 sends a strong message to Baptist's managers regarding the acceptability of CHP's $35 PMPM contract offer. If Baptist were to accept the offer, and then loosely manage utilization for the enrollee population, it would lose $55.99 − $35 = $20.99 PMPM on the contract. The costs in Table 7.9 represent full costs as opposed to only variable (marginal) costs. Baptist may therefore be able to carry the contract in the short run, but it would not be able to sustain the contract over time. On the other hand, if Baptist could manage the enrollee population in accordance with "best-observed practices," it would make a profit of $35 − $26.95 = $8.05 PMPM on the contract.

A common practice when analyzing contracts is to express the PMPM premium as a percentage of PMPM costs, which is often defined as the *target premium*. Thus, under loosely managed utilization, the proposed premium is $35 / $55.99 = 0.625 = 62.5% of the target, while under tightly managed utilization, the premium is $35 / $26.95 = 1.30 = 130% of the target. To be acceptable over the long term, the premium-to-costs ratio must be greater than 100 percent, which indicates that the premium is greater than the estimated full costs of providing the service.

The contract also can be analyzed in accounting rather than actuarial terms. This format, along with the required worksheet, is shown in Table 7.10. Again, focus on the loosely managed utilization section. In Table 7.10, instead of showing inpatient days per 1,000 enrollees as in Table 7.9, inpatient days are expressed in terms of the total number of enrollees, which is expected to be 40,000 for this contract. Thus, using utilization data from Table 7.9, the total number of patient days of general medical services is 157 × 40,000 = 6,280. With an estimated cost of $1,500 per day, total costs for general medical services amount to 6,280 × $1,500 = $9,420,000. The costs for all service categories were calculated in the same way and total $24,192,000. Each nonmedical service cost was calculated as 40,000 × $2.80 × 12 = $1,344,000, which results in total costs under loosely managed utilization of $26,880,000.

Regardless of the level of utilization management, revenues from the contract are expected to total 40,000 × $35 × 12 = $16,800,000. Thus, the proforma P&L statements, in simplified form, consist of this revenue amount minus total costs under each utilization scenario. The end result is an expected net income of −$10,080,000 under loosely managed utilization, and $3,864,000 under tightly managed utilization.

Note that the actuarial data presented in Table 7.9 could also have been used to determine expected net income. To illustrate, consider the loosely managed utilization scenario. With a premium of $35 PMPM and estimated costs of $55.99 PMPM, the net income spread is $35 − $55.99 = −$20.99 PMPM on each enrollee. With 40,000 enrollees and 12 months in a year, total net income must be 40,000 ×−$20.99 × 12 = −$10,075,200, which, except for a rounding difference, is the same amount shown in Table 7.10.

TABLE 7.10
CHP/Baptist
Memorial Hospital:
Pro-Forma Cost
Worksheets and
P&L Statements

COST WORKSHEETS:
Loosely Managed (Sub-optimal) Utilization:

Service Category	Inpatient Days per 40,000 Enrollees	Average Cost per Day	Total Annual Cost
General	6,280	$1,500	$ 9,420,000
Surgical	5,280	1,800	9,504,000
Psychiatric	2,840	700	1,988,000
Alcohol/Drug abuse	1,520	500	760,000
Maternity	1,680	1,500	2,520,000
Total medical costs	17,600	$1,374	$24,192,000
Administrative costs			1,344,000
Risk (profit) margin			1,344,000
Total			$26,880,000

Tightly Managed (Optimal) Utilization:

Service Category	Inpatient Days per 40,000 Enrollees	Average Cost per Day	Total Annual Cost
General	3,160	$1,600	$ 5,056,000
Surgical	2,320	1,900	4,408,000
Psychiatric	520	800	416,000
Alcohol/Drug abuse	160	600	96,000
Maternity	1,040	1,600	1,664,000
Total medical costs	7,200	$1,617	$ 11,640,000
Administrative costs			648,000
Risk (profit) margin			648,000
Total			$12,936,000

P&L STATEMENTS:
Loosely Managed (Sub-optimal) Utilization:

Total revenues	$16,800,000
Total costs	26,880,000
Net income	($10,080,000)

Tightly Managed (Optimal) Utilization:

Total revenues	$16,800,000
Total costs	12,936,000
Net income	$ 3,864,000

Note: Some rounding differences occur in the table.

What should Baptist's managers do regarding the contract? For now, the decision appears simplistic: accept the contract if the hospital can tightly manage utilization or reject the contract if it cannot. Unfortunately, the base case contract analysis, like many financial analyses, raises more questions than it answers. This demonstrates that analyses conducted to help with pricing and service decisions tend more to raise managers' awareness of potential consequences than offer simple solutions.

Sensitivity Analysis

Suppose that Baptist's managers believe that, right now, the hospital's utilization management is poor and that utilization and costs during the first year of the contract are likely to be those associated with loosely managed utilization. However, utilization management would so improve over time that by the third year, utilization and costs would likely be those associated with tightly managed utilization. During the second year, utilization and costs would fall between the two extremes. Under these assumptions, how does the contract look?

Table 7.11 contains the same information shown in Table 7.9, except that a middle section is added to reflect moderately managed utilization.[5] Using the PMPM spread approach discussed in the last section, the projected annual and average net incomes are as follows:

$$\text{Year 1: } 40{,}000 \times (\$35 - \$55.99) \times 12 = -\$10{,}075{,}200$$

$$\text{Year 2: } 40{,}000 \times (\$35 - \$43.46) \times 12 = -\$\ 4{,}060{,}800$$

$$\text{Year 3: } 40{,}000 \times (\$35 - \$26.95) \times 12 = \quad \$\ 3{,}864{,}000$$

Three-year average =	$-\$\ 3{,}423{,}733$
Five-year average =	$-\$\quad 508{,}800$
Six-year average =	$\$\quad 220{,}000$

When considering the long-term consequences of the contract, Baptist would, on average, lose money on the contract over five years, but profit if the contract continued for six or more years.[6]

What else would Baptist's managers want to know prior to making the decision? One key element of information is the cost structure (fixed versus variable) associated with the contract. Even though the analyses indicate that the contract is unprofitable in the short term, the analysis has been on a full-cost basis. If the costs associated with the contract consist of 50 percent fixed costs and 50 percent variable costs, the variable cost PMPM in the worst case (loosely managed utilization) would be $0.50 \times \$55.99 = \$28.00$. At a premium of $35, the PMPM contribution margin is $\$35 - \$28 = \$7$. Thus, even under loose utilization management, the premium would at least cover the contract's variable costs. If Baptist cannot afford to lose the market share associated with CHP's members, its managers may deem the contract acceptable in the short run. Assuming that the hospital can improve its utilization management over time, it will be able to eventually cover the total costs associated with the contract.

TABLE 7.11

CHP/Baptist
Memorial Hospital:
Contract Analysis
Under Three
Utilization
Management
Scenarios

Loosely Managed Utilization:

Service Category	Inpatient Days per 1,000 Enrollees	Average Cost per Day	Average Cost Per Member Per Month*
General	157	$1,500	$19.62
Surgical	132	1,800	19.80
Psychiatric	71	700	4.14
Alcohol/Drug abuse	38	500	1.58
Maternity	42	1,500	5.25
Total medical costs	440	$1,374	$50.39
Administrative costs			2.80
Risk (profit) margin			2.80
Total			$55.99

Moderately Managed Utilization:

Service Category	Inpatient Days per 1,000 Enrollees	Average Cost per Day	Average Cost Per Member Per Month*
General	118	$1,550	$15.24
Surgical	95	1,850	14.65
Psychiatric	42	750	2.62
Alcohol/Drug abuse	21	550	0.96
Maternity	34	1,550	4.39
Total medical costs	310	$1,466	$37.86
Administrative costs			2.80
Risk (profit) margin			2.80
Total			$43.46

Tightly Managed Utilization:

Service Category	Inpatient Days per 1,000 Enrollees	Average Cost per Day	Average Cost Per Member Per Month*
General	79	$1,600	$10.53
Surgical	58	1,900	9.18
Psychiatric	13	800	0.87
Alcohol/Drug abuse	4	600	0.20
Maternity	26	1,600	3.47
Total medical costs	180	$1,617	$24.25
Administrative costs			2.08
Risk (profit) margin			2.08
Total			$26.95

*Assuming 40,000 members (enrollees).

Note: Some rounding differences occur in the table.

Cost structure is not the only variable that can change over time. Perhaps Baptist can demonstrate superior quality and negotiate a higher premium over time. On the down side, perhaps CHP will gain additional market power over time and push the premium lower. These are just a few of the imponderables that Baptist's managers must consider when making the service decision.

Self-Test Questions

1. Why does utilization management play such an important role in pricing and service decisions under capitation?
2. Why are nonmedical costs included in the analysis?
3. What would you do regarding the contract if you were the CEO of Baptist Memorial Hospital?
4. What other factors should Baptist's managers consider when making the capitation contract decision?

Key Concepts

Managers rely on managerial accounting and actuarial information to help make pricing and service decisions. Pricing decisions involve setting prices on services for which the provider is a price setter, while service decisions involve whether or not to offer a service when the price is set by the payor (the provider is a price taker). The key concepts of this chapter are:

- *Pricing* and *service strategies* are linked to an organization's financial statements and the need for revenues to (1) cover the full cost of doing business, and (2) provide the profits necessary to acquire new technologies and offer new services.
- *Price takers* are healthcare providers that have to accept, more or less, the prices set in the marketplace for their services, including the prices set by governmental insurers.
- *Price setters* are healthcare providers whose services can be differentiated from others either by market share or by quality or other differences such that they have the ability to set the prices on some or all of their services.
- *Full-cost pricing* permits businesses to recover all costs, including both fixed and variable and direct and indirect, whereas *marginal-cost pricing* recovers only variable costs, and *direct-cost pricing* recovers only direct costs.
- In *competitive pricing*, a health services organization sets prices as dictated by market conditions, regardless of its internal cost structure.
- Purchasers of healthcare services are now exercising considerable market power, thereby restricting the ability of providers to *cross subsidize* (*price shift*).
- *Target costing* is a concept that takes the prices paid for healthcare services as a given and then determines the cost structure necessary for financial survival given the set prices.
- Three primary techniques are used to develop capitation rates: *fee-for-service equivalent method, budgetary* or *cost approach,* and the *demographic based approach.*

- Pricing and service decisions are supported by a variety of analyses that use both actuarial and accounting data. Typically, such analyses include a *base case*, which uses the best estimates for all input values, plus *sensitivity analyses* that consider the effects of alternative assumptions.

In the next chapter the coverage of managerial accounting turns to planning and budgeting.

Questions

7.1 a. Using a healthcare provider (e.g., a hospital) to illustrate your answer, explain the difference between a price setter and a price taker.
b. Can most providers be classified strictly as price setters or a price takers?

7.2 Explain the essential differences among the following four pricing strategies: full-cost, marginal-cost, direct-cost, and competitive pricing.

7.3 What would happen financially to a health services organization over time if its prices were set at:
a. Full costs
b. Marginal costs
c. Direct costs
d. Competitive rates

7.4 a. What is cross subsidization (price shifting)?
b. Is it as prevalent today as it has been in the past?

7.5 a. What is target costing?
b. Suppose a hospital was offered a capitation rate for a covered population of $40 per member per month (PMPM). Briefly explain how target costing would be applied in this situation.

7.6 What is the role of information systems in pricing decisions?

7.7 Compare and contrast the following three methods for developing capitation rates: fee-for-service equivalent method, budgetary or cost approach, and the demographic based approach.

7.8 a. What is sensitivity analysis as applied to pricing and service decisions?
b. Why is it such an important part of the process?

Problems

7.1 Assume that the managers of Fort Winston Hospital are setting the price on a new outpatient service. Here are relevant data estimates:

Variable cost per visit	$5.00
Annual direct fixed costs	$500,000
Annual overhead allocation	$50,000
Expected annual utilization	10,000 visits

a. What per visit price must be set for the service to break even? To earn an annual profit of $100,000?

b. Repeat Part a, but assume that the variable cost per visit is $10.

c. Return to the data given in the problem. Again repeat Part a, but assume that direct fixed costs are $1,000,000.

d. Repeat Part a assuming both a $10 variable cost and $1,000,000 in direct fixed costs.

7.2 The Audiology Department at Randall Clinic offers many services to the clinic's patients. The three most common, along with cost and utilization data, are:

Service	Variable Cost per Service	Annual Direct Fixed Costs	Annual Number of Visits
Basic examination	$ 5	$50,000	3,000
Advanced examination	7	30,000	1,500
Therapy session	10	40,000	500

a. What is the fee schedule for these services, assuming that the goal is to cover only variable and direct fixed costs?

b. Assume that the Audiology Department is allocated $100,000 in total overhead by the clinic and the department director has allocated $50,000 of this amount to the three services listed above. What is the fee schedule assuming that these overhead costs must be covered? (To answer this question, assume that the allocation of overhead costs to each service is made on the basis of number of visits.)

c. Assume that these services must make a combined profit of $25,000. Now what is the fee schedule? (To answer this question, assume that the profit requirement is allocated in the same way as overhead costs.)

7.3 Allied Laboratories is combining some of its most common tests into one-price packages. One such package will contain three tests having the following variable costs:

	Test A	Test B	Test C
Disposable syringe	$3.00	$3.00	$3.00
Blood vial	0.50	0.50	0.50
Forms	0.15	0.15	0.15
Reagents	0.80	0.60	1.20
Sterile bandage	0.10	0.10	0.10
Breakage/losses	0.05	0.05	0.05

When the tests are combined, only one syringe, form, and sterile bandage will be used. Furthermore, only one charge for breakage/losses will apply. Two blood vials are required and reagent costs will remain the same (reagents from all three tests are required).

a. As a starting point, what is the price of the combined test assuming marginal-cost pricing?

b. Assume that Allied wants a contribution margin of $10 per test. What price must be set to achieve this goal?

c. Allied estimates that 2,000 of the combined tests will be conducted during the first year. The annual allocation of direct fixed and overhead costs total $40,000. What price must be set to cover full costs? What price must be set to produce a profit of $20,000 on the combined test?

7.4 Assume that Valley Forge Hospital has only the following three payor groups:

Payor	Number of Admissions	Average Revenue per Admission	Variable Cost per Admission
PennCare	1,000	$5,000	$3,000
Medicare	4,000	4,500	4,000
Commercial	8,000	7,000	2,500

The hospital's fixed costs are $38 million.

a. What is the hospital's net income?
b. Assume that half of the 100,000 covered lives in the commercial payor group will be moved into a capitated plan. All utilization and cost data remain the same. What PMPM rate will the hospital have to charge to retain their Part a net income?
c. What overall net income would be produced if the admission rate of the capitated group were reduced from the commercial level by 10 percent?
d. Assuming that the utilization reduction also occurs, what overall net income would be produced if the variable cost per admission for the capitated group were lowered to $2,200?

7.5 Bay Pines Medical Center estimates that a capitated population of 50,000 would have the following base case utilization and total cost characteristics:

Service Category	Inpatient Days per 1,000 Enrollees	Average Cost per Day
General	150	$1,500
Surgical	125	1,800
Psychiatric	70	700
Alcohol/Drug abuse	38	500
Maternity	42	1,500
Total	440	$1,374

In addition to medical costs, Bay Pines allocates 10 percent of the total premium for administration/reserves.

a. What is the PMPM rate that Bay Pines must set to cover medical costs plus administrative expenses?
b. What would be the rate if a utilization management program would reduce utilization within each patient service category by 10 percent? By 20 percent?
c. Return to the initial base case utilization assumption. What rate would be set if the average cost on each service were reduced by 10 percent?

d. Assume that both utilization and cost reductions were made. What would the premium be?

Notes

1. The values in Tables 7.1 and 7.3 were obtained from a spreadsheet analysis, which does not round to the nearest dollar when performing calculations. Thus, some minor rounding differences occur when the calculations are made by hand.

2. In Chapter 15, a point is made to distinguish between sensitivity analysis and scenario analysis. However, for purposes here, the terms are used interchangeably. Essentially, when input values are changed to create alternative scenarios, the determination being made is how sensitive the results are to changes in underlying assumptions.

3. The two cost savings amounts total $490,616 + $232,754 = $723,370, which is greater than the $696,794 savings realized if both efforts were undertaken. This apparent anomaly occurs because a reduction in admissions lowers the value of the reduction in variable costs by $258 \times \$103 = \$26,574$, which, except for a rounding difference, equals $723,370 − $696,794 = $26,576.

4. Baptist's managers use the same 10 percent nonmedical cost allocation for both the loosely and tightly managed utilization scenarios. One could argue that the greater the utilization management effort, the higher the administrative costs. Thus, it may be better to allocate a greater percentage for administrative costs in the tightly managed scenario than in the loosely managed scenario. In fact, administrative costs could require a higher dollar allocation under tightly managed utilization, even though the overall premium amount is lower.

5. This analysis, although useful, ignores two very important points. First, it is likely that both costs and premiums will change over time because of inflation, if not changes in technology. Second, by merely averaging the forecasted net incomes, the time value of money, an important finance concept that is discussed in Chapter 9, is being ignored.

6. Total costs under moderately managed utilization ($43.46) do **not** equal the average of the total costs under the loosely and tightly managed utilization scenarios ([$55.99 + $26.95]/2 = $41.47). The difference occurs because the two variables that change (inpatient days per 1,000 enrollees and average cost per day) are multiplied together to get PMPM costs. If only one of the variables changes or if the two variables were added together instead of multiplied, total costs under moderately managed utilization would be the average of the other two scenarios.

References

Anderson, G. F., et al. 1990. "Setting Payment Rates for Capitated Systems: A Comparison of Various Alternatives." *Inquiry* (Fall): 225–233.

Baker, J. J., P. Chiverton, and V. Hines. 1998. "Identifying Costs for Capitation in Psychiatric Case Management." *Journal of Health Care Finance* (Spring): 41–44.

Benz, P. D. and R. V. Nagelhout. 1986. "Evaluating Pricing for Health Care Service Contracts." *Journal of Health Care Finance* (Winter): 59–78.

Horowitz, J. L. and M. A. Kleinman. 1994. "Advanced Pricing Strategies for Hospitals in Contracting with Managed Care Organizations." *Journal of Health Care Finance* (Fall): 90–100.

Jacobs, P. and C. R. Franz. 1985. "Developing Pricing Policies by Diagnostic Group." *Healthcare Financial Management* (January): 50–52.

Pickard, J. G., R. A. Friedman, and T. J. Johnson. 1991. "Repricing Plan Yields Realistic Revenue Enhancement." *Healthcare Financial Management* (May): 45–52.

Rosko, M. D. and C. E. Carpenter. 1994. "Hospital Markups: Responses to Environmental Pressures in Pennsylvania." *Hospital & Health Services Administration* (Spring): 3–16.

PLANNING AND BUDGETING

Learning Objectives

After studying this chapter, readers will be able to:

- Describe the overall planning process and the key components of the financial plan.
- Discuss briefly the format and use of several types of budgets.
- Explain the difference between a static budget and a flexible budget.
- Create a simple operating budget.
- Use variance analysis to assess financial performance and identify operational areas of concern.
- Explain the format and use of a cash budget.

Introduction

Planning and budgeting play a critical role in the finance function of all health services organizations. In fact, one could argue—and usually win—that planning and budgeting are the most important of all finance related tasks. *Planning* encompasses the overall process of preparing for the future. Because of its importance to organizational success, most health services managers, especially at large organizations, spend a great deal of time on activities related to planning.

Budgeting is an offshoot of the planning process. A set of *budgets* is the basic accounting tool used to tie together managerial planning and control functions. In general, organizational plans focus on the long-term big picture, whereas budgets address the details of both planning for the immediate future and, through the control mechanism, ensuring that current performance is consistent with organizational plans and goals.

This chapter includes an introduction to the planning process and a discussion of how budgets are used within health services organizations. In particular, the chapter focuses on how managers can use flexible budgets and variance analysis to help exercise control over current operations. Unfortunately, in an introductory textbook, only the surface of these very important topics can be scratched.[1]

The Planning Process

The *strategic plan* is the foundation of any organization's planning process. It begins with the organization's mission statement, scope, and objectives. The strategic plan then outlines the broad strategies to be followed to achieve the plan's stated objectives. Although the strategic plan is the lynchpin of the planning and budgeting process, it does not provide managers with detailed operational guidance. The "how to" or perhaps "how we expect to" portion of the planning process is contained in the *operating plan*.

Operating plans can be developed for any time horizon, but most organizations use a five-year horizon. Thus, the term *five-year plan* is often used in place of *operating plan*. In a five-year plan, the plans are most detailed for the first year, with each succeeding year's plan becoming less specific. Unlike the strategic plan, which is short on specifics, the five-year plan contains considerable detail concerning who is responsible for what particular function and when specific tasks are to be accomplished.

Table 8.1 contains Bayside Memorial Hospital's annual planning schedule. This schedule illustrates the fact that for most organizations, the planning process is essentially continuous. Next, Table 8.2 outlines the key elements of the hospital's five-year plan with an expanded section for the financial plan (Part 7 of the operating plan). A full outline would require several pages, but Table 8.2 at least provides insights into the format and contents of a five-year plan. Note that the first two chapters of the operating plan are drawn from the organization's strategic plan.

For Bayside, much of the planning function takes place at the department level, with technical assistance from the marketing, planning, and financial staffs. Larger firms with divisions would begin the planning process at the divisional level. Each division would have its own mission and goals as well as objectives and budgets designed to support its goals; these plans are then consolidated to form the overall corporate plan.

Section A of the financial plan (Part 7 of the operating plan) focuses on long-term financial planning at the organizational level. Its first component is a review of the business' current financial condition, which provides the basis or starting point for the remainder of the financial plan. (Insights into how this is accomplished are presented in Chapter 17.) Next, the capital budget, which outlines future capital acquisitions (i.e., long-term asset purchases), is presented. (Capital budgeting procedures are discussed in Chapters 14 and 15.) This information feeds into the pro-forma financial statements, which are projected for the next five years.[2] Finally, the organization's external financing requirements are listed, along with a plan for obtaining these funds. (Financing decisions will be covered in Chapters 11, 12, and 13.) As can be seen from its content, Section A of the financial plan provides an overview of the financial future of the organization.

Section B of the financial plan concerns current asset and current liability management, which often is called *working capital management*. Here, the financial staff receives overall guidance regarding day-to-day, short-term financial operations. (The cash budget is discussed later in the chapter. The remainder of working capital management is covered in Chapter 16.) Section C of the financial plan provides short-term operating benchmarks for all levels of management. For example, the accounting plan provides financial goals at the micro level by

Months	Action	
April–May	Marketing department analyzes national and local economic factors likely to influence Bayside's patient volume and reimbursement rates. At this time, a preliminary volume forecast is prepared for each service line.	**TABLE 8.1** Bayside Memorial Hospital: Annual Planning Schedule
June–July	Operating departments prepare new project (long-term asset) requirements, as well as operating cost estimates based on the preliminary volume forecast.	
August–September	Financial analysts evaluate proposed capital expenditures and department operating plans. Preliminary forecasted financial statements are prepared with emphasis on Bayside's overall sources and uses of funds and forecasted financial condition.	
October–November	All previous input is reviewed and the hospital's five-year plan is drafted by the planning, financial, and departmental staffs. At this stage, the operating and cash budgets are finalized. Any changes that have occurred since the beginning of the planning process are incorporated into the plan.	
December	The five-year plan, including all budgets for the coming year, is approved by the hospital's executive committee, and then submitted to the board of directors for final approval.	

division, contract, or diagnosis, and is used to control operations through frequent comparisons with actual results.

If financial planning were compared to planning a cross-country road trip, Section A could be thought of as a roadmap of the United States, which provides the overview, while Section C could be thought of as the state maps, which provide the details. The bulk of this chapter is devoted to a discussion of Section C, specifically, the preparation and use of budgets.

Self-Test Questions

1. What is the primary difference between strategic and operating plans?
2. What is the most common time horizon for operating plans?
3. Briefly describe the contents of a typical financial plan.
4. What is the primary difference between Sections A and C of the financial plan?

Introduction to Budgeting

Budgeting involves detailed plans, expressed quantitatively in dollar terms, that specify how resources will be obtained and used during a specified period of time. In general, budgets rely heavily on revenue and cost estimates, so the budgeting process applies many of the managerial accounting concepts that were presented in Chapters 5, 6, and 7.

TABLE 8.2

Bayside Memorial
Hospital: Five-Year
Plan Outline

Part 1	Corporate mission, scope, and objectives
Part 2	Corporate strategies
Part 3	Projected business environment
Part 4	Summary of projected business results
Part 5	Marketing plan
Part 6	Operating plan
Part 7	Financial plan

    A. Long-term plan
        1. Financial condition analysis
        2. Capital budget
        3. Pro-forma financial statements
        4. External financing requirements
    B. Working capital management plan
        1. Overall working capital policy
        2. Cash budget
        3. Cash and marketable securities management
        4. Inventory management
        5. Credit policy and receivables management
        6. Short-term financing
    C. Accounting plan (first year only)
        1. Revenue budget
        2. Expense budget
        3. Operating budget
        4. Control procedures

Part 8   Administration and human resources plan

To be of greatest usefulness, managers must think of budgets not as accounting tools, but as managerial tools. Budgets are more important to managers than to accountants because budgets provide the means to plan and communicate operational expectations within an organization. Every manager within an organization must be aware of the plans made by other managers and by the organization as a whole, and budgets provide the means of communication. In addition, the budgeting process and the resultant final budget provide the means for senior managers to allocate limited resources among competing demands within an organization.

Although planning, communication, and allocation are important purposes of the budgeting process, perhaps the greatest value of budgeting is that it establishes financial benchmarks for control. When compared to actual results, budgets provide managers with feedback about the relative financial performance of the enterprise, whether it is a department, diagnosis, contract, or the organization as a whole. Such comparisons help managers evaluate the performance of individuals, departments, product lines, reimbursement contracts, and so on.

Furthermore, budgets provide managers with information about what needs to be done to improve performance. When actual results are not as good as those specified in the budget, managers use *variance analysis* to identify the areas causing the sub-par performance. In this way, managerial resources can be brought to bear on those areas of operations that offer the most promise for financial improvement. Finally, the information developed by comparing actual results with planned results (i.e., the control process) is useful in improving the overall accuracy of the planning process. Managers want to meet budget targets, and hence most managers will think long and hard when those targets are being developed.

1. What is budgeting?
2. What are its benefits to the organization?

Self-Test Questions

Budget Types

Although an organization's immediate financial expectations are expressed in a document called *the budget*, typically the document is composed of several different budgets. Unlike financial statements, budget formats are not controlled by external requirements, so a great deal of room exists in the budgeting process for managerial innovation and creativity. The specific types and contents of the budget are dictated by the organization's mission, structure, and managerial preferences. Nevertheless, several primary types of budgets are used, either formally or informally, at virtually all health services organizations.

Statistics Budget

The *statistics budget* is the foundation budget in that it develops the data used in the other budgets. In general, the statistics budget identifies the volume of services to be provided and the resources necessary to provide those services. Because the statistics budget feeds into all other budgets, accuracy is particularly important. The statistics budget does not provide detailed data on required resources such as staffing or short-term operating asset requirements, but rather it provides general guidance.

Some organizations, especially smaller ones, may not have a separate statistics budget, but instead may incorporate its data directly into the revenue and expense budgets, or perhaps into a single operating budget. The advantage of having a separate statistics budget is that it forces all forecasting within the organization to begin with the same set of volume and resource assumptions. Unfortunately, volume estimates, which are the heart of the statistics budget and which drive all other forecasts, are among the most difficult to make.

To illustrate the complexities of volume forecasting, consider the volume forecast procedures followed by Bayside Memorial Hospital. To begin, the demand for services is divided into four major groups: inpatient, outpatient, ancillary, and other services. Volume trends in each of these areas over the past five years are plotted and a first approximation forecast is made, assuming a continuation of past trends. Next, the level of population growth and disease trends are forecasted. For example, what will be the growth in the over-65 population in the hospital's service area? These forecasts are used to develop volume by major diagnoses and to differentiate between normal services and critical care services.

Bayside's managers then analyze the competitive environment. Consideration is given to such factors as the hospital's inpatient and outpatient capacities, its competitors' capacities, and new services or service improvements that either Bayside or its competitors may institute. Next, Bayside's managers consider the effect of the hospital's planned pricing actions on volume. For example, does the hospital have plans to raise outpatient charges to boost profit margins or to lower charges to gain market share and utilize excess capacity? If such actions are expected to affect volume forecasts, these estimates must be revised.

Marketing campaigns and contracts or loss of contracts with managed care plans also affect volume, so probable developments in these areas must be considered. This facet of the forecast is particularly important to Bayside, which is in the process of buying physician group practices and creating an integrated delivery system. The success or failure of this venture could have a significant impact on future volume estimates.

If the hospital's volume forecast is off the mark, the consequences can be serious. First, if the market for any particular service expands more than Bayside has expected and planned for, the hospital will not be able to meet its patients' needs. Potential patients will end up going to competitors, and Bayside will lose market share and perhaps miss a major opportunity. However, if its projections are overly optimistic, Bayside could end up with too much capacity, which means higher than necessary costs because of excess equipment, inventory, and staff. All this would result in low profitability, which could degrade the hospital's ability to compete in the future.

Revenue Budget

Detailed information from the statistics budget feeds into the *revenue budget*, which combines volume data with reimbursement data to develop revenue forecasts. Bayside's managers consider the hospital's pricing strategy for managed care plans, conventional fee-for-service contracts, and private-pay patients, as well as trends in inflation and third-party payor reimbursement, all of which affect operating revenues. Also, price changes related to other income, such as lease rates to tenant physicians, must be considered.

The end result is a compilation of revenue forecasts by service, both in the aggregate—for example, inpatient operating revenue—and on an individual diagnosis basis. The individual diagnosis forecasts are summed and then compared with the aggregate service group forecasts. Differences are reconciled and the result is a revenue forecast for the hospital as a whole, but with breakdowns by service categories and by individual diagnoses. Finally, both the amount and the **timing** of future revenues are important. Thus, the revenue budget must forecast not only the amount of revenue expected, but also when it is likely to be received, typically by month.

Expense Budget

Like the revenue budget, the *expense budget* is derived from data in the statistics budget. The focus here is on the costs of providing services, rather than the resulting revenues. The expense budget typically is divided into labor (salaries, wages, and fringe benefits) and nonlabor components. The nonlabor components include expenses associated with such items as depreciation, leases, administrative and medical supplies, and medical training and education. Expenses normally will be broken down into fixed and variable components. (As discussed later in this chapter, cost structure information is required if an organization uses flexible budgeting techniques.) Finally, at larger organizations, the expense budget may be composed of several component budgets, each one focusing on a single category of expense such as labor, supplies, or utilities.

Operating Budget

For larger organizations, the *operating budget* is a combination of the revenue and expense budgets. For smaller businesses, the statistics, revenue, and expense budgets often are combined into a single operating budget. Because the operating budget (and, by definition, the revenue and expense budgets) is prepared using accrual accounting methods, it can be roughly thought of as a pro-forma (or forecasted) income statement. However, unlike the income statement, which is typically prepared at the organizational level, operating budgets are prepared at the unit level, say, a department or product line. Because of its overall importance to the budgeting process, especially for managers, most of this chapter focuses on the operating budget.

Cash Budget

Finally, the *cash budget* focuses on the organization's cash position. Because the operating budget and its component budgets use accrual accounting, they do not provide cash flow information. Like the statement of cash flows, which recasts the income statement to focus on cash, the cash budget recasts the operating budget to focus on the actual flow of cash into and out of a business. Thus, the cash budget tells managers whether the business will be generating excess cash, which will have to be invested, or experiencing a cash shortfall, which will have to be covered in some way.

The primary difference between a cash budget and the statement of cash flows is time period. The statement of cash flows generally is prepared on an annual (and perhaps quarterly) basis, and is used for long-term cash planning. The cash budget is prepared on a monthly, weekly, or daily basis, and is used for short-term cash management. Cash budgeting will be discussed later in this chapter, while its implications for cash management will be discussed in Chapter 16.

1. What are some of the budget types used within health services organizations?
2. Briefly describe the purpose and use of each.

Self-Test Questions

3. How are the statistics budget, revenue and expense budgets, and operating budget related?
4. How does the cash budget differ from the operating budget? From the statement of cash flows?

Budget Decisions

In addition to the types of budgets used within an organization, managers must make several other decisions regarding the budget process.

Timing

Virtually all health services organizations have annual budgets, which set the standards for the coming year. However, it would take too long for managers to detect adverse trends if budget feedback were solely on an annual basis, so most organizations also have quarterly budgets, while some even have monthly, weekly, or daily budgets. Not all budget types have to use the same timing pattern. Additionally, many organizations prepare budgets for one or more *out years*, or years beyond the next budget year. Out year budgets are more closely aligned to financial planning than to operational control.

Conventional Versus Zero-Based Budgeting

Traditionally, health services organizations have used the *incremental/decremental*, or *conventional, approach* to budgeting. In this approach, the previous budget is used as the starting point for creating the new budget. Each line on the old budget is examined, and typically, minor changes are made to reflect changes in circumstances. Also, in the conventional approach, it is common for most budget changes to be applied more or less equally across departments and programs. For example, labor costs may be assumed to increase at the same inflation rate for all departments within an organization. In essence, the traditional approach to budgeting assumes that prior budgets are based on operational rationality, so the main issue is determining what changes (typically minor) must be made to the previous budget to account for changes in the operating environment.

As its name implies, *zero-based budgeting* starts with a clean slate.[3] For example, departments begin with a budget of zero. Department heads, then, must fully justify every line item in their budgets. In effect, departments and programs must justify their very existence each budget period. Often, budgets must be created that show the type and amount of department or program services that could be offered at alternative funding levels. Senior management, then, can use this information to make rational decisions about what budgets should be cut in the event of funding constraints.

Conceptually, zero-based budgeting is superior to incremental/decremental budgeting. Indeed, when zero-based budgeting was first introduced in the 1970s, it was widely embraced. However, what should be obvious is that the managerial resources required for zero-based budgeting far exceed those required for conventional budgeting. Therefore, many organizations that initially adopted zero-based budgeting soon concluded that its benefits were not as great as its costs. There is evidence, however, that zero-based budgeting is making a comeback among health services organizations because of the fact that market forces now require providers to continually apply cost-control efforts.

Top-Down Versus Bottom-Up Budgeting

There is no other area of accounting in which behavioral implications are more important than in budgeting. A budget affects virtually everyone in the organization, and individuals' reactions to the budgeting process can have considerable influence on an organization's overall effectiveness. One of the most important decisions regarding budget preparation is whether the budget should be created top down or bottom up.

In the *bottom-up*, or *participatory*, *approach*, budgets are developed by department or program managers first. Presumably, such individuals are most knowledgeable regarding their departments' or programs' financial needs. These budgets, then, are submitted to the finance department for review and compilation into the organizational budget, which must be approved by top management. Unfortunately, the aggregation of department or program budgets often results in an organizational budget that is not financially feasible. In such cases, the component budgets must be sent back to the original preparers for revision, which starts a negotiation process aimed at creating a budget acceptable to all parties or at least to as many parties as possible.

A more authoritarian approach to budgeting is the *top-down approach* in which little negotiation takes place between junior and senior managers. This approach has the advantages of being relatively expeditious and reflecting top management's perspective from the start. However, by limiting involvement and communication, the top-down approach often results in less commitment among junior managers and employees than does the participatory approach. Most people will perform better and make greater attempts to achieve budgetary goals if they have been consulted in setting those goals. The idea of participatory budgeting is to involve as many managers, and even employees, as possible in the budgetary process.

Fixed Versus Flexible Budgeting

As its name implies, the dollar amounts in a *fixed budget* are set in stone. A fixed budget, once it is approved, ignores the fact that revenues and expenses are tied to volume. One can think of a fixed budget as assuming no uncertainty in the volume forecast. Conversely, a *flexible budget* explicitly recognizes that rarely will the forecasted volume be realized. In essence, the flexible budget assumes perfect foresight **after the fact** because it adjusts the initial budget to recognize the actual volume of services provided. Flexible budgeting is discussed in detail in later sections of this chapter.

1. What time periods are used in budgeting?
2. What are the primary differences between conventional and zero-based budgeting?
3. What are the primary differences between top-down and bottom-up budgeting?
4. What is the difference between fixed and flexible budgeting?

Constructing a Simple Operating Budget

Table 8.3 contains the 1998 operating budget for Carroll Clinic, a large inner-city primary care facility. As with most financial forecasts, the starting point for the operating budget, which was developed in October of 1997, is volume. *A volume projection* gives managers a sense of the extent of business to be performed, and hence a starting point for making revenue and cost estimates. As shown in Part I of Table 8.3, Carroll Clinic's expected patient volume for 1998 comes from two sources: a fee-for-service (FFS) population expected to generate 36,000 visits and a capitated population expected to average 30,000 members. Historically, annual utilization by the capitated population has averaged 0.15 visits per member-month, so this population is expected to generate $30,000 \times 12 \times 0.15 = 54,000$ visits in 1998. Therefore, in total, Carroll's patient base is expected to produce $36,000 + 54,000 = 90,000$ visits. Armed with this Part I volume projection, Carroll's managers can proceed with revenue and cost projections.

Part II contains revenue data. The clinic's net collection for each FFS visit averages $25. Some visits will generate greater revenues and some will generate less. On average, though, expected revenue is $25 per visit. Thus, 36,000 visits would produce $\$25 \times 36,000 = \$900,000$ in FFS revenues. Additionally, the capitated population will produce a revenue of $3 PMPM, for total revenues of $\$3 \times 30,000 \times 12 = \$3 \times 360,000$ member months $= \$1,080,000$. Considering both patient sources, total revenues for the clinic are forecasted to be $\$900,000 + \$1,080,000 = \$1,980,000$ in 1998.

Because of the uncertainty inherent in the clinic's volume estimates, it is useful to recognize that total revenues will be $1,980,000 only if the volume forecast holds. In reality, Total revenues = ($25 × Number of FFS visits) + ($3 × Number of capitated member-months). If the actual number of FFS visits is more or less than 90,000 in 1998 or the number of capitated lives is something other than 30,000, the resulting revenues will be different from the $1,980,000 forecast.

Part III of Table 8.3 focuses on expenses. To provide the quantity and quality of care to support the forecasted 90,000 visits, the clinic is expected to use 48,000 hours of medical labor, at an average cost of $25 per hour, for a total medical staffing expense of $48,000 \times \$25 = \$1,200,000$. Thus, medical staffing costs are expected to average $\$1,200,000 / 90,000 = \$13.33$ per visit in 1998. In reality, all medical staffing costs are not variable, but there are a sufficient number of part-time clinical workers such that medical labor hours are closely related to the number of visits.

TABLE 8.3

Carroll Clinic: 1998
Operating Budget

I.   *Volume Assumptions:*

   A.   FFS   36,000   visits

   B.   Capitated lives   30,000   members

         Number of member months   360,000

         Expected utilization per member-month   0.15

           Number of visits   54,000   visits

   C.   Total expected visits   90,000   visits

II.   *Revenue Assumptions:*

   A.   FFS $ 25   per visit

                                × 36,000   expected visits

                             $ 900,000

   B.   Capitated lives $ 3   PMPM

                             × 360,000   actual member months

                         $ 1,080,000

   C.   Total expected revenues $ 1,980,000

III.   *Cost Assumptions:*

   A.   Variable Costs:

         Medical staffing $ 1,200,000   (48,000 hours at $25/hour)

         Supplies   150,000   (100,000 units at $1.50/unit)

           Total variable costs $ 1,350,000

         Variable cost per visit $ 15   ($1,350,000/90,000)

   B.   Fixed Costs:

         Overhead, plant,

           and equipment $ 500,000

   C.   Total expected costs $ 1,850,000

IV.   *Pro-Forma Profit and Loss (P&L) Statement:*

        Revenues:

           FFS $ 900,000

           Capitated   1,080,000

           Total $ 1,980,000

        Costs:

           Variable:

              FFS $ 540,000

              Capitated   810,000

              Total $ 1,350,000

           Contribution margin $ 630,000

           Fixed costs   500,000

           Projected profit $ 130,000

Supplies expense, the bulk of which is inherently variable in nature, historically has averaged about $1.50 per bundle (unit) of supplies, with 100,000 units expected to be used to support 90,000 visits. (A unit of supplies is a more or less standard package that contains both administrative and clinical supplies.) Thus, supplies expense is expected to total $150,000, or $150,000 / 90,000 = $1.67

per visit. Taken together, Carroll's variable costs are forecasted to be $133.33 + $1.67 = $15 per visit in 1998. The same amount can be calculated by dividing total variable costs by the number of visits: $1,350,000 / 90,000 = $15.

Finally, the clinic is expected to incur $500,000 of fixed costs for 1998, primarily administrative overhead labor costs, depreciation, and lease expense. Therefore, to serve the anticipated 90,000 visits in 1998, costs are expected to consist of $1,350,000 in variable costs plus $500,000 in fixed costs, for a total of $1,850,000. Again, it is important to recognize that some costs (in Carroll's case, a majority of costs) are tied to volume. Thus, total costs can be expressed as ($15 × Number of visits) + $500,000. If the actual number of visits in 1998 comes in at more or less than 90,000 in total, then total costs will differ from the $1,850,000 budget estimate.

The final section (Part IV) of Table 8.3 contains Carroll Clinic's budgeted 1998 *profit and loss (P&L) statement*, the heart of the operating budget. A P&L statement is, in reality, a simplified pro-forma income statement. The difference between the projected revenues of $1,980,000 and the projected variable costs of $1,350,000 produces a contribution margin of $630,000, which when compared to forecasted fixed costs of $500,000 produces a budgeted profit of $130,000. The amount of data (the number of lines) shown in an operating budget varies considerably. Most budgets are more complex than the Carroll Clinic example shown in Table 8.3. The illustration has purposely been kept simple for ease of discussion.

Although the format of the P&L statement encourages sensitivity analysis (i.e., "what if" scenarios), the purpose of an operating budget is not so much to forecast profits as it is to set financial goals for the clinic. Although this first step in the operating budget very much resembles a typical pro-forma analysis, the significance of the budgeted bottom line number of $130,000 and its underlying volume, revenue, and expense assumptions become much more important in terms of managerial accountability. In effect, the operating budget can be thought of as a psychological contract between the organization and its managers. Thus, the $130,000 profit forecast becomes the overall financial benchmark for the clinic in 1998, and individual managers will be held accountable for the revenues and expenditures needed to meet the budget.

Self-Test Questions

1. What are some of the key assumptions required to prepare an operating budget?
2. Do the required assumptions depend on the type of organization and the nature of its reimbursement contracts?
3. What is a profit and loss (P&L) statement? Why is it so important?

Variance Analysis

Variance analysis is an important technique for controlling financial performance. This section includes a discussion of the basics of variance analysis, including flexible budgeting, as well as an illustration of the process.

Variance Analysis Basics

In accounting, a *variance* is the difference between a budgeted value, often called a *standard*, and the actual value. Thus, *variance analysis* is an examination and interpretation of differences between what has actually happened and what was planned. If the budget is based on realistic expectations, variance analysis can provide managers with very useful information. Variance analysis does not provide all the answers, but it does help managers ask the right questions. (Note that the accounting definition of variance is different from the statistical definition, although both meanings connote a difference from some base value.)

Variance analysis is essential to the managerial control process. Actions taken in response to variance analysis often have the potential to dramatically improve the operations and financial performance of the organization. For example, many variances are controllable, so managers can take actions to avoid unfavorable variances in the future. The primary focus of variance analysis should not be to assign blame for unfavorable results. Rather, the goal of variance analysis is to uncover the cause of operational problems so that these problems can be avoided, or at least minimized, in the future. Unfortunately, not all variances are controllable by management. Nevertheless, knowledge of such variances is essential to the overall management and well-being of the organization. It may be necessary to revise plans, for example, to tighten controllable costs in an attempt to offset unfavorable cost variances in areas that are beyond managerial control.

Static Versus Flexible Budgets

To be of maximum value to managers, variance analysis must be approached systematically. The starting point for such analysis is the *static budget,* which is the original approved budget unadjusted for differences between planned and actual (i.e., realized) volumes. However, at the end of a budget period, it is not likely that realized volume will equal budgeted volume, so any resulting variances will be based on an apples-to-oranges comparison.

To illustrate the comparison problems that arise with static budgets, consider Carroll Clinic's 1998 operating budget contained in Table 8.3. The profit projection, $130,000, is predicated upon specific volume assumptions: 36,000 visits for the FFS population and 360,000 member months, which results in 54,000 visits for the capitated population. At the end of 1998, the clinic's managers will compare actual profits with budgeted profits. The problem, of course, is that it is highly unlikely that actual profits will be based upon 36,000 fee-for-service visits and 360,000 member months (with 54,000 visits) for the capitated population. Thus, if Carroll's managers were to merely compare the realized profit with the $130,000 in the budget, they would not know whether any profit difference is caused by volume differences or underlying operational differences.

To provide an explanation of what is driving the profit variance, managers must adopt a flexible budget. A *flexible budget* is one in which the static budget has been adjusted to reflect the actual volume achieved in the budget period. Essentially, flexible budgets are an after-the-fact device to tell managers what the results would have been under the volume level actually attained, **assuming all**

other budgeting assumptions held. The flexible budget permits a much more in-depth variance analysis than is possible with a static budget. However, a flexible budget requires the identification of variable and fixed costs, and hence places a larger burden on the organization's managerial accounting system.

Variance Analysis Illustration

To illustrate variance analysis, consider Carroll's static budget for 1998 (Table 8.3), which projects a profit of $130,000. Data used for variance analysis is tracked in various parts of Carroll's managerial accounting information system throughout the year, and variance analyses are performed monthly. This allows managers to take necessary actions during the year to positively influence annual results. For purposes of this illustration, however, the monthly feedback is not shown. Rather, the focus is on the year-end results, which are contained in Table 8.4.

Total Variance, Volume Variance, and Management Variance

The variance analysis begins with a calculation of Carroll's *total variance*. Total variance is merely the difference between the realized profit (Table 8.4) and the static profit (Table 8.3): Total variance = Actual profit − Static profit, or −$212,000 − $130,000 = −$342,000. Although this large negative value should generate considerable concern among Carroll's managers, a variance analysis based on the static budget is not capable of providing any insights into why profit expectations were not met. For this, a flexible budget variance analysis is required.

Table 8.5 contains three profit and loss statements (budgets) for 1998. The static budget taken from Table 8.3 is the forecast made at the beginning of 1998, while the actual budget taken from Table 8.4 reflects after-the-fact results. The flexible budget in the center column of Table 8.5 reflects projected revenues and costs at the realized (actual) volume as opposed to the projected volume, but incorporating all other assumptions that went into the static budget in Table 8.3. By analyzing differences in these three budgets, Carroll's managers can gain insights into why the clinic ended the year with a profit shortfall (from budget) of $342,000.

Before the total variance is decomposed for analysis, it is useful to examine the flexible budget in more detail. The flexible budget maintains the original budget parameters of Revenues = ($25 × Number of FFS visits) + ($3 × Number of capitated member-months), and Expenses = ($15 × Number of FFS visits) + ($15 × Number of capitated visits) + $500,000. However, the flexible budget *flexes* (adjusts) revenue and costs to reflect actual volume levels. Thus, in the flexible budget column, Revenues = ($25 × 40,000) + ($3 × 360,000) = $1,000,000 + $1,080,000 = $2,080,000, and Expenses = ($15 × 40,000) + ($15 × 72,000) + $500,000 = $600,000 + $1,080,000 + $500,000 = $2,180,000.

The flexible budget can be described as follows. The $2,080,000 in total revenues is what the clinic **would have expected** for 40,000 FFS visits and a capitated membership of 30,000. The total variable costs of $1,680,000 are the costs that Carroll **would have expected** for 40,000 FFS visits and 72,000 capitated

TABLE 8.4
Carroll Clinic:
1998 Results

I.   Volume:
   A.   FFS   40,000   visits
   B.   Capitated lives   30,000   members
       Number of member months   360,000
       Actual utilization per member-month   0.20
          Number of visits   72,000   visits

   C.   Total actual visits   112,000   visits

II.   Revenues:
   A.   FFS $ 25   per visit
                            × 40,000   actual visits
                        $ 1,000,000
   B.   Capitated lives $ 3   PMPM
                          × 360,000   actual member months
                        $ 1,080,000

   C.   Total actual revenues $ 2,080,000

III.   Costs:
   A.   Variable Costs:
       Medical staffing $ 1,557,400   (59,900 hours at $26/hour)
       Supplies   234,600   (124,800 units at $1.88/unit)
          Total variable costs $ 1,792,000

       Variable cost per visit $ 16   ($1,792,000/112,000)

   B.   Fixed Costs:
       Overhead, plant,
         and equipment $ 500,000

   C.   Total actual costs $ 2,292,000

IV. Profit and Loss Statement:
       Revenues:
         FFS $ 1,000,000
         Capitated   1,080,000
         Total $ 2,080,000

       Costs:
         Variable:
           FFS $ 640,000
           Capitated   1,152,000
           Total $ 1,792,000
        Contribution margin $ 288,000
        Fixed costs   500,000
        Actual profit   ($ 212,000)

visits (based on a membership of 30,000). By definition, the fixed costs should be the same, within a reasonable range, no matter what the volume level. Thus, the $100,000 loss shown on the flexible budget represents the profit expected given the initial assumed revenue, cost, and volume relationships coupled with a forecasted volume equal to the realized volume.

TABLE 8.5

Carroll Clinic: Static, Flexible, and Actual Budgets for 1998

	Static Budget	Flexible Budget	Actual Budget
Assumptions:			
FFS visits	36,000	40,000	40,000
Capitated visits	54,000	72,000	72,000
Total	90,000	112,000	112,000
Revenues:			
FFS	$ 900,000	$1,000,000	$1,000,000
Capitated	1,080,000	1,080,000	1,080,000
Total	$1,980,000	$2,080,000	$2,080,000
Costs:			
Variable:			
FFS	$ 540,000	$ 600,000	$ 640,000
Capitated	810,000	1,080,000	1,152,000
Total	$1,350,000	$1,680,000	$1,792,000
Contribution margin	$ 630,000	$ 400,000	$ 288,000
Fixed costs	500,000	500,000	500,000
Profit	$ 130,000	($ 100,000)	($ 212,000)

Table 8.6 breaks down the total variance of −$342,000 into its two component variances. The total variance is the difference between actual profit and static profit, so it represents changes caused by all factors including volume differences and management factors. But, the flexible budget profit is the profit expected under the realized volume, assuming all other budget assumptions hold. Thus, the difference between the flexible budget profit and the original static budget profit, which is called the *volume variance*, is solely caused by volume differences. Carroll's 1998 volume variance is −$100,000 − $130,000 = −$230,000.

Any profit differences not caused by volume must be caused by factors that are controllable management, and the *management variance* is defined as the actual profit less the flexible profit. In Carroll's case, Management variance = −$212,000 − (−$100,000) = −$112,000. Because all differences are classified as either volume differences or management differences, the sum of the volume variance and the management variance must equal the total variance: −$230,000 + (−$112,000) = −$342,000.

Variance analysis, along with the flexible budget, has helped Carroll's managers better understand the clinic's 1998 operating results. If they did not have a budget process, they simply would have received a year-end profit and loss statement that would have told them that they lost $212,000. The budget data and variance analysis contained in Tables 8.5 and 8.6 disclose several important operational issues. First, the overall situation is **worse** than the $212,000 loss reported for 1998 because Carroll's managers had reason to believe that the

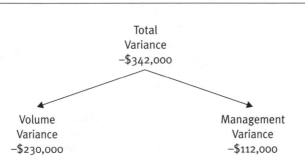

TABLE 8.6

Variance Summary
Under Flexible
Budgeting

Total variance	= Actual profit − Static profit
Volume variance	= Flexible profit − Static profit
Management variance	= Actual profit − Flexible profit

clinic would realize a profit of $130,000 in 1998. The total variance of −$342,000 shows the true magnitude of the problem and provides a starting point for further analysis.

Carroll's managers also know that the total variance of −$342,000 consists of a $230,000 shortfall caused by volume differences and a $112,000 shortfall caused by managerial control problems. About 67 percent of the total variance ($230,000 / $342,000) is caused by volume differences, over which Carroll's managers have limited control. Of course, volume is an issue of management concern at the clinic. Carroll's managers want more capitated lives with a utilization rate that is the same or less than the current rate, as well as more FFS visits. The bad news, however, is that their ability to influence volume is limited.

The good news is that Carroll's managers have a much better chance of attacking that portion of the total variance (33 percent) caused by management variables. With improved efficiency of operations at least up to the standards assumed in the static budget, the clinic would have suffered a shortfall from projections in 1998 of only $230,000, rather than the actual total variance of $342,000. Put another way, operating at standard efficiency would have resulted in a loss on the actual budget of only $100,000, not the $212,000 that actually occurred. Further variance analysis is needed to determine precisely where the managerial efficiency problem lies.

Volume Variance Breakdown

As shown in Table 8.7, volume variance typically has two components. Although the Carroll Clinic example contains a mix of FFS and capitated patients, planned capitated enrollment is equal to actual enrollment (360,000 member months), so there is no enrollment component to the volume variance. In general, with a capitated population, the volume variance breakdown shows both the difference from budget caused by utilization rate changes and the difference caused by changes in the size of the population served.[4]

TABLE 8.7
Volume Variance
Components

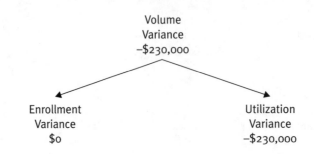

Volume variance	= Flexible profit − Static profit
Enrollment variance	= Static profit − Static profit
Utilization variance	= Flexible profit − Static profit

Note: In our example, there were no enrollment differences. However, if some patients are capitated, and there are enrollment differences between expected and realized budgets, the situation becomes more complex. Then, it is necessary to create two flexible budgets: one flexed for both enrollment and utilization, and one flexed only for enrollment. With two flexible budgets, the volume variances are calculated as follows:

Volume variance	= Flexible (enrollment and utilization) profit− Static profit.
Enrollment variance	= Flexible (enrollment) profit − Static profit.
Utilization variance	= Flexible (enrollment and utilization) profit− Flexible (enrollment) profit.

In general, the utilization variance (−$230,000) is the difference in the volume (i.e., the number of visits) multiplied by the contribution margin on each visit. Because Carroll Clinic has two different patient populations (FFS and capitated), there are two different contribution margins. For the capitated population, there were 18,000 more visits realized in 1998 than were planned (72,000 actual visits versus 54,000 budgeted). The contribution margin for this population using budgeted rather than actual costs is −$15 per visit. This is the budgeted variable cost per visit because there are no incremental revenues associated with visits by capitated patients. Thus, the 18,000 additional visits for this population resulted in a reduction in profits of −$15 × 18,000 = −$270,000, which, of course, is only one component of the utilization variance of −$230,000.

The overall effect of this −$270,000 can be understood by examining the static and flexible budget columns in Table 8.5. Moving from the static to the flexible budget, essentially adjusting for volume differences, shows no change on the capitated revenue line; revenue remains at $1,080,000. However, variable costs for the capitated population increased from $810,000 to $1,080,000, or by $270,000. This amount is the expected budgeted cost increase caused by the additional 18,000 visits. The fact that variable costs for the capitated population increased to $1,152,000 in the actual budget is caused by reasons other than utilization changes.

The other subcomponent of the utilization variance is related to the FFS population. There were 4,000 FFS visits above the static budget, each with a budgeted contribution margin of $25 revenue − $15 variable cost = $10. Thus, the volume variance for the FFS population is $10 × 4,000 = $40,000, a positive number. The +$40,000 reflects the fact that the clinic's profitability is positively related to the number of FFS visits. Again, the +$40,000 can be understood by examining the static and flexible budget columns of Table 8.5. Moving from the static budget to the flexible budget, FFS revenues increase by $100,000. At the same time, FFS variable costs increase by only $60,000, which results in a profit increase of $40,000. The positive $40,000 utilization variance caused by FFS patients partially offsets the negative $270,000 utilization variance caused by the capitated population. Combining the utilization variances of the two populations gives +$40,000 − $270,000 = −$230,00, which is the overall utilization variance and, with no enrollment variance, the overall volume variance.

What did Carroll's managers learn from the volume variance analysis? A major portion, $230,000, of the overall profit shortfall from standard of $342,000 can be explained by volume discrepancies. Within the volume variance, the problem is actually a little worse within the capitated population than the aggregate variance data reveal. That is, there was a $270,000 shortfall caused by utilization control problems within the capitated population, which was partially offset (i.e., disguised) by the benefits (+$40,000) of increased FFS utilization. Thus, the breakdown of volume variance reveals a major issue that Carroll's managers must address—its utilization management of the capitated population. Either utilization management must be tightened or utilization forecasts need to be revised (i.e., increased), which may cause Carroll to reconsider its pricing on this managed care contract.

Management Variance Breakdown

Now consider the management variance of −$112,000.[5] This value represents the profit shortfall from standard that results not from volume assumption errors, but from cost factors that presumably are more controllable by management.

For Carroll, the realized cost per visit was $16, while the standard budgeted cost was only $15. Thus, total costs in 1998 to handle 112,000 visits (40,000 FFS plus 72,000 capitated) amounted to $1 × 112,000 = $112,000 more than budgeted. Table 8.5 shows the $112,000 cost overrun as the difference between actual total costs of $1,792,000 and flexible budget costs of $1,680,000.[6] This management variance, which results from production (i.e., cost) inefficiencies, can be broken down according to population served. However, in Carroll's situation, it costs the same on a per visit basis to treat both FFS and capitated patients, so the cost overruns are the same proportionally for each population: $40,000 on FFS and $72,000 on capitated patients.

As previously stated, the management variance of −$112,000 indicates that Carroll has cost-control problems. Furthermore, the major resources involved in operating costs are medical staffing and supplies, so it would be valuable to Carroll's managers to learn which of the two areas contributed most to the management variance. Perhaps an even deeper investigation can be made within staffing and supplies: Is too much of each resource being used or is too much money being paid for what is being used? Table 8.8 examines the components of the management variance. Most of the budget data required to calculate the component variances are contained in Part III of Table 8.3 (the static budget) and Table 8.4 (the actual results).

First, consider medical staffing, which represents labor utilization. The original static budget of $1,200,000 was based on the expectation that it would require 48,000 hours of work at $25 per hour to treat 90,000 visits. However, actual staffing amounted to 59,900 hours at $26 per hour to treat 112,000 visits, for a total cost of $1,557,400. If 48,000 hours are expected to be sufficient to provide for 90,000 visits, a labor efficiency ratio of 90,000 / 48,000 = 1.875 visits per hour results. In effect, for every hour of labor expended, the expectation is that the clinic can serve 1.875 patients. With this productivity assumption, the clinic would expect a staffing requirement of 112,000 / 1.875 = 59,733 hours to provide for the 112,000 visits realized in 1998. The flexed value for labor hours when combined with the standard labor cost of $25 per hour produced a flexible, volume adjusted labor cost of $25 × 59,733 = $1,493,325. The difference between the flexible and actual budget staffing costs produces a medical staffing variance of $1,493,325 − $1,557,400 = −$64,075.

Of the management variance of −$112,000, −$64,075 is caused by medical staffing and the remainder is caused by supplies; there is no fixed cost variance. The $64,075 medical staffing variance can be decomposed into that portion caused by productivity (the efficiency variance) and that portion caused by wage rates (the rate variance). As suggested previously, the flexible hours allowed based upon the initial productivity assumption were 59,733. However, the actual hours required were 59,900. The difference between the number of hours suggested by the flexible budget and the actual number needed is 59,733 − 59,900 = −167. An overage of 167 hours, coupled with a budgeted hourly rate of $25, produces a staffing efficiency variance of −167 × $25 = −$4,175. Thus, of the $64,075 overrun in medical staffing costs, $4,175 is caused by productivity inefficiencies and the remainder ($59,900) must be caused by paying more for labor than the clinic had originally planned (rate variance). The rate variance can be calculated directly by first comparing the actual labor rate of $26 per hour to the budgeted rate of $25 per hour, for a cost rate of $1 per hour above standard. When this additional cost is multiplied by the actual number of hours worked in 1998 (59,900), the rate variance of −$59,900 is obtained.

What can Carroll's managers learn from the medical staffing variance data? The numbers indicate that only a very small portion of the cost overrun was caused by productivity problems; the vast majority of the overrun was caused by higher-than-expected wages. This suggests that Carroll's managers have to take a close look at the clinic's wage rates to ensure that they are not paying more than the local

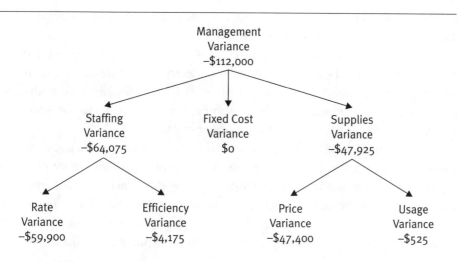

TABLE 8.8

Detailed Analysis of the Management Variance

Management variance   = Actual profit − Flexible (enrollment and utilization) profit
Fixed cost variance   = Flexible fixed costs − Actual fixed costs
Staffing variance   = Flexible staffing costs − Actual staffing costs
Rate variance   = (Static rate − Actual rate) × Actual labor hours
Efficiency variance = (Flexible hours − Actual hours) × Static rate
Supplies variance   = Flexible supplies costs − Actual supplies costs
Price variance   = (Static price − Actual price) × Actual units
Usage variance   = (Flexible units − Actual units) × Static price

market for labor dictates. Of course, Carroll wants to have quality employees, but at the same time, management needs to be concerned about labor costs.

How did Carroll do in 1998 regarding supplies costs? At the beginning of the year, Carroll estimated supplies costs of $150,000, based on the assumption that 100,000 units at $1.50 per unit would be needed for 90,000 visits. However, actual usage was 124,800 units that cost a total of $234,600, or about $1.88 per unit, to accommodate 112,000 visits. If 100,000 units were budgeted for 90,000 visits, then supplies usage was forecasted to be 100,000 / 90,000 = 1.11 units per visit. Thus, with an actual number of visits of 112,000 in 1998, Carroll should have used 1.11 × 112,000 = 124,450 units according to standard usage. (There are some rounding differences in these calculations.) At a budgeted cost of $1.50 per unit, total supplies costs should have been $1.50 × 124,450 = $186,675 for the 112,000 visits that occurred in 1998. However, $234,600 was actually spent on supplies, for a variance of $186,675 − $234,600 = −$47,925.

If −$47,925 of the management variance of −$112,000 is caused by supplies, the remainder, as discovered previously, must be caused by staffing. Within the −$47,925 supplies variance, the amount caused by excess utilization (the usage variance) and the amount caused by price differentials (the price variance) can be determined. The flexible budget suggests that the appropriate usage was 124,450 units. However, in 1998, 124,800 units were actually consumed. The difference between the flexed usage and the actual usage produces a usage overage of $124,450 - 124,800 = -350$ units. At a budgeted cost of $1.50 per unit, the usage variance is $-350 \times \$1.50 = -\$525$.

If $-\$525$ of the supplies variance of $-\$47,925$ is caused by usage differences, the remainder ($-\$47,400$) must be caused by price differences. To find the price variance directly, Carroll paid $\$1.50 - \$1.88 = -\$0.38$ above budget for each of the 124,800 units actually consumed, for a price variance of $-\$0.38 \times 124,800 = -\$47,400$, with a small rounding error.

What did Carroll's managers learn from the supplies variance analysis? They know that the supplies cost overrun was caused almost totally by price increases; supplies usage was almost on target when volume differences are accounted for. Thus, it would be prudent for management to investigate the clinic's purchasing policy to see if prices can be lowered through such actions as changing vendors, making larger purchases at a single time, or joining a purchasing alliance.

Final Comments on Variance Analysis

In summary, variance analysis, combined with flexible budgeting, helps managers identify the factors that cause realized profits to be different from those expected. If profits are higher than expected, managers can see why and then try to exploit those factors even further in the future. If profits are lower than expected, managers can identify the causes and then embark on a plan to correct the deficiencies. Larger health services organizations have made significant improvements in their use of flexible budgeting and variance analysis. The benefit from expanding the level of information detail is that it is easier for managers to isolate and presumably rectify problem areas. Fortunately, the marginal cost of obtaining such detailed information is lower now than ever before because detailed managerial accounting information is being generated both to support cost-control efforts and to aid in pricing and service decisions.

Self-Test Questions

1. What is variance analysis and what is its value to healthcare providers?
2. What is the difference between a static budget and a flexible budget?
3. What are the two components of volume variance?
4. What are the three components of management variance?

The Cash Budget

Thus far, our discussion of budgeting has focused on the operating budget. As shown in the Carroll Clinic illustration, the operating budget, along with the budgetary control process, provides managers with numerous insights into the efficiency of an organization's operations. However, the operating budget is based on accrual accounting principles, and hence does not provide managers with much information about a business' cash position. This situation is corrected by the *cash budget*.

To create a cash budget, managers forecast both fixed asset and inventory requirements, along with the times when such payments must be made. This information is combined with projections about the delay in collecting accounts receivable, wage payment dates, interest payment dates, and so on. All this information is then combined to show the organization's projected cash inflows and outflows over some specified period. Generally, businesses use a monthly cash budget forecasted over the next year, plus a more detailed daily or weekly cash budget for the coming month. The monthly cash budget is used for liquidity planning purposes and the daily or weekly budget for actual cash control.

Creating a cash budget does not require the application of a complex set of accounting rules. Rather, all the entries in a cash budget represent the actual movement of cash into or out of the organization. Table 8.9 contains a monthly cash budget that covers six months of 1999 for Madison Homecare, a small, for-profit home health care company. Madison's cash budget, which is broken down into three sections, is typical, although there is a great deal of variation in formats used by different organizations.

The first section of the cash budget contains the *collections worksheet,* which translates the billing for services provided into cash revenues. Because of its location in a summer resort area, Madison's patient volume, and hence billings, peak in July. However, like most health services organizations, Madison rarely collects when services are provided. What is relevant from a cash budget perspective is not when services are provided or when billings occur, but rather when cash is collected. Based on previous experience, Madison's managers know that most collections occur 30 to 60 days after billing. In fact, Madison's managers have a collections table that allows them to forecast, with some precision, the timing of collections. This table was used to convert the billings shown on Line 1 of Table 8.9 into the collection amounts shown on Lines 2 and 3.

The next section of Madison's cash budget is the *supplies worksheet,* which accounts for timing differences between when supplies are ordered and when they are paid for. Madison's patient volume forecasts, which are used to predict the billing amounts shown on Line 1, are also used to forecast the supplies (primarily medical) needed to support patient services. These supplies are ordered and received one month prior to expected usage, as shown on Line 4. However, Madison's suppliers do not demand immediate payment. Rather, Madison has, on average, 30 days to pay for supplies after they are received. Thus, the actual payment occurs one month after purchase, as shown on Line 5.

The next section combines data from the collections and supplies worksheets with other projected cash outflows to show the *net cash gain (loss)* for each month. Cash from collections is shown on Line 6. Lines 7 through 12 list cash payments that are expected to be made during each month including payments for supplies. Then, all payments are summed, with the total shown on Line 13. The difference between expected cash receipts and cash payments, Line 6 minus Line 13, is the net cash gain or loss during the month, which is shown on Line 14. For May, there is a forecasted net cash flow of −$13,900, where the parentheses indicate a negative cash flow (loss).

Although Line 14 contains the meat of the cash budget, Lines 15 through 18 (the *borrowing/surplus summary*) extend the basic budget data to show Madison's forecasted cash position for each month. Line 15 shows the forecasted cash

TABLE 8.9

Madison
Homecare:
May through
October Cash
Budget

	Mar	Apr	May	June	July	Aug	Sept	Oct
Collections Worksheet:								
1. Billed charges	$50,000	$50,000	$100,000	$150,000	$200,000	$100,000	$100,000	$50,000
2. Collections:								
a. Within 30 days			19,600	29,400	39,200	19,600	19,600	9,800
b. 30–60 days			35,000	70,000	105,000	140,000	70,000	70,000
c. 60–90 days			5,000	5,000	10,000	15,000	20,000	10,000
3. Total collections			$ 59,600	$104,400	$154,200	$174,600	$109,600	$ 89,800
Supplies Worksheet:								
4. Amount of supplies ordered	$10,000	$ 15,000	$ 20,000	$ 10,000	$ 10,000	$ 5,000		
5. Payments made for supplies		$ 10,000	$ 15,000	$ 20,000	$ 10,000	$ 10,000	$ 5,000	
Net Cash Gain (Loss):								
6. Total collections (from Line 3)			$ 59,600	$104,400	$154,200	$174,600	$109,600	$ 89,800
7. Total purchases (from Line 5)			$ 10,000	$ 15,000	$ 20,000	$ 10,000	$ 10,000	$ 5,000
8. Wages and salaries			60,000	70,000	80,000	60,000	60,000	60,000
9. Rent			2,500	2,500	2,500	2,500	2,500	2,500
10. Other expenses			1,000	1,500	2,000	1,000	1,000	500
11. Taxes				20,000			20,000	
12. Payment for capital assets						50,000		
13. Total payments			$ 73,500	$109,000	$104,500	$123,500	$ 93,500	$ 68,000
14. Net cash gain (loss)			($ 13,900)	($ 4,600)	$ 49,700	$ 51,100	$ 16,100	$ 21,800
Borrowing/Surplus Summary:								
15. Cash at beginning with no borrowing			$ 15,000	$ 1,100	($ 3,500)	$ 46,200	$ 97,300	$113,400
16. Cash at end with no borrowing			$ 1,100	($ 3,500)	$ 46,200	$ 97,300	$113,400	$135,200
17. Target cash balance			10,000	10,000	10,000	10,000	10,000	10,000
18. Cumulative surplus cash (loan balance)			($ 8,900)	($ 13,500)	$ 36,200	$ 87,300	$103,400	$125,200

on hand at the beginning of each month, assuming that no borrowing takes place. Madison is expected to enter the budget period, the beginning of May, with $15,000 of cash on hand. For each succeeding month, Line 15 is merely the value shown on Line 16 for the previous month. The values on Line 16, which are obtained by adding Lines 14 and 15, show the cash on hand at the end of each month assuming no borrowing takes place. For May, Madison expects a cash loss of $13,900 on top of a starting balance of $15,000, for an ending cash balance of $1,100 in the absence of any borrowing. This amount is the cash at beginning with no borrowing amount for June, which is shown on Line 15.

To continue, Madison's target cash balance (i.e., the amount that it wants on hand at the beginning of each month), which is shown on Line 17, is $10,000. The target cash balance is subtracted from the forecasted ending cash with no borrowing amount to determine the firm's borrowing requirements (shown in parentheses) or surplus cash (shown without parentheses). Because Madison expects to have ending cash, as shown on Line 16, of only $1,100 in May, it will have to borrow $1,100 − $10,000 = −$8,900 to bring the cash account up to the target balance of $10,000. Assuming that this amount is indeed borrowed, the total loan outstanding will be $8,900 at the end of May. (The assumption is that Madison will not have any loans outstanding on May 1 because the beginning cash balance exceeds the firm's target balance.)

The cumulative cash surplus or required loan balance is shown on Line 18; a positive value indicates a cash surplus, while a negative value indicates a loan requirement. The surplus cash or loan requirement shown on Line 18 is a **cumulative amount**. Thus, Madison is projected to borrow $8,900 in May; it has a cash shortfall during June of $4,600, as reported on Line 14, so its total loan requirement projected for the end of June is $8,900 + $4,600 = $13,500, as shown on Line 18.

The same procedures are followed in subsequent months. Patient volume and billings are projected to peak in July, accompanied by increased payments for supplies, wages, and other items. However, collections are projected to increase by a greater amount than costs and Madison expects a $49,700 net cash inflow during July. This amount is sufficient to pay off the cumulative loan of $13,500 and have a $36,200 cash surplus on hand at the end of the month.

Patient volume and the resulting operating costs are expected to fall sharply in August, but collections will be the highest of any month because they will reflect the high June and July billings. As a result, Madison would normally be forecasting a healthy $101,100 net cash gain during the month. However, the company expects to make a cash payment of $50,000 to purchase a new computer system during August, so the forecasted net cash gain is reduced to $51,100. This net gain adds to the surplus, so August is projected to end with $87,300 in surplus cash. If all goes according to the forecast, later cash surpluses will enable Madison to end this budget period with a surplus of $125,200.

The cash budget is used by Madison's managers for liquidity planning purposes. For example, the Table 8.9 cash budget indicates that Madison will need to obtain $13,500 in total to get through May and June. Thus, if the firm does not have any marketable securities to convert to cash, it will have to arrange a loan, typically a line of credit, to cover this period. Furthermore, the budget indicates a $125,200 cash surplus at the end of October. Madison's managers will have to consider how these funds can best be utilized. Perhaps the money should be paid out to shareholders as dividends, or be used for fixed asset acquisitions or be temporarily invested in marketable securities for later use within the business. This decision will be made on the basis of Madison's overall financial plan.

This brief illustration shows the mechanics and managerial value of the cash budget. However, before concluding this discussion of the cash budget, several additional points need to be made. First, if cash inflows and outflows are not uniform during the month, a monthly cash budget could seriously understate a business' peak financing requirements. The data in Table 8.9 show the situation expected on the last day of each month, but on any given day during the month it could be quite different. If all payments had to be made on the fifth of each month, but collections came in uniformly throughout the month, Madison would need to borrow cash to cover within-month shortages. For example, August's $123,500 of cash payments may occur before the full amount of the $174,600 in collections have been made. In this situation, some amount of cash would have to be obtained to cover shortfalls in August, even though the end of month cash flow after all collections have been made is positive. In this case, Madison would have to prepare a weekly or daily cash budget to indicate such borrowing needs.

Also, because the cash budget represents a forecast, all the values in the table are **expected** values. If actual patient volume, collection times, supplies purchases, wage rates, and so on, differ from forecasted levels, the projected cash deficits and surpluses will be incorrect. Thus, there is a reasonable chance that Madison may end up needing to obtain a larger amount of funds than is indicated on Line 18. Because of the uncertainty of the forecasts, spreadsheet programs are particularly well-suited for constructing and analyzing cash budgets. For example, Madison's managers could change any assumption, say, projected monthly volume or the time third-party payors take to pay, and the cash budget would automatically and instantly be recalculated. This would show Madison's managers exactly how the firm's cash position would change under alternative operating assumptions. Typically, such an analysis is used to determine how large a credit line to establish to cover temporary cash shortages.[7] In Madison's case, such an analysis indicated that a $20,000 line is sufficient.

Self-Test Questions
1. Considering all the information in the operating budget, why do organizations need a cash budget?
2. Does the cash budget require an extensive knowledge of accounting principles?
3. In your view, what is the most important line of the cash budget?

Key Concepts

Planning and budgeting are important managerial activities. In particular, budgets allow health services managers to assess financial performance and to ensure that operations are carried out in a manner consistent with expectations. The key concepts of this chapter are:

- *Planning* encompasses the overall process of preparing for the future, while *budgeting* is the accounting process that ties together planning and control functions.
- The *strategic plan*, which provides broad guidance for the future, is the foundation of any organization's planning process. More detailed managerial guidance is contained in the *operating plan*, often called the *five-year plan*.
- The *financial plan*, which is the financial portion of the operating plan, contains a *long-term plan*, *working capital management plan*, and *accounting plan*.
- *Budgeting* provides a means for communication and coordination of organizational expectations and allocation of scarce resources. In addition, budgeting establishes benchmarks for control.

- There are several types of budgets including the *statistics budget*, *revenue budget*, *expense budget*, *operating budget*, and *cash budget*.
- The *conventional*, or *incremental/decremental*, *approach* to budgeting uses the previous budget as the basis for constructing the new budget. *Zero-based budgeting* begins each budget as a clean slate, and hence all entries have to be justified each budget period.
- *Bottom-up budgeting*, which begins at the unit level, encourages maximum involvement by junior managers. Conversely, *top-down budgeting*, which is less participatory in nature, is a more efficient way to communicate senior management's views.
- The *operating budget* is the basic budget of an organization, in that it sets the profit expectations for the budget period. A critical element of the operating budget is the *profit and loss (P&L) statement*, which is a simplified income statement.
- A *variance* is the difference between a budgeted (planned) value, or *standard*, and the actual (realized) value. *Variance analysis* examines differences between budgeted and realized amounts, with the goal of finding out why things went either badly or well.
- A budget that fully reflects realized results is called the *actual budget*. When the original budget, or *static budget*, is recast to reflect the actual volume of patients treated, but with all other static budget assumptions unchanged, the result is called a *flexible budget*. To be most useful, variance analysis examines differences between the actual, flexible, and static budgets.

This chapter concludes the discussion of managerial accounting. Chapter 9 begins the examination of basic financial analysis concepts.

Questions

8.1 Why is planning and budgeting so important to an organization's success?

8.2 Briefly describe the planning process. Be sure to include summaries of the strategic, operating, and financial plans.

8.3 Describe some of the components of a financial plan.

8.4 How are the statistics, revenue, expense, and operating budgets related?

8.5 a. What are the advantages and disadvantages of conventional budgeting versus zero-based budgeting?
   b. What organizational characteristics create likely candidates for zero-based budgeting?

8.6 If you were the CEO of Bayside Memorial Hospital, would you advocate a top-down or bottom-up approach to budgeting? Explain the rationale behind your answer.

8.7 What is a profit and loss (P&L) statement?

8.8 a. Explain the relationships among the static budget, flexible budget, and actual budget.

b. Assume that a group practice has both capitated and fee-for-service (FFS) patients. Furthermore, the number of capitated enrollees has changed over the budget period. In order to calculate the volume variance and break it down into enrollment and utilization components, how many flexible budgets must be constructed?

8.9 a. What is a cash budget and how is it used?

b. Should depreciation expense appear on a cash budget? Explain your answer.

Problems

8.1 Consider the following three years of profit data for Newark General Hospital (in millions of dollars):

Year	Static Budget	Flexible Budget	Actual Budget
1996	$4.7	$3.6	$2.2
1997	2.4	3.1	3.8
1998	1.6	0.9	(1.3)

a. Calculate and interpret the total variance for each year.
b. Calculate and interpret the volume variance for each year.
c. Calculate and interpret the management variance for each year.
d. How are the variances calculated in Parts a, b, and c related?

8.2 Here are the 1998 profits for the Wendover Group Practice Association for four different budgets, in thousands of dollars:

Static Budget	Flexible (Enrollment/Utilization) Budget	Flexible (Enrollment) Budget	Actual Budget
$425	$200	$180	$300

a. What does the budget data tell you about the nature of Wendover's patients? (Hint: Are they capitated or fee-for-service?)
b. Calculate and interpret the following variances:
   (1) Total variance
   (2) Volume variance
   (3) Management variance
   (4) Enrollment variance
   (5) Utilization variance

8.3 Here are the budgets of Brandon Surgery Center for the most recent historical quarter, in thousands of dollars:

	Static	Flexible	Actual
Number of surgeries	1,200	1,300	1,300
Patient revenue	$2,400	$2,600	$2,535
Salary expense	1,200	1,300	1,365

Non-salary expense	600	650	585
Profit	$ 600	$ 650	$ 585

The center assumes that all revenues and costs are variable, and hence tied directly to patient volume.

a. Explain how each amount in the flexible budget was calculated. (Hint: Examine the static budget to determine the relationship of each budget line to volume.)

b. Determine the variances for each line of the profit and loss statement, both in dollar terms and in percentage terms. (Hint: Each line has a total variance, a volume variance, and a management variance.)

c. What do the Part b results tell Brandon's managers about the surgery center's operations for the quarter?

8.4 Refer to Carroll Clinic's 1998 operating budget contained in Table 8.3. Instead of the actual results reported in Table 8.4, assume the results reported below:

Carroll Clinic: New 1998 Results

I. *Volume:*

A.	FFS	34,000	visits
B.	Capitated lives	30,000	members
	Number of member months	360,000	
	Actual utilization per member-month	0.12	
	Number of visits	43,200	visits
C.	Total actual visits	77,200	visits

II. *Revenues:*

A.	FFS	$ 28	per visit
		× 34,000	actual visits
		$ 952,000	
B.	Capitated lives	$ 2.75	PMPM
		× 360,000	actual member months
		$ 990,000	
C.	Total actual revenues	$1,942,000	

III. *Costs:*

A.	Variable Costs:		
	Medical staffing	$1,242,000	(46,000 hours at $27/hour)
	Supplies	126,000	(90,000 units at $1.40/unit)
	Total variable costs	$1,368,000	
	Variable cost per visit	$ 17.72	($1,368,000/77,200)
B.	Fixed Costs:		
	Overhead, plant, and equipment	$ 525,000	
C.	Total actual costs	$1,893,000	

IV. *Profit and Loss Statement:*

Revenues:	
FFS	$ 952,000
Capitated	990,000
Total	$1,942,000
Costs:	
Variable:	
FFS	$ 602,487
Capitated	765,513
Total	$1,368,000
Contribution margin	$ 574,000
Fixed costs	525,000
Actual profit	$ 49,000

a. Construct Carroll's flexible budget for 1998.

b. What are the total variance, volume variance, and management variance?

c. What is the enrollment variance? The utilization variance?

d. Break down the management variance into staffing, supplies, fixed costs, and revenues variances.

e. Break down the staffing variance into rate and efficiency components.

f. Break down the supplies variance into price and usage components.

g. Interpret your results. In particular, focus on the differences between the variance analysis here and the Carroll Clinic illustration presented in the chapter.

8.5 Refer to Problem 8.4. Assume the results reported in that problem hold, except that a difference existed among budgeted, static enrollment, and realized enrollment. The corrected results are:

Carroll Clinic: Corrected 1998 Results

I.	*Volume:*		
	A. FFS	34,000	visits
	B. Capitated lives	31,000	members
	Number of member months	372,000	
	Actual utilization per member-month	0.11613	
	Number of visits	43,200	visits
	C. Total actual visits	77,200	visits
II.	*Revenues:*		
	A. FFS	$ 28	per visit
		× 34,000	actual visits
		$ 952,000	
	B. Capitated lives	$ 2.75	PMPM
		× 372,000	actual member months
		$1,023,000	
	C. Total actual revenues	$1,975,000	

III. *Costs:*
  A. Variable Costs:

Medical staffing	$1,242,000	(46,000 hours at $27/hour)
Supplies	126,000	(90,000 units at $1.40/unit)
Total variable costs	$1,368,000	
Variable cost per visit	$ 17.72	($1,368,000/77,200)

  B. Fixed Costs:

Overhead, plant, and equipment	$ 525,000
  C. Total actual costs | $1,893,000 |

IV. *Profit and Loss Statement:*
  Revenues:

FFS	$ 952,000
Capitated	1,023,000
Total	$1,975,000
Costs:	
Variable:	
FFS	$ 602,487
Capitated	765,513
Total	$1,368,000
Contribution margin	$ 607,000
Fixed costs	525,000
Actual profit	$ 82,000

a. Construct Carroll's flexible budgets for 1998. (Hint: Because of a change in enrollment, creating three flexible budgets is necessary. See the note to Table 8.7.)

b. What are the total variance, volume variance, and management variance?

c. What is the enrollment variance? The utilization variance? How does your answer here differ from your corresponding answer to Problem 8.5.

d. Break down the management variance into staffing, supplies, fixed costs, and revenues variances.

e. Break down the staffing variance into rate and efficiency components.

f. Break down the supplies variance into price and usage components.

g. Interpret your results. In particular, focus on the differences between the variance analysis here and the one in Problem 8.5.

Notes

1. For an in-depth treatment of budgeting within health services organizations, see A. G. Herkimer, Jr., *Understanding Health Care Budgeting* (Rockville, MD: Aspen, 1988).

2. Financial statement forecasting is an important function of any business' financial staff. However, this discussion will be left to other texts. For more information, see L. C. Gapenski, *Understanding Health Care Financial Management* (Chicago: AUPHA Press/Health Administration Press, 1996).

3. For an extensive discussion on zero-based budgeting within hospitals, see M. M. Person, III, *The Zero-Base Hospital* (Chicago: Health Administration Press, 1997).

4. By assuming no change in enrollment, the example has been simplified to make variance analysis easier to understand at the introductory level. In essence, the Carroll

Clinic analysis is similar to a variance analysis in which all patients are under FFS. Without enrollment variance, only one flexible budget is required. However, had enrollment differences been built into the illustration, two different flexible budgets would have been required. See the note to Table 8.7 and Problems 8.2 and 8.5.

5. Variances can be defined such that the resulting value is either a positive or a negative number. For example, when cost variances are calculated, they can be defined so that a negative variance implies costs less than standard, which is good, or costs greater than standard, which is bad, depending on which budget value is subtracted from the other. In this example, all variances have been defined such that a negative number indicates an undesirable variance and not necessarily that the realized value is less than the standard. For example, a higher-than-standard wage rate would be a negative variance, even though realized wages were higher than standard.

6. In this illustration, no difference exists in revenues between the flexible and actual budgets, so the management variance is also the difference in profit between these two budgets.

7. A *credit line* is an agreement between a borrower and a financial institution that obligates the institution to furnish credit over a time period, typically a year, up to the agreed-on amount. The borrower may use some, all, or none of the credit line. Usually, credit lines require borrowers to pay an up-front fee for the credit guarantee called a *commitment fee*.

References

Gapenski, L. C. 1996. *Understanding Health Care Financial Management*. Chicago: AUPHA Press/Health Administration Press.

Herkimer, A. G., Jr. 1988. *Understanding Health Care Budgeting*. Rockville, MD: Aspen.

Person, M. M., III. 1997. *The Zero-Base Hospital*. Chicago: Health Administration Press.

BASIC FINANCIAL ANALYSIS CONCEPTS

TIME VALUE ANALYSIS

Learning Objectives

After studying this chapter, readers will be able to:

- Explain why time value analysis is so important to healthcare financial management.
- Find the present and future values for lump sums, annuities, and uneven cash flow streams.
- Solve for interest rate and number of periods.
- Explain and apply the opportunity cost principle.
- Describe and apply stated, periodic, and effective annual interest rates.

Introduction

The financial value of any asset, whether a *financial asset*, such as a stock or a bond, or a *real asset*, such as a piece of diagnostic equipment or an ambulatory surgery center, is based on future cash flows. However, a dollar to be received in the future is worth less than a current dollar because a dollar in hand today can be invested, perhaps in a bank savings account, can earn interest, and hence can be worth more than one dollar in the future.[1] Because current dollars are worth more than future dollars, valuation analyses must account for cash flow timing differences.

The process of assigning proper values to cash flows that occur at different points in time is called *time value analysis*. It is an important part of many healthcare financial decisions because many financial analyses involve the valuation of future cash flows. In fact, of all the financial analysis techniques that are discussed in this book, none is more important than time value analysis. The concepts presented here are the cornerstones of financial analysis, so a thorough understanding of time value concepts is essential to good financial decision making.

Time Lines

One important tool used in time value analysis is the *time line*. Time lines make it easier to visualize when the cash flows in a particular analysis occur. To illustrate the time line concept, consider the following five-period time line:

```
0        1        2        3        4        5
|--------|--------|--------|--------|--------|
```

Time 0 is any starting point; Time 1 is one period from the starting point, or the end of Period 1; Time 2 is two periods from the starting point, or the end of Period 2, and so on. Thus, the numbers on top of the tick marks represent end-of-period values. Often, the periods are years, but other time intervals such as quarters, months, or days are also used when needed to fit the timing of the cash flows being evaluated. If the time periods are years, the interval from 0 to 1 would be Year 1, and the tick mark labeled 1 would represent both the end of Year 1 and the beginning of Year 2. Also, in many time value analyses, Time 0 (the starting point) is considered to be today.

Cash flows are shown on a time line directly below the tick marks, and interest rates are sometimes shown directly above the time line. Additionally, unknown cash flows—the ones to be determined in the analysis—are sometimes indicated by question marks. To illustrate, consider the following time line:

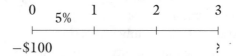

In this case, the interest rate for each of the three periods is 5 percent; a *lump sum* (single amount) investment of $100 is made at Time 0 and the Time 3 value is unknown. The $100 is an *outflow* because it is shown as a negative cash flow. (Outflows are often designated by parentheses rather than by minus signs.)

Time lines are essential when learning time value concepts, but even experienced analysts use time lines when dealing with complex problems. The time line may be an actual line, as illustrated above, or it may be a series of columns (or rows) on a spreadsheet. Time lines will be used extensively in the remainder of this book, so get into the habit of creating time lines when conducting analyses that involve future cash flows.

Self-Test Question

1. Draw a three-year time line that illustrates the following situation:
   • an investment of $10,000 at Time 0;
   • inflows of $5,000 at the end of Years 1, 2, and 3; and
   • an interest rate during the entire three years of 10 percent.

Future Value of a Lump Sum (Compounding)

The process of going from today's values, or *present values*, to future values is called *compounding*. To illustrate *lump sum* compounding, which deals with a single starting cash flow, suppose that the manager of Meridian Clinics deposits $100 in a bank account that pays 5 percent interest each year. How much would be in the account at the end of one year? To begin, here are some terms that are used in the solution:

- PV = $100 = present value, or beginning amount, of the account.
- I   = 5% = interest rate the bank pays on the account per year. The interest amount, which is paid at the end of the year, is based on the balance at the beginning of each year. Expressed as a decimal, I = 0.05.
- INT = dollars of interest earned during each year, which equals the beginning amount multiplied by the interest rate. Thus, INT = PV × I.
- FV_N = future value, or ending amount, of the account at the end of N years. Whereas PV is the value now, or *present value*, FV_N is the value N years into the *future* after the interest earned has been added to the account.
- N   = number of years involved in the analysis.

In the preceding example, N = 1, so FV_N can be calculated as follows:

$$FV_N = FV_1 = PV + INT$$
$$= PV + (PV \times I)$$
$$= PV \times (1 + I).$$

The future value at the end of one year, FV_1, equals the present value multiplied by 1.0 plus the interest rate. This future value relationship can be used to find how much $100 will be worth at the end of one year, if it is invested in an account that pays 5 percent interest:

$$FV_1 = PV \times (1 + I) = \$100 \times (1 + 0.05) = \$100 \times 1.05 = \$105.$$

What would be the value of the $100 if Meridian Clinics left its money in the account for five years? Here is a time line that shows the amount at the end of each year:

	0	1	2	3	4	5
	5%					
Beginning amount	−$100	?	?	?	?	?
Interest earned		$ 5	$ 5.25	$ 5.51	$ 5.79	$ 6.08
End of year amount		105	110.25	115.76	121.55	127.63.

Note the following points:

- The account is opened with a deposit of $100. This is shown as an outflow at Year 0.
- Meridian earns $100 × 0.05 = $5 of interest during the first year, so the amount in the account at the end of Year 1 is $100 + $5 = $105.
- At the start of the second year, the account balance is $105. Interest of $105 × 0.05 = $5.25 is earned on the now larger amount, and the account balance at the end of the second year is $105 + $5.25 = $110.25. The Year 2 interest,

$5.25, is higher than the first year's interest, $5, because $5 \times 0.05 = \$0.25$ in interest was earned on the first year's interest.

- This process continues, and because the beginning balance is higher in each succeeding year, the interest earned increases in each year.
- The total interest earned, $27.63, is reflected in the final balance at the end of Year 5, $127.63.

The Year 2 value, $110.25, is equal to:

$$FV_2 = FV_1 \times (1 + I)$$
$$= PV \times (1 + I) \times (1 + I)$$
$$= PV \times (1 + I)^2$$
$$= \$100 \times (1.05)^2 = \$110.25.$$

Continuing, the balance at the end of Year 3 is:

$$FV_3 = FV_2 \times (1 + I)$$
$$= PV \times (1 + I)^3$$
$$= \$100 \times (1.05)^3 = \$115.76,$$

and

$$FV_5 = \$100 \times (1.05)^5 = \$127.63.$$

In general, the future value of a lump sum at the end of N years can be found by applying this equation:

$$FV_N = PV \times (1 + I)^N.$$

Future values, as well as most other time value problems, can be solved three ways:

1. *Use a regular calculator.* Use a regular calculator, either by multiplying the PV by $(1 + I)$ for N times or by using the exponential function to raise $(1 + I)$ to the Nth power, and then multiplying the result by the PV. The easiest way to find the future value of $100 after five years when compounded at 5 percent is to enter $100, then multiply this amount by 1.05 five times. If the calculator is set to display two decimal places, the answer would be $127.63:

0	1	2	3	4	5
$100 × 1.05	× 1.05	× 1.05	× 1.05	× 1.05	$127.63

As denoted by the arrows, compounding involves moving to the **right** along the time line.

2. *Use a financial calculator.* Financial calculators have been programmed to solve many types of time value problems. In effect, the future value equation is programmed directly into the calculator. Using a financial calculator, the future value is found using these time value input keys[2]:

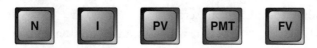

Note that these keys correspond to the five time value variables that are commonly used:

- N = number of periods;
- I = interest rate per period;
- PV = present value;
- PMT = payment (This key is used only if the cash flows involve a series of equal payments—an annuity.); and
- FV = future value.

This chapter deals with time value problems that involve only four of the variables at any one time. Three of the variables will be known and the calculator will solve for the fourth, unknown variable. In Chapter 11, when bond valuation is discussed, all five variables will be included in the analysis.

To find the future value of $100 after five years at 5 percent interest using a financial calculator, just enter PV = 100, I = 5, and N = 5 and then press the FV key. The answer, 127.63 (rounded to two decimal places), will appear. Many financial calculators require that cash flows be designated as either inflows or outflows (entered as either positive or negative values). Applying this logic to the illustration, Meridian deposits the initial amount, which is an outflow to the firm, and takes out or receives the ending amount, which is an inflow to the firm. If the calculator requires this sign convention, the PV would be entered as −100. (If the PV was entered as 100, a positive value, the calculator would display —127.63 as the answer.)

Also, some calculators require the user to press a *Compute* key before pressing the FV key. Finally, financial calculators permit specifying the number of decimal places that are displayed, even though 12 (or more) significant digits are actually used in the calculations. Two places are generally used for answers in dollars or percentages and four places for decimal answers. The final answer, however, should be rounded to reflect the accuracy of the input values; it makes no sense to say that the return on a particular investment is 14.63827 percent when the cash flows are highly uncertain. The nature of the analysis dictates how many decimal places should be displayed.

3. *Use a spreadsheet.* Personal computer spreadsheet programs such as Excel, Lotus 1-2-3, and Quattro Pro are frequently used to solve time value problems. Many common time value solutions are preprogrammed in the spreadsheet software and users can create their own formulas to perform

tasks that have not been preprogrammed. The time value formulas that are preprogrammed in spreadsheets are called *functions* (or in some software, @ functions [pronounced "at functions"]). Like any formula, a time value function consists of a number of arithmetic calculations combined into one statement. By using functions, spreadsheet users can save the time and tedium of building formulas from scratch.

Each function begins with a unique function name that identifies the calculation to be performed, along with one or more *arguments* (the input values for the calculation) enclosed in parentheses. There is no spreadsheet function for finding the future value of a lump sum because it can be quickly calculated by formula. For example, the Excel formula for solving the Meridian Clinic example over five years is:

$$= 100 * (1.05)^\wedge 5$$

where = tells the spreadsheet that a formula is being entered into the cell, * is the spreadsheet multiplication sign, and ^ is the spreadsheet exponential (or power) sign. When this formula is entered into a spreadsheet cell, the value 127.63 appears in the cell.[3]

The most efficient way to solve most problems involving time value is to use a financial calculator or a spreadsheet.[4] However, the basic mathematics behind the calculations must be understood to set up complex problems before solving them. In addition, the underlying logic must be understood to comprehend stock and bond valuation, lease analysis, capital budgeting analysis, and other important healthcare financial management topics.

Self-Test Questions

1. What is a lump sum?
2. What is compounding?
3. What is meant by the term *interest on interest*?
4. What are three solution techniques for solving lump sum compounding problems?
5. How does the future value of a lump sum change as the time is extended and as the interest rate increases?

Present Value of a Lump Sum (Discounting)

Suppose that GroupWest Health Plans, which has premium income reserves to invest, has been offered the chance to purchase a low-risk security from a local broker that will pay $127.63 at the end of five years. A local bank is currently offering 5 percent interest on a five-year certificate of deposit (CD), and GroupWest's managers regard the security offered by the broker as being as safe as the bank CD. The 5 percent interest rate available on the bank CD is GroupWest's *opportunity cost rate*. (Opportunity costs are discussed in detail in the next section.) How much would GroupWest be willing to pay for the security that promises to pay $127.63 in five years?

The future value example presented in the previous section showed that an initial amount of $100 invested at 5 percent per year would be worth $127.63 at the end of five years. Thus, GroupWest should be indifferent to the choice between $100 today and $127.63 at the end of five years. Today's $100 is defined as the *present value*, or *PV*, of $127.63 due in five years when the opportunity cost rate is 5 percent. If the price of the security being offered is anything less than $100, GroupWest should buy it. If the price is greater than $100, GroupWest should turn the offer down. If the price is exactly $100, GroupWest could buy it or turn it down because that is the security's "fair value."

In general, the present value of a cash flow due N years in the future is the amount which, if it were on hand today, would grow to equal the future amount when compounded at the opportunity cost rate. Because $100 would grow to $127.63 in five years at a 5 percent interest rate, $100 is the present value of $127.63 due five years in the future when the opportunity cost rate is 5 percent.

Finding present values is called *discounting*, and it is simply the reverse of compounding: if the PV is known, compound to find the FV; if the FV is known, discount to find the PV. Here are the solution techniques used to solve this discounting problem.

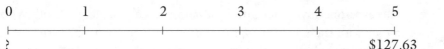

Time Line

To develop the discounting equation, solve the compounding equation for PV:

Compounding: $FV_N = PV \times (1 + I)^N$

Discounting: $PV = \dfrac{FV_N}{(1 + I)^N}$

Enter $127.63 and divide it five times by 1.05:

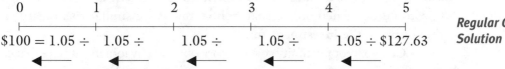

Regular Calculator Solution

As shown by the arrows, discounting is moving to the left along a time line.

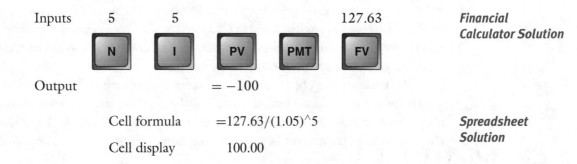

Financial Calculator Solution

Inputs	5	5			127.63
	N	I	PV	PMT	FV
Output			= −100		

Cell formula	=127.63/(1.05)^5
Cell display	100.00

Spreadsheet Solution

1. What is discounting? How is it related to compounding?
2. What are the three techniques for solving lump sum discounting problems?
3. How does the present value of an amount to be received in the future change as the time is extended and as the interest rate increases?

Opportunity Costs

In the last section, the *opportunity cost* concept was used to set the discount rate on GroupWest's investment. This concept plays a very important role in time value analysis. To illustrate, suppose that a person found the winning ticket for the Florida lottery and now has $1 million to invest. Should the person assign a cost to these funds? At first blush, it may appear that this money has zero cost because its acquisition was purely a matter of luck. However, as soon as he or she thinks about what to do with the $1 million, the person has to think in terms of the opportunity costs involved. By using the funds to invest in one alternative, for example Columbia/HCA stock, the person forgoes the opportunity to make some other investment, for example buying U.S. Treasury bonds. Thus, there is an opportunity cost associated with any investment planned for the $1 million even though the lottery winnings were "free."

Because one investment decision automatically negates all other possible investments with the same funds, the cash flows expected to be earned from any investment must be discounted at a rate that reflects the return that could be earned on forgone opportunities **regardless of the source of the funds**. The problem is that the number of forgone opportunities is virtually infinite, so which one should be chosen to establish the opportunity cost rate? The opportunity cost rate to be applied in time value analysis is the rate that could be earned on alternative investments of similar risk. It would not be logical to assign a very low opportunity cost rate to a series of very risky cash flows or vice versa. This concept is one of the cornerstones of financial management, so it is worth repeating. **The opportunity cost rate (i.e., the discount rate) applied to investment cash flows is the rate that could be earned on alternative investments of similar risk regardless of the source of the investment funds.**

Generally, opportunity cost rates are obtained by looking at rates that could be earned (or more precisely, rates that are expected to be earned) on securities such as stocks or bonds. Securities are usually chosen to set opportunity cost rates because their expected returns are more easily estimated than rates of return on real assets such as HMOs, group practices, hospital beds, MRI machines, and the like. Furthermore, as discussed in Chapter 12, securities generally provide the minimum return appropriate for the amount of risk assumed, so securities returns provide a good benchmark for other investments.

To illustrate the opportunity cost concept, assume that Oakdale Community Hospital is considering building a nursing home. The first step in the financial analysis is to forecast the cash flows that the nursing home is expected to produce. These cash flows, then, must be discounted at some opportunity cost rate. Would the hospital's opportunity cost rate be (1) the expected rate of return on Treasury bonds; (2) the expected rate of return on the stock of Beverly Enterprises, which owns some 850 nursing homes; or (3) the expected rate of return on pork belly futures? (Pork belly futures are investments that involve commodity contracts for delivery at some future time.) The answer is the expected rate of return on Beverly Enterprises' stock because that is the rate of return available to the hospital on alternative investments of similar risk. Treasury securities are low-risk investments, so they would understate the opportunity cost rate in owning a nursing home. Conversely, pork belly futures are very high-risk investments, so that rate of return is probably too high to apply to Oakdale's nursing home investment.[5]

The source of the funds used for the nursing home investment is **not relevant** to the analysis. Oakdale may obtain the needed funds by issuing tax-exempt debt or by soliciting contributions, or it may have excess cash accumulated from profit retention. The discount rate applied to the nursing home cash flows depends only on the riskiness of those cash flows and the returns available on alternative investments of similar risk, not on the source of the investment funds.

The bottom line is that some opportunity cost rate has to be applied to discount future cash flows. The proper rate is the rate available on foregone investments of risk similar to the flows being discounted; this rate is normally established by looking at expected returns on securities. (Chapter 13 contains a discussion of how baseline opportunity cost rates are established for capital investments; Chapter 15 presents a detailed discussion on how the riskiness of a cash flow stream can be assessed.)

<table>
<tr><td>

1. Why does an investment have an opportunity cost rate even when the funds employed have no explicit cost?
2. How are opportunity cost rates established?
3. Does the opportunity cost rate depend on the source of the investment funds?

</td><td>

Self-Test Questions

</td></tr>
</table>

Solving for Interest Rate and Time

At this point, it should be obvious that compounding and discounting are recipro-cal processes. Furthermore, four time value analysis variables have been presented: PV, FV, I, and N. If the values of three of the variables are known, with the help of a financial calculator or spreadsheet the value of the fourth can be found. Thus far, the interest rate, I, and the number of years, N, plus either PV or FV have been given in the illustrations. In some situations, however, the analysis may require solving for either I or N.[6]

Solving for Interest Rate (I)

Suppose that Family Practice Associates (FPA), a primary care physicians' group practice, can buy a bank CD for $78.35 that will return $100 after five years. In this case PV, FV, and N are known, but I, the interest rate that the bank is paying, is not known. These types of problems are solved as follows.

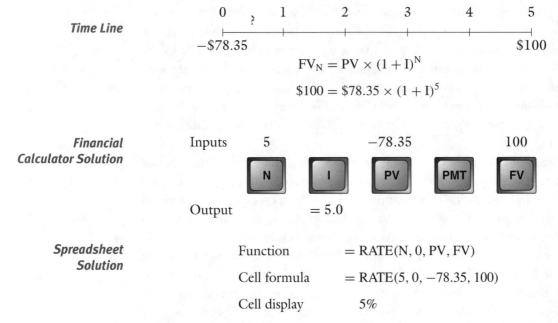

Time Line

$$FV_N = PV \times (1 + I)^N$$

$$\$100 = \$78.35 \times (1 + I)^5$$

Financial Calculator Solution

Inputs   5   −78.35   100

Output   = 5.0

Spreadsheet Solution

Function   = RATE(N, 0, PV, FV)

Cell formula   = RATE(5, 0, −78.35, 100)

Cell display   5%

In this case, a spreadsheet function named RATE is used to solve for I. Note that some spreadsheet programs display the answer in decimal form, unless the cell is formatted to display in percent

Solving for Time (N)

Suppose that the bank told FPA that a certificate of deposit pays 5 percent interest each year, that it costs $78.35, and that at maturity the group would receive $100. How long must the funds be invested in the CD? In this case, PV, FV, and I are known, but N, the number of periods, is not known. Following are ways to solve this type of problem.

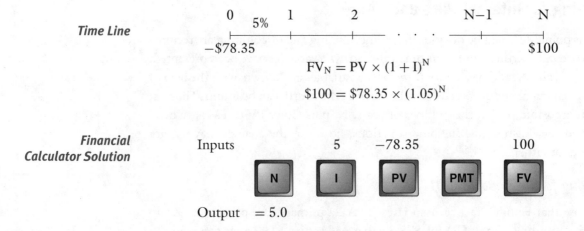

Time Line

$$FV_N = PV \times (1 + I)^N$$

$$\$100 = \$78.35 \times (1.05)^N$$

Financial Calculator Solution

Inputs   5   −78.35   100

Output   = 5.0

Spreadsheet Solution

Function	= NPER(I, 0, PV, FV)
Cell formula	= NPER(0.05, 0, 78.35, 100)
Cell display	5.00

Note in this example that interest rates are entered as decimals in function arguments.

Self-Test Questions

1. What are a few real-world situations that may require you to solve for interest rate or time?
2. Can financial calculators and spreadsheets easily solve for interest rate or time?

Annuities

Whereas lump sums are single values, an *annuity* is a series of **equal payments** at **fixed intervals** for a specified number of periods. Annuity cash flows, which are given the symbol PMT, can occur at the beginning or end of each period. If the payments occur at the end of each period as they typically do, the annuity is an *ordinary*, or *deferred*, *annuity*. If payments are made at the beginning of each period, the annuity is an *annuity due*. Because ordinary annuities are far more common in time value problems when the term *annuity* is used in this book, assume that payments occur at the end of each period.

Ordinary Annuities

A series of equal payments at the end of each period constitute an ordinary annuity. If Meridian Clinics were to deposit $100 at the end of each year for three years in an account that paid 5 percent interest per year, how much would Meridian accumulate at the end of three years? The answer to this question is the future value of the annuity.

Time Line

```
0        1        2        3
   5%
 |--------|--------|--------|
     -$100   -$100   -$100
                        ?
```

The future value of any annuity occurs at the end of the last period. Thus, for regular annuities, the future value coincides with the final payment.

One approach to the problem is to compound each individual cash flow to Year 3.

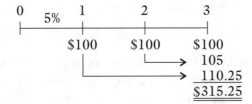

Regular Calculator Solution

Financial Calculator Solution

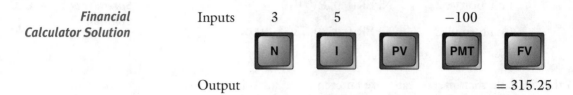

Inputs   3   5   −100

Output   = 315.25

In annuity problems, the PMT key is used in conjunction with either the PV or FV key.

Spreadsheet Solution

Function	$= FV(I, N, PMT)$
Cell formula	$= FV(0.05, 3, -100)$
Cell display	\$315.25

Suppose that Meridian Clinics was offered the following alternatives: a three-year annuity with payments of \$100 at the end of each year, or a lump sum payment today. Meridian has no need for the money during the next three years. If it accepts the annuity, it would deposit the payments in an account that pays 5 percent interest per year. Similarly, the lump sum payment would be deposited into the same account. How large must the lump sum payment be today to make it equivalent to the annuity?

Regular Calculator Solution

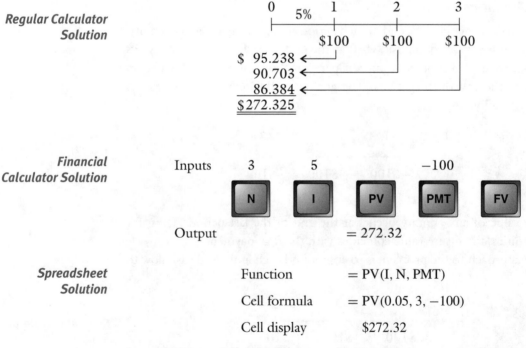

Financial Calculator Solution

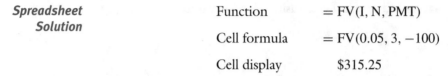

Inputs   3   5   −100

Output   = 272.32

Spreadsheet Solution

Function	$= PV(I, N, PMT)$
Cell formula	$= PV(0.05, 3, -100)$
Cell display	\$272.32

One especially important application of the annuity concept relates to loans with constant payments such as mortgages, auto loans, and many bank loans to businesses. Such loans are examined in more depth in a later section on amortization.

Annuities Due

If the three $100 payments in the previous example had been made at the beginning of each year, the annuity would have been an *annuity due*. Each payment would be shifted to the left one year, so each payment would be discounted for one less year. Because its payments come in faster, an annuity due is more valuable than an ordinary annuity.

The future value of our example, assuming an annuity due, is found as follows:

```
0       1       2       3
   5%
├───────┼───────┼───────┤
-$100   -$100   -$100     ?
```
Time Line

The future value of an annuity due occurs one period after the final payment, while the future value of a regular annuity coincides with the final payment.

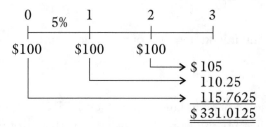

Regular Calculator Solution

In the case of an annuity due, as compared with an ordinary annuity, all the cash flows are compounded for one additional period, and hence the future value of an annuity due is greater than the future value of a similar ordinary annuity by $(1 + I)$. Thus, the future value of an annuity due also can be found as follows:

$$\text{FV (Annuity due)} = \text{FV of a regular annuity} \times (1 + I)$$

$$= \$315.25 \times 1.05 = \$331.01.$$

Most financial calculators have a switch or key marked DUE or BEGIN that permits the switching of the mode from end-of-period payments (ordinary annuity) to beginning-of-period payments (annuity due). When the beginning-of-period mode is activated, the display will normally indicate the changed mode with the word BEGIN or another symbol. To deal with annuities due, change the mode to beginning of period and proceed as before. Because most problems will deal with end-of-period cash flows, do not forget to switch the calculator back to the END mode.

Financial Calculator Solution

Function	$= \text{FV}(I, N, PMT) * (1 + I)$
Cell formula	$= \text{FV}(0.05, 3, -100) * (1.05)$
Cell display	$331.01

Spreadsheet Solution

The present value of an annuity due is found in a similar manner.

Time Line and Regular Calculator Solution

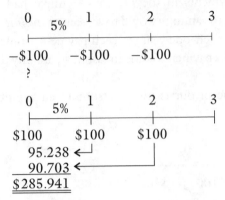

The present value of an annuity due can be thought of as the present value of an ordinary annuity that is compounded for one period, so it also can be found as follows:

$$PV(\text{Annuity due}) = PV \text{ of a regular annuity} \times (1 + I)$$

$$= \$272.32 \times 1.05 = \$285.94.$$

Financial Calculator Solution Activate the beginning of period mode (i.e., the BEGIN mode) and then proceed as before. Again, because most problems will deal with end-of-period cash flows, do not forget to switch the calculator back to the END mode.

Spreadsheet Solution

Function	$= PV(I, N, PMT) * (1 + I)$
Cell formula	$= PV(0.05, 3, -100) * (1.05)$
Cell display	$285.94

Self-Test Questions

1. What is an annuity?
2. What is the difference between an ordinary annuity and an annuity due?
3. Which annuity has the greater future value: an ordinary annuity or an annuity due? Why?
4. Which annuity has the greater present value: an ordinary annuity or an annuity due? Why?

Perpetuities

Most annuities call for payments to be made over some finite period of time—for example, $100 per year for three years. However, some annuities go on indefinitely, or perpetually. Such annuities are called *perpetuities*. The present value of a perpetuity is found as follows:

$$PV \text{ (Perpetuity)} = \frac{\text{Payment}}{\text{Interest rate}} = \frac{PMT}{I}.$$

Perpetuities can be illustrated by some securities issued by General Healthcare, Inc. Each security promises to pay $100 annually in perpetuity (forever). What would each security be worth if the opportunity cost rate, or discount rate, was 10 percent? The answer is $1,000:

$$PV \text{ (Perpetuity)} = \frac{\$100}{0.10} = \$1,000.$$

Suppose interest rates, and hence the opportunity cost rate, rose to 15 percent. What would happen to the security's value? The interest rate increase would lower its value to $666.67:

$$PV \text{ (Perpetuity)} = \frac{\$100}{0.15} = \$666.67.$$

Assume that interest rates fell to 5 percent. The rate decrease would increase the perpetuity's value to $2,000:

$$PV \text{ (Perpetuity)} = \frac{\$100}{0.05} = \$2,000.$$

The value of a perpetuity changes dramatically when interest rates change. All securities' values are affected by interest rate changes, but some, like perpetuities, are more sensitive to interest rate changes than others, such as short-term government bonds. The risks associated with interest rate changes are discussed in more detail in Chapter 11.

Self-Test Questions

1. What is a perpetuity?
2. What happens to the value of a perpetuity when interest rates increase or decrease?

Uneven Cash Flow Streams

The definition of an annuity includes the words "constant amount," so annuities involve payments that are the same in every period. Although some financial decisions, such as bond valuation, do involve constant payments, most important healthcare financial analyses involve uneven, or nonconstant, cash flows. For example, the financial evaluation of a proposed outpatient clinic or MRI facility rarely involves constant cash flows.

In general, the term *payment (PMT)* is reserved for annuity situations, in which the cash flows are constant, and the term *cash flow (CF)* denotes uneven cash flows. Financial calculators are set up to follow this convention. When dealing with uneven cash flows, CF functions rather than the PMT key are used.

Present Value

The present value of an uneven cash flow stream is found as the sum of the present values of the individual cash flows of the stream. For example, suppose the Medical Practice of San Diego is considering opening a new office in a rapidly developing suburban area. The firm's medical director forecasts that the new office would produce the following stream of cash flows in thousands of dollars:

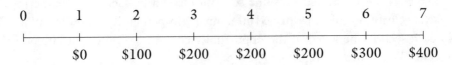

What is the present value of the new office investment if the appropriate discount rate (i.e., the opportunity cost rate) is 10 percent?

Regular Calculator Solution   The PV of each individual cash flow can be found using a regular calculator, and then these values are summed to find the present value of the stream, $868.28[7]:

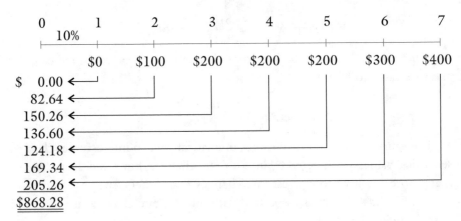

Financial Calculator Solution   Problems involving uneven cash flows can be solved in one step with most financial calculators. In this case:

1. Input the individual cash flows in chronological order into the *cash flow registers*, usually designated as CF_0 and CF_j (CF_1, CF_2, CF_3, and so on) or just CF_j (CF_0, CF_1, CF_2, CF_3, and so on).
2. Enter the discount rate.
3. Push the *NPV* key.

For this problem, enter 0, 0, 100, 200, 200, 200, 300, and 400 in that order into the calculator's cash flow registers; enter I = 10; and then push NPV to obtain the answer, 868.30. A rounding difference occurs because each PV on the time line above was rounded to two decimal places. Also, note that an implied cash flow of zero is entered for CF.

　　　Three points should be noted about the calculator solution technique. First, when dealing with the cash flow registers, the term *NPV* is used to represent present value rather than *PV*. The letter N in *NPV* stands for the word *net*, so *NPV* is the abbreviation for net present value. Net present value means the sum or net of the present values of a cash flow stream that generally contains both positive and negative cash flows—both inflows and outflows. In effect, the inflows and outflows are netted out on a present value basis. This example has no negative cash flows, but if it did, they would be input into the cash flow registers as negative numbers.

Second, the annuity cash flows can be entered into the cash flow registers more efficiently on most calculators by using the N_j key. This key allows the user to specify the number of times a constant payment occurs within an uneven cash flow stream. (Some calculators prompt the user to enter the number of times the cash flow occurs.) In this illustration, enter $CF_0 = 0$, $CF_1 = 0$, $CF_2 = 100$, $CF_3 = 200$, $N_j = 3$, $CF_6 = 300$, and $CF_7 = 400$. Enter $I = 10$, press the NPV key and 868.30 appears in the display.

Finally, amounts entered into the cash flow registers remain in those registers until they are cleared. Thus, if a problem had been previously worked with eight cash flows and then a problem is worked with only four cash flows, the calculator would assume that the final four cash flows from the first calculation belonged to the second calculation. Be sure to clear the cash flow registers before starting a new problem.

Spreadsheet Solution

The NPV function calculates the present value of a series called a spreadsheet *range* of cash flows. First, the cash flow values must be entered into consecutive cells in the spreadsheet. For example:

Cell Address:	A10	B10	C10	D10	E10	F10	G10
Value:	0	100	200	200	200	300	400.

The NPV function then is placed in an empty cell, for example, A5:

Function	$= NPV(I, range)$
Cell formula	$= NPV(0.10, A10 : G10)$
Cell display	$868.30

The NPV function assumes that cash flows occur at the **end** of each period, so NPV is calculated as of the **beginning** of the period of the first cash flow specified in the range. Because the cash flow specified as the first flow in the range was a Year 1 value, the calculated NPV occurs at the beginning of Year 1 (or the end of Year 0), which is correct for this problem. However, many situations include a Year 0 cash flow, which means that the NPV would be calculated at the beginning of Year 0 (or the end of Year -1), which would be incorrect.

This problem has two solutions. One solution is to compound the calculated present value one period at 10 percent. The effect is to move the PV one year to the right along the time line. The spreadsheet cell would look like this:

$$\text{Function} \quad = NPV(I, \text{range including } CF_0) * (1 + I)$$

Another solution is to change the range in the argument to force the first payment in the range to occur at Year 1, so the present value will be calculated at Year 0. However, because there is a Year 0 cash flow that must enter into the calculation, the Year 0 cash flow must be added to the spreadsheet-calculated NPV. This approach would look like this:

$$\text{Function} = \text{NPV(I, modified range without } CF_0) + \text{Year 0 Cell}$$

Future Value

The future value of an uneven cash flow stream is found by compounding each payment to the end of the stream and then summing the future values.

Regular Calculator Solution The future value of each individual cash flow can be found using a regular calculator, and then summing these values to find the future value of the stream, $1,692.07:

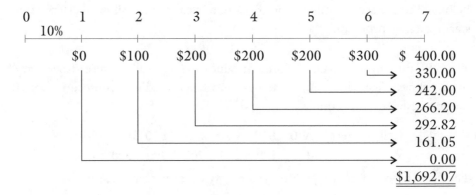

Financial Calculator Solution Some financial calculators have a net future value key (NFV) which, after the cash flows have been entered into the cash flow registers, can be used to obtain the future value of an uneven cash flow stream. However, there is generally more interest in the present value of a cash flow stream than in its future value because the present value represents today's value, which can be compared to the cost of the asset, be it a stock, bond, or a new group practice office.

Spreadsheet Solution Most spreadsheet programs do not have a function that computes the future value of an uneven cash flow stream. However, future values can be found by building a formula in a cell that replicates the regular calculator solution.

Solving for the Interest Rate (I)

Although solving for I is relatively easy when the cash flows are lump sums or annuities, solving for I is more difficult when the present or future value is given and the cash flows are uneven. One can use a trial and error technique in which various values of I are chosen until the one is found that forces the correct value for the PV or FV. Alternatively, a financial calculator's internal rate of return (IRR) function can be used when the present value is known. IRR will be discussed further in Chapter 14 in connection with capital investment decisions.

1. Give two examples of financial decisions that typically involve uneven cash flows.
2. What is meant by the term *net present value*?

Semiannual and Other Compounding Periods

In all the examples thus far, the assumption was that interest is compounded once a year, or annually. This is called *annual compounding*. Suppose, however, that Meridian Clinics puts $100 into a bank account that pays 6 percent annual interest, but it is compounded *semiannually*. How much would the clinic accumulate at the end of one year, two years, or some other period? Semiannual compounding means that interest is paid each six months, so interest is earned more often than under annual compounding.

To illustrate semiannual compounding, assume that the $100 is placed into the account for three years. The following situation occurs under **annual** compounding:

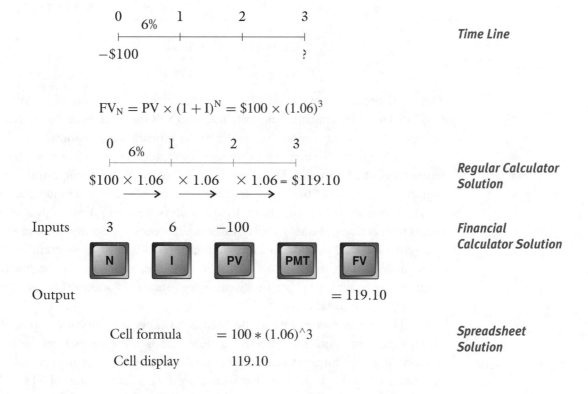

$$FV_N = PV \times (1 + I)^N = \$100 \times (1.06)^3$$

Time Line

Regular Calculator Solution

Financial Calculator Solution

Spreadsheet Solution

Now consider what happens under **semiannual** compounding. Because interest rates usually are stated as annual rates, this situation would be described as 6 percent interest, compounded semiannually. With semiannual compounding, N = 2 × 3 = 6 semiannual periods and I = 6 / 2 = 3% per semiannual period. Here is the solution:

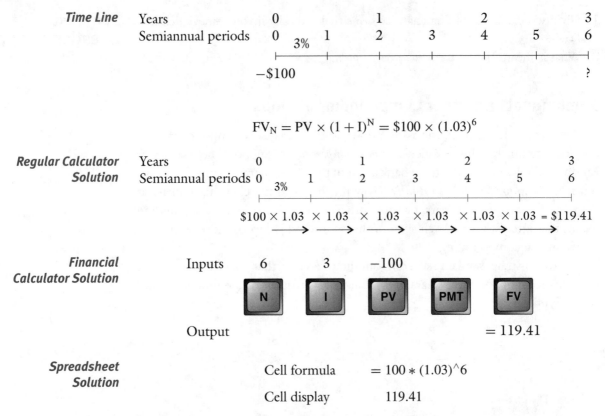

Time Line

$$FV_N = PV \times (1 + I)^N = \$100 \times (1.03)^6$$

Regular Calculator Solution

Financial Calculator Solution

Spreadsheet Solution

| Cell formula | $= 100 * (1.03)^6$ |
| Cell display | 119.41 |

The $100 deposit grows to $119.41 under semiannual compounding, but only to $119.10 under annual compounding. This result occurs because interest on interest is being earned more frequently under semiannual compounding.

Throughout the economy, different compounding periods are used for different types of investments. For example, bank accounts often compound interest monthly or daily, most bonds pay interest semiannually, and stocks generally pay quarterly dividends.[8] Furthermore, the cash flows stemming from capital investments such as hospital wings or diagnostic equipment can be analyzed in monthly, quarterly or annual periods, or even another interval. To properly compare time value analyses with different compounding periods, they need to be put on a common basis, which leads to a discussion of *stated*, or *nominal*, *interest rates* versus *effective annual rates*.

The stated interest rate in the Meridian Clinics semiannual compounding example is 6 percent. The effective annual rate is the rate that produces the same ending (i.e., future) value under annual compounding. In the example, the effective annual rate is the rate that would produce a future value of $119.41 at the end of Year 3 under **annual compounding**. The solution is 6.09 percent:

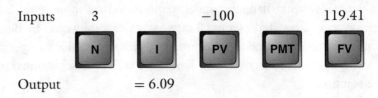

Thus, if one bank offered to pay 6 percent interest with semiannual compounding on a savings account while another offered 6.09 percent with annual compounding, they would both be paying the same effective annual rate because the ending value is the same under both sets of terms:

Years   0   1   2   3
Semiannual periods 0   1   2   3   4   5   6

3%

$$\$100 \times 1.03 \times 1.03 \times 1.03 \times 1.03 \times 1.03 \times 1.03 = \$119.41$$

Years   0   1   2   3

6.09%

$$\$100 \times 1.0609 \times 1.0609 \times 1.0609 = \$119.41$$

In general, the effective annual rate (EAR) can be determined, given the stated rate and number of compounding periods per year, by using this equation[9]:

$$\text{Effective annual rate (EAR)} = (1 + I_{Stated}/M)^M - 1.0.$$

In this case, I_{Stated} is the stated (i.e., the annual) interest rate and M is the number of compounding periods per year. The term I_{Stated}/M is the *periodic* interest rate, so the EAR equation can be restated as:

$$\text{Effective annual rate (EAR)} = (1 + \text{Periodic rate})^M - 1.0.$$

To illustrate use of the EAR equation, the effective annual rate when the stated rate is 6 percent and semiannual compounding occurs is 6.09 percent:

$$\begin{aligned} \text{EAR} &= (1 + 0.06/2)^2 - 1.0 \\ &= (1.03)^2 - 1.0 \\ &= 1.0609 - 1.0 = 0.0609 = 6.09\%. \end{aligned}$$

As shown in the preceding calculations, semiannual compounding, or for that matter any compounding that occurs more than once a year, can be handled two ways. First, the input variables can be expressed as periodic variables rather than annual variables. In the Meridian Clinics example, use N = 6 periods rather than N = 3 years, and I = 3% per period rather than I = 6% per year. Second, find the effective annual rate and then use this rate as an annual rate over the number of years. In the example, use I = 6.09% and N = 3 years.

For another illustration, consider the interest rate charged on credit cards. Many banks charge 1.5 percent per month and in their advertising state that the annual percentage rate (APR) is 18.0 percent.[10] However, the true cost rate to credit card users is the effective annual rate of 19.6 percent:

$$EAR = (1 + \text{Periodic rate})^M - 1.0$$

$$= (1.015)^{12} - 1.0 = 0.196 = 19.6\%.$$

Compounding periods, other than annually, also can occur when dealing with annuities. To illustrate, first consider the case of an ordinary annuity of $100 per year for three years discounted at 8 percent, compounded annually.

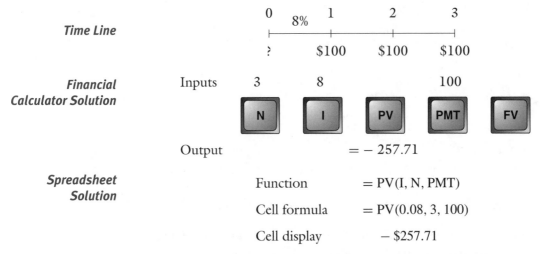

Time Line

Financial Calculator Solution

Spreadsheet Solution

Suppose that the annuity calls for payments of $50 every six months for three years and the interest rate is 8 percent, compounded semiannually:

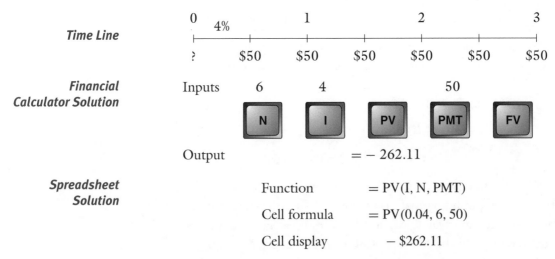

Time Line

Financial Calculator Solution

Spreadsheet Solution

Semiannual payments come in earlier than annual payments, so the $50 semiannual annuity is a little more valuable than the $100 annual annuity. However, an annuity with annual payments, but with semiannual compounding, cannot be treated in the same way. The discount rate period must match the annuity period, so if there are annual payments, an annual discount rate must be used. Under semiannual compounding, the correct rate to apply to annual payments is not the stated rate, but rather the effective annual rate.

Self-Test Questions

1. What changes must be made in the calculations to determine the future value of an amount being compounded at 8 percent semiannually versus one being compounded annually at 8 percent?
2. Why is semiannual compounding better than annual compounding from an investor's standpoint?
3. How does the effective annual rate differ from the stated rate?

Amortized Loans

One important application of time value analysis involves loans that are to be paid off in equal installments over time. Included are automobile loans, home mortgage loans, and most business debt other than very short-term loans and long-term bonds. If a loan is to be repaid in equal periodic amounts (monthly, quarterly, or annually), it is said to be an *amortized loan*. The word *amortize* comes from the Latin *mors* meaning *death*, so an amortized loan is one that is killed off over time.

To illustrate, suppose Santa Fe Healthcare System borrows $1 million from the Bank of New Mexico to be repaid in three equal installments at the end of each of the next three years. The bank is to receive 6 percent interest on the loan balance that is outstanding at the beginning of each year. The first task in analyzing the loan is to determine the amount Santa Fe must repay each year, or the annual payment. To find this amount, recognize that the loan represents the present value of an annuity of PMT dollars per year for three years, discounted at 6 percent.

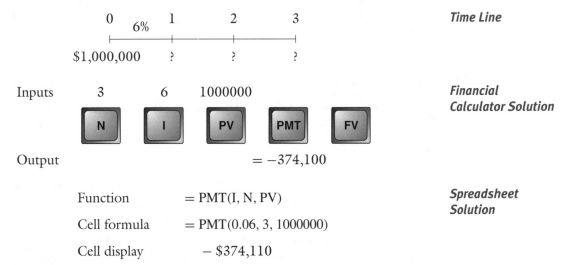

Time Line

Financial Calculator Solution

Spreadsheet Solution

Therefore, if Santa Fe pays the bank $374,110 at the end of each of the next three years, the percentage cost to the borrower and the rate of return to the lender will be 6 percent.

Each payment consists partly of interest and partly of repayment of principal. This breakdown is given in the *amortization schedule* shown in Table 9.1. The interest component is largest in the first year and it declines as the outstanding

TABLE 9.1
Loan Amortization
Schedule

Year	Beginning Amount (1)	Payment (2)	Interest[a] (3)	Repayment of Principal[b] (4)	Remaining Balance (5)
1	$1,000,000	$ 374,110	$ 60,000	$ 314,110	$685,890
2	685,890	374,110	41,153	332,957	352,933
3	352,933	374,110	21,177	352,933	0
		$1,122,330	$122,330	$1,000,000	

[a]Interest is calculated by multiplying the loan balance at the beginning of each year by the interest rate. Therefore, interest in Year 1 is $1,000,000 × 0.06 = $60,000; in Year 2 is $685,890 × 0.06 = $41,153; and in Year 3 is $352,933 × 0.06 = $21,177.
[b]Repayment of principal is equal to the payment of $374,110 minus the interest charge for each year.

balance of the loan is reduced over time. For tax purposes, a taxable business borrower reports the interest payments in Column 3 as a deductible cost each year, while the lender reports these same amounts as taxable income.

Financial calculators are often programmed to calculate amortization schedules; simply key in the inputs and then press one button to get each entry in Table 9.1.

Self-Test Questions

1. When constructing an amortization schedule, how is the periodic payment amount calculated?
2. Does the periodic payment remain constant over time?
3. Do the principal and interest components remain constant over time? Explain your answer.

A Final Discussion of Interest Rate Types

This chapter has covered many time value concepts including three different types of interest rate. In closing, it may be useful to review these three rates.

Stated Rate

The stated rate is the rate that is typically stated in financial contracts; it is usually an annual rate. Convention in the stock, bond, mortgage, commercial loan, consumer loan, and other markets calls for terms to be expressed in stated rates. A banker, broker, or mortgage lender will normally quote the stated rate. However, to be meaningful, the stated rate must indicate the number of compounding periods per year. For example, a bank savings account may offer 10 percent interest compounded quarterly, or a money market mutual fund may offer a 12 percent rate with interest paid monthly. The stated rate is **not** used for calculations (i.e., never use I_{Stated} on a time line, in the calculator, or in a spreadsheet formula or function) **unless compounding occurs once a year** (M = 1). In this case, I_{Stated} = Periodic rate = Effective annual rate.

Periodic Rate

The periodic rate is the rate charged by a lender or paid by a borrower, or any other time value rate that is expressed on a per period basis. It can be a rate per year, per six months, per quarter, per month, per day, or per any other time interval. For example, a bank may charge 1 percent per month on its credit card loans or a finance company may charge 3 percent per quarter on consumer loans. Periodic rate = I_{Stated} / M, which implies that I_{Stated} = Periodic rate × M, where M is the number of compounding periods per year. To illustrate, consider the finance company loan at 3 percent per quarter:

$$I_{Stated} = \text{Periodic rate} \times M = 3\% \times 4 = 12\%,$$

and

$$\text{Periodic rate} = I_{Stated}/M = 12\%/4 = 3\% \text{ per quarter.}$$

The periodic rate often is used when payments or cash flows occur more frequently than once a year, and when the number of payments or cash flows per year corresponds to the number of compounding periods per year. Thus, if dealing with a retirement annuity that provides monthly payments, a semiannual payment bond, a consumer loan with quarterly payments, or with a credit card loan with monthly payments, the calculations would use Periodic rate = I_{Stated} / M. The implication in all these examples is that the interest compounding period is the same as the payment or cash flow period. **The periodic rate can only be used directly in calculations when the cash flow period coincides with the interest rate compounding period (e.g., quarterly payments and quarterly compounding).**

To illustrate use of the periodic rate, assume that eight quarterly payments of $100 are made into an account that pays 12 percent, compounded quarterly. What amount would be accumulated after two years?

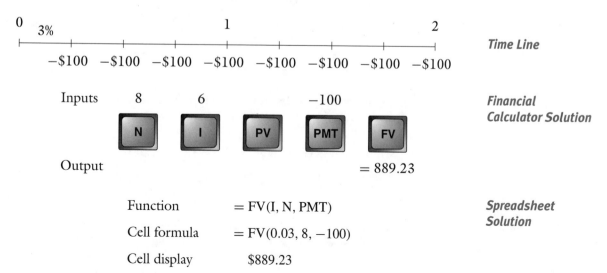

Function	= FV(I, N, PMT)			
Cell formula	= FV(0.03, 8, −100)			
Cell display	$889.23			

Time Line

Financial Calculator Solution

Spreadsheet Solution

Effective Annual Rate

This is the rate that, under annual compounding (M = 1), would produce the same results as a given stated rate with compounding more frequently than annual (M > 1). The effective annual rate (EAR) is found as follows:

$$\text{Effective annual rate (EAR)} = (1 + I_{\text{Stated}}/M)^M - 1.0$$
$$= (1 + \text{Periodic rate})^M - 1.0.$$

For example, suppose that either the 1 percent per month credit card loan or the 3 percent per quarter consumer loan could be used to make a purchase. Which one should be chosen? To answer this question, the cost rate of each alternative must be expressed as an EAR.

$$\text{Credit card loan: EAR} = (1 + 0.01)^{12} - 1.0 = (1.01)^{12} - 1.0$$
$$= 1.126825 - 1.0 = 0.126825 = 12.6825\%.$$
$$\text{Consumer loan: EAR} = (1 + 0.03)^4 - 1.0 = (1.03)^4 - 1.0$$
$$= 1.125509 - 1.0 = 0.125509 = 12.5509\%.$$

Thus, the consumer loan is slightly less costly than the credit card loan. This result should have been intuitive because both loans have the same 12 percent stated rate, but monthly payments would have to be made on the credit card; under the consumer loan terms, only quarterly payments would have to be made.

The EAR is also used when the interest-rate compounding period occurs more often than the period between payments or cash flows. For example, if payments occur semiannually, but interest is compounded quarterly, then the EAR must be used. In this case, the EAR is really an "effective semiannual rate" calculated as $(1 + I_{\text{Stated}} / 4)^2 - 1.0$, which is then applied to the semiannual payment stream. Assume that four semiannual payments of $100 are made into an account that pays 12 percent, compounded quarterly. How much would be accumulated after two years?

Time Line

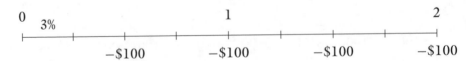

Calculate the *semiannual EAR* because although the compounding is quarterly, the payments occur semiannually:

$$\text{Semiannual EAR} = (1 + 0.03)^2 - 1.0 = (1.03)^2 - 1.0$$
$$= 1.0609 - 1.0 = 0.0609 = 6.09\%$$

Financial Calculator Solution

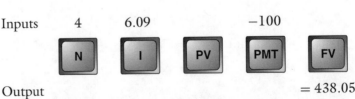

Output   = 438.05

Function	$= FV(I, N, PMT)$
Cell formula	$= FV(0.0609, 4, -100)$
Cell display	$438.05

The number of periods, N, must equal the number of payments when using the annuity formulas and the financial calculator PMT key. If the value for N that is being used in a calculation does not match the number of payments, something is wrong.

1. Define the stated rate, the periodic rate, and the effective annual rate.
2. How are these three rates related?
3. Can you think of a situation where all three of these rates are the same?

Key Concepts

Financial decisions often involve situations in which future cash flows must be valued. The process of valuing future cash flows is called *time value analysis*. The key concepts of this type of analysis are:

- *Compounding* is the process of determining the *future value (FV)* of a lump sum or a series of payments.
- *Discounting* is the process of finding the *present value (PV)* of a future lump sum or series of payments.
- An *annuity* is a series of equal periodic *payments (PMT)* for a specified number of periods.
- An annuity that has payments occurring at the end of each period is called an *ordinary* annuity.
- If each annuity payment occurs at the beginning of the period rather than at the end, the annuity is an *annuity due*.
- A *perpetuity* is an annuity that lasts forever.
- If an analysis involving more than one cash value does not meet the definition of an annuity, it is called an *uneven cash flow stream*.
- The *stated rate* is the annual rate normally quoted in financial contracts.
- The *periodic rate* equals the stated rate divided by the number of compounding periods per year.
- If compounding occurs more frequently than once a year, it is often necessary to calculate the *effective annual rate*, which is the rate that produces the same results under annual compounding, as opposed to more frequent compounding.
- An *amortized* loan is one that is paid off in equal amounts over some specified number of periods. An *amortization schedule* shows how much of each payment represents interest, how much is used to reduce the principal, and the remaining balance on each payment date.

Time value analysis will be applied in subsequent chapters, so the contents of this chapter are very important. Readers should feel comfortable with this material before moving ahead.

Questions

9.1 a. What is an opportunity cost rate?
   b. How is this rate used in time value analysis?
   c. Is this rate a single number that is used in all situations?

9.2 What is the difference between a lump sum, an annuity, and an unequal cash flow stream?

9.3 Great Lakes Health Network's net income increased from $3.2 million in 1988 to $6.4 million in 1998. The total growth rate over the ten years is 100 percent, while the annual growth rate is only about 7.2 percent, which is much less than 100 percent divided by ten years.
   a. Why does this relationship hold?
   b. Which growth rate has more meaning: the total rate over ten years or the annualized rate?

9.4 Would you rather have a savings account that pays 5 percent compounded semiannually or one that pays 5 percent compounded daily? Explain your answer.

9.5 The present value of a perpetuity is equal to the payment divided by the opportunity cost (interest) rate: $PV = PMT/I$. What is the future value of a perpetuity?

9.6 When a loan is amortized, what happens over time to the size of the total payment, interest payment, and principal payment?

9.7 Explain the difference between the stated rate, periodic rate, and effective annual rate.

9.8 What are three techniques for solving time value problems?

Problems

9.1 Find the following values for a lump sum assuming annual compounding:
   a. The future value of $500 invested at 8 percent for one year
   b. The future value of $500 invested at 8 percent for five years
   c. The present value of $500 to be received in one year when the opportunity cost rate is 8 percent
   d. The present value of $500 to be received in five years when the opportunity cost rate is 8 percent

9.2 Repeat Problem 9.1 above, but assume the following compounding conditions:
   a. Semiannual
   b. Quarterly

9.3 What is the effective annual rate (EAR) if the stated rate is 8 percent and compounding occurs semiannually? Quarterly?

9.4 Find the following values assuming a regular, or ordinary, annuity:
  a. The present value of $400 per year for ten years at 10 percent
  b. The future value of $400 per year for ten years at 10 percent
  c. The present value of $200 per year for five years at 5 percent
  d. The future value of $200 per year for five years at 5 percent

9.5 Repeat Problem 9.4, but assume the annuities are annuities due

9.6 Consider the following uneven cash flow stream:

Year	Cash Flow
0	$ 0
1	250
2	400
3	500
4	600
5	600

  a. What is the present (Year 0) value if the opportunity cost (discount) rate is 10 percent?
  b. Add an outflow (or cost) of $1,000 at Year 0. What is the present value (or net present value) of the stream?

9.7 Consider another uneven cash flow stream:

Year	Cash Flow
0	$2,000
1	2,000
2	0
3	1,500
4	2,500
5	4,000

  a. What is the present (Year 0) value of the cash flow stream if the opportunity cost rate is 10 percent?
  b. What is the value of the cash flow stream at the end of Year 5 if the cash flows are invested in an account that pays 10 percent annually?
  c. What cash flow today (Year 0), in lieu of the $2,000 cash flow, would be needed to accumulate $20,000 at the end of Year 5? (Assume that the cash flows for Years 1 through 5 remain the same.)
  d. Time value analysis involves either discounting or compounding cash flows. Many healthcare financial management decisions such as bond refunding, capital investment, and lease versus buy involve discounting projected future cash flows. What factors must executives consider when choosing a discount rate to apply to forecasted cash flows?

9.8 What is the present value of a perpetuity of $100 per year if the appropriate discount rate is 7 percent? Suppose that interest rates doubled in the economy and the appropriate discount rate is now 14 percent. What would happen to the present value of the perpetuity?

9.9 Assume that you just won $35 million in the Florida lottery, and hence the state will pay you 20 annual payments of $1.75 million each beginning immediately. If the rate of return on securities of similar risk to the lottery earnings (e.g., the rate on 20-year U.S. Treasury bonds) is 6 percent, what is the present value of your winnings?

9.10 An investment that you are considering promises to pay $2,000 semiannually for the next two years beginning six months from now. You have determined that the appropriate opportunity cost (discount) rate is 8 percent, compounded quarterly. What is the value of this investment?

9.11 Epitome Healthcare has just borrowed $1,000,000 on a five-year, annual payment term loan at a 15 percent rate. The first payment is due one year from now. Construct the amortization schedule for this loan.

Notes

1. Even if no investment opportunities existed, a dollar in hand would still be worth more than a dollar to be received in the future because a dollar today can be used for immediate consumption, whereas a future dollar cannot.

2. On some financial calculators, the keys are buttons on the face of the calculator; on others, the time value variables are shown on a display after accessing the time value menu. Also, some calculators use different symbols to represent the number of periods and interest rate. For example, both lower and upper cases are used for N and I, while other calculators use N/YR and I percent/YR or similar variations. Finally, financial calculators today are quite powerful in that they can easily solve relatively complex time value of money problems such as when intraperiod cash flows occur. To focus on concepts rather than mechanics, all the illustrations in this chapter and the remainder of the book assume that cash flows occur at the end or beginning of a period and that there is only one cash flow per period. Thus, to follow the illustrations, financial calculators must be set to **one period per year**; it is not necessary to use the calendar function.

3. In constructing spreadsheets, normally a formula that can accommodate changing inputs must be created, so a more useful approach would be a formula such as:

$$= A1 * (1 + B1)^\wedge C1$$

where the equal sign tells the spreadsheet that a formula is being used, the present value ($100) would be contained in Cell A1, the interest rate (0.05) in Cell B1, and the number of periods (5) in Cell C1. With this formula, the future value over 1, 2, 3, or more years can be calculated, as shown in the example. Finally, different spreadsheet programs use slightly different syntax in their time value functions. The examples presented in this book use Excel syntax.

4. Time value problems also can be solved using mathematical multipliers obtained from tables. Using this technique to find lump sum future values, the present value is multiplied by a table-derived interest factor that matches the combination of N and I needed for the problem. At one time, tables were the most efficient way to solve time value problems, but calculators and spreadsheets have superseded tabular solutions.

5. Owning a single nursing home is riskier than owning a chain that has geographical diversification, so the true opportunity cost is probably somewhat higher than the return expected on Beverly Enterprises stock. Also, an owner of Beverly Enterprises stock can easily sell the stock if circumstances dictate, whereas it would be much more difficult for Oakdale to sell a nursing home. These differences in risk and liquidity suggest that the true opportunity cost is higher than the return that is expected from owning the stock of Beverly Enterprises.

6. The *Rule of 72* gives a simple and quick method for judging the effect of different interest rates on the growth of a lump sum deposit. To find the number of years required to double the value of a lump sum, merely divide the number 72 by the interest rate paid. For example, if the interest rate is 10 percent, it would take 72 / 10 = 7.2 years for the money in an account to double in value. The calculator solution is 7.27 years, so the Rule of 72 is relatively accurate, at least when reasonable interest rates are applied. In a similar manner, the Rule of 72 can be used to determine the interest rate required to double the money in an account in a given number of years. To illustrate, an interest rate of 72 / 5 = 14.4 percent is required to double the value of an account in five years. The calculator solution in this case is 14.9 percent, so the Rule of 72 again gives a reasonable approximation of the precise answer.

7. Because the cash flows in Years 3, 4, and 5 represent an annuity, the present value of the entire stream could be found by finding the PV of the ordinary annuity at Year 2 and then discounting this value, along with the lump sum values for Years 1, 2, 6, and 7, back to Year 0, and then summing. Indeed, there are numerous ways of organizing the cash flows to be discounted. These nuances, however, are of little real-world value because the actual present value calculation would be done with a financial calculator's cash flow registers or a spreadsheet.

8. Some financial institutions even have saving accounts that pay interest that is compounded *continuously*. However, continuous compounding is not relevant to most healthcare financial management situations, so it will not be discussed here.

9. Most financial calculators are programmed to calculate the EAR or given the EAR, to find the stated rate. This is called *interest rate conversion*. Enter the stated rate and the number of compounding periods per year and then press the EFF percent key to find the EAR.

10. The *annual percentage rate (APR)* and *annual percentage yield (APY)* are terms defined in Truth in Lending and Truth in Savings laws. APR is defined as Periodic rate × Number of periods per year, so it ignores the consequences of compounding. For example, the APR on a credit card with interest charges of 1.5 percent per month is 1.5% × 12 = 18.0%. Conversely, APY is defined in the same way as the EAR. Banks are required to use APR when they advertise loan rates and APY when they advertise savings rates. Although the APY accurately reflects savings rates, APR understates the true cost of loans.

References

The owner's manual for your calculator.

The reference manual for your spreadsheet software or any of the after-market spreadsheet manuals.

FINANCIAL RISK AND RETURN

Learning Objectives

After studying this chapter, readers will be able to:

- Define and calculate financial returns.
- Explain the concept of financial risk in general terms.
- Define and differentiate between stand-alone risk and portfolio risk.
- Define and differentiate between corporate risk and market risk.
- Explain the CAPM relationship between risk and required rate of return.

Introduction

Two of the most important concepts in healthcare financial management are financial risk and return. How are financial returns measured? What is financial risk, how is it measured, and what effect, if any, does it have on required rates of return, and hence on managerial decisions? Because so much of financial decision making involves risk and return, it is impossible to gain a good understanding of healthcare finance without having a solid appreciation of risk and return concepts.

If investors—both individuals and businesses—viewed risk as a benign fact of life, it would have little impact on decision making. However, decision makers are for the most part averse to risk; they believe that risk is to be avoided. Furthermore, if risks must be taken, there must be a reward for doing so. Thus, investments of higher risk, whether an individual investor's security investment or a radiology group's investment in diagnostic equipment, must offer higher returns to make the investment financially worthwhile. This characteristic of good financial decision making makes risk concepts important.

Two factors come into play that complicate any discussion of financial risk. First, financial risk is seen both by businesses and the investors in businesses. There is some risk inherent in the business itself that depends on the type of business. For example, pharmaceutical firms are generally acknowledged to face a great deal of risk, while healthcare providers typically have less risk. The investors in any business (i.e., stockholders and creditors) then must bear the riskiness inherent in the business, but as modified by the nature of the securities they hold. For example, the stock of Beverly Enterprises is more risky than its debt, although the risk of both securities depends on the inherent risk of operating a business in the long-term care industry. Not-for-profit firms have the same partitioning of risk with debtholders, but now the inherent riskiness of the business is split between creditors and the implied stockholders who generally are considered to be the community at large.

The second complicating factor results because the riskiness of any asset changes with the context in which it is held. For example, a stock held alone is riskier than the same stock held as part of a large portfolio of stocks. Similarly, a MRI system operated independently is riskier than the same system operated as part of a large, geographically dispersed company that owns numerous types of diagnostic equipment.

In this chapter, basic risk and return concepts are presented from the perspective of both individual investors and businesses. Health services managers must be familiar with both contexts because investors supply the capital that businesses need to function. The chapter begins with a discussion of financial returns, which provide a rational way to express the performance of an investment. Such measures are needed before risk can be considered. Then, the chapter describes several measures of financial risk. Finally, the chapter examines a simple model that tells investors how much return is required to compensate for a given amount of risk.

Investment Returns

In most investments, an individual or business spends money today with the expectation of receiving money in the future. To illustrate, suppose that an individual buys ten shares of stock for $1,000. The stock pays no dividends, but at the end of one year, the stock is sold for $1,100. What is the *return* on the $1,000 investment? One way of expressing an investment return is in *dollar terms*. The dollar return is simply the total dollars received from the investment less the amount invested:

$$\text{Dollar return} = \text{Amount received} - \text{Amount invested}$$

$$= \$1,100 - \$1,000$$

$$= \$100.$$

At the end of the year, if the stock is sold for only $900, the dollar return would be −$100.

Although expressing returns in dollars is simple to do, two problems arise:

- *The scale problem.* To make a meaningful judgment about the adequacy of the return, the size of the investment must be known. A $100 return on a $500 investment is a good return, assuming that the investment is held for one year, while a similar dollar return on a $5,000 investment is a poor return.
- *The timing problem.* The timing of the return also must be known. A $100 return on a $500 investment is a good return if held for one year, but the same dollar return in ten years is a poor return.

The solution to the scale and timing problems of dollar returns is to express investment returns as a *rate of return*, or *percentage return*. For example, the rate of return on the one-year stock investment when sold for $1,100 is 10 percent:

$$\text{Rate of return} = \frac{\text{Amount received} - \text{Amount invested}}{\text{Amount invested}} = \frac{\text{Dollar return}}{\text{Amount invested}}$$

$$= \frac{\$1,100 - \$1,000}{\$1,000} = \frac{\$100}{\$1,000}$$

$$= 0.10 = 10\%.$$

Rate of return normalizes return by considering the return per unit of investment. In this example, the return of 0.10, or 10 percent, indicates that each dollar invested will earn $0.10 \times \$1.00 = \$0.10$, or 10 cents. A negative rate of return signifies that the original investment will not even be recovered. For example, selling the stock for only $900 results in a -10 percent rate of return, which means that each dollar invested will lose ten cents. A $100 return on a $500 investment produces a 20 percent rate of return, while a $100 return on a $5,000 investment results in a rate of return of only 2 percent. Percentage return, therefore, takes into account the size of the investment, and hence solves the scale problem.

Expressing rate of return on an *annual basis*, which is typically done in practice, solves the timing problem. A $100 return after one year on a $500 dollar investment results in a 20 percent annual rate of return, while a $100 return after ten years only yields a 1.9 percent annual rate of return. Because annual returns contain more information about an investment's true value, most rates of return are expressed in annual terms.

Rate of return is an application of time value analysis discussed in Chapter 9. In the preceding one-year investment example, the present value is $-\$1,000$ (it is negative because it is an investment outflow), the future value is $1,100 and the number of periods (years in this case) is 1. Here are the solutions:

	0		1
	├──	?	──┤
	$-\$1,000$		$\$1,100$

Time Line

Inputs	1		-1000		1100
	N	I	PV	PMT	FV
Output		= 10.0			

Financial Calculator Solution

Formula	$= (1100/1000)^{(1/1)} - 1$
Cell display	0.100

Spreadsheet Solution

In the spreadsheet formula, the exponential term is $(1/N)$. Because $N = 1$ in this example, the term becomes $1/1$.

When the return is after five years, the following situation exists:

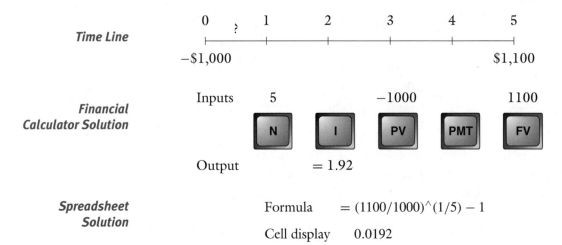

Time Line

Financial Calculator Solution

Spreadsheet Solution

Formula $= (1100/1000)^{\wedge}(1/5) - 1$

Cell display   0.0192

Note that rate of return concepts can easily be applied to situations where multiple cash flows occur. An example would be an investment in a new x-ray machine that is expected to generate net cash inflows over a number of years. The discussion of returns involving multiple cash flows, which are called internal rates of return (IRRs), can be found in Chapter 14.

Self-Test Questions

1. Differentiate between dollar return and rate of return.
2. Why is rate of return superior to dollar return?
3. Is rate of return an application of time value analysis? Explain your answer.

Introduction to Financial Risk

Generically, *risk* is defined as "a hazard; a peril; exposure to loss or injury." Thus, risk refers to the chance that an unfavorable event will occur. If a person engages in skydiving, he or she is taking a chance with injury or death; skydiving is risky. If a person gambles at roulette, he or she is not risking injury or death, but is taking a *financial risk*. Even when a person invests in stocks or bonds, he or she is taking a risk in the hope of earning a positive rate of return. Similarly, when a healthcare business invests in new assets, such as diagnostic equipment, new hospital beds, or a new managed care plan, it is taking a financial risk.

To illustrate financial risk, consider two potential personal investments. The first investment consists of a one-year, $1,000 face value U.S. Treasury bill that is bought for $950. Treasury bills are short-term federal debt that are sold at a *discount* (i.e., less than face value) and return *face*, or *par*, *value* at maturity. The investor expects to receive $1,000 at maturity in one year, so the anticipated rate of return on the T-bill investment is ($1,000 − $950) / $950 = $50 / $950 = 0.053, or 5.3%. Using a financial calculator:

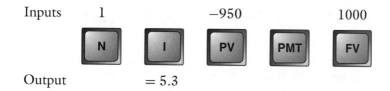

Inputs   1   −950   1000

Output   = 5.3

The $1,000 payment is fixed by contract (the T-bill promises to pay this amount) and the U.S. government is certain to make the payment, except in the case a national disaster—a very unlikely event. Thus, there is virtually a 100 percent probability that the investment will actually earn the 5.3 percent rate of return that is expected. In this situation, the investment is defined as being *riskless*, or *risk free*.

Now assume that the $950 is invested in a biotechnology partnership that will be terminated in one year. If the partnership develops a new commercially valuable product, its rights will be sold and $2,000 will be received from the partnership for a rate of return of ($2,000 − $950)/$950 = $1,050 / $950 = 1.1053 = 110.53%:

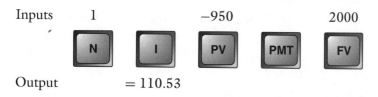

Inputs   1   −950   2000

Output   = 110.53

But if nothing worthwhile is developed, the partnership would be worthless; no money would be received and the rate of return would be ($0 − $950) / $950 = −1.00 = −100%:

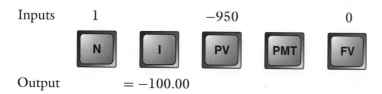

Inputs   1   −950   0

Output   = −100.00

Note that most financial calculators give no solution when the future value is zero, but if a very small number, for example 0.0001, is entered for the future value, the solution for interest rate is −100.00.

Now assume that there is a 50 percent chance that a valuable product will be developed. In this admittedly unrealistic situation, the expected rate of return, a statistical concept that will be discussed shortly, is the same 5.3 percent as on the T-bill investment: (0.50 × 110.53%) + (0.50 × −100%) = 5.3%. However, the biotechnology partnership is a far cry from being riskless. If things go poorly, the realized rate of return will be −100 percent; the entire $950 investment will be lost. Because there is a significant chance of actually earning a return that is far less than expected, the partnership investment is described as being very risky.

Thus, financial risk is related to the probability of earning a return less than expected. The greater the chance of low or negative returns, the greater the amount of financial risk.[1]

Self-Test Questions

1. What is a generic definition of risk?
2. Explain the general concept of financial risk.

Risk Aversion

Why is it so important to define and measure financial risk? The reason is that, for the most part, both individual and business investors dislike risk. Suppose that a person was given the choice between a sure one million dollars and the flip of a coin for either zero or two million dollars. That person, and just about everyone else, would take the million and run. A person that takes the sure million dollars is said to be *risk averse*; a person who is indifferent between the two alternatives is *risk neutral*; and an individual who prefers the gamble to the sure thing is a *risk seeker*.

Of course, people and businesses do gamble and take other financial chances, so all of us at some time typically exhibit risk-seeking behavior. However, most individuals would never put a sizable portion of their wealth at risk and most health services managers would never "bet the business"; most people are risk averse when it really matters.

What are the implications of risk aversion for financial decision making? First, given two investments with similar returns but differing risk, investors will favor the lower-risk alternative. Second, investors will require higher returns on higher-risk investments. These simple outcomes of risk averse behavior have a significant impact on many facets of financial management. Thus, the implications of risk aversion will appear again in this and later chapters.

Self-Test Questions

1. What does the term *risk aversion* mean?
2. What are the implications of risk aversion for financial decision making?

Probability Distributions

The chance that an event will occur is called its *probability of occurrence*, or just *probability*. For example, a weather forecast might predict a 40 percent chance of rain. Or, when rolling a single die, the probability of rolling a two is one out of six, or $1 / 6 = 0.1667 = 16.67\%$. If all possible outcomes related to a particular event are listed and a probability is assigned to each outcome, the result is a *probability distribution*. In the example of the weather forecast, the probability distribution looks like this:

Outcome	Probability
Rain	$0.40 = 40\%$
No rain	$0.60 = 60\%$
	$1.00 = 100\%$

In the example of the role of a die, the probability distribution looks like this:

Outcome	Probability
1	0.1667 = 16.67%
2	0.1667 = 16.67%
3	0.1667 = 16.67%
4	0.1667 = 16.67%
5	0.1667 = 16.67%
6	0.1667 = 16.67%
	1.0000 = 100.00%

The possible outcomes (i.e., the number of dots showing after the roll on the dice distribution) are listed in the left column, while the probability of each outcome is listed in the right column expressed as both decimals and percentages. For a complete probability distribution that includes all possible outcomes for an event, the probabilities must sum to 1.0, or 100 percent.

Probabilities can also be assigned to possible outcomes—in this case, returns—on both personal and business investments. If a person buys stock, the return will usually come in the form of *dividends* and *capital gains* (selling the stock for more than the person paid for it), or *losses* (selling the stock for less than the person paid for it). Because all stock returns are uncertain, there is some chance that the dividends will not be as high as expected and that the stock price will not increase as much as expected or that it will even decrease. The higher the probabilities of dividends and stock price well below those expected, the higher the probability that the return will be significantly less than expected, and hence the greater the risk.

To illustrate the concept using a business investment, consider a hospital evaluating the purchase of a new MRI system. The cost of the system is an investment, and the net cash inflows that stem from patient utilization provide the return. The net cash inflows, in turn, depend on the number of procedures, charge per procedure, payor discounts, operating costs, and so on. These values typically are not known with certainty, but rather depend on factors such as patient demographics, physician acceptance, local market conditions, labor costs, and so on. Thus, the hospital actually faces a probability distribution of returns rather than a single return known with certainty. The greater the probability of returns well below the return anticipated, the greater the risk of the MRI investment.

1. What is a probability distribution?
2. How are probability distributions used in financial decision making?

Self-Test Questions

Expected and Realized Rates of Return

To be most useful, the concept of financial risk must be defined more precisely than just the chances of a return well below that anticipated. Table 10.1 contains the estimated return distributions developed by the financial staff of Norwalk Community Hospital for two proposed projects: a MRI system and a walk-in clinic. Here, each economic state reflects a combination of factors that dictate each project's profitability. For example, for the MRI project, the very poor economic state signifies very low physician acceptance and hence very low utilization, very high discounts on reimbursements, very high operating costs, and so on. The economic states are defined in a similar fashion for the walk-in clinic.

The *expected rate of return*, as defined in the statistical sense, is the weighted average of the return distribution where the weights are the probabilities of occurrence. For example, the expected rate of return on the MRI system, $E(R_{MRI})$, is 10 percent:

$$
\begin{aligned}
E(R_{MRI}) =\ & \text{Probability of Return 1} \times \text{Return 1} \\
& + \text{Probability of Return 2} \times \text{Return 2} \\
& + \text{Probability of Return 3} \times \text{Return 3 and so on} \\
=\ & (0.10 \times [-10\%]) + (0.20 \times 0\%) + (0.40 \times 10\%) \\
& + (0.20 \times 20\%) + 0.10 \times 30\% \\
=\ & 10.0\%.
\end{aligned}
$$

Calculated in a similar manner, the expected rate of return on the walk-in clinic is 15 percent.

The expected rate of return is the average return that would result, given the return distribution, if the investment were randomly repeated many times. In this illustration, if 1,000 clinics were built in different areas, each of which faced the return distribution given in Table 10.1, the average return on the 1,000 investments would be 15 percent, assuming the returns in each area are independent of one another (random). However, only one clinic would actually be built and the realized rate of return may be less than the expected 15 percent. Therefore, the clinic investment (as well as the MRI investment) is risky.

Expected rate of return expresses expectations for the future. When the managers at Norwalk Community Hospital analyzed the MRI project, they ex-

TABLE 10.1
Norwalk Community Hospital: Estimated Returns for Two Proposed Projects

Economic State	Probability of Occurrence	Rate of Return if State Occurs MRI	Rate of Return if State Occurs Clinic
Very poor	0.10	−10%	−20%
Poor	0.20	0	0
Average	0.40	10	15
Good	0.20	20	30
Very good	0.10	30	50
	1.00		

pected it to earn 10 percent. However, assume that economic conditions took a turn for the worse and the very poor economic scenario actually occurred. In this case, the *realized rate of return*, which is the rate of return that the project actually produced as measured at termination, would be a negative 10 percent. It is the potential of realizing a return of −10 percent on an investment that has an expected return of +10 percent that produces risk.[2]

1. How is the expected rate of return calculated?
2. What is the economic interpretation of the expected rate of return?
3. What is the difference between the expected rate of return and the realized rate of return?

Stand-Alone Risk

One may intuitively conclude from looking at the two distributions in Table 10.1 that the clinic is more risky than the MRI system because the clinic has a chance of a 20 percent loss, while the worst possible loss on the MRI system is 10 percent. This intuitive risk assessment is looking at the *stand-alone risk* of the two investments. That is, the risk assessment focuses on the riskiness that is relevant if the MRI system or the walk-in clinic were Norwalk's only asset (i.e., operated in isolation). In the next section, portfolio effects will be introduced, but for now, the discussion will focus on stand-alone risk.

Stand-alone risk depends on the "tightness" of the investment's return distribution, that is, on the amount of dispersion of the distribution about its expected value. If an investment has a tight return distribution, with returns that fall close to the expected return, it has relatively low stand-alone risk. Conversely, an investment with a return distribution that is loose, and hence that has values well below the expected return, is relatively risky.

It is important to recognize that risk and return are **separate** attributes of an investment. An investment may have a very tight distribution of returns, and hence very low stand-alone risk, but its expected rate of return may be only 2 percent. In this situation, the investment probably would not be financially attractive, in spite of its low risk. Similarly, a high-risk investment with a sufficiently high expected rate of return would be attractive.

To be truly useful, any definition of risk must have a numerical measure, so a way to measure the "degree of tightness" of an investment's return distribution is needed. One such measure is *standard deviation*, which is often given the symbol of the Greek, lower-case sigma, σ. Standard deviation is a common statistical measure of the dispersion of a distribution about its mean, or expected, value; the smaller the standard deviation, the tighter the return distribution, and hence the lower the stand-alone risk of the investment.

The following steps illustrate the calculation of standard deviation of the MRI project's estimated returns listed in Table 10.1:

- The expected rate of return on the MRI, $E(R_{MRI})$, is 10 percent.
- The *variance* of the return distribution is determined as follows:

$$
\begin{aligned}
\text{Variance} &= (\text{Probability of Return 1} \times [\text{Rate of Return 1} - E(R_{MRI})]^2) \\
&\quad + (\text{Probability of Return 2} \times [\text{Rate of Return 2} - E(R_{MRI})]^2)\text{and so on} \\
&= (0.10 \times [-10\% - 10\%]^2) + (0.20 \times [0\% - 10\%]^2) + (0.40 \times [10\% - 10\%]^2) \\
&\quad + (0.20 \times [20\% - 10\%]^2) + (0.10 \times [30\% - 10\%]^2) \\
&= 120.00.
\end{aligned}
$$

Variance, like standard deviation, is a measure of the dispersion of a distribution about its expected value, but it is less useful than standard deviation because its measurement unit is percent or dollars **squared**, which has no economic meaning.

- The standard deviation is defined as the square root of the variance:

$$
\begin{aligned}
\text{Standard deviation } (\sigma) &= \sqrt{\text{Variance}} \\
&= \sqrt{120.00} = 10.95\% \approx 11.0\%.
\end{aligned}
$$

In practice, standard deviations are usually calculated by formulas constructed within a spreadsheet model or sometimes by using a calculator. The mathematical work, therefore, is relatively easy.[3]

Using the same procedure as listed above, the clinic project from Table 10.1 was found to have a standard deviation of returns of about 18 percent. Because the clinic project's standard deviation of returns is larger than that of the MRI project, the clinic project has more stand-alone risk than the MRI project.[4]

Self-Test Questions

1. What is stand-alone risk?
2. How is it measured?

Portfolio Risk and Return

The preceding section developed a risk measure—standard deviation—that applies to investments held in isolation. However, most investments are not held in isolation, but rather are held as part of a collection, or *portfolio*, of investments. Individual investors typically hold portfolios of **securities** (i.e., stocks and bonds), while businesses generally hold portfolios of **projects** (i.e., product or service lines). When investments are held in portfolios, the primary concern of investors is not the realized rate of return on an individual investment, but rather the realized rate of return on the entire portfolio. Similarly, the riskiness of each individual asset in the portfolio is not important to the investor; what matters is the aggregate riskiness of the portfolio. Thus, the whole nature of risk and how it is defined and measured changes when one recognizes that investments are not held in isolation, but rather as parts of portfolios.

Portfolio Returns

Consider the returns estimated for the seven investment alternatives listed in Table 10.2. The individual investment alternatives (Investments A, B, C, and D) could be projects under consideration by South West Clinics, Inc., or they could be stocks that are being evaluated as personal investments. The remaining three alternatives in Table 10.2 are portfolios. Portfolio AB consists of 50 percent invested in Investment A and 50 percent in Investment B (e.g., $10,000 invested in A and $10,000 invested in B), while Portfolio AC is an equal-weighted portfolio of Investments A and C and Portfolio AD is an equal-weighted portfolio of Investments A and D. As shown in the bottom of the table, Investments A and B have 10 percent expected rates of return, while the expected rates of return for Investments C and D are 15 percent and 12 percent, respectively. Investments A and B have identical stand-alone risk (i.e., standard deviation), while Investments C and D have greater stand-alone risk than A and B.

The *expected rate of return on a portfolio*, $E(R_{Portfolio})$, is the weighted average of the expected returns on the assets that make up the portfolio, with the weights being the proportion of the total portfolio invested in each asset:

$$E(R_{Portfolio}) = (w_1 \times E[R_1]) + (w_2 \times E[R_2]) + (w_3 \times E[R_3]) \text{ and so on.}$$

In this case, w_1 is the proportion of Investment 1 in the overall portfolio and $E(R_1)$ is the expected rate of return of Investment 1, and so on. Thus, the expected rate of return on Portfolio AB is 10 percent:

$$E(R_{AB}) = (0.5 \times 10\%) + (0.5 \times 10\%) = 5\% + 5\% = 10\%$$

while the expected rate of return on Portfolio AC is 12.5 percent and on AD is 11.0 percent.

Alternatively, the expected rate of return on a portfolio can be calculated by looking at the portfolio's return distribution. To illustrate, consider the return distribution for Portfolio AC contained in Table 10.2. The portfolio return in

Economic State	Probability of Occurrence	Rate of Return if State Occurs						
		A	B	C	D	AB	AC	AD
Very poor	0.10	−10%	30%	−25%	15%	10%	−17.5%	2.5%
Poor	0.20	0	20	−5	10	10	−2.5	5.0
Average	0.40	10	10	15	0	10	12.5	5.0
Good	0.20	20	0	35	25	10	27.5	22.5
Very good	0.10	30	−10	55	35	10	42.5	32.5
	1.00							
Expected rate of return		10.0%	10.0%	15.0%	12.0%	10.0%	12.5%	11.0%
Standard deviation		11.0%	11.0%	21.9%	12.1%	0.0%	16.4%	10.1%

TABLE 10.2

Estimated Returns for Four Individual Investments and Three Portfolios

each economic state is the weighted average of the returns on Investments A and C in that state. For example, the return on Portfolio AC in the very poor state is $(0.5 \times [-10\%]) + (0.5 \times [-25\%]) = -17.5\%$. Portfolio AC's return in each other state is calculated similarly. Portfolio AC's return distribution now can be used to calculate its expected rate of return:

$$E(R_{AC}) = (0.10 \times [-17.5\%]) + (0.20 \times [-2.5\%]) + (0.40 \times 12.5\%)$$
$$+ (0.20 \times 27.5\%) + (0.10 \times 42.5\%)$$
$$= 12.5\%.$$

This is the same value as calculated from the expected rates of return of the two portfolio components:

$$(0.5 \times 10\%) + (0.5 \times 15\%) = 12.5\%.$$

After the fact, the actual, or realized, returns on Investments A and C will probably be different from their expected values, and hence the realized rate of return on Portfolio AC will likely be different from its 12.5 percent expected return.

Portfolio Risk: Two Assets

When an investor holds a portfolio of assets, the portfolio is in effect a stand-alone investment, so the riskiness of the **portfolio** is measured by the standard deviation of portfolio returns, the previously discussed measure of stand-alone risk. How does the riskiness of the individual investments in a portfolio combine to create the overall riskiness of the portfolio? Although the rate of return on a portfolio is the weighted average of the returns on the component investments, a portfolio's standard deviation (i.e., riskiness) is generally **not** the weighted average of the standard deviations of the individual components. The portfolio's riskiness may be smaller than the weighted average of each component's riskiness. Indeed, the riskiness of a portfolio may be less than the least risky portfolio component; under certain conditions, a portfolio of risky assets may be even riskless.

A simple example can be used to illustrate this concept. Suppose that a person is given the opportunity to flip a coin once; if it comes up heads, the person wins $10,000, but if it comes up tails, he or she loses $8,000. This is a reasonable bet; the expected dollar return is $(0.5 \times \$10,000) + (0.5 \times [-\$8,000]) = \$1,000$. However, it is a highly risky proposition; the person has a 50 percent chance of losing $8,000. Thus, because of risk aversion, most people would refuse to make the bet, especially if the $8,000 potential loss would result in financial hardship.

Alternatively, suppose that person is given the opportunity to flip the coin 100 times, and he or she would win $100 for each head but lose $80 for each tail. It is possible, although extremely unlikely, that the person would flip all heads and win $10,000. It is also possible, and also extremely unlikely, that he or she would flip all tails and lose $8,000. But the chances are very high that the person would actually flip close to 50 heads and 50 tails and net about $1,000. Even if he or she flipped a few more tails than heads, the person would still make money on the gamble.

Although each individual flip is a very risky bet in the stand-alone sense, collectively the person has a low-risk proposition. In effect, the multiple flipping has created a portfolio of investments; each flip of the coin can be thought of as one investment, so the person now has a 100-investment portfolio. Furthermore, the return on each investment is independent of the returns on the other investments; the person has a 50 percent chance of winning on each flip of the coin, regardless of the results of the previous flips. By combining the flips into a single gamble (i.e., into an investment portfolio), he or she can reduce the risk associated with each individual bet. In fact, if the gamble consisted of a very large number of flips, almost all risk would be eliminated; the probability of a near-equal number of heads and tails would be extremely high and the result would be a sure profit. The key to the risk reduction inherent in the portfolio is the fact that the negative consequences of tossing a tail can now be offset by the positive consequences of tossing a head.

To examine portfolio effects in more depth, consider Portfolio AB in Table 10.2. Each individual investment (A and B) is quite risky when held in isolation; each has a standard deviation of returns of 10 percent. However, a portfolio of the two investments has a rate of return of 10 percent in every possible state of the economy, and hence it offers a riskless 10 percent return. This result is verified by the value of zero for Portfolio AB's standard deviation of return. The reason Investments A and B can be combined to form a riskless portfolio is that their returns move exactly opposite to one another. Thus, in economic states when A's returns are relatively low, those of B are relatively high and vice versa, so the gains on one investment in the portfolio exactly offset losses in the other.

The movement relationship of two variables (i.e., their tendency to move either together or in opposition) is called *correlation*. The *correlation coefficient*, *r*, measures this relationship. Investments A and B can be combined to form a riskless portfolio because the returns on A and B are *perfectly negatively correlated*, which is designated by $r = -1.0$. In every state where Investment A has a return higher than its expected return, Investment B has a return lower than its expected return and vice versa.

The opposite of perfect negative correlation is *perfect positive correlation*, with $r = +1.0$. Returns on two perfectly positively correlated investments move up and down together as the economic state changes. When the returns on two investments are perfectly positively correlated, combining the investments into a portfolio will not lower risk; the standard deviation of the portfolio is merely the weighted average of the standard deviations of the two components.

To illustrate the impact of perfect positive correlation, consider Portfolio AC in Table 10.2:

- Its expected rate of return, $E(R_{AC})$, is 12.5 percent
- The variance of the portfolio is 270:

$$\text{Variance} = (\text{Probability of Return 1} \times [\text{Rate of Return 1} - \text{E}(\text{R}_{\text{AC}})]^2)$$

$$+ (\text{Probability of Return 2} \times [\text{Rate of Return 2} - \text{E}(\text{R}_{\text{AC}})]^2) \text{ and so on}$$

$$= (0.10 \times [-17.5\% - 12.5\%]^2) + (0.20 \times [-2.5\% - 12.5\%]^2)$$

$$+ (0.40 \times [12.5\% - 12.5\%]^2) + (0.20 \times [27.5\% - 12.5\%]^2)$$

$$+ (0.10 \times [42.5\% - 12.5\%]^2)$$

$$= 270.00.$$

- Finally, Portfolio AC's standard deviation is 16.4 percent:

$$\sigma_{\text{AC}} = \sqrt{\text{Variance}}$$

$$= \sqrt{270.00} = 16.4\%.$$

Because of perfect positive correlation between the returns on A and C, Portfolio AC's standard deviation is the weighted average standard deviation of its components:

$$\sigma_{\text{AC}} = (0.5 \times 11.0\%) + (0.5 \times 21.9\%)$$

$$= 16.4\%.$$

There is no risk reduction in this situation. The risk of the portfolio is less than the risk of Investment C, but it is more than the risk of Investment A. Forming a portfolio does not reduce risk when the returns on the two components are perfectly positively correlated; the portfolio merely **averages** the risk of the two investments.

What happens when a portfolio is created with two investments that have positive, but not perfectly positive, correlation? Combining the two investments can eliminate some—but not all—risk. To illustrate, consider Portfolio AD in Table 10.2. This portfolio has a standard deviation of returns of 10.1 percent, so it is risky. However, Portfolio AD's standard deviation is not only less than the weighted average of its components' standard deviations, $(0.5 \times 11\%) + (0.5 \times 12.1\%) = 11.6\%$, but also less than the standard deviation of each component. The correlation coefficient between the return distributions for A and D is 0.53, which indicates that the two investments are positively correlated, but the correlation is less than +1.0. Thus, combining two investments that are positively but not perfectly correlated lowers risk, but does not eliminate it.[5]

What is the correlation among the returns on "real-world" investments? Generalizing about the correlations among real-world investment alternatives is difficult. However, it is safe to say that the return distributions of two randomly selected investments—whether they are real assets in a hospital's portfolio of projects or financial assets in an individual's investment portfolio—are virtually never perfectly correlated, and hence correlation coefficients are never −1.0 or

+1.0. In fact, it is almost impossible to find actual investment opportunities with returns that are negatively correlated with one another, or even to find investments with returns that are uncorrelated ($r = 0$). Because all investment returns are affected to a greater or lesser degree by general economic conditions, investment returns tend to be positively correlated with one another. However, because investment returns are not affected identically by general economic conditions, returns on most real-world investments are not perfectly positively correlated.

The correlation coefficient between the returns of two randomly chosen investments will usually fall in the range of +0.4 to +0.8. Returns on investments that are similar in nature, such as two inpatient projects in a hospital or two stocks in the same industry, will typically have return correlations at the upper end of this range. Conversely, returns on dissimilar projects or securities will tend to have correlations at the lower end of the range.

Portfolio Risk: Many Assets

Businesses are not restricted to two projects and individual investors are not restricted to holding two-security portfolios. Most companies have tens, or even hundreds or thousands, of individual projects (i.e., product or service lines), and most individual investors hold many different securities or mutual funds, which themselves may be composed of hundreds of individual securities. Thus, what is most relevant to financial decision making is not what happens when two investments are combined into portfolios, but rather what happens when many investments are combined.

To illustrate the risk impact of creating large portfolios, consider Figure 10.1. The figure illustrates the riskiness inherent in holding randomly selected portfolios of one asset, two assets, three assets, four assets, and so on, considering the correlations that occur among real-world investments. The plot is based on **historical** annual returns on common stocks traded on the New York Stock Exchange (NYSE), but the conclusions reached are applicable to portfolios made up of any type of investment including healthcare providers that offer many different types of services.

The riskiness inherent in holding an average one-asset portfolio is relatively high, as measured by the standard deviation of annual returns. The average two-asset portfolio has a lower standard deviation, so holding an average two-asset portfolio, then, is less risky than holding a single asset of average risk. The average three-asset portfolio has an even lower standard deviation of returns, so an average three-asset portfolio is even less risky than an average two-asset portfolio. As more assets are randomly added to create larger portfolios, the average riskiness of the portfolio decreases. However, as more and more assets are added, the incremental risk reduction of adding even more assets decreases; regardless of how many assets are added, some risk always remains in the portfolio; substantial risk remains even with a portfolio of thousands of assets.

The reason why all risk cannot be eliminated by creating a very large portfolio is that the returns on the component investments, although not perfectly

FIGURE 10.1
Portfolio Size
and Risk

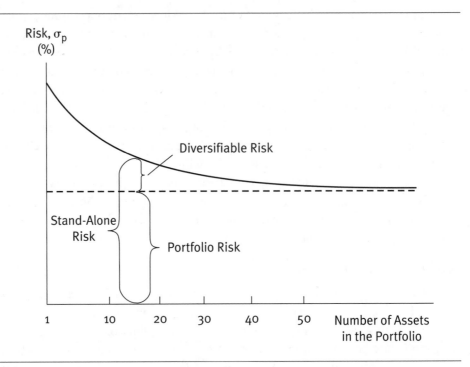

so, are still positively correlated with one another. In other words, all investments, both real and financial, are affected to a lesser or greater degree by
general economic conditions. If the economy booms, all investments tend to do
well; in a recession, all investments tend to do poorly. It is the positive correlation among real-world asset returns that prevents investors from creating riskless
portfolios.[6]

Diversifiable Risk Versus Portfolio Risk

Figure 10.1 shows what happens as investors create ever larger portfolios. As
the size of a randomly created portfolio increases, the riskiness of the portfolio
decreases. Thus, a large proportion of the stand-alone risk inherent in an individual
investment can be eliminated if it is held as part of a large portfolio. For example, if
a stock investor wanted to eliminate as much stand-alone risk inherent in owning
NYSE stocks as possible, he or she would have to own over 2,000 stocks. Such
a portfolio is called the *market portfolio* because it consists of the entire stock
market, or at least one entire segment of the stock market.

Recent studies have found that the market portfolio has only about one-
half the standard deviation of an average stock. However, it is not necessary for
individual investors to own 2,000 or so stocks to gain the risk-reducing benefit
that is inherent in holding large portfolios. As illustrated in Figure 10.1, most
of the benefit of diversification can be obtained by holding about 50 randomly
selected stocks.[7] Such a large, randomly chosen portfolio is called a *well-diversified
portfolio*. (A portfolio of 50 healthcare stocks, for example, is not well diversified

because the stocks are in the same sector of the economy, and hence are not randomly chosen.)

That part of the stand-alone riskiness of an individual investment that can be eliminated by diversification (i.e., by holding it as part of a well-diversified portfolio) is called *diversifiable risk*. That part of the riskiness of an individual investment that cannot be eliminated by diversification is called *portfolio risk*. Thus, every investment, whether it be the stock of Beverly Enterprises held by an individual investor or an MRI system operated by a hospital, has some diversifiable risk that can be eliminated and some portfolio risk that cannot be diversified away. Not all investments benefit to the same degree from portfolio risk-reducing effects, and some portfolios are not truly well diversified. In general, however, any investment will have some of its stand-alone risk eliminated when it is held as part of a portfolio.

Diversifiable risk, as seen by individuals investing in stocks, is caused by events that are unique to a single firm such as new product or service introductions, strikes, and lawsuits. Because these events are essentially random, their effects can be eliminated by diversification. When one stock in a portfolio does worse than expected because of a negative event unique to that firm, another stock in the portfolio will do better than expected because of a firm-unique positive event. On average, bad events in some companies will be offset by good events in others, so lower than expected returns will be offset by higher than expected returns, which leaves the investor with an overall portfolio return closer to that expected than would be the case if only a single stock were held.

The same logic can be applied to a firm with a portfolio of projects. Perhaps hospital returns generated from inpatient surgery are less than expected because of the trend toward outpatient procedures, but this may be offset by returns that are greater than expected on state-of-the-art diagnostic services. (If the hospital offered both inpatient and outpatient surgery, it would be *hedging* itself against the trend toward more outpatient procedures because reduced demand for inpatient surgery would be offset by increased demand for outpatient surgery.)

The point to be made here is that the negative impact of random events that are unique to a particular firm, or to a particular product or service within a firm, can be offset by positive events in other firms, or in other products or services. Thus, the risk caused by random, unique events can be eliminated by portfolio diversification. Individual investors can diversify by holding many securities, while businesses can diversify by operating many projects.

Unfortunately, not all risk can be diversified away. Portfolio risk, the risk that remains in portfolios, stems from factors, such as wars, inflation, recessions, and high interest rates, that systematically affect all stocks in a portfolio or all products or services produced by a business. For example, the increasing power of managed care organizations could lower reimbursement levels for all services offered by a hospital. Portfolio risk cannot be eliminated, so even well-diversified investors, whether they are individuals with large securities portfolios or diversified health companies with many different service lines, must deal with this type of risk.

Implications for Investors

The ability to eliminate a portion of the stand-alone riskiness inherent in individual investments has two significant implications for investors, whether the investor is an individual who holds securities or a business that offers products or services.

• Holding a single investment is **not** rational. Holding a portfolio can eliminate much of the stand-alone riskiness inherent in individual investments. Investors who are risk averse should seek to eliminate all diversifiable risk. Individual investors can easily diversify their personal investment portfolios by buying either many individual securities or mutual funds that hold diversified portfolios. Businesses cannot diversify their investments as easily as individuals, but businesses that offer a diverse line of products or services are less risky than businesses that rely on a single product or service.

• Because an asset held in a portfolio has less risk than when held in isolation, the traditional stand-alone risk measure of standard deviation is no longer appropriate for individual assets. Thus, it is necessary to rethink the definition and measurement of financial risk for such assets. (Note, though, that standard deviation remains the correct measure for the riskiness of an investor's portfolio because the portfolio is, in effect, a single asset held in isolation.)

Self-Test Questions

1. What is a portfolio of assets?
2. What is a well-diversified portfolio?
3. What happens to the risk of a single asset when it is held as part of a portfolio of assets?
4. Explain the differences between stand-alone risk, diversifiable risk, and portfolio risk.
5. Why should all investors hold portfolios rather than individual assets?
6. Is standard deviation the appropriate risk measure for an individual asset?
7. Is standard deviation the appropriate risk measure for an investor's portfolio of assets?

Measuring the Risk of Individual Assets Held in Portfolios

The stand-alone risk of individual assets is reduced when the assets are held as part of a portfolio, so standard deviation is no longer the relevant risk measure for such assets. Because investors are concerned with the overall riskiness of the portfolio, which is measured by standard deviation, the appropriate measure of risk for individual assets in the portfolio is the contribution of each asset to overall portfolio risk. How can this risk be measured?

The Beta Coefficient

The most widely used measure of risk for assets held in portfolios is called the *beta coefficient*, or just *beta*. It measures the volatility of an asset's returns relative to the overall volatility of the portfolio. To illustrate the concept of beta, consider

Table 10.3, which contains **historical** annual returns for three individual assets—H, M, and L—and for a large portfolio of assets, P. Five years of annual returns are displayed in the table, but three years of monthly returns, or some other combination, could have been chosen. Because the returns are historical (i.e., realized) rather than projected, the probability of occurrence of each return is the same; for five years of returns, each return has a probability of $100\%/5 = 20\%$. For now, the context does not matter; H, M, and L could be stocks that an individual investor is considering as an addition to Portfolio P, a stock portfolio, or they could be projects that are being evaluated by a hospital, and hence would be added to the hospital's portfolio of services, Portfolio P.

Figure 10.2 plots the historical annual returns on the three individual investments on the Y axis versus returns on the portfolio on the X axis. Investment M has the same volatility as the portfolio. When the portfolio return increased by 10 percentage points, as it did in Year 5 from a 25 percent return to a 35 percent return, the return on Investment M also increased by 10 percentage points. However, Investment H is more volatile than the portfolio; when the portfolio return increased by 10 percentage points, H increased by 15 percentage points. Conversely, Investment L only increased by 5 percentage points from Year 4 to Year 5, so it is less volatile than the portfolio.

Investments that are more volatile than a portfolio increase the riskiness of the portfolio when they are added, while investments that are less volatile decrease the riskiness of the portfolio. Thus, the amount of volatility of an investment, relative to the portfolio, measures the contribution of the investment to the overall riskiness of the portfolio, and hence relative volatility measures an individual investment's portfolio risk. Remember that an individual investment's **stand-alone risk** is defined as volatility about its mean (expected) return, so a completely different concept is being used to assess the **portfolio risk** of an individual investment.

How should the risks of Investments H, M, and L be measured, considering that they would be held as part of Portfolio P? In fact, the lines that are plotted on Figure 10.2 are regression lines in the statistical sense, and the slope of each line measures the volatility of that investment **relative to** the volatility of the portfolio. (The slope of a regression line is a measure of its steepness and is defined as rise

TABLE 10.3 Beta Coefficient Illustration

| Year | \multicolumn{4}{c}{Rate of Return} | | | |
	H	M	L	Portfolio (P)
1	20%	15%	10%	15%
2	5	5	5	5
3	−10	−5	0	−5
4	35	25	15	25
5	50	35	20	35

FIGURE 10.2

Relative Volatility of
Assets H, M, and L

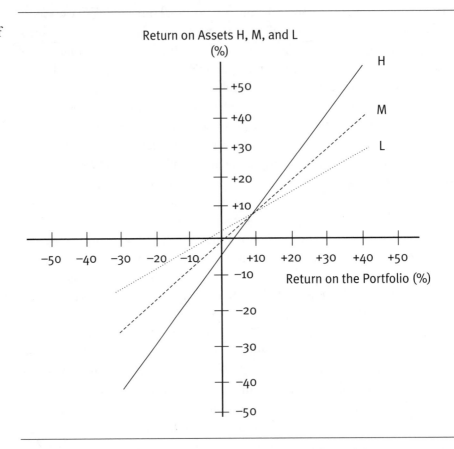

over run.) The regression line for Investment M has a slope, or beta coefficient, of 1.0, which shows that M has the same volatility as the portfolio, and hence has average risk, where average is defined as the riskiness of the portfolio. Investment H has a beta of 1.5, hence it is 1.5 times as risky as the average investment in the portfolio, while L with a beta of 0.5 is only half as risky as the average investment in Portfolio P.

A U.S. Treasury security that had a 5 percent realized return in each year over the same five years as shown in Table 10.3 would have a horizontal regression line, and hence a slope of zero. Such an investment would have a beta of zero, which signifies no portfolio risk. In fact, such a Treasury security would have no stand-alone risk because a 5 percent rate of return in each year would result in a standard deviation of zero.

Theoretically, an investment could have a negative beta; the regression line for such an investment would slope downward. In this case, the investment's return would move opposite to the portfolio's return. In years when the portfolio's return increased, the investment's return would decrease and vice versa. Such an investment has negative portfolio risk, which means that it would have a significant risk-reducing impact on the portfolio. Although it is possible to find investments in the real world that have negative betas based on **historical returns**, it is much more difficult to find an investment that is expected to have a negative beta on the basis of **future returns**. The reason is that the returns on all assets in a portfolio are typically affected in a similar manner by most external economic forces.

Portfolio Risk Seen By Businesses (Corporate Risk)

Firms typically offer a myriad of products or services, and thus can be thought of as having a large number (hundreds or even thousands) of individual activities. For example, most managed care organizations offer numerous healthcare plans to diverse groups of enrollees in numerous service areas. And many hospitals and hospital systems offer a large number of inpatient, outpatient, and even home health services that cover a wide geographical area and treat a wide range of illnesses and injuries. Thus, healthcare businesses operate a portfolio of individual products or services, so they consist of a portfolio of *projects*.

What is the riskiness of an individual project to a business with many projects? Because the project is part of the business' portfolio of assets, its stand-alone risk is not relevant—the project is not held in isolation. The relevant risk of any project to a business with many projects is its contribution to the business' overall risk, or the impact of the project on the variability of the firm's overall rate of return. Some of the stand-alone riskiness of the project will be diversified away by combining the project with the firm's other projects. The remaining risk, which is the portfolio risk in a business context, is called *corporate risk*.

The quantitative measure of corporate risk is a project's *corporate beta*, or *corporate b*, which is the slope of the regression line that results when the project's returns are plotted on the Y axis and the overall returns on the firm are plotted on the X axis. If Table 10.3 and Figure 10.2 represented returns on three projects and the overall returns for AtlantiCare, a not-for-profit HMO, the betas for H, M, and L would be corporate betas. They would measure the contribution of each project to AtlantiCare's overall risk.

A project's corporate beta measures the volatility of returns on the project relative to the business as a whole, which has a corporate beta of 1.0.[8] If a project's corporate beta is 1.5, such as for Project H, its returns are 1.5 times as volatile as the firm's returns. Such a project increases the volatility of AtlantiCare's overall returns, and hence increases the riskiness of the business. A corporate beta of 1.0, such as for Project M, indicates that the project's returns have the same volatility as the firm. Hence, the project has the same risk as AtlantiCare's *average project*, which is a hypothetical project that has the same risk as the aggregate business. A corporate beta of 0.5, such as for Project L, indicates that the project's returns are less volatile than the firm's returns, so the project reduces AtlantiCare's overall risk.

In closing the discussion of corporate risk (the risk of individual projects within a business with many projects), it must be noted that the concepts presented here are important to health services managers. The fact that a project's **corporate risk** depends on its context—that is, where it is held—has important implications for managerial decision making. However, the discussion has glossed over the problems inherent in implementing the concept in practice. That discussion will take place in Chapter 15.

Portfolio Risk Seen by Stock Investors (Market Risk)

The previous section discussed the riskiness of business projects to an organization. This section discusses the riskiness of business projects to common stock investors. Why should health services managers be concerned about how stock investors view risk? The answer is simple: stock investors are the suppliers of equity capital to investor-owned businesses, so they set the rates of return that such businesses must pay to raise that form of capital. In turn, these rates set the minimum profitability that investor-owned businesses must earn on the equity portion of their real asset investments. Even managers of not-for-profit firms should have an understanding of how stock investors view risk because market-set required rates of return can influence the opportunity cost rates used in making real asset investments within not-for-profit businesses. Chapter 13 discusses this topic in detail.

Because stock investors hold well-diversified portfolios of stocks, the relevant riskiness of an individual project undertaken by a company whose stock is held in the stock portfolio is the project's contribution to the riskiness of that portfolio. Some of the stand-alone riskiness of the project will be diversified away by combining the project with all the other projects in the stock portfolio. The remaining portfolio risk is called *market risk*, which is defined as the contribution of the project to the riskiness of a well-diversified stock portfolio.

How should a project's market risk be measured? A project's *market beta*, or *market b*, measures the volatility of the project's returns relative to the returns on a well-diversified portfolio of stocks, which represents a very large portfolio of individual projects. If Table 10.3 and Figure 10.2 represented returns on three projects and the overall returns on a well-diversified stock portfolio, the betas for H, M, and L would be *market betas*, which would measure the market risk of the projects. The only difference between the discussion of market risk and the previous discussion of corporate risk is what defines the relevant portfolio. When focusing on **corporate risk**, the relevant portfolio is the firm's overall portfolio of projects. When discussing **market risk**, the relevant portfolio is a well-diversified stock portfolio (i.e., the market portfolio).[9]

A project with a market beta of 1.5, such as for Project H, has returns that are 1.5 times as volatile as the returns on the market and, hence, increases the riskiness of a well-diversified stock portfolio. A market beta of 1.0 indicates that the project's returns have the same volatility as the market—such a project has the same market risk as the market portfolio. A market beta of 0.5 indicates that the project's returns are half as volatile as the returns on the market—such a project reduces the riskiness of a well-diversified stock portfolio.

In these illustrations, the same probability distributions are being used to illustrate both corporate risk and market risk. In reality, it is unlikely that returns on a particular firm and returns on the market portfolio would be the same. (The portfolio returns in the right column of Table 10.3 would not be identical for both a given firm and for the market portfolio.) This reality would cause the lines plotted in Figure 10.2 to have different slopes, and hence different corporate and market betas. For example, Project H may have a corporate beta of 1.5 and a market beta of 1.2. In general, a project's corporate beta and market beta will differ.

The two types of portfolio risk—corporate and market—are identical in concept. Both types of risk are measured by the contribution of the asset—in this case, a business project—to the overall riskiness of the portfolio. Also, both types of risk are measured by the volatility of the asset's returns relative to the volatility of the portfolio. The only difference between corporate and market risk is what defines the portfolio. In corporate risk, the portfolio is defined as the collection of projects held within a business; in market risk, the portfolio is defined as the collection of projects held within a well-diversified stock portfolio.

Finally, even though an individual investor's stock portfolio can be thought of as a portfolio of many separate projects, the portfolio actually consists of the stocks of firms. Individual investors, therefore, are most concerned with the aggregate risk and return characteristics of the companies they own rather than the risk and return characteristics of each company's projects. This logic leads investors to be more concerned with the company's (stock's) market beta than they are with the market betas of individual projects.

A stock's market beta is the slope of the line formed by regressing the individual firm's stock returns against the aggregate returns on the market. For example, the market beta of Columbia/HCA Healthcare Corporation, as recently reported in the *Value Line Investment Survey*, is 1.1. This means that an equity investment in Columbia/HCA is slightly more risky to well-diversified stock investors than an average stock, which has a beta of 1.0. Columbia/HCA's corporate beta, like all other company's corporate betas, is 1.0 by definition. What is relevant to stock investors, because they hold portfolios of common stocks, is the firm's market beta and not its corporate beta.

Self-Test Questions

1. What is the definition of portfolio risk?
2. How is portfolio risk measured?
3. What is a corporate beta and how is it estimated?
4. What is a market beta and how is it estimated?
5. Briefly, what is the difference between corporate risk and market risk?
6. What is the difference between a project's market beta and the firm's market beta?

Portfolio Betas

Individual investors hold portfolios of stocks, each with its own market risk as measured by the stock's market beta, while businesses hold portfolios of projects, each with its own corporate and market betas. What impact does the beta of a portfolio component have on the overall portfolio's beta? The beta of any portfolio of investments is simply the weighted average of the individual component betas:

$$b_{Portfolio} = (w_1 \times b_1) + (w_2 \times b_2) \text{ and so on.}$$

In this equation, $b_{Portfolio}$ is the beta of the portfolio, which measures the volatility of the entire portfolio; w_1 is the fraction of the portfolio in Investment 1; b_1 is the beta coefficient of Investment 1, and so on.

To illustrate, the stock of Columbia/HCA has a market beta of 1.1, which indicates that its returns to stockholders are slightly more volatile than the returns on a well-diversified stock portfolio (i.e., the market portfolio with a beta of 1.0). Hence, the stock is somewhat riskier than an average stock. However, each project within Columbia/HCA has its own market risk, as measured by its market beta. Some projects may have very high market betas (e.g., over 1.5), while other projects may have very low market betas (e.g., under 0.5). When all the thousands of projects are combined, the overall market beta of the company is 1.1.

For ease of discussion, assume that Columbia/HCA Healthcare only has the following three projects:

Project	Market Beta	Dollar Investment	Proportion
A	0.4	$ 15,000	15.0%
B	0.9	30,000	30.0
C	1.4	55,000	55.0
		$100,000	100.0%

The weighted average of the project market betas, which is the firm's market beta, is 1.1:

$$\text{Market } b_{Columbia/HCA} = (w_1 \times b_1) + (w_2 \times b_2) + (w_3 \times b_3)$$
$$= (0.15 \times 0.4) + (0.30 \times 0.9) + (0.55 \times 1.4)$$
$$= 1.1.$$

Each project's market beta reflects its volatility relative to the market portfolio. Note that each of Columbia/HCA's fictitious projects also has a corporate beta that measures the volatility of the project's returns relative to that of the corporation as a whole. The weighted average of these project corporate betas must equal 1.0, which is the corporate beta of any business.

Self-Test Questions
1. How is the beta of a portfolio related to the betas of the components?
2. What is the value of the weighted average of all project corporate betas within a business?

Relevance of the Three Risk Measures

So far, this chapter has discussed in some detail three measures of financial risk—stand alone, corporate, and market—but what is still unclear is which risk is most relevant in financial decision making. **The risk that is relevant to any financial**

decision depends on the particular situation at hand. When the decision involves a single investment that will be held in isolation, stand-alone risk is the relevant risk. Here, the risk and return on the portfolio is the same as the risk and return on the single asset in the portfolio. In this situation, the riskiness faced by the investor, whether an individual considering a stock purchase or a business considering an MRI system investment, is defined in terms of returns less than expected, and the appropriate risk measure is the standard deviation of the return distribution.

In most investment decisions, however, the asset under consideration will not be held in isolation, but will be held as part of an investment portfolio. Individual investors typically hold portfolios of stocks, while businesses typically hold portfolios of real asset investments. For individual investors who hold stock portfolios, the most relevant risk is the asset's contribution to the overall riskiness of a well-diversified stock portfolio. This risk is market risk, and it is measured by the asset's market beta.

For businesses, the most relevant risk depends on whether the business is for profit or not for profit. For investor-owned businesses, the goal is shareholder wealth maximization, so risk must be measured in shareholder terms. Because stockholders tend to hold large portfolios of securities, and hence a very large portfolio of individual projects, the most relevant risk of a project under consideration by a for-profit firm is its contribution to a well-diversified stock portfolio (i.e., the market portfolio), which is the project's market risk.

Not-for-profit firms do not have stockholders, and their goals stem from a mission statement that generally involves service to the community. In this situation, market risk is irrelevant. The concern to managers is the impact of the project on the riskiness of the business, which is measured by a project's corporate risk. Thus, the risk measure most relevant to projects in not-for-profit firms is a project's corporate beta.

Self-Test Questions

1. Explain the situations in which stand-alone, corporate, and market risk are the most relevant.
2. How often would stand-alone risk be relevant?

The Relationship Between Risk and Return

This chapter contains a great deal of discussion that focuses on defining and measuring financial risk and return. However, being able to define and measure financial risk is of no value in financial decision making unless risk can be related to return. That is, the answer to this question is needed: How much return is required to compensate investors for assuming a given level of risk? In this section, the focus is on setting required rates of return on stock investments, but in other chapters the focus is on setting required rates of return on individual projects within companies.

The relationship between the market risk of a stock, as measured by its market beta, and its required rate of return is given by the *Capital Asset Pricing Model (CAPM)*.[10]

To begin, some basic definitions are needed:

$E(R_i)$ = Expected rate of return on Stock i, any stock.

$R(R_i)$ = Required rate of return on Stock i. If $E(R_i)$ is less $R(R_i)$, the stock would not be purchased, or it would be sold if it was owned. If $E(R_i)$ was greater than $R(R_i)$, the stock should be bought, and a person would be indifferent about the purchase if $E(R_i) = R(R_i)$.

RF = Risk-free rate of return. In a CAPM context, RF is generally measured by the return on long-term U.S. Treasury bonds.

b_i = Market beta coefficient of Stock i. The market beta of an average-risk stock is $b_A = 1.0$.

$R(R_M)$ = Required rate of return on a portfolio that consists of all stocks, which is the market portfolio. $R(R_M)$ is also the required rate of return on an average ($b_A = 1.0$) stock.

RP_M = Market risk premium = $R(R_M) - RF$. This is the additional return over the risk-free rate required to compensate investors for assuming average ($b_A = 1.0$) risk.

RP_i = Risk premium on Stock i = $[R(R_M) - RF] \times b_i = RP_M \times b_i$. Stock i's risk premium is less than, equal to, or greater than the premium on an average stock, depending on whether its beta is less than, equal to, or greater than 1.0. If $b_i = b_A = 1.0$, then $RP_i = RP_M$.

Using these definitions, the CAPM relationship between risk and required rate of return is given by the following equation, which is called the *Security Market Line (SML)*:

$$R(R_i) = RF + (R[R_M] - RF) \times b_i$$

$$= RF + (RP_M \times b_i).$$

To illustrate use of the SML, assume that the risk-free rate (RF) is 6 percent and the required rate of return on the market, $R[R_M]$, is 10 percent. The market beta of Columbia/HCA stock is 1.1. According to the SML, Columbia/HCA stock's required rate of return is 10.4 percent:

$$R(R_{Columbia/HCA}) = 6\% + (10\% - 6\%) \times 1.1$$

$$= 6\% + (4\% \times 1.1)$$

$$= 6\% + 4.4\% = 10.4\%.$$

If the expected rate of return, $E(R_{Columbia/HCA})$, were 15 percent, investors should buy the stock because $E(R_{Columbia/HCA})$ is greater than $R(R_{Columbia/HCA})$.

Conversely, if the expected rate of return were $E(R_{Columbia/HCA}) = 8\%$, investors should sell the stock because $E(R_{Columbia/HCA})$ is less than $R(R_{Columbia/HCA})$.

A stock with a beta of 2.0, one that is riskier than Columbia/HCA, would have a required rate of return of 14 percent:

$$R(R_{b=2.0}) = 6\% + (4\% \times 2.0)$$

$$= 6\% + 8\% = 14\%$$

while an average-risk stock, with $b_i = 1.0$, would have a required return of 10 percent, which is the same as the market return:

$$R(R_{b=1.0}) = 6\% + (4\% \times 1.0)$$

$$= 6\% + 4\% = 10\% = R(R_M).$$

A stock with below-average risk, for example, $b_i = 0.5$, would have a required return of 8 percent:

$$R(R_{b=0.5}) = 6\% + (4\% \times 0.5)$$

$$= 6\% + 2\% = 8\%.$$

The market risk premium, RP_M, depends on the degree of aversion that investors in the aggregate have to risk. In this example, T-bonds yielded $RF = 6\%$ and an average share of stock had a required rate of return of $R(R_M) = 10\%$, so RP_M is 4 percentage points. If the degree of risk aversion increased, $R(R_M)$ may increase to 12 percent, which would cause RP_M to increase to 6 percentage points. Thus, the greater the overall degree of risk aversion, the higher the required rate on the market, and hence the higher the required rates of return on all stocks.

Also, values for the risk-free rate, RF, and the required rate of return on the market, $R(R_M)$, are influenced by inflation expectations. The higher the expectations of investors regarding inflation, the greater these values; hence, the greater the required rates of return on all stocks.

The SML is often expressed in graphical form, as in Figure 10.3, which shows the SML when $RF = 6\%$ and $R(R_M) = 10\%$. Here are the relevant points concerning Figure 10.3:

- Required rates of return are shown on the vertical axis, while risk as measured by market beta is shown on the horizontal axis.
- Riskless securities have $b_i = 0$; therefore, RF is the vertical axis intercept.
- The slope of the SML reflects the degree of risk aversion in the economy. The greater the average investor's aversion to risk, (1) the steeper the slope of the SML, (2) the greater the risk premium for any stock, and (3) the higher the required rate of return on stocks.
- The Y intercept reflects the level of expected inflation. The higher the inflation

expectations, the greater both RF and $R(R_M)$; thus, the higher the SML plots on the graph.
- The values previously calculated for the required rates of return on stocks with $b_i = 0.5$, $b_i = 1.0$, and $b_i = 2.0$ agree with the values shown on the graph.

FIGURE 10.3

The Security
Market Line

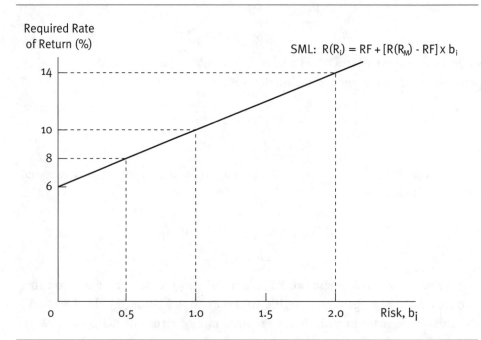

Both the SML and a company's position on it change over time because of changes in interest rates, investors' risk aversion, and individual companies' betas. Thus, the SML, as well as a company's risk, must be evaluated on the basis of current information. The SML, its use, and how its input values are estimated are covered in greater detail in Chapter 13.

How Good is the CAPM?

A word of caution about betas and the Capital Asset Pricing Model (CAPM) is in order. To begin, the CAPM is based on a very restrictive set of assumptions that does not conform well to real-world conditions. Second, although these concepts are logical, the entire theory is based on expectations, yet only historical data are available. Thus, the market betas that are calculated and reported in practice show how volatile a stock has been in the *past*. However, conditions may change, and a stock's *future volatility*—the item of real concern to investors—may be quite different from its past volatility. Although the CAPM represents a very important contribution to risk and return theory, it does have potentially serious problems when applied in practice. This point is addressed again in Chapter 13.

Self-Test Questions

1. What is the Capital Asset Pricing Model (CAPM)?
2. What is the appropriate measure of risk in the CAPM?
3. Write out the equation for the Security Market Line (SML) and graph it.
4. Describe the SML in words.

Key Concepts

This chapter has covered the very important concepts of financial risk and return. The key concepts of this chapter are:

- *Investment returns* can be measured on either a dollar basis or a rate of return (percentage) basis.
- Risk definition and measurement is very important in financial management because decision makers, in general, are *risk averse*, and hence require higher returns from investments that have higher risk.
- *Financial risk* is associated with the prospect of returns less than anticipated. The higher the probability of a return being far less than anticipated, the greater the risk.
- The riskiness of investments held in isolation, called *stand-alone risk*, can be measured by the dispersion of the rate of return distribution about its *expected value*. One commonly used measure of stand-alone risk is the *standard deviation* of the return distribution.
- Most investments are not held in isolation, but rather as part of *portfolios*. Individual investors hold portfolios of securities and businesses hold portfolios of projects (i.e., products and services).
- When investments with returns that are less than perfectly positively correlated are combined in a portfolio, risk is reduced. The risk reduction occurs because less-than-expected returns on some investments are offset by greater-than-expected returns on other investments. However, among real-world investments, it is impossible to eliminate all risk because the returns on all assets are influenced to a greater or lesser degree by overall economic conditions.
- That portion of the stand-alone risk of an investment that can be eliminated by holding the investment in a portfolio is called *diversifiable risk*, while the risk that remains is called *portfolio risk*.
- There are two different types of portfolio risk. *Corporate risk* is the riskiness of business projects when they are considered as part of a business' portfolio of projects. *Market risk* is the riskiness of business projects (or of the stocks of entire businesses) when they are considered as part of an individual investor's well-diversified portfolio of securities.
- Corporate risk is measured by a project's *corporate beta*, which reflects the volatility of the project's returns relative to the volatility of returns of the aggregate business.

- Market risk is measured by a project's or stock's *market beta*, which reflects the volatility of a project's or stock's returns relative to the volatility of returns on a well-diversified stock portfolio.
- *Stand-alone risk* is most relevant to investments held in isolation; *corporate risk* is most relevant to projects held by not-for-profit firms; and *market risk* is most relevant to projects held by investor-owned firms.
- The *overall beta coefficient of a portfolio* is the weighted average of the betas of the components of the portfolio where the weights are the proportion of the overall investment in each component. Therefore, the weighted average of corporate betas of all projects in a business must equal 1.0, while the weighted average of all projects' market betas must equal the market beta of the firm's stock.
- The *Capital Asset Pricing Model (CAPM)* is an equilibrium model that describes the relationship between market risk and required rates of return.
- The *Security Market Line (SML)* provides the actual risk/required rate of return relationship. The required rate of return on any Stock i is equal to the risk-free rate plus the market risk premium times the stock's market beta coefficient: $R(R_i) = RF + [R(R_M) - RF] \times b_i = RF + (RP_M \times b_i)$.

This concludes the discussion of basic financial management concepts. The next chapter begins the coverage of long-term financing.

Questions

10.1 When considering stand-alone risk, the return distribution of a less risky investment is more peaked than that of a riskier investment. What shape would the return distribution have for an investment with (a) completely certain returns and (b) completely uncertain returns?

10.2 Stock A has an expected rate of return of 8 percent, a standard deviation of 20 percent, and a market beta of 0.5. Stock B has an expected rate of return of 12 percent, a standard deviation of 15 percent, and a market beta of 1.5. Which investment is riskier? Why? (Hint: Remember that the risk of an investment depends on its context.)

10.3 a. What is risk aversion?
  b. Why is risk aversion so important to financial decision making?

10.4 Explain why holding investments in portfolios has such a profound impact on the concept of financial risk.

10.5 Assume that two investments are combined in a portfolio.
  a. In words, what is the expected rate of return on the portfolio?
  b. What condition must be present for the portfolio to have lower risk than the weighted average of the two investments?
  c. Is it possible for the portfolio to have lower risk than that of either investment?

d. Is it possible for the portfolio to be riskless? What condition is necessary to create a riskless portfolio?

10.6 Explain the difference between portfolio risk and diversifiable risk.

10.7 What are the implications of portfolio theory for investors?

10.8 a. What are the two types of portfolio risk?
   b. How is each type defined?
   c. How is each type measured?

10.9 Under what circumstances is each type of risk—stand alone, corporate, and market—relevant?

Problems

10.1 Assume that $10,000 was invested in the stock of General Medical Corporation with the intention of selling after one year. The stock pays no dividends, so the entire return will be based on the price of the stock when sold.
   a. To begin, assume that the stock sale nets $11,500. What is the dollar return on the stock investment? What is the rate of return?
   b. Assume that the stock price falls, and the net is only $9,500 when the stock is sold. What is the dollar return and rate of return?

10.2 Consider the following probability distribution of returns estimated for a proposed project involving a new ultrasound machine:

State of the Economy	Probability of Occurrence	Rate of Return
Very poor	0.10	−10.0%
Poor	0.20	0.0
Average	0.40	10.0
Good	0.20	20.0
Very good	0.10	30.0

   a. What is the expected rate of return on the project?
   b. What is the project's standard deviation of returns?
   c. What type of risk does the standard deviation measure?
   d. In what situation is this risk relevant?

10.3 Suppose that a person won the Florida lottery and was offered a choice of two prizes: (1) $500,000 or (2) a coin-toss gamble in which he or she would get $1 million if a head were flipped and zero for a tail.
   a. What is the expected dollar return on the gamble?
   b. Would the person choose the sure $500,000 or the gamble?
   c. If he or she chose the sure $500,000, is the person a risk averter or a risk seeker?

10.4 Suppose that the risk-free rate, RF, were 8 percent and the required rate of return on the market, $R(R_M)$, were 14 percent.
   a. Write out the Security Market Line (SML) and explain each term.
   b. Plot the SML on a sheet of paper.

c. Suppose that inflation expectations increase such that the risk-free rate, RF, increases to 10 percent and the required rate of return on the market, $R(R_M)$, increases to 16 percent. Write out and plot the new SML.

d. Return to the original assumptions in this problem. Now, suppose that investors' risk aversion increases, and the required rate of return on the market, $R(R_M)$, increases to 16 percent. (There is no change in the risk-free rate because RF reflects the required rate of return on a riskless investment.) Write out and plot the new SML.

10.5 The *Value Line Investment Survey* reported the following market betas for the stocks of selected healthcare providers:

Company	Beta
Quorum Health Group	0.90
Beverly Enterprises	1.20
HEALTHSOUTH Corporation	1.45
United Healthcare	1.70

At the time these betas were developed, reasonable estimates for the risk-free rate, RF, and required rate of return on the market, $R(R_M)$, were 6.5 percent and 13.5 percent, respectively.

a. What are the required rates of return on the four stocks?

b. Why do their required rates of return differ?

c. Suppose that a person is planning to invest in only one stock, rather than hold a well-diversified stock portfolio. Are the required rates of return calculated above applicable to the investment? Explain your answer.

10.6 Suppose that Apex Health Services has four different projects. These projects are listed below, along with the amount of capital invested and estimated corporate and market betas:

Project	Amount Invested	Corporate Beta	Market Beta
Walk-in clinic	$ 500,000	1.5	1.1
MRI facility	2,000,000	1.2	1.5
Clinical laboratory	1,500,000	0.9	0.8
X-ray laboratory	1,000,000	0.5	1.0
	$5,000,000		

a. Why do the corporate and market betas differ for same project?

b. What is the overall corporate beta of Apex Health Services? Is the calculated beta consistent with corporate risk theory?

c. What is the overall market beta of Apex Health Services?

d. How does the riskiness of Apex's stock compare with the riskiness of an average stock?

e. Would stock investors require a rate of return on Apex that is greater than, less than, or the same as the return on an average-risk stock?

10.7 Assume that Columbia/HCA Healthcare is evaluating the feasibility of building a new hospital in an area not currently served by the company. The company's analysts estimate a market beta for the hospital project of 1.1, which is the same market risk as the company's average project. Financial forecasts for the new hospital indicate an expected rate of return on the equity portion of the investment of 20 percent. If the risk-free rate, RF, is 7 percent and the required rate of return on the market, R(R_M), is 12 percent, is the new hospital in the best interest of Columbia/HCA's shareholders? Explain your answer.

Notes

1. Defining financial risk as the probability of earning a return far below that expected is somewhat simplistic. There are many different ways of viewing financial risk. For example, a person saving for old age may define financial risk as the probability of not achieving some specified standard of living at retirement. However, the narrow definition presented here is a good starting point for discussing the types of risk that are most relevant to decisions made within health services organizations.

2. In certain situations, the expected rate of return may not be achievable. For example, an investment that has a 50 percent chance of a 5 percent return and a 50 percent chance of a 15 percent return has an expected rate of return of $(0.5 \times 5\%) + (0.5 \times 15\%) = 7.5\%$, which has a zero probability of occurrence.

3. Most financial calculators and spreadsheet programs have built-in functions that calculate the standard deviation of a specified distribution. However, such built-in functions assume that the values entered have equal probabilities of occurrence, and hence these functions **cannot** be used with the types of distributions contained in Table 10.1. The functions built into calculators and spreadsheet programs deal with *historical* distributions such as returns for each year over the past five years and not *forecasted* distributions with unequal probabilities of occurrence.

4. Standard deviation can provide useful information about the values that lie within the distribution. For example, if the distribution is *normal* (i.e., a specific type of bell-shaped distribution), just about all values in the distribution fall within three standard deviations above and below the expected value.

5. A portfolio of two assets will have lower risk than that of either asset only when the correlation coefficient between the assets is less than the ratio of the assets' standard deviations where the ratio is constructed with the lower standard deviation in the numerator. Thus, for Portfolio AD to have less risk than both A and D, the correlation coefficient between the returns on A and D must be less than $\sigma_A/\sigma_D = 11.0\% / 12.1\% = 0.91$. The actual correlation coefficient is 0.53, so the condition is met in this example.

6. If there is zero correlation among investment returns, as in the multiple coin toss example, then a very large portfolio would be riskless (standard deviation of returns of 0 percent), or close to it. Because this is not the case among most real-world investments, even very large portfolios are risky. Although stocks can be combined

with complex investments called derivatives (i.e., options) to form riskless portfolios, for the purposes of healthcare finance in which asset returns tend to have positive correlations, some risk remains even in very large portfolios.

7. Today, investors can buy index mutual funds that own all the stocks in a particular index or a subset selected to mimic the returns on the index. Thus, investors can create a completely diversified stock portfolio, as defined by a particular index, with only a single purchase.

8. Consider what the slope of the line would be if Portfolio P's returns were plotted on both the X and Y axes. The regression line would be a 45-degree line, which has a slope of 1.0. Thus, an average risk investment, as defined by the risk of the portfolio, has a slope of 1.0.

9. In practice, some stock index, for example, the S&P 500 Index or the NYSE Index, is used as a proxy for the market portfolio. (The Standard & Poor's 500 is an index made up of 500 stocks across many industries, while the New York Stock Exchange Index is made up of the over 2,000 common stocks traded on the NYSE.)

10. The CAPM is a relatively complex subject; only the basic concepts are presented in this text. For a more detailed discussion, see E. F. Brigham and L. C. Gapenski, *Intermediate Financial Management* (Fort Worth, TX: Dryden Press, 1996), chapter 3.

References

Brigham, E. F. and L. C. Gapenski. 1997. *Financial Management: Theory and Practice.* Fort Worth, TX: Dryden Press.

Gapenski, L. C. 1992. "'Project Risk Definition and Measurement in a Not-for-Profit Setting." *Health Services Management Research* (November): 216–24.

LONG-TERM FINANCING

LONG-TERM DEBT FINANCING

Learning Objectives

After studying this chapter, readers will be able to:

- Describe how interest rates are set in the economy.
- Discuss the various types of long-term debt instruments and their features.
- Discuss the components that make up the interest rate on a debt security.
- Value debt securities.

Introduction

If a business is to operate, it must have assets. To acquire assets, it must raise *capital*. Capital comes in two basic forms: debt and equity. Historically, capital furnished by the owners of investor-owned businesses (i.e., stockholders of for-profit corporations) was called *equity* capital, while capital obtained by not-for-profit businesses from grants, contributions, and retained earnings was called *fund* capital. Both types of capital serve the same purpose in financing businesses—providing a permanent financing base without a contractually fixed cost—so today the term *equity* is often used to represent nonliability capital regardless of ownership type.

In addition to equity financing, most healthcare businesses use a considerable amount of *debt* financing, which is provided by *creditors*. To illustrate debt usage, *Value Line* reports that, on average, healthcare providers finance their assets with 5 percent short-term debt, 30 percent long-term debt, and 65 percent equity. Thus, over one-third of providers' financing comes from debt. In this chapter, many facets of debt financing are discussed including important background material related to how interest rates are set in the economy. The discussion here focuses on long-term debt; short-term debt is discussed in Chapter 16.

The Cost of Money

Capital in a free economy is allocated through the price system. The *interest rate* is the price paid to obtain debt capital, whereas in the case of equity capital in for-profit firms, investors' returns come in the form of *dividends* and *capital gains* or *losses*. The four most fundamental factors that affect the supply of and demand for investment capital, and hence the cost of money, are investment opportunities, time preferences for consumption, risk, and inflation.

To see how these factors operate, visualize the situation facing Lori Gibbs, an entrepreneur who is planning to found a new home health agency. Lori does not have sufficient personal funds to start the business, so she must go to the debt markets for additional capital. If Lori estimates that the business will be highly profitable, she will be able to pay creditors a higher interest rate than if it is barely profitable. Thus, her ability to pay for borrowed capital depends on the business' *investment opportunities*. The higher the profitability of the business, the higher the interest rate that Ms. Gibbs can afford to pay lenders for use of their savings.

The interest rate that lenders will charge depends, in large part, on their *time preferences for consumption*. For example, one potential lender, Jane Wright, may be saving for retirement, so she may be willing to loan funds at a relatively low rate because her preference is for future consumption. Another person, John Davis, may have a wife and several young children to clothe and feed, so he may be willing to lend funds out of current income, and hence forgo consumption, only if the interest rate is very high. Mr. Davis is said to have a high time preference for consumption and Ms. Wright a low time preference. If the entire population of an economy were living right at the subsistence level, time preferences for current consumption would necessarily be high, aggregate savings would be low, interest rates would be high, and capital formation would be difficult.

The *risk* inherent in the prospective home health care business, and thus in Ms. Gibbs' ability to repay the loan, would also affect the return lenders would require; the higher the perceived risk, the higher the interest rate. Investors would be unwilling to lend to high-risk businesses unless the interest rate was higher than on loans to low-risk businesses.

Finally, because the value of money in the future is affected by *inflation*, the higher the expected rate of inflation, the higher the interest rate demanded by savers. Note that to simplify matters, the illustration implied that savers would lend directly to businesses that need capital, but in most cases the funds would actually pass through a *financial intermediary* such as a bank or a mutual fund.

Self-Test Questions
1. What is the "price" of debt capital?
2. What four factors affect the cost of money?

Common Long-Term Debt Instruments

There are many types of long-term debt: amortized and nonamortized, publicly issued and privately placed, taxable and tax exempt, secured and unsecured, marketable and nonmarketable, callable and noncallable, and so on. In this section, the long-term debt instruments that are most commonly used by healthcare businesses are briefly discussed.

Term Loans

A *term loan* is a contract under which a borrower agrees to make a series of interest and principal payments on specified dates to a lender. Investment bankers are generally not involved; term loans are negotiated directly between the borrowing business and the lender. Typically, the lender is a financial institution such as a bank, a mutual fund, an insurance company, or a pension fund, but it can also be a wealthy private investor. Most term loans have maturities of three to 15 years.

Term loans are usually amortized in equal installments over the life of the loan, so part of the principal of the loan is retired with each payment. For example, Sacramento Cardiology Group has a $100,000 five-year term loan with Bank of America to fund the purchase of new diagnostic equipment. The interest rate on the fixed-rate loan is 10 percent, which obligates the Group to five end-of-year payments of $26,379.75. Thus, loan payments total $131,898.75, of which $31,898.75 is interest and $100,000 is repayment of principal (i.e., the amount borrowed).

Term loans have three major advantages over bonds (which are typically sold to the general public): speed, flexibility, and low issuance costs. Because term loans are negotiated directly between the lender and the borrower, formal documentation is minimized. The key provisions of the loan can be worked out much more quickly, and with more flexibility, than can those for a public issue. It is not necessary for a term loan to go through the Securities and Exchange Commission (SEC) registration process. Also, after a term loan has been negotiated, changes can be renegotiated more easily than with bonds if financial circumstances so dictate.

The interest rate on a term loan either can be fixed for the life of the loan or variable. If it is fixed, the rate used will be close to the rate on equivalent maturity bonds issued by businesses of comparable risk. If the rate is variable, it is usually set at a certain number of percentage points over an index rate such as the prime rate.[1] When the index rate goes up or down, so does the interest rate that must be paid on the outstanding balance of the loan.

Bonds

Like a term loan, a *bond* is a long-term contract under which a borrower agrees to make payments of interest and principal on specific dates to the debtholder. Although bonds are similar to term loans, a bond issue is generally registered with the SEC, advertised, offered to the public through investment bankers, and sold to many different investors. Thousands of individual and institutional investors may participate when a firm such as Columbia/HCA Healthcare sells a bond issue, while there is generally only one lender in the case of a term loan. Occasionally, however, a bond issue can be sold to one lender or to just a few. In this situation, the bond is said to be *privately placed*. (Private placements are discussed in more depth in a later section.)

Although bonds are generally issued with maturities in the range of 20 to 30 years, shorter maturities, such as seven to ten years, are occasionally used, as are longer maturities. In 1995, Columbia/HCA Healthcare issued $200 million of noncallable 100-year bonds following the issuance of 100-year bonds by Disney and Coca-Cola in 1993. These ultra long-term bonds had not been used by any company since the 1920s.

Unlike term loans, a bond's interest rate is generally fixed, although in recent years there has been an increase in the use of various types of floating rate bonds. Also unlike term loans, bonds typically pay only interest over the life of the bond; the entire amount of principal is returned to lenders at maturity. The most common types of bonds are mortgage bonds, debentures, subordinated debentures, and municipal bonds, which are discussed in the following sections.

Mortgage Bonds

With a *mortgage bond*, the issuer pledges certain real property as security for the bond. To illustrate, Mid-Texas Healthcare System recently needed $30 million to purchase land and to build a new hospital. *First mortgage bonds* in the amount of $15 million, secured by a mortgage on the property, were issued. If Mid-Texas *defaults* on the bonds (i.e., fails to make a promised interest or principal payment), the bondholders could foreclose on the hospital and sell it to satisfy their claims.

If it so chooses, Mid-Texas could also issue *second mortgage bonds,* secured by the same $30 million hospital. In the event of bankruptcy and liquidation, the holders of these second mortgage bonds would have a claim against the property only after the first mortgage bondholders had been paid off in full. Thus, second mortgages are sometimes called *junior mortgages*, or *junior liens*, because they are junior in priority to claims of senior (i.e., first) mortgage bonds.

Debentures

A *debenture* is an unsecured bond. As such, it has no lien against specific property as security for the obligation. For example, in addition to its mortgage bonds, Mid-Texas Healthcare System has $5 million of debentures outstanding. These bonds are not secured by real property, but are backed instead by the revenue-producing power of the corporation. Therefore, debenture holders are general creditors whose claims are protected by property not otherwise pledged.

In practice, the use of debentures depends on the nature of the firm's assets and its general credit strength. If a firm's credit position is exceptionally strong, it can issue debentures; it does not need specific collateral. Companies with only a small amount of assets suitable as collateral also issue debentures. Finally, companies that have used up their capacity to borrow in the lower-cost mortgage market may be forced to use higher-cost debentures.

Subordinated Debentures

The term *subordinate* means below or inferior. Thus, *subordinated debt* has a claim on assets in the event of bankruptcy only after senior debt has been paid off. Debentures may be subordinated either to designated notes payable—usually bank loans—or to all other debt. In the event of liquidation, holders of subordinated debentures cannot be paid until all senior debt obligations named in the bond agreement have been paid. The subordinated debentures of a company that has used up its ability to employ other bonds (mortgage bonds and unsubordinated debentures) are normally quite risky, and such debentures carry interest rates that are much higher than the rate on top quality debt.

Municipal, or *muni, bonds* are long-term debt obligations issued by states and their political subdivisions such as counties, cities, port authorities, toll road or bridge authorities, and so on. Short-term municipal securities are used primarily to meet temporary cash needs, while municipal bonds are usually used to finance capital projects.

Municipal Bonds

There are several types of municipal bonds. For example, *general obligation bonds* are secured by the full faith and credit of the issuing municipality (i.e., they are backed by the full taxing authority of the issuer). Conversely, *special tax bonds* are secured by a specified tax such as a tax on utility services. *Revenue bonds* are bonds that are not backed by taxing power, but rather by the revenues derived from such projects as roads or bridges, airports, and water and sewage systems. Revenue bonds are of particular interest to not-for-profit healthcare providers because they are legally entitled to issue such securities through government-sponsored healthcare financing authorities.

Not-for-profit healthcare firms issue large amounts of municipal debt. To illustrate, healthcare providers issued over $30 billion of municipal bonds in 1998. Recently, about 20 percent of the dollar volume of healthcare muni debt has had floating rates, while the remaining 80 percent has had fixed rates. Floating rate bonds are riskier to the issuer because interest rates could rise in the future. However, virtually all such municipal debt has call provisions that permit issuers to replace the floating rate debt with fixed rate debt if interest rates rise substantially.

Most municipal bonds are sold in *serial* form, that is, a portion of the issue comes due periodically, anywhere from six months after issue to 30 years or more. Thus, a single issue actually consists of a series of sub-issues of different maturities. In effect, the bond issue is amortized, with a portion of the issue being retired every year. The purpose of structuring a bond issue in this way is to match the overall maturity of the issue to the maturity of the assets being financed. For example, a new hospital wing having a predicted useful life of about 30 years may be financed with a 30-year serial issue. Over time, some of the revenues associated with the new wing will be used to meet the *debt service requirements* (i.e., the interest and principal payments). At the end of 30 years, the entire issue will be paid off, and the issuer can plan for a replacement facility or major renovation that would be funded, at least in part, by another debt issue.

Whereas the vast majority of federal government and corporate bonds are held by institutions, close to half of all municipal bonds outstanding are held by individual investors. The primary attraction of most municipal bonds is their exemption from federal and state (in the state of issue) taxes. To illustrate, the interest rate on an AAA-rated, long-term corporate bond recently was 7.1 percent, while the rate on a similar risk healthcare muni was 5.5 percent. To an individual investor in the 40 percent federal-plus-state tax bracket, the corporate bond's after-tax yield was $7.1\% \times (1 - 0.40) = 7.1\% \times 0.6 = 4.3\%$, while the muni's after-tax yield was the same as its before-tax yield, 5.5 percent. This yield differential on otherwise similar securities illustrates why investors in high tax brackets are so enthusiastic about municipal bonds.

Private Versus Public Placement

Most bonds, including Treasury, corporate, and municipal, are sold through investment bankers to the public at large. For example, the New York State Medical Care Facilities Financing Agency recently sold a $675 million municipal mortgage revenue issue for New York Hospital. The issue was marketed to the public at large, including institutional investors, by Goldman Sachs & Co., one of the top underwriters of tax-exempt healthcare issues. However, smaller bond issues, typically $10 million or less, often are sold directly to a single buyer or a small group of buyers. Issues placed directly with lenders, or *private placements*, have the same advantages as term loans, which were discussed in a previous section.

Although the interest rate on private placements is generally higher than the interest rate set on public issues, the up-front costs of placing an issue, such as legal, accounting, printing, and selling fees, are less for private placements than for public issues. Moreover, because there is direct negotiation between the borrower and lender, the opportunity is greater to structure bond terms that are more favorable to the borrower than the terms routinely contained in public debt issues.

To illustrate a private placement, Pacific Shores Hospital recently sold $5 million of ten-year municipal bonds to a regional bank at an interest rate of 6.4 percent. When the up-front costs were added in, the *all-in cost* rate of the issue was 6.5 percent. The interest rate on a public issue would have been only 6 percent, but the addition of selling fees, bond insurance, and other up-front costs would raise the all-in cost rate of the public issue to 6.75 percent. Thus, the bank received an interest rate that was 40 *basis points* above the rate it would have earned if it had bought the bonds in a public sale, and the hospital saved 25 basis points on the issue when all costs are considered. (A basis point is $1/100^{th}$ of a percentage point. Thus, 40 basis points equal 0.40 percentage points.) The reason why private placements can be structured so that both borrower and lender win is that the savings in issuance costs can be allocated to the benefit of both parties.

Self-Test Questions

1. Describe the primary features of the following long-term debt securities:
   a. Term loan
   b. Bond
   c. First mortgage bond
   d. Junior mortgage
   e. Debenture
   f. Subordinated debenture
   g. Municipal bond
2. What are the key differences between a private placement and a public issue?

Debt Contract Provisions

Health services managers are most concerned about the overall cost of debt, including issuance costs, and any provisions which may restrict the organization's future actions. In this section, some contract features that could affect either the business' future flexibility or its cost of the debt issue are discussed.

Bond Indentures

An *indenture*, which is a legal document that may be several hundred pages in length, spells out the rights of both bondholders and the issuing businesses. (For term loans, a similar but much shorter document called a *loan agreement* is used.) The indenture includes a set of *restrictive covenants*, which is designed to protect bondholders from managerial actions that would be detrimental to the bond's value. Examples of such covenants include the financial condition that the company must maintain to issue additional debt and, for investor-owned businesses, restrictions against the payment of dividends unless earnings meet specified levels. If an issuer violates any of the restrictive covenants, as opposed to missing a required debt payment, the issue is said to be in *technical default.*

The *trustee* is an official or institution—usually a bank—that represents the bondholders and ensures that the terms of the indenture are being carried out. The trustee is responsible for trying to keep the covenants from being violated and for taking appropriate action if a violation does occur. What constitutes appropriate action varies with the circumstances. Insisting on immediate compliance may result in bankruptcy and possibly large losses on the bonds. In such a case, the trustee may decide that the bondholders would be better served by giving the business a chance to work out its problems, and thus avoid forcing it into bankruptcy.

Call Provisions

A *call provision* gives the issuer the right to call a bond for *redemption* prior to maturity. That is, the issuer can pay off the bondholders in entirety and *redeem,* or *retire,* the issue. If it is used, the call provision generally states that the company must pay an amount greater than the initial amount borrowed. The additional sum required is defined as the *call premium.*

Many callable bonds offer a period of call protection, which protects investors from a call just a short time after the bonds are issued. For example, the 20-year callable bonds issued by Vanguard Healthcare in 1997 are not callable until 2007, which is ten years after the original issue date. This type of call provision is known as a *deferred call.*

The call privilege is valuable to the issuer but potentially detrimental to bondholders, especially if the bond is issued in a period when interest rates are cyclically high. In general, bonds are called when interest rates have fallen because the issuer usually replaces the old high-interest issue with a new lower-interest issue, and hence reduces annual interest expense. When this occurs, investors are forced to reinvest the principal returned in new securities at the then current (lower) rate. As readers will see later, the added risk to investors of a call provision causes the interest rate on a new issue of callable bonds to exceed that on a similar new issue of noncallable bonds.

Sinking Funds

A *sinking fund* is a provision that provides for the systematic retirement of a bond issue. Typically, sinking fund provisions require the issuer to retire (i.e., redeem) a portion of the issue in each year. (A serial issue of municipal bonds can be thought of as a type of sinking fund.)

On some occasions, the issuer of bonds with a sinking fund may be required to deposit money with a trustee who invests the funds and then uses the accumulated sum to retire the entire bond issue when it matures. Sometimes, the stipulated sinking fund payment is tied to the level of revenues or earnings in each year, but usually it is a mandatory fixed amount. If it is mandatory, a failure to meet the sinking fund requirement causes the bond issue to be thrown into default, which could force the issuer into bankruptcy.

Although a sinking fund is designed to protect the bondholders by assuring that the issue is retired in an orderly fashion, it must be recognized that, like a call provision, a sinking fund may at times work to the detriment of bondholders. However, securities that provide for a sinking fund are regarded as being safer than bonds without sinking funds, which tend to balance the risk of a sinking fund call. Thus, sinking fund provisions tend to have little effect on an issue's interest rate.

Self-Test Questions

1. Describe the following bond features:
   a. Bond indenture
   b. Restrictive covenant
   c. Call provision
   d. Sinking fund
2. What impact does a call provision have on an issue's interest rate?
3. How do sinking fund provisions differ from call provisions?

Bond Ratings

Since the early 1900s, bonds have been assigned quality ratings that reflect their probability of going into default. The two major rating agencies are Moody's Investors Service (Moody's) and Standard & Poor's Corporation (S&P), which rate both corporate and municipal bonds. These agencies' rating designations are shown in Table 11.1. In the discussion to follow, reference to the S&P code is intended to imply the Moody's code as well. For example, triple B signifies both BBB and Baa bonds, double B signifies both BB and Ba bonds, and so on.

Bonds with a BBB and higher rating are called *investment grade*, which are the lowest rated bonds that many institutional investors are permitted by law to hold. Double B and lower bonds, called *junk bonds*, are more speculative in nature because they have a much higher probability of going into default than do higher rated bonds.

TABLE 11.1
Bond Ratings

Credit Risk	Moody's	Standard & Poor's
Prime	Aaa	AAA
Excellent	Aa	AA
Upper medium	A	A
Lower medium	Baa	BBB
Speculative	Ba	BB
Very speculative	B	B
	Caa	CCC
		CC
Default	Ca	D
	C	

Note: Both Moody's and S&P use "modifiers" for bonds ratings below triple A. S&P uses a plus and minus system. Thus, A+ designates the strongest A-rated bond and A– the weakest. Moody's uses a 1, 2, or 3 designation, with 1 denoting the strongest and 3 the weakest; thus, within the double-A category, Aa1 is the best, Aa2 is average, and Aa3 is the weakest. Triple-A bonds have no modifiers in either system.

Bond Rating Criteria

Although the rating assignments are subjective, they are based on both qualitative characteristics, such as quality of management, and quantitative factors, such as a firm's financial strength. Analysts at the rating agencies have consistently stated that no precise formula is used to set a firm's rating—many factors are taken into account, but not in a mathematically precise manner. Statistical studies have supported this contention. Researchers who have tried to predict bond ratings on the basis of quantitative data have had only limited success, which indicates that the agencies do indeed use a good deal of subjective judgment to establish a firm's rating.

Importance of Bond Ratings

Bond ratings are important both to businesses and to investors. First, a bond's rating is an indicator of its default risk, so the rating has a direct, measurable influence on the interest rate required by investors, and hence on the firm's cost of debt capital. Second, most corporate (i.e., taxable) bonds are purchased by institutional investors rather than by individuals. Many of these institutions are restricted to investment-grade securities. Also, most individual investors who buy municipal bonds are unwilling to take high risks in their bond purchases. Thus, if an issuer's bonds fall below BBB, it will have a harder time trying to sell new bonds because the number of potential purchasers is reduced. As a result of their higher risk and more restricted market, low-grade bonds typically carry much higher interest rates than do high-grade bonds.

Changes in Ratings

A change in a firm's bond rating will have a significant effect on its ability to borrow long-term capital and on the cost of that capital. Rating agencies review outstanding bonds on a periodic basis; occasionally, they upgrade or downgrade a bond as a result of the issuer's changed circumstances. Also, an announcement that a company plans to sell a new debt issue or to merge with another company and pay for the acquisition by exchanging bonds for the stock of the acquired company will trigger an agency review and possibly lead to a rating change. If a firm's situation has deteriorated somewhat, but its bonds have not been reviewed and downgraded, it may choose to use a term loan or short-term debt rather than to finance through a public bond issue. This will perhaps postpone a rating agency review until the situation has improved.

To illustrate a ratings change, on November 7, 1997, Fitch Investor Services, another large rating agency, lowered its rating on Columbia/HCA Healthcare's $4.2 billion of senior debt from A to BBB+. In the announcement, Fitch stated that the downgrade reflected its concern over the possible negative impact that the then current federal government investigation regarding Medicare fraud could have on operating results.

Self-Test Questions

1. What are the two major rating agencies?
2. What are some criteria that the rating agencies use when assigning ratings?
3. What impact do bond ratings have on the cost of debt to the issuing firm?

Credit Enhancement

Credit enhancement, or *bond insurance*, which is available only for municipal bonds, is a relatively recent development for upgrading a bond's rating to AAA. Credit enhancement is offered by several credit insurers; the three largest are the Municipal Bond Investors Assurance (MBIA) Corporation, AMBAC Indemnity Corporation, and Financial Guaranty Insurance Corporation, a subsidiary of General Electric Capital Corporation. Currently, almost 60 percent of all new healthcare municipal issues carry bond insurance.

Here is how credit enhancement works. Regardless of the inherent credit rating of the issuer, the bond insurer guarantees that bondholders will receive the promised interest and principal payments. Thus, bond insurance protects investors against default by the issuer. Because the insurer gives its guarantee that payments will be made, the bond carries the credit rating of the insurance company rather than that of the issuer. For example, Sabal Palms Medical Center has an A rating, so new bonds issued by the hospital without credit enhancement would be rated A. However, in 1998, Sabal Palms Medical Center issued $50 million of hospital revenue bonds with an AAA rating because of MBIA insurance.

Credit enhancement gives the issuer access to the lowest possible interest rate, but not without a cost. Bond insurers typically charge an up-front fee of about 45 to 75 basis points of the total debt service over the life of the bond. The lower the hospital's inherent credit rating, the higher the cost of bond insurance. Most of the newly issued insured municipal bonds have an underlying credit rating of AA or A. The remainder are still of investment grade, rated BBB.

Thus far, municipal bond issuers have defaulted on very few insured issues. For example, in its 20-year existence, MBIA has had to cover only two defaults: a $30 million hospital issue and a $12 million housing issue. However, many insurance analysts question the ability of the bond insurers to cover default payments should a severe recession occur. Furthermore, the market as a whole has some reservations about bond insurance because interest rates on AAA insured issues tend to be slightly higher than rates on otherwise similar bonds that carry an uninsured AAA rating.

1. What does the term "credit enhancement" mean?
2. Why would healthcare issuers seek bond insurance?

Self-Test Questions

Interest Rate Components

The rate of return (i.e., the interest rate) required by investors on a debt security consists of several components. By understanding the components, it is possible to gain insights on why interest rates change over time, differ among borrowers, and even differ on separate issues by the same borrower.

Real Risk-Free Rate (RRF)

The base on which all interest rates are built is the *real risk-free rate (RRF)*. This is the rate that investors would demand on a debt security that is totally **riskless** when there is **no inflation**. Although difficult to measure, the RRF is thought to fall somewhere in the range of 2 to 4 percent. In the real world, inflation is rarely zero and most debt securities have some risk; thus, the actual interest rate on a given debt security will be typically higher than the real risk-free rate.

Inflation Premium (IP)

Inflation has a major impact on interest rates because it erodes the purchasing power of the dollar, and hence lowers the value of investment returns. Creditors, who are the suppliers of debt capital, are well aware of the impact of inflation. Thus, they build an *inflation premium (IP)* into the interest rate that is equal to the expected inflation rate over the life of the security.

For example, suppose that the real risk-free rate was RRF = 3% and that inflation was expected to be 4 percent (and hence IP = 4%) during the next year. The rate of interest on a one-year riskless debt security would be 3% + 4% = 7%. The combination of the RRF and IP is called the *risk-free rate (RF)*. Thus, the risk-free rate incorporates inflation expectations, but it does not incorporate any risk factors. In this example, RF = 7%.

The rate of inflation built into interest rates is the rate of inflation **expected in the future** not the rate experienced in the past. Thus, the latest reported figures may show an annual inflation rate of 3 percent, but that is for a past period. If investors expect a 6 percent inflation rate in the future, then 6 percent would be built into the current rate of interest. Also, the inflation rate reflected in any interest rate is the average rate of inflation expected **over the life of the security**. Thus, the inflation rate built into a one-year bond is the expected inflation rate for the next year, but the inflation rate built into a 30-year bond is the average rate of inflation expected over the next 30 years.

Default Risk Premium (DRP)

The risk that a borrower will default (not make the payments promised) has a significant impact on the interest rate set on a debt security. This risk along with the possible consequences of default are captured by a *default risk premium (DRP)*. Treasury securities have no default risk; thus, they carry the lowest interest rates on taxable securities in the United States.[2] For corporate and municipal bonds, the higher the bond's rating, the lower its default risk. All else the same, the lower the default risk, the lower the DRP and interest rate.

In addition to the probability of default, the DRP incorporates a second risk factor called *recovery risk*. To illustrate recovery risk, consider an issuer that has both mortgage bonds and subordinated debentures outstanding, each carrying the same default rating. Yet, if default occurred, the mortgage bondholders would have a better chance of recovering the full amount due to them than would the debenture holders. Thus, the DRP would be higher on the debenture than on the mortgage bond, even though both bonds had the same default rating.

Liquidity Premium (LP)

A *liquid* asset is one that can be sold quickly at a predictable fair market price, and thus can be converted to a known amount of cash on short notice. Active markets, which provide liquidity, exist for Treasury securities and for the stocks and bonds of larger corporations. Securities issued by small companies, including healthcare providers that issue municipal bonds, are *illiquid;* they can be sold to raise cash, but not quickly and not at a predictable price. Furthermore, illiquid assets are normally difficult to sell, and hence have relatively high *transactions costs*. (Transactions costs include commissions, fees, spreads between asking and selling prices, and other expenses associated with selling an asset.)

If a security is illiquid, investors will add a *liquidity premium (LP)* when they set their required interest rate. It is very difficult to measure liquidity premiums with precision, but a differential of at least two percentage points is thought to exist between the least liquid and the most liquid financial assets of similar default risk and maturity.

Price Risk Premium (PRP)

As will be demonstrated later in the bond valuation section, the market value (price) of a long-term bond declines sharply when interest rates rise. Because interest rates can and do rise, all long-term bonds including Treasury bonds have an element of risk called *price risk*. For example, if a person bought a 30-year Treasury bond in 1972 for $1,000 when the long-term interest rate on Treasury securities was 7 percent and held it until 1981 when T-bond rates were about 14.5 percent, the value of the bond would have declined to about $514. That would represent a loss of almost half the investment, which demonstrates that long-term bonds—even U.S. Treasury bonds—are not riskless.

As a general rule, the bonds of any organization, from the U.S. government to Columbia/HCA Healthcare to St. Vincent's Community Hospital, have more price risk the longer the maturity of the bond. Therefore, a *price risk premium (PRP)*, which is higher the longer the years to maturity, must be included in the interest rate. The effect of price risk premiums is to raise interest rates on long-term bonds relative to those on short-term bonds. This premium, like the others, is extremely difficult to measure, but it seems to vary over time; it rises when interest rates are more volatile and uncertain, and falls when they are more stable. In recent years, the price risk premium on 30-year T-bonds appears to have been generally in the range of one-half to two percentage points.

Call Risk Premium (CRP)

Bonds that are callable are riskier for investors than those that are noncallable because callable bonds have uncertain maturities. To compensate for bearing call risk, investors charge a *call risk premium (CRP)* on callable bonds. The amount of the premium depends on such factors as the interest rate on the bond, current interest rate levels, and time to first call. Historically, call risk premiums have been in the range of 30 to 50 basis points.

Combining the Components

When all the interest rate components listed above are taken into account, the interest rate on any debt security is expressed as follows:

$$\text{Interest rate} = \text{RRF} + \text{IP} + \text{DRP} + \text{LP} + \text{PRP} + \text{CRP}.$$

To illustrate, assume that RRF is 2 percent, and inflation is expected to average 3 percent in the coming year. Because T-bills have no default, liquidity or call risk, and almost no price risk, the interest rate on a 1-year T-bill would be 5 percent:

$$\text{Interest rate}_{\text{T-bill}} = \text{RRF} + \text{IP} + \text{DRP} + \text{LP} + \text{PRP} + \text{CRP}$$
$$= 2\% + 3\% + 0 + 0 + 0 + 0 = 5\%.$$

As discussed previously, the combination of RRF and IP is the risk-fee rate, so RF = 5%. In general, the rate of interest on short-term Treasury securities (T-bills) is used as a proxy for the **short-term** risk-free rate.

Consider another illustration: the callable 30-year bonds issued by Columbia/HCA. Assume that these bonds have an inflation premium of 4 percent; default risk, liquidity, and price risk premiums of 1 percent each; and a call risk premium of 40 basis points. Under these assumptions, the Columbia/HCA bonds would have an interest rate of 9.4 percent:

$$\text{Interest rate}_{\text{30-yearbonds}} = \text{RRF} + \text{IP} + \text{DRP} + \text{LP} + \text{PRP} + \text{CRP}$$
$$= 2\% + 4\% + 1\% + 1\% + 1\% + 0.4\% = 9.4\%.$$

When interest rates are viewed as the sum of a base rate plus premiums for inflation and risk, it is easy to visualize the underlying economic forces that cause interest rates to vary among different issues and over time.

Self-Test Questions

1. Write out an equation for the required interest rate on a debt security.
2. What is the difference between the real risk-free rate, RRF, and the risk-free rate, RF?
3. Do the interest rates on Treasury securities include a default risk premium? A liquidity premium? A price risk premium? Explain your answer.
4. Does the default risk premium incorporate only the probability of default? Explain your answer.
5. What is price risk? What type of debt securities would have the largest price risk premium?

The Term Structure of Interest Rates

At certain times, such as in 1998, short-term interest rates are lower than long-term rates. At other times, such as in 1980, short-term rates are higher than long-term rates. The relationship between long- and short-term rates, which is called the *term structure of interest rates*, is important to health services managers who must decide whether to borrow by issuing long- or short-term debt, and to investors who must decide whether to buy long- or short-term bonds. Thus, it is important to understand how interest rates on long- and short-term bonds are related to one another and what causes shifts in their relative positions.

To examine the current term structure, look up the interest rates on bonds of various maturities by a single issuer (usually the U.S. Treasury) in a source such as the *Wall Street Journal* or the *Federal Reserve Bulletin*. For example, the tabular section of Figure 11.1 presents interest rates for Treasury securities of different maturities on two dates. The set of data for a given date when plotted on a graph is called a *yield curve*. As shown in the figure, the yield curve changes both in position and in shape over time. Had the yield curve been drawn during January of 1982, it would have been essentially horizontal because long-term and short-term bonds at that time had about the same rate of interest.

Figure 11.1 shows yield curves for U.S. Treasury securities, but the curves could have been constructed for similarly rated corporate or municipal (i.e., tax-exempt) bonds if the data were available. In each case, the yield curve would be approximately the same shape, but would differ in vertical position. For example, had the yield curve been constructed for Beverly Enterprises, a for-profit nursing home operator, it would fall above the Treasury curve because interest rates on corporate bonds include default risk premiums, while Treasury rates do not. Conversely, the curve for Baptist Medical Center, a not-for-profit hospital, would probably fall below the Treasury curve because the tax-exemption benefit, which lowers the interest rate on tax-exempt securities, generally outweighs the default

FIGURE 11.1

U.S. Treasury Bond
Interest Rates on
Two Dates

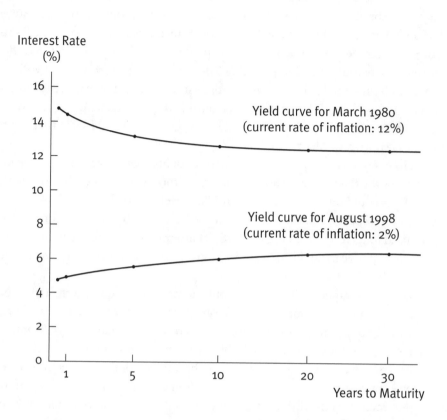

Term to Maturity	Interest Rate	
	March 1980	*August 1998*
6 months	15.0%	5.2%
1 year	14.0	5.3
5 years	13.5	5.4
10 years	12.8	5.5
20 years	12.5	5.6
30 years	12.4	5.7

risk premium. In every case, however, the riskier the issuer (i.e., the lower the bonds are rated), the higher the yield curve plots on the graph.

Historically, long-term rates have generally been above short-term rates, so usually the yield curve has been upward sloping. An *upward-sloping curve* would be expected if the inflation premium is relatively constant across all maturities because the price risk premium applied to long-term issues will push long-term rates above short-term rates. Because an upward-sloping yield curve is most prevalent, this shape is also called a *normal yield curve*. Conversely, a yield curve that slopes downward is called an *inverted*, or *abnormal, yield curve*. Thus, in Figure 11.1, the yield curve for March 1980 is inverted, but the one for August 1998 is normal.[3]

Health services managers use yield curve information to help make decisions regarding debt maturities. To illustrate, assume for the moment that it is August 1998 and that the yield curve for that month in Figure 11.1 applies to Baptist Medical Center. Now, assume that the hospital plans to issue $10 million of debt to finance a new outpatient clinic with a 20-year life. If it borrowed in 1998 on a short-term basis—say for one year—Baptist's interest cost for that year would be 5.3 percent, or $530,000. If it used long-term (30-year) financing, its cost would be 5.7 percent, or $570,000. Therefore, at first glance, it would seem that Baptist should use short-term debt.

However, if the hospital uses short-term debt, it will have to renew the loan every year at the then current short-term rate. Although unlikely, it is possible that interest rates could return to their March 1980 levels. If this happened, by 2000 or so the hospital could be paying 14 percent, or $1,400,000, per year. Conversely, if Baptist used long-term financing in 1998, its interest costs would remain constant at $570,000 per year, so an increase in interest rates in the economy would not hurt the hospital.

Does this suggest that firms should always avoid short-term debt? Not necessarily. If Baptist had borrowed on a long-term basis for 5.7 percent in August 1998, it would be at a major disadvantage if interest rates remained low. Its interest expense would be locked in at $570,000 a year, while any competitors that used short-term debt that cost 5.3 percent would be able to continually renew the debt at the lower rate or even less. Conversely, inflation expectations could push interest rates up to record levels. If that situation occurred, all borrowers would wish that they had borrowed on a long-term basis in 1998.

Financing decisions would be easy if managers could develop accurate forecasts of future interest rates. Unfortunately, predicting future interest rates with consistent accuracy is somewhere between difficult and impossible—people who make a living by selling interest rate forecasts say it is difficult, but many others say it is impossible. Sound financial policy, therefore, calls for using a mix of long- and short-term debt, as well as equity, in such a manner that the business can survive in all but the most severe, and hence unlikely, interest rate environments. Furthermore, the optimal financing policy depends in an important way on the maturities of the firm's assets; in general, to reduce risk, managers try to match the maturities of the financing with the maturities of the assets being financed. This issue will be addressed again in Chapter 16 when current asset financing policies are discussed.

Self-Test Questions

1. What is a yield curve and what information is needed to create this curve?
2. What is the difference between a normal yield curve and an abnormal one?
3. If short-term rates are lower than long-term rates, why may a business still choose to finance with long-term debt?
4. Explain the following statement: "A firm's financing policy depends in large part on the nature of its assets."

Debt Valuation

Now that the basics of long-term debt financing have been discussed, the next step is to understand how investors value debt securities. Security valuation concepts are important to health services managers for many reasons. Here are just a few:

- The lifeblood of any business is capital. In fact, one of the most common reasons for business failures is insufficient capital. Therefore, it is vital that health services managers understand how investors make investment allocation decisions.
- For investor-owned firms, stock price maximization is the primary goal, so health services managers of for-profit firms must know how investors value the firm's securities to understand how managerial actions affect stock price.
- For health services managers to make financially sound investment decisions regarding real assets (e.g., plant and equipment), it is necessary to estimate the business' cost of capital. Security valuation is a necessary skill in this process, which is covered in detail in Chapter 13.
- Real assets are valued in the same general way as securities. Thus, security valuation provides managers with an excellent foundation to learn real asset valuation, the heart of capital investment decision making within health services organizations. The concepts presented here are crucial to a good understanding of Chapters 14 and 15.

General Valuation Model

In the financial sense, the value of any asset stems from the same source: the cash flows that the asset is expected to produce. Thus, all assets are valued financially in the same way:

- *Estimate the expected cash flow stream.* Estimating the cash flow stream involves estimating the expected cash flow in each period during the productive life of the asset. For some assets, such as Treasury securities, the estimation process is quite easy; the interest and principal repayment stream is specified by contract. For other assets, such as the stock of a biotechnology start-up company that is not yet paying dividends, the estimation process can be very difficult.
- *Assess the riskiness of the stream.* The next step is to estimate the riskiness of the cash flows. The cash flows of most assets are not known with certainty, but rather are best represented by probability distributions. The more uncertain these distributions, the greater the riskiness of the cash flow stream. Again, in some situations it will be fairly easy to assess the riskiness of the estimated cash flow stream; in other situations it may be quite difficult.
- *Set the required rate of return.* The required rate of return on the cash flow stream is established on the basis of the stream's riskiness and the returns available on alternative investments of similar risk. In essence, the *opportunity cost* principle discussed in Chapter 9 is applied here. By investing in one asset,

the funds are no longer available to invest in alternative assets of similar risk. This opportunity cost sets the required rate of return on the asset being valued.
* *Discount and sum the expected cash flows.* Each expected cash flow is now discounted at the asset's required rate of return. Then, the final step is to sum the present values of the cash flows to find the value of the asset.

The following time line formalizes the valuation process:

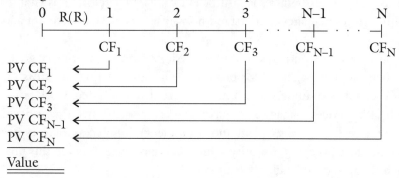

Here, CF_t is the expected cash flow in each Period t, $R(R)$ is the required rate of return (i.e., the opportunity cost rate) on the asset, and N is the number of periods for which cash flows are expected. The periods can be months, quarters, semiannual periods, or years, depending on the frequency of the cash flows expected from the asset.

The general valuation model can be applied to both *financial assets* (i.e., *securities*), such as stocks and bonds, and *real* (i.e., *physical*) *assets,* such as buildings, equipment, and even whole businesses. Each asset type requires a somewhat different application of the general valuation model, but the basic approach remains the same. In this chapter, the general valuation model is applied to a specific type of security: bonds. In the chapters that follow, the model is applied to other types of securities and to real assets.

Definitions

To begin the discussion of bond (debt) valuation, it is necessary to present some basic bond concepts:

* *Par value.* The par value, also called *par*, is the stated face value of the bond. It is often set at $1,000 or $5,000. The par value generally represents the amount of money the firm borrows (per bond) and promises to repay at some future date.
* *Maturity date.* Bonds generally have a specified maturity date on which the par value will be repaid. For example, Big Sky Healthcare, a for-profit hospital system, issued $50 million worth of $1,000 par value bonds on January 1, 1998. The bonds will mature on December 31, 2012, so they had a 15-year

maturity at the time they were issued. The effective maturity of a bond declines each year after it was issued. Thus, at the beginning of 1999, Big Sky's bonds will have a 14-year maturity and so on.

- *Coupon rate.* A bond requires the issuer to pay a specific amount of interest each year or, more typically, each six months. The rate of interest is called the *coupon interest rate*, or just *coupon rate*. The rate may be variable, in which case it is tied to some index, such as two percentage points above the prime rate. More commonly, the rate will be fixed over the life (maturity) of the bond. For example, Big Sky's bonds have a 10 percent coupon rate, so each $1,000 par value bond pays $0.10 \times \$1,000 = \$100$ in interest each year. The dollar amount of annual interest, in this case $100, is called the *coupon payment.* The term *coupon* goes back to the time when all bonds were *bearer bonds.* Such bonds had small coupons attached, one for each interest payment. To collect an interest payment, bondholders would remove (i.e., "clip") a coupon and send it to the issuer, or take it to a bank, where it would be exchanged for the dollar payment. Today, all bonds are *registered bonds*; the issuer (through an *agent*) automatically sends interest payments to the registered owner.

- *New issues versus outstanding bonds.* As readers will discover, a bond's value is determined by its coupon payment—the higher the coupon payment, with other things held constant, the higher its value. At the time a bond is issued, its coupon rate is generally set at a level that will cause the bond to sell at its par value. In other words, the coupon rate is set at the rate that investors require to buy the bond (i.e., the *going rate*). A bond that has just been issued is called a *new issue.* After the bond has been on the market for a while, about a month, it is classified as an *outstanding bond*, or a *seasoned issue.* New issues sell close to par, but because a bond's coupon payment is generally fixed, changing economic conditions (and hence interest rates) will cause a seasoned bond to sell for more or less than its par value.

- *Debt service requirements.* Firms that issue bonds are concerned with their total debt service requirements, which include both interest expense and repayment of principal. For Big Sky, the debt service requirement (payment) is $0.10 \times \$50$ million $= \$5$ million per year until maturity. In 2012, the firm's debt service payment will be $5 million in interest plus $50 million in principal repayment, for a total of $55 million. In Big Sky's case, only interest is paid until maturity, so the entire principal amount must be repaid at that time. As discussed earlier, many municipal bonds are serial issues structured so that the debt service requirements are relatively constant over time. In this situation, the issuer pays back a portion of the principal during each year.

The Basic Bond Valuation Model

Bonds call for the payment of a specific amount of interest for a specific number of years and for the repayment of par on the bond's maturity date. Thus, a bond represents an annuity plus a lump sum, and its value is found as the present value of this cash flow stream:

$$
\begin{array}{ccccccc}
0 & 1 & 2 & 3 & & & N \\
\vdash & + & + & + & \cdots & & \dashv \\
& \text{INT} & \text{INT} & \text{INT} & & & \text{INT} + \text{M}
\end{array}
$$

$$
\text{Value} = \frac{\text{INT}}{[1 + \text{R(R)}]^1} + \frac{\text{INT}}{[1 + \text{R(R)}]^2} + \cdots + \frac{\text{INT} + \text{M}}{[1 + \text{R(R)}]^N}.
$$

Here

INT = dollars of interest paid each year = Coupon rate × Par value.
M   = par, or maturity, value.
R(R) = required rate of return on the bond, which, in general, depends on the returns available on alternative investments of similar risk. For bonds, these returns depend on the real risk-free rate, inflation expectations, and the riskiness of the security.
N   = number of years until maturity. N declines each year after the bond is issued.

Here are the cash flows from Big Sky's bonds on a time line:

$$
\begin{array}{ccccccc}
0 & 1 & 2 & & 13 & 14 & 15 \\
\vdash & + & + & \cdots & + & + & \dashv \\
& \$100 & \$100 & & \$100 & \$100 & \$\ \ 100 \\
& & & & & & 1{,}000
\end{array}
$$

If the bonds had just been issued and the coupon rate was set at the current interest rate for bonds of this risk, then R(R) = 10%. Because the value of the bond is merely the present value of the bond's cash flows, discounted to Time 0 at a 10 percent discount rate, the value of the bond at issue was $1,000:

Present value of a 15-year, $100 payment annuity at 10 percent = $ 760.61

Present value of a $1,000 lump sum discounted 15 years =   239.39

Value of bond = $1,000.00

The value of the bond can be found using most financial calculators as follows:

Inputs   15   10   −100   −1000

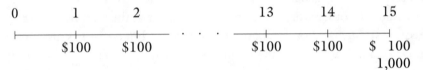

       N   I   PV   PMT   FV

Output   = 1,000

Input N = 15, I = 10, PMT = −100, and FV = −1000, and then press the PV key to get the answer, 1,000. (The cash flows were treated as outflows so that the value would be displayed as a positive number.) Also, in bond valuation, all five time-value-of-money keys on a financial calculator are used because bonds involve both an annuity and a lump sum.

If R(R) remained constant at 10 percent over time, what would be the value of the bond one year after it was issued? Now, the term to maturity is only 14 years, that is, N = 14. As seen below, the bond's value remains at $1,000:

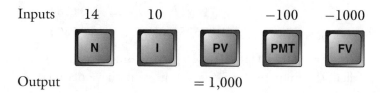

Suppose that interest rates in the economy fell after the Big Sky bonds were issued, and as a result, R(R) decreased from 10 percent to 5 percent. The coupon rate and par value are fixed by contract so they remain unaffected by changes in interest rates, but now the discount rate is 5 percent rather than 10 percent. At the end of the first year, with 14 years remaining, the value of the bond would be $1,494.93:

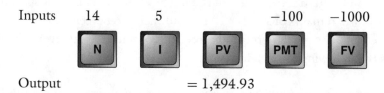

The arithmetic of the bond value increase should be clear (lower discount rates lead to higher present values), but what is the logic behind it? The fact that R(R) has fallen to 5 percent means that if a person had $1,000 to invest, that person could buy new bonds like Big Sky's (every day some 10 to 20 companies sell new bonds), except that these new bonds would only pay $50 in interest each year. Naturally, he or she would favor $100 to $50 and would be willing to pay more than $1,000 for Big Sky's bonds. All investors would recognize this; as a result, the Big Sky bonds would be bid up in price to $1,494.93, at which point they would provide the same rate of return as new bonds of similar risk, 5 percent.

Assuming that interest rates stay constant at 5 percent over the next 14 years, what would happen to the value of a Big Sky bond? It would fall gradually from $1,494.93 at present to $1,000 at maturity when the company will redeem each bond for $1,000. This point can be illustrated by calculating the value of the bond one year later when it has only 13 years remaining to maturity:

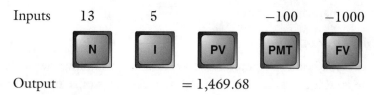

The value of the bond with 13 years to maturity is $1,469.68.

If a person purchased the bond at a price of $1,494.93 and then sold it one year later with interest rates still at 5 percent, he or she would have a capital loss of $25.25. The rate of return on the bond over the year consists of an *interest*, or *current*, *yield* plus a *capital gains yield*:

Current yield	=	$100/$1,494.93	=	0.0669	=	6.69%
Capital gains yield	=	−$25.25/$1,494.93	=	−0.0169	=	−1.69%
Total rate of return, or yield	=	$74.75/$1,494.93	=	0.0500	=	5.00%

Had interest rates risen from 10 to 15 percent during the first year after issue rather than fallen, the value of Big Sky's bonds would have declined to $713.78 at the end of the first year. If interest rates held constant at 15 percent, the bond would have a value of $720.84 at the end of the second year, so the total yield to investors would be:

Current yield	=	$100/$713.78	=	0.1401	=	14.01%
Capital gains yield	=	$7.06/$713.78	=	0.0099	=	0.99%
Total rate of return, or yield	=	$107.06/$713.78	=	0.1500	=	15.00%

Figure 11.2 graphs the values of the Big Sky bond over time, assuming that interest rates will remain constant at 10 percent, fall to 5 percent and then remain at that level, and rise to 15 percent and remain constant at that level. The figure illustrates the following important points:

- Whenever the required rate of return on a bond equals its coupon rate, the bond will sell at its par value.
- When interest rates, and hence required rates of return, fall after a bond is issued, the bond's value rises above its par value and the bond sells at a *premium*.
- When interest rates, and hence required rates of return, rise after a bond is issued, the bond's value falls below its par value and the bond sells at a *discount*.
- Bond prices on outstanding issues and interest rates are inversely related. Increasing rates lead to falling prices and decreasing rates lead to increasing prices.
- The price of a bond will always approach its par value as its maturity date approaches, provided the issuer does not default on the bond.

Note, however, that interest rates do **not** remain constant over time, so in reality a bond's price fluctuates both as interest rates in the economy fluctuate and the bond's term to maturity decreases.

Yield to Maturity on a Bond

Up to this point, a bond's required rate of return and cash flows have been used to determine its value. In reality, investors' required rates of return on securities are not observable, but security prices can be easily determined—at least on those

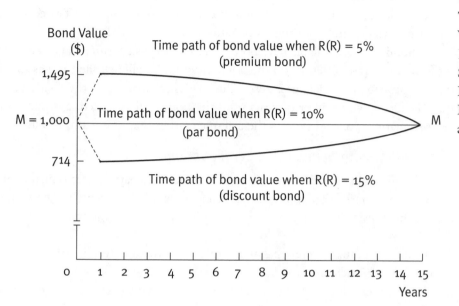

FIGURE 11.2

Time Path of the Value of a 15-Year, 10% Coupon, $1,000 Par Value Bond When Interest Rates are 5%, 10%, and 15%

	Bond Value at a Required Rate of Return of		
Year	5%	10%	15%
0	—	$1,000.00	—
1	$1,494.93	1,000.00	$ 713.78
2	1,469.68	1,000.00	720.84
3	1,443.16	1,000.00	728.97
.	.	.	.
.	.	.	.
.	.	.	.
13	1,092.97	1,000.00	918.71
14	1,047.62	1,000.00	956.52
15	1,000.00	1,000.00	1,000.00

securities that are actively traded—by looking in the local newspaper or the *Wall Street Journal*. Suppose that the Big Sky bond had 14 years remaining to maturity and the bond was selling at a price of $1,494.93. What percentage rate of return, or *yield to maturity (YTM)*, would be earned if the bond was bought at this price and held to maturity? To find the answer, 5 percent, use a financial calculator as follows:

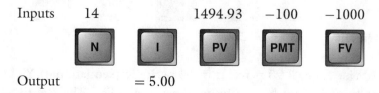

Inputs   14   1494.93   −100   −1000

N   I   PV   PMT   FV

Output   = 5.00

The YTM is the expected rate of return on a bond, assuming it is held to maturity and no default occurs. It is similar to the total rate of return discussed in the previous section. For a bond that sells at par, the YTM consists entirely of an interest yield, but if the bond sells at a discount or premium, the YTM consist of the current yield, plus a positive or negative capital gains yield.

Bonds that are callable have both a YTM and a *yield to call (YTC)*. The YTC is the expected rate of return on the bond assuming it will be called and assuming that the probability of default is zero. The YTC is calculated like the YTM, except that N reflects the number of years until the bond will be called, as opposed to years to maturity, and M reflects the call price rather than the maturity value.

Bond Values with Semiannual Compounding

Virtually all bonds issued in the United States actually pay interest semiannually, or every six months. To apply the preceding valuation concepts to semiannual bonds, the bond valuation procedures must be modified as follows:

1. Divide the annual interest payment, INT, by two to determine the dollar amount paid **each six months**.
2. Multiply the number of years to maturity, N, by two to determine the number of **semiannual interest periods**.
3. Divide the annual required rate of return, R(R), by two to determine the **semiannual required rate of return**.

To illustrate the use of the semiannual bond valuation model, assume that the Big Sky bonds pay $50 every six months rather than $100 annually. Thus, each interest payment is only half as large, but there are twice as many of them. When the going rate of interest is 5 percent annually, the value of Big Sky's bonds with 14 years left to maturity is $1,499.12:

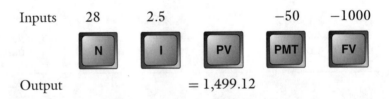

Output = 1,499.12

Similarly, if the bond were actually selling for $1,400 with 14 years to maturity, its YTM would be 5.80 percent:

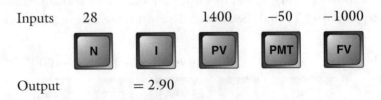

Output = 2.90

The value for I, 2.90 percent, is the **periodic (semiannual) YTM**, so it is necessary to multiply it by two to get the annual YTM. The effective annual YTM on the bond is somewhat greater than the 5.80 percent that was calculated.[4]

However, it is convention in the bond markets to quote all rates on a stated annual basis, so the procedures outlined in this section are correct when bonds—all of which have semiannual coupons—are being compared. However, when the returns on securities that have different periodic payments are being compared, all rates of return should be expressed as effective annual rates.

Interest Rate Risk

Interest rates change over time, which causes two types of risk that fall under the general classification of *interest rate risk*. First, an increase in interest rates leads to a decline in the values of outstanding bonds. Because interest rates can rise, bondholders face the risk of losses on their holdings. This risk is called *price risk*. Second, many bondholders buy bonds to build funds for future use. These bondholders reinvest the interest and principal cash flows as they are received. If interest rates fall, bondholders will earn a lower rate on the reinvested cash flows, which will have a negative impact on the future value of their holdings. This risk is called *reinvestment rate risk*.

To illustrate price risk, suppose you bought some of Big Sky's 10 percent bonds when they were issued at a price of $1,000. As illustrated earlier, if interest rates rise, the value of the bonds will fall. An investor's exposure to price risk depends on the maturity of the bonds. Figure 11.3, which shows the values of one-year and 14-year bonds at several different market interest rates, illustrates price risk. Notice how much more sensitive the price of the 14-year bond is to changes in interest rates. For bonds with similar coupons, the longer the maturity of the bond, the greater its price change in response to a given change in interest rates. Thus, bonds with longer maturities are exposed to more price risk.

Although a one-year bond exposes the buyer to less price risk than a 14-year bond, the one-year bond carries with it more reinvestment rate risk. That is, if the holding period is more than one year, investing in a one-year bond means that the principal and interest will have to be reinvested at the end of the first year. If interest rates fall, the return earned during the second year will be less than the return earned during the first year. Reinvestment rate risk is the second dimension of interest rate risk.

Clearly, bond investors face both price risk and reinvestment rate risk as a result of interest rate fluctuations over time. Which risk is most meaningful to a particular investor depends on the circumstances, but in general, interest rate risk, including both price and reinvestment rate risk, is reduced by matching the maturity of the bond with the anticipated *investment horizon*. For example, suppose Hilldale Community Hospital received a $5 million contribution that it will use in five years to build a new neonatal care center. By investing the contribution in five-year bonds, the hospital would minimize its interest rate risk because it would be matching its investment horizon. Price risk would be minimized because the bond will mature in five years, and hence investors will receive par value regardless of the level of interest rates at that time. Reinvestment rate risk is also minimized

FIGURE 11.3

Value of Long-Term and Short-Term 10% Annual Coupon Rate Bonds at Different Market Interest Rates

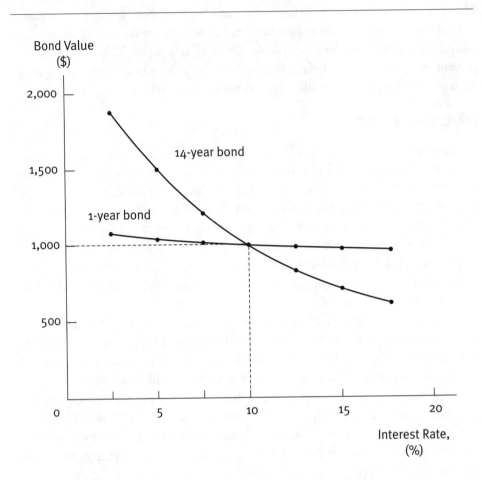

Current Market	Bond Value	
Interest Rate	1-Year Bond	14-Year Bond
2.5%	$1,073.17	$1,876.82
5.0	1,047.62	1,494.93
7.5	1,023.26	1,212.23
10.0	1,000.00	1,000.00
12.5	977.78	838.45
15.0	956.52	713.78
17.5	936.17	616.25

because only the interest on the bond would have to be reinvested, which is a less risky situation than if both principal and interest had to be reinvested.

Self-Test Questions

1. What is the general valuation model?
2. How are bonds valued?
3. What is meant by a bond's yield to maturity (YTM)?
4. Differentiate between price risk and reinvestment rate risk.

Key Concepts

This chapter provides an overview of long-term debt financing including how interest rates are determined, the characteristics of the major types of debt securities, and how such securities are valued. The key concepts of this chapter are:

- Any business must have assets if it is to operate and, in order to acquire assets, the business must raise *capital*. Capital comes in two basic forms: *debt* and *equity (or fund)* capital.
- Capital is allocated through the price system; a price is charged to "rent" money. Lenders charge *interest* on funds they lend, while equity investors receive *dividends* and *capital gains* in return for letting the firm use their money.
- Four fundamental factors affect the cost of money: *investment opportunities, time preferences for consumption, risk,* and *inflation.*
- *Term loans* and *bonds* are long-term debt contracts under which a borrower agrees to make a series of interest and principal payments on specific dates to the lender. A term loan is generally sold to one (or a few) lenders, while a bond is typically offered to the public and sold to many different investors.
- Many different types of bonds exist including *mortgage bonds, debentures, subordinated debentures,* and *municipal bonds.* Prevailing interest rates, the bond's riskiness, and tax consequences determine the return required on each type of bond.
- *Revenue bonds* are municipal bonds in which the revenues derived from such projects as roads or bridges, airports, water and sewage systems, and not-for-profit healthcare facilities are pledged as security for the bonds.
- A bond's *indenture* is a legal document that spells out the rights of the bondholders and of the issuing business. A *trustee* is assigned to make sure that the terms of the indenture are carried out.
- A *call provision* gives the issuer the right to redeem the bonds prior to maturity under specified terms, usually at a price greater than the maturity value (the difference is a *call premium*). A firm will call a bond issue and refund it if interest rates fall sufficiently after the bond has been issued.
- A *sinking fund* is a provision that requires the issuer to retire a portion of the bond issue each year. The purpose of the sinking fund is to provide for the orderly retirement of the issue. No call premium is paid to the holders of bonds called for sinking fund purposes.
- Bonds are assigned *ratings* that reflect the probability of their going into default. The higher a bond's rating and the greater the probability of recovering bondholder capital should default occur, the lower its interest rate.
- *Credit enhancement,* or *bond insurance,* upgrades a municipal bond rating to AAA. Regardless of the inherent credit rating of the issuer, the bond insurance company guarantees that bondholders will receive the promised interest and principal payments.

- The *interest rate* on a debt security is composed of the real risk-free rate (RRF) plus premiums that reflect inflation (IP), default risk (DRP), liquidity (LP), price risk (PRP), and call risk (CRP):

$$\text{Interest rate} = RRF + IP + DRP + LP + PRP + CRP.$$

- The relationship between the yields on securities and the securities' maturities is known as the *term structure of interest rates*. The *yield curve* is a graph of this relationship.
- Bonds call for the payment of a specific amount of *interest* for a specific number of years and for the *repayment of par* on the bond's maturity date. Like most assets, a bond's value is simply the present value of the expected cash flow stream.
- The annual rate of return on a bond consists of an *interest*, or *current, yield* plus a *capital gains yield*. Assuming constant interest rates, if the bond is selling at a *discount*, the capital gains yield is positive; if the bond is selling at a *premium*, the capital gains yield is negative.
- A bond's *yield to maturity (YTM)* is the rate of return earned on a bond if it is held to maturity and no default occurs. The YTM for a bond that sells at par consists entirely of an interest yield, but if the bond sells at a discount or premium, the YTM consists of the current yield plus a positive or negative capital gains yield.
- Bondholders face *price risk* because bond values change when interest rates change. An investor's exposure to price risk depends on the maturity of the bonds.
- Bondholders face *reinvestment rate risk* when the investment horizon exceeds the maturity of the bond issue.

Long-term debt is a major source of capital for health services organizations. Thus, it is necessary for health services managers to be familiar with debt concepts. Furthermore, learning how to value long-term debt provides an excellent introduction to asset valuation. The topics covered in this chapter will be useful throughout the remainder of the text.

Questions

11.1 The four fundamental factors that affect the supply of and demand for investment capital, and hence interest rates, are productive opportunities, time preferences for consumption, risk, and inflation. Explain how each of these factors affects the cost of money.

11.2 The interest rate required by investors on a debt security can be expressed by the following equation:

$$\text{Interest rate} = RRF + IP + DRP + LP + PRP + CRP.$$

Define each term of the equation, and explain how it affects the interest rate.

11.3 a. What is a yield curve?

    b. Is the yield curve static or does it change over time?

    c. What is the difference between a normal yield curve and an inverted yield curve?

    d. What impact does the yield curve have on debt financing decisions?

11.4 Briefly describe the following types of debt:

    a. Term loan

    b. Bond

    c. Mortgage bond

    d. Senior debt; junior debt

    e. Debenture

    f. Subordinated debenture

    g. Municipal bond

11.5 Briefly explain the following debt features:

    a. Indenture

    b. Restrictive covenant

    c. Trustee

    d. Call provision

    e. Sinking fund

11.6 a. (1) What are the two major bond rating agencies?

       (2) What do bond ratings measure?

       (3) How do investors interpret bond ratings?

       (4) What is the difference between an A-rated bond and a B-rated bond?

    b. (1) Why are bond ratings important to investors?

       (2) Why are ratings important to businesses that issue bonds?

11.7 What is credit enhancement?

11.8 a. What is price risk?

    b. What is reinvestment rate risk?

11.9 State whether this statement is true or false: "The values of outstanding bonds change whenever the going rate of interest changes. In general, short-term interest rates are more volatile than long-term rates, so short-term bond prices are more sensitive to interest rate changes than are long-term bond prices." Explain your answer.

Problems

11.1 Assume Venture Healthcare sold bonds that have a ten-year maturity, a 12 percent coupon rate with annual payments, and a $1,000 par value.

    a. Suppose that two years after the bonds were issued, the required interest rate fell to 7 percent. What would be the bonds' value?

    b. Suppose that two years after the bonds were issued, the required interest rate rose to 13 percent. What would be the bonds' value?

   c. What would be the value of the bonds three years after issue in each
      scenario above, assuming that interest rates stayed steady at either 7
      percent or 13 percent?

11.2 Twin Oaks Health Center has a bond issue outstanding with a coupon rate
     of 7 percent and four years remaining until maturity. The par value of the
     bond is $1,000 and the bond pays interest annually.
     a. Determine the current value of the bond if present market conditions
        justify a 14 percent required rate of return.
     b. Now suppose Twin Oaks' four-year bond had semiannual coupon
        payments. Now what would be its current value? (Assume a 7 percent
        semiannual required rate of return. However, the actual rate would be
        slightly less than 7 percent because a semiannual coupon bond is slightly
        less risky than an annual coupon bond.)
     c. Assume that Twin Oaks' bond had a semiannual coupon, but 20 years
        remaining to maturity. What is the current value under these conditions?
        (Again, assume a 7 percent semiannual required rate of return, although
        the actual rate would probably be greater than 7 percent because of
        increased price risk.)

11.3 Tidewater Home Health Care, Inc., has a bond issue outstanding with
     eight years remaining to maturity, a coupon rate of 10 percent with interest
     paid annually, and a par value of $1,000. The current market price of the
     bond is $1,251.22.
     a. What is the bond's yield to maturity?
     b. Now assume that the bond has semiannual coupon payments. What is
        its yield to maturity in this situation?

11.4 Pacific Homecare has three bond issues outstanding. All three bonds pay
     $100 in annual interest plus $1,000 at maturity. Bond S has a maturity of
     five years, Bond M has a 15-year maturity, and Bond L matures in 30 years.
     a. What is the value of each of these bonds when the required interest rate
        is 5 percent, 10 percent, and 15 percent?
     b. Why is the price of Bond L more sensitive to interest rate changes than
        the price of Bond S?

11.5 Minneapolis Health System has bonds outstanding that have 4 years
     remaining to maturity, a coupon interest rate of 9 percent paid annually,
     and a $1,000 par value.
     a. What is the yield to maturity on the issue if the current market price is
        $829?
     b. If the current market price is $1,104?
     c. Would you be willing to buy one of these bonds for $829 if you required
        a 12 percent rate of return on the issue? Explain your answer.

11.6 Six years ago, Bradford Community Hospital issued 20-year municipal
     bonds with a 7 percent annual coupon rate. The bonds were called today
     for a $70 call premium, that is, bondholders received $1,070 for each

bond. What is the realized rate of return for those investors who bought the bonds for $1,000 when they were issued?

11.7 A few years ago, Regal Health Plans issued a 12 percent annual coupon bond that currently has 10 years remaining to maturity. The bond now sells for $1,100. The bond has a call provision that allows Regal to call the bond in four years at a call price of $1,060.

a. What is the bond's yield to maturity?

b. What is the bond's yield to call?

Notes

1. The *prime rate* is the interest rate that banks charge their very best (most creditworthy) customers. Theoretically, the prime rate is set separately by every bank, but in practice all banks follow the lead of the major New York City banks, so there is usually a single prime rate in the United States. The prime rate is changed—sometimes quite rapidly—in response to changing inflation expectations. In August 1998, the prime rate was set at 8.5 percent.

2. *Treasury securities* are debt obligations of the U. S. government. Because such securities are issued with different maturities, they have different names. *Treasury bonds*, or *T-bonds*, have maturities when issued of greater than 10 years; *T-notes* have maturities from one to 10 years; and *T-bills* have maturities of less than one year. Although the maturities of such securities decline over time after the date of issue, they retain the name appropriate to their **original** maturity.

3. For a discussion of the forces that influence the shape of the yield curve, see E. F. Brigham and L. C. Gapenski, *Financial Management: Theory and Practice* (Fort Worth, TX: Dryden Press, 1997), 110–115.

4. The effective annual YTM is $(1.029)^2 - 1.0 = 1.0588 - 1.0 = 0.0588 = 5.88\%$, as compared with the stated rate of 5.80%.

References

Aderholdt, J. M. and C. R. Pardue. 1989. "A Guide to Taxable Debt Financing Alternatives." *Healthcare Financial Management* (July): 58–66.

Carlile, L. L. and B. M. Serchuk. 1995. "The Coming Changes in Tax-Exempt Health Care Finance." *Journal of Health Care Finance* (Fall): 1–42.

Cleverley, W. O. and P. C. Nutt. 1984. "The Decision Process Used for Bond Rating—and Its Implications." *Health Services Research* (December): 615–637.

Culler, S. D. 1993a. "Assessing Hospital Credit Risk: A Banker's View." *Topics in Health Care Financing* (Summer): 35–43.

———. 1993b. "A Creditor's Perspective on the Hospital Industry." *Topics in Health Care Financing* (Summer):12–20.

Elrod, J. L., Jr. 1986. "Can Municipal Bond Futures Contracts Minimize Financial Risk?" *Healthcare Financial Management* (April): 40–44.

Harris, J. P. and J. B. Price. 1988. "Finding Money Under Your Nose Using New Capital Techniques." *Healthcare Financial Management* (July): 24–30.

Kaufman, K. and M. L. Hall. 1990. *The Capital Management of Health Care Organizations.* Chicago: Health Administration Press.

LeBuhn, J. 1994. "Primary Market Derivatives: Satisfying Investor Appetites." *Journal of Health Care Finance* (Winter): 11–21.

Mullner, R., D. Matthews, J. D. Kubal, and S. Andes. 1983. "Debt Financing: An Alternative for Hospital Construction Funding." *Healthcare Financial Management* (April): 18–24.

Nemes, J. 1991. "Dealing with the Authorities." *Modern Healthcare* (October 14): 22–29.

Odegard, B. M. 1988. "Tax-Exempt Financing Under the Tax Reform Act of 1986." *Topics in Health Care Financing* (Summer): 35–45.

Prince, T. R. and R. Ramanan. 1994. "Bond Ratings, Debt Insurance, and Hospital Operating Performance." *Topics in Health Care Financing* (Fall): 36–50.

Sims, W. B. 1984. "Financing Strategies for Long-Term Care Facilities." *Healthcare Financial Management* (March): 42–54.

Smith, S. D. 1994. "The Use of Interest Rate Swaps in Hospital Capital Finance." *Journal of Health Care Finance* (Winter): 35–44.

Sterns, J. B. 1994. "Emerging Trends in Health Care Finance." *Journal of Health Care Finance* (Winter): 1–10.

West, D. A. 1983. "Debt Financing in the 1980s: Is the Risk for Non-Profit Hospitals Too Great?" *Healthcare Financial Management* (April): 56–62.

Woodward, M. A. 1993. "Interest Rate Swaps: Financial Tool of the '90s." *Healthcare Financial Management* (November): 56–64.

EQUITY FINANCING, INVESTMENT BANKING, AND MARKET EFFICIENCY

Learning Objectives

After studying this chapter, readers will be able to:

- Describe the key features associated with equity financing.
- Discuss the investment banking process.
- Conduct simple valuation analyses of common stock.
- Explain the concepts of market equilibrium and efficiency.

Introduction

Long-term debt financing was discussed in Chapter 11 including how interest rates are set in the economy, the features of various long-term debt securities, and how debt securities, particularly bonds, are valued. The second primary source of capital to healthcare firms is *equity financing*. Within investor-owned, or for-profit, firms, equity financing is obtained from shareholders through the sale of *common stock* and by retaining earnings within the business.[1] The equivalent financing in not-for-profit firms is often called *fund capital*, which is raised through contributions, grants, and by retaining earnings. From a financial perspective, common stock and fund financing serve the same basic purpose, so the generic term *equity* will be used to refer to all nondebt capital regardless of a business' ownership.

In this chapter, we cover the same general issues as in Chapter 11, but the focus here is on equity rather than debt financing. In addition, supplemental information is provided on how securities are sold (the investment banking process). The chapter closes with a discussion of two very important financing concepts: market equilibrium and market efficiency.

Equity in For-Profit Businesses

In for-profit businesses, equity financing is supplied by the owners of the business, either directly through the purchase of an equity interest in the business or indirectly through earnings retention. Because most large for-profit businesses are organized as corporations, the discussion here focuses on corporate stockholders as opposed to proprietors or partners. Stockholders are the owners of for-profit corporations, and as such they have certain rights and privileges. The most important of these rights and privileges are discussed in this section.

Claim on Residual Earnings

The reason why most people buy common stock is to gain the right to a proportionate share of the *residual earnings* of the firm. A firm's net income, which is the residual earnings after all expenses have been paid, belongs to the firm's common stockholders. Some portion of net income will typically be paid out in *dividends* each quarter, so stockholders often receive quarterly cash payments. In addition, the portion of net income that is retained within the firm will be invested in new assets, which presumably will increase the firm's earnings, and hence dividends, over time.

An increasing dividend stream means that the firm's stock will be more valuable in the future than it is today because dividends will be higher, for example, in five years than they are today. Thus, common stockholders typically expect to be able to sell the stock they purchased at some time in the future at a higher price than they paid for it, and hence to realize a *capital gain*. To illustrate the payment of dividends, consider Table 12.1, which lists the annual per share dividend payment and earnings, as well as the average annual stock price, for Big Sky Healthcare from 1988 through 1998. Over the ten growth periods, Big Sky's dividend grew by 275 percent or at an average annual growth rate of 14.1 percent. At the same time, the firm's stock price grew by 247 percent, which is an average annual rate of 13.2 percent.

Although Big Sky's dividend growth **averaged** 14.1 percent annually over the period, it was not a **constant** 14.1 percent each year. Firms often hold the dividend constant for several years to allow earnings to climb to a point where it is clear that a higher dividend payment is warranted. For example, Big Sky kept its dividend at $0.23 a share from 1989 through 1991, while earnings per share were flat at about $0.55.

In general, managers are very reluctant to reduce dividends because investors interpret lower dividends as a signal that management forecasts poor

TABLE 12.1
Big Sky Healthcare: Selected Financial Data

Year	Annual Per Share Dividend	Annual Per Share Earnings	Average Annual Stock Price
1988	$0.20	$0.48	$ 7.70
1989	0.23	0.55	10.95
1990	0.23	0.52	11.00
1991	0.23	0.58	10.40
1992	0.48	0.85	15.30
1993	0.52	1.10	18.70
1994	0.58	1.25	20.60
1995	0.58	0.45	19.50
1996	0.65	1.35	23.20
1997	0.70	1.50	24.40
1998	0.75	1.55	26.70

earnings ahead. Thus, when Big Sky saw its earnings per share temporarily tumble from $1.25 in 1994 to $0.45 in 1995, it maintained its $0.58 per share dividend. Big Sky was able to pay a cash dividend that exceeded earnings in 1995 because the firm's cash flow, which generally exceeds net income, easily supported the dividend.[2] When earnings picked up again in 1996, Big Sky increased its dividend to $0.65.

Over the entire period, Big Sky has proved to be a good investment for stockholders. For example, assume that the stock was purchased for $7.70 in 1988, a $0.20 dividend payment was paid and then the stock was sold one year later for $10.95. For simplicity, assume that the dividend payment, rather than occurring quarterly, was paid at the end of the one-year holding period. Thus, $7.70 was paid and one year later $10.95 + $0.20 = $11.15 was received. The rate of return earned was ($11.15 − $7.70) / $7.70 = $3.45 / $7.70 = 0.448 = 44.8%. (Using a financial calculator, enter PV = 7.70 [or −7.70], FV = 11.15, N = 1 and press I to get 44.8 percent.) However, investors who bought Big Sky's stock in 1990 or 1994 and then sold it one year later would have had a capital loss rather than a capital gain on the sale, even though they would have received quarterly dividends over each one-year holding period. Stock valuation is addressed in more detail later in the chapter.

Control of the Firm

Common stockholders have the right to elect the firm's directors who in turn elect the officers who will manage the business. In small firms, the major stockholder often assumes the positions of chief executive officer (CEO) and chairman of the board of directors. In large, publicly owned firms, managers typically own some stock, but their personal holdings are insufficient to allow them to exercise voting control. Thus, stockholders can remove the management of most publicly owned firms if they decide a management team is ineffective.

Various state and federal laws stipulate how stockholder control is to be exercised. First, corporations must hold an election of directors periodically, usually once a year, with the vote taken at the annual meeting. Frequently, one third of the directors are elected each year for a three-year term. Each share of stock has one vote; thus, the owner of 1,000 shares has 1,000 votes. Stockholders can appear at the annual meeting and vote in person, but typically they transfer their right to vote to a second party by means of a *proxy*. Management always solicits stockholders' proxies and usually gets them. However, if the common stockholders are dissatisfied with current management, an outside group may solicit the proxies in an effort to overthrow management and take control of the business. Such a bid for control is known as a *proxy fight*.

The Preemptive Right

Common stockholders often have the right, called the *preemptive right*, to purchase any new shares sold by the firm. In some states, the preemptive right is mandatory, while in others, it can be specified in the corporate charter to be in force.

The purpose of the preemptive right is twofold. First, it protects the present stockholders' power of control. If it were not for this safeguard, the management of a corporation under criticism from stockholders could secure its position by issuing a large number of additional shares and purchasing the shares themselves or selling them to a friendly party. Management would thereby gain control of the corporation and frustrate current stockholders.

The second, and more important, reason for the preemptive right is that it protects stockholders against dilution of value should new shares be issued at less than the market price. For example, suppose HealthOne HMO has 1,000 shares of common stock outstanding, each with a price of $100, which makes a total market value of $100,000. If an additional 1,000 shares were sold to friends and relatives of management at $50 a share, or for $50,000, this would presumably raise the total market value of HealthOne's stock to $150,000. When the new market value is divided by the new number of shares outstanding, a share price of $75 is obtained. HealthOne's old stockholders thus lose $25 per share and the new stockholders have an instant profit of $25 per share. As demonstrated by this example, selling common stock at a price below the current market price dilutes value and transfers wealth from the present stockholders to those who purchase the new shares. The preemptive right, which gives current stockholders the first opportunity to buy any new shares, protects them against such dilution of value.

Self-Test Questions
1. In what forms do common stock investors receive returns?
2. How do common stockholders exercise their right of control?
3. What is the preemptive right and what is its purpose?

Types of Common Stock

Although most for-profit corporations issue only one type of common stock, in some instances several types of stock are used to meet the special needs of the company. Generally, when special classifications of stock are used, one type is designated *Class A*, another *Class B*, and so on. For this reason, such stock is called *classified stock*.

Small, new companies that seek to obtain funds from outside sources frequently use classified stock. For example, when Genetic Research, Inc., went public in 1995, its Class A stock was sold to the public and paid a dividend, but carried no voting rights for five years. Its Class B stock was retained by the organizers of the company and carried full voting rights for five years, but dividends could not be paid on the Class B stock until the company had established its earning power by building up retained earnings to a designated level. The firm's use of classified stock allowed the public to take a position in a conservatively financed growth company without sacrificing income, while the founders retained absolute control during the crucial early stages of the firm's development. At the same time, outside investors were protected against excessive withdrawals of funds by the original owners. As is often the case in such situations, the Class B stock was also called *founders' shares*.

Class A, Class B, and so on, have no standard meanings. Most firms have no classified shares, but a firm that does could designate its Class B shares as founders' shares and its Class A shares as those sold to the public. Other firms could use the A and B designations for entirely different purposes.

1. What is meant by the term *classified stock*?
2. Give one reason for using classified stock.

The Market for Common Stock

Some for-profit corporations are so small that their common stock is not actively traded, it is owned by only a few people, usually the companies' managers. Such companies are said to be *privately held*, or *closely held*, and the stock is said to be *closely held stock*.

The stocks of smaller, publicly owned firms are not listed on any exchange; they trade in the *over-the-counter (OTC)* market. This market is composed of brokers and dealers who belong to a trade group called the *National Association of Securities Dealers (NASD)*, which licenses brokers and oversees their trading practices. The computerized trading network that is used for the OTC market is known as the NASD Automated Quotation System, or *NASDAQ*. Thus, over-the-counter transactions are listed in the *Wall Street Journal* and other publications under the title NASDAQ. Stocks traded on the OTC market (and their companies) are said to be *unlisted*.

Most larger, publicly owned companies apply for listing on an exchange. These companies and their stocks are said to be *listed*. As a general rule, companies are first listed on a regional exchange, such as the *Pacific* or *Midwest*, then they move up to the *American (AMEX)*, and finally—if they grow large enough—to the "Big Board," the *New York Stock Exchange (NYSE)*. For example, American Healthcare Management, a King of Prussia, Pennsylvania-based company that owns or manages 16 hospitals in nine states recently listed on the NYSE. The stock had previously traded on the AMEX, but the firm's managers believed that listing on the NYSE would increase the trading of its shares and make the company more visible to the investment community, which presumably would have a positive impact on stock price. Many more stocks are traded in the OTC market than on the NYSE, and daily trading volume in the OTC market typically exceeds that of the NYSE. However, in terms of the market value of daily transactions, the NYSE dominates with about 60 percent of the total trading business in the United States.

Institutional investors such as pension funds, insurance companies, and mutual funds own about 40 percent of all common stocks. However, the institutions buy and sell relatively actively, so they account for about 80 percent of all transactions. Thus, the institutions have a heavy influence on the prices of individual stocks; in a real sense, institutional investors determine the price levels of individual stocks.

Stock market transactions can be classified into three distinct categories:

- *Initial public offerings by privately held firms: the new issue market.* A small company is typically owned by its management and a handful of private investors. At a certain point in its life, if the company is to grow further, its stock must be sold to the general public. This action is defined as *going public.* The market for stock that is in the process of going public is often called the *new issue market* and the issue is called an *initial public offering (IPO).* For example, American Oncology Resources, a Houston-based company that manages 12 oncology practices with 90 physicians in nine states, recently raised $100 million in equity financing by going public.
- *Additional shares sold by established, publicly owned companies: the primary market.* Evergreen Healthcare, which operates 79 nursing homes in ten states, recently sold 3.1 million shares of new common stock, thereby raising $31.2 million of new equity financing. Because the shares sold were newly created, Evergreen's issue was defined as a *primary market* offering, but because the firm was already publicly held, the offering was **not** an IPO. Firms generally prefer to obtain equity by retaining earnings because of the high insurance costs associated with new common stock sales, as well as the pressure on stock price brought about by adding to the supply. Still, if a company requires more equity funds than can be generated from retained earnings, a stock sale may be required.
- *Outstanding shares of established, publicly owned companies: the secondary market.* If the owner of 100 shares of Columbia/HCA Healthcare sells his or her stock, the trade is said to have occurred in the *secondary market.* Thus, the market for outstanding shares, or *used shares,* is defined as the secondary market. Over 15 million shares of Columbia/HCA were bought and sold on the NYSE in 1997, but the company did not receive a dime from these transactions.

Self-Test Questions

1. What is an initial public offering (IPO)?
2. What are the differences between Columbia/HCA Healthcare shares that are sold in the primary market versus its shares that are sold in the secondary market?

Procedures for Selling New Common Stock

For-profit corporations can sell new common stock in six primary ways:

- rights offerings;
- public offerings;
- private placements;

- employee stock purchase plans;
- dividend reinvestment plans; and
- direct purchase plans.

In this section, each method is briefly described.

Rights Offerings

As discussed previously, common stockholders often have the *preemptive right* to purchase any additional shares sold by the firm. If the preemptive right is contained in a particular firm's charter, the company must offer any newly issued common stock to existing stockholders. If the charter does not prescribe a preemptive right, the firm can choose to sell to its existing stockholders or to the public at large. If it sells its newly issued shares to the existing stockholders, the stock sale is called a *rights offering*. Each existing stockholder is issued an *option*, which gives the holder the right to buy a certain number of the new shares, typically at a price below the existing market price. The precise terms of the option are listed on a certificate called a *stock purchase right*, or simply a *right*. If the stockholder does not wish to purchase any additional shares in the company, he or she can sell the rights to another person who does want to buy the stock.[3]

Public Offerings

If the preemptive right exists in a company's charter, it must sell new stock through a rights offering. If the preemptive right does not exist, the company may choose to offer the new shares to the general public through a *public offering*. Procedures for public offerings are discussed in detail in a later section.

Private Placements

In a *private placement*, securities are sold to one or a few investors, generally institutional investors. As discussed in Chapter 11, private placements are most common with bonds, but they also occur with stock. The primary advantages of private placements are lower issuance costs and greater speed because the shares do not have to go through the SEC registration process.

The primary disadvantage of a private placement is that the securities, because they are unregistered, must be sold to a large, sophisticated investor, usually an insurance company, mutual fund, or pension fund. Furthermore, in the event that the original purchaser wants to sell privately placed securities, they must be sold to other large, sophisticated investors. However, the SEC currently allows any institution with a portfolio of $100 million or more to buy and sell private placement securities. Because thousands of institutions have assets that exceed this limit, there is a large market for the resale of private placements, and hence they are becoming more popular with issuers.

Employee Stock Purchase Plans

Many companies have plans that allow employees to purchase stock of the employing firm on favorable terms. Under executive-incentive *stock option plans*, key managers are given options to purchase stock at a fixed price. These managers generally have a direct, material influence on the company's fortunes, so if they perform well, the stock price will go up and the options will become valuable.

Also, many companies have *stock purchase plans* for lower-level employees. For example, Texas HealthPlans, Inc., a regional investor-owned HMO, permits employees who are not participants in its stock option plan to allocate up to 10 percent of their salaries to its stock purchase plan The funds are then used to buy newly issued shares at 85 percent of the market price on the purchase date. The company's contribution, the 15 percent discount, is not vested in an employee until five years after the purchase date. Thus, the employee cannot realize the benefit of the company's contribution without working an additional five years. This type of plan is designed both to improve employee performance and to reduce employee turnover.

Dividend Reinvestment Plans

During the 1970s, many large companies instituted *dividend reinvestment plans (DRIPs)* whereby stockholders can automatically reinvest their dividends in the stock of the paying corporation. There are two basic types of DRIPs: plans that involve only old stock that is already outstanding and plans that involve newly issued stock. In either case, the stockholder must pay income taxes on the dollar amount of the dividends, even though stock rather than cash is received.

Under both types of DRIP, stockholders must choose between continuing to receive cash dividends or using the cash dividends to buy more stock in the corporation. Under the *old stock* type of plan, a bank, acting as a trustee, takes the total funds available for reinvestment from each quarterly dividend, purchases the corporation's stock on the open market, and allocates the shares purchased to the participating stockholders on a pro rata basis. The brokerage costs of buying the shares are low because of volume purchases, so these plans benefit small stockholders who do not need cash for current consumption.

The *new stock* type of DRIP provides for dividends to be invested in newly issued stock; hence, these plans raise new capital for the firm. No fees are charged to participating stockholders, and some companies offer the new stock at a discount of 3 to 5 percent below the prevailing market price. The companies absorb these costs as a trade-off against the issuance costs that would be incurred if the stock were sold through investment bankers rather than through the DRIP.

Direct Purchase Plans

In recent years, many companies have established *direct purchase plans,* which allow individual investors to purchase stock directly from the company. Many of these plans grew out of DRIPs, which were expanded to allow participants to purchase shares in excess of the dividend amount. In direct purchase plans, investors usually pay little or no brokerage fees, and many plans offer convenient features such as fractional share purchases, automatic purchases by bank debit, and quarterly statements. Although employee purchase plans, DRIPs, and direct purchase plans are an excellent way for employees and individual investors to purchase stock, they typically do not raise large sums of new capital for the firm, so other methods must be used when equity needs are great.

1. What is a rights offering?
2. What is a private placement and what are its primary advantages over a public offering?
3. Briefly, what are employee stock purchase plans?
4. What is a dividend reinvestment plan?
5. What is a direct purchase plan?

Self-Test Questions

Regulation of Securities Markets

Sales of securities are regulated by the *Securities and Exchange Commission (SEC)* and, to a lesser extent, by each of the 50 states. Here are the primary elements of SEC regulation:

- The SEC has jurisdiction over all interstate offerings of new securities to the public in amounts of $1.5 million or more.
- Newly issued securities must be registered with the SEC at least 20 days before they are offered to the public. The *registration statement* provides financial, legal, and technical information about the company to the SEC; the *prospectus* summarizes this information for investors. SEC lawyers and accountants analyze both the registration statement and the prospectus; if the information is inadequate or misleading, the SEC will delay or stop the public offering.
- After the registration has become effective, new securities may be offered, but any sales solicitation must be accompanied by the prospectus. *Preliminary*, or *red herring, prospectuses* may be distributed to potential buyers during the 20-day waiting period, but no sales may occur during this time. The red herring prospectus contains all the key information that will appear in the final prospectus except the price, which is generally set after the market closes the day before the new securities are actually offered to the public.
- If the registration statement or prospectus contains misrepresentations or omissions of material facts, any purchaser who suffers a loss may sue for damages. Severe penalties may be imposed on the issuer or its officers, directors, accountants, engineers, appraisers, underwriters, and all others who participated in the preparation of the registration statement or prospectus.
- The SEC also regulates all national stock exchanges. Companies whose securities are listed on an exchange must file annual reports with both the SEC and the exchange.
- The SEC has control over corporate *insiders*. Officers, directors, and major stockholders must file monthly reports of changes in their holdings of the stock of the corporation.

- The SEC has the power to prohibit manipulation by such devices as *pools* (i.e., large amounts of money used to buy or sell stocks to artificially affect prices) or *wash sales* (i.e., sales between members of the same group to record artificial transaction prices).
- The SEC has control over the form of the proxy and the way the company uses it to solicit votes.

States also exercise control over the issuance of new securities within their boundaries. Such control is usually supervised by a corporation commissioner or someone with a similar title. State laws relating to security sales are called *blue sky laws* because they were put into effect to keep unscrupulous promoters from selling securities that offered the "blue sky" (something wonderful), but that actually had no assets or earnings to back up the promises.

The securities industry itself realizes the importance of stable markets, sound brokerage firms, and the absence of price manipulation. Therefore, the various exchanges, as well as other industry trade groups, work closely with the SEC to police transactions and to maintain the integrity and credibility of the system. These industry groups also cooperate with regulatory authorities to set net worth and other standards for securities firms, to develop insurance programs that protect the customers of brokerage houses, and the like.

In general, government regulation of securities trading, as well as industry self-regulation, is designed to ensure that investors receive information that is as accurate as possible, that no one artificially manipulates the market price of a given security, and that corporate insiders do not take advantage of their position to profit in their companies' securities at the expense of others. Neither the SEC, nor the state regulators, nor the industry itself can prevent investors from making foolish decisions, but they can and do help investors obtain the best information possible, which is the first step in making sound investment decisions.

Self-Test Questions

1. What is the purpose of securities markets regulation?
2. What agencies and groups are involved in such regulation?
3. What is a prospectus?
4. What are "blue sky" laws?

The Investment Banking Process

Investment banks are the companies—such as Salomon Smith Barney and Merrill Lynch—that help businesses sell securities to the public. The procedures followed in issuing new securities are called the *investment banking process*. Generally, the following key decisions regarding the issuance of new securities are made jointly by the issuing company's managers and the investment bankers that will handle the deal.

- *Dollars to be raised.* How much new capital is needed?

- *Type of securities used.* Should common stock, bonds, another security, or a combination of securities be used? Furthermore, if common stock is to be issued, should it be done as a rights offering, by a direct sale to the general public, or by a private placement?

- *Selection of an investment banker.* If the issue is to be sold to the public, the firm must select an investment banker. This can be an important decision for a firm that is going public. However, an older firm that has already "been to market" will have an established relationship with an investment banker. Changing bankers is easy, though, if the firm is dissatisfied.

- *Contractual basis of issue.* If an investment banker is used, will the banker work on a *best efforts* basis or will it *underwrite* the issue? In a best efforts sale, the banker guarantees neither the price nor the sale of the securities, only that it will put forth its best efforts to sell the issue. On an underwritten issue, the company does get a guarantee because the banker agrees to buy the entire issue and then resell the securities to its customers. Bankers bear significant risk in underwritten offerings because the banker must bear the loss if the price of the security falls between the time the security is purchased from the issuer and the time of resale to the public.

- *Banker's compensation and other expenses.* The investment banker's compensation (if used) must be negotiated. Also, the firm must estimate the other issuance expenses that it will incur in connection with the issue such as lawyers' fees, accountants' costs, printing and engraving, and so on. In an underwritten issue, the banker will buy the issue from the company at a discount below the price at which the securities are to be offered to the public, with this spread set to cover the banker's costs and to provide a profit. In a best efforts sale, fees to the investment banker are normally set as some percentage of the dollar volume sold. Issuance costs as a percentage of the proceeds are higher for stocks than for bonds, and costs are higher for small than for large issues. The relationship between size of issue and issuance cost is caused primarily by the existence of fixed costs; certain costs must be incurred regardless of the size of the issue, so the percentage cost is quite high for small issues. To illustrate, issuance costs for a $5 million bond issue are about 5 percent, while the costs drop to about 1 percent for issues over $50 million. For a stock issue, the costs are about 12 percent and 4 percent, respectively.

- *Setting the offering price.* If the company is already publicly owned, the offering price will be based on the existing market price of its stock or the yield to maturity (YTM) on its bonds. On initial public offerings, however, pricing decisions are much more difficult because there is no existing market price for guidance. The investment banker will have an easier job if the issue is priced relatively low, but the issuer of the securities naturally wants as high a price as possible. Conflict of interest on price, therefore, arises between the investment banker and the issuer. If the issuer is financially sophisticated and makes comparisons with similar security issues, the investment banker will be forced to price the new security close to its true value.

After the company and its investment banker have decided how much money to raise, the types of securities to issue, and the basis for pricing the issue, they will prepare and file a registration statement and a prospectus (if needed). The final price of the stock or the interest rate on a bond issue is set at the close of business the day the issue clears the SEC, and the securities are offered to the public the following day.

Investors are required to pay for securities within ten days, and the investment banker must pay the issuing firm within four days of the official commencement of the offering. Typically, the banker sells the securities within a day or two after the offering begins. However, on occasion, the banker miscalculates, sets the offering price too high, and thus is unable to move the issue. At other times, the market declines during the offering period, which forces the banker to reduce the price of the stock or bonds. In either instance, on an underwritten offering, the firm receives the agreed-upon dollar amount, so the banker must absorb any losses incurred.

Because they are exposed to large potential losses, investment bankers typically do not handle the purchase and distribution of issues single handedly, unless the issue is a very small one. If the sum of money involved is large, investment bankers form *underwriting syndicates* in an effort to minimize the risk that each banker carries. The banking house that sets up the deal is called the *lead*, or *managing, underwriter.*

In addition to the underwriting syndicate, on larger offerings, even more investment bankers are included in a *selling group*, which handles the distribution of securities to individual investors. The selling group includes all members of the underwriting syndicate plus additional dealers who take relatively small percentages of the total issue from members of the underwriting syndicate. Thus, the underwriters act as *wholesalers*, while members of the selling group act as *retailers*. The number of investment banks in a selling group depends partly on the size of the issue, but also on the number and types of buyers. For example, the selling group that handled a recent $92 million municipal bond issue for Adventist Health System/Sunbelt consisted of three members, while the one that sold $1 billion in B-rated junk bonds for National Medical Enterprises consisted of eight members.[4]

Self-Test Questions

1. What types of decisions must the issuer and its investment banker make?
2. What is the difference between an underwritten and a best efforts issue?
3. Are there any conflicts that may arise between the issuer and the investment banker when setting the offering price on a securities issue?

Equity in Not-for-Profit Businesses

Investor-owned firms have two sources of equity financing: retained earnings and new stock sales. Not-for-profit businesses can and do retain earnings, but they do not have access to the equity markets, that is, they cannot sell common stock to raise equity capital.[5] Not-for-profit firms can, however, raise equity capital through *government grants* and *charitable contributions*. Federal, state, and local governments are concerned about the provision of healthcare services to the general population. Therefore, these public entities often make grants to not-for-profit providers to help offset the costs of services rendered to patients who cannot pay for those services. Sometimes these grants are nonspecific, but often they are to provide specific services such as neonatal intensive care to needy infants.

As for charitable contributions, individuals, as well as companies, are motivated to contribute to not-for-profit health services organizations for a variety of reasons including concern for the well-being of others, the recognition that often accompanies large contributions, and tax deductibility. Because only contributions to not-for-profit firms are tax deductible, this source of funding is, for all practical purposes, not available to investor-owned health services organizations. Although charitable contributions are not a substitute for profit retentions, charitable contributions can be a significant source of fund capital. For example, in 1997, the Association for Health Care Philanthropy reported total gifts of over $4 billion to not-for-profit hospitals.

Most not-for-profit hospitals received their initial, start-up equity capital from religious, educational, or governmental entities, and today some hospitals continue to receive funding from these sources. However, since the 1970s, these sources have provided a much smaller proportion of hospital funding, which forces not-for-profit hospitals to rely more on profits and outside contributions. Furthermore, federal programs such as the Hill-Burton Act, which provided large amounts of funds for hospital expansion following World War II, have been discontinued. Additionally, state and local governments, which are also facing significant financial pressures, are finding it more and more difficult to fund grants to healthcare providers.

Finally, as discussed in Chapter 2, a growing trend among legislative bodies and tax authorities is to force not-for-profit hospitals to "earn" their favorable tax treatment by providing a certain amount of charity care. Even more severe, some cities have pressured not-for-profit hospitals to make "voluntary" payments to the city to make up for the lost property tax revenue. These trends tend to reduce the ability of not-for-profit health services organizations to raise equity capital by grants and contributions; hence, the result is increased reliance on making money the old fashioned way—by earning it.

On the surface, investor-owned firms may appear to have a significant advantage in raising equity capital. In theory, new common stock can be issued at any time and in any reasonable amount. Conversely, charitable contributions are much less certain. The planning, solicitation, and collection periods can take years, and pledges are not always collected. Therefore, charitable contributions that were counted on may not materialize. Also, the proceeds of new stock sales may be used for any purpose, but charitable contributions may be *restricted*, in which case they can be used only for a designated purpose.

In reality, however, managers of investor-owned firms do **not** have complete freedom to raise capital by selling new common stock. First, the issuance expenses associated with a new common stock issue are not trivial. Second, if market conditions are poor and the stock is selling at a low price, a new stock issue can dilute the value of existing shares, and hence be harmful to current stockholders. Finally, new stock issues are often viewed by investors as a signal that the firm's stock is overvalued, and hence new issues often drive the stock price lower.

For all these reasons, managers of investor-owned firms would rather not issue new common stock. The key point here is that yes, for-profit health services organizations do have greater access to equity capital than do not-for-profit organizations. However, the differential access to equity capital may not be as great an advantage as it initially appears. The greatest advantage is for young, growing businesses that need a great deal of new capital. More mature companies have much less flexibility in raising new equity capital.

Self-Test Questions

1. What are the sources of equity (i.e., fund capital) to not-for-profit firms?
2. Are not-for-profit firms at a disadvantage when it comes to raising equity capital? Explain your answer.

Common Stock Valuation

Common stocks provide expected future cash flows and, hence, a stock's value is found in the same way as the values of most other assets—namely, as the present value of the expected future cash flow stream. The expected cash flows consist of two elements: the dividends expected in each year and the price investors expect to receive when they sell the stock.

The valuation discussion begins with definitions of the following terms:

- $E(D_t)$ = Dividend the stockholder **expects** to receive at the end of Year t. D_0 is the most recent dividend, which has already been paid and is known with certainty; $E(D_1)$ is the first dividend expected, and for valuation purposes is assumed to be paid **at the end** of one year; $E(D_2)$ is the dividend expected at the end of two years; and so forth. $E(D_1)$ represents the **first** cash flow a new purchaser of the stock will receive. D_0, the dividend that has just been paid, is known with certainty, but all future dividends are expected values, so the estimate of any $E(D_t)$ may differ among investors.[6]
- P_0 = Actual *market price* of the stock today.
- $E(P_t)$ = Expected price of the stock at the end of each Year t. $E(P_0)$ is the *intrinsic value* of the stock today, as seen by a particular investor based on his or her estimate of the stock's expected dividend stream and riskiness; $E(P_1)$ is the price expected at the end of one year; and so on. Thus, whereas P_0 is fixed and is identical for all investors, $E(P_0)$ will differ among investors depending on each investor's assessment of the stock's riskiness and dividend stream. $E(P_0)$, each investor's estimate of the intrinsic value today, could be above or below P_0, the current stock price, but an investor would buy the stock only if his or her estimate of $E(P_0)$ were equal to or greater than P_0.

- $E(g_t)$ = Expected growth rate in dividends in each future Year t. Different investors may use different $E(g_t)$s to evaluate a firm's stock. In reality, $E(g_t)$ is normally different for each Year t. However, the valuation process will be simplified by assuming that $E(g_t)$ is constant across time.
- $R(R_i)$ = Required rate of return on Stock i, considering both its riskiness and the returns available on other investments. In Chapter 10, the Capital Asset Pricing Model (CAPM) was introduced including an illustration of how the Security Market Line (SML) can be used to estimate $R(R_i)$.
- $E(R_i)$ = Expected rate of return on Stock i. $E(R_i)$ could be above or below $R(R_i)$, but an investor would buy the stock only if his or her $E(R_i)$ were equal to or greater than $R(R_i)$. Note that $E(R_i)$ is an **expectation**. A return of $E(R_i)$ = 15% may be expected if Columbia/HCA Healthcare stock were purchased today. If either conditions in the market or prospects at Columbia/HCA take a turn for the worse, however, the realized return may be much lower than that expected—perhaps even negative.
- $E(D_1)/P_0$ = Expected *dividend yield* on a stock during the first year. If a stock is expected to pay a dividend of $1 during the next 12 months and if its current price is $10, then its expected dividend yield is $1 / $10 = 0.10 = 10%.
- $[E(P_1) - P_0] / P_0$ = Expected *capital gains yield* on the stock during the first year. If the stock sells for $10 today and if it is expected to rise to $10.50 at the end of the year, then the expected capital gain is $E(P_1) - P_0$ = $10.50 - $10.00 = $0.50 and the expected capital gains yield is $[E(P_1) - P_0] / P_0$ = $0.50 / $10 = 0.050 = 5%.

Expected Dividends as the Basis for Stock Values

In the discussion of long-term debt in Chapter 11, the value of a bond was found by adding the present value of the interest payments over the life of the bond to the present value of the bond's maturity, or par, value. In essence, a bond's value is the present value of the cash flows expected from the bond. Stock prices are likewise determined as the present value of a stream of cash flows, and the basic stock valuation equation is similar to the bond valuation equation. What are the cash flows that stocks provide to their holders? First, consider an investor who buys a stock with the intention of holding it in his or her family forever. In this situation, all the investor and his or her heirs will receive is a stream of dividends, and the value of the stock today is calculated as the present value of an infinite stream of dividends.[7]

Consider the more typical case in which an investor expects to hold the stock for a finite period and then sell it. What would be the value of the stock in this case? The value of the stock is again the present value of the expected dividend stream. To see this, recognize that for any individual investor, expected cash flows consist of expected dividends plus the expected price of the stock when it is sold. However, the sale price received by the current investor will depend on the dividends some future investor expects to receive. Therefore, for all present and future investors in total, expected cash flows must be based on expected future dividends. To put it another way, unless a business is liquidated or sold to another concern, the cash flows it provides to its stockholders consist only of a stream of dividends; therefore, the value of a share of its stock must be the present value of that expected dividend stream.

The validity of this concept can also be confirmed by asking the following question: Suppose that an investor buys a stock and expects to hold it for one year? He or she will receive dividends during the year plus the value $E(P_1)$ when selling out at the end of the year, but what will determine the value of $E(P_1)$? It will be determined as the present value of the dividends during Year 2 plus the stock price at the end of that year, which in turn will be determined as the present value of another set of future dividends and an even more distant stock price. This process can be continued ad infinitum, and the ultimate result is that the value of a stock is the present value of its expected dividend stream regardless of the holding period of the investor who performs the analysis. Occasionally, stock shares could have additional value, such as the value of a controlling interest when an investor buys 51 percent of a company's outstanding stock, or the added value brought about by a takeover bid. However, in most situations, the sole value inherent in stock ownership stems from the dividends expected to be paid by the company to its shareholders.

Investors periodically lose sight of the long-run nature of stocks as investments and forget that in order to sell a stock at a profit, one must find a buyer who will pay the higher price. Suppose that a stock's value is analyzed on the basis of expected future dividends, and the conclusion is that the stock's market price exceeded a reasonable value. If an investor buys the stock anyway, he or she would be following the "bigger fool" theory of investment: The investor may be a fool to buy the stock at its excessive price, but he or she believes that when ready to sell, an even bigger fool can be found.

The concept of the value of a stock being the present value of the expected dividend stream holds regardless of the pattern of growth. Dividends can be rising, falling, constant, or can fluctuate more or less randomly. Thus, stocks can always be valued by projecting the expected dividend stream and then finding the present value of that stream. It is not even necessary to project the stream for more than 40 or 50 years. Because of the time value of money, dividends beyond that point contribute an insignificant amount to a stock's value today. Needless to say, it is generally not possible to have much confidence in dividend values projected over a 40- or 50-year period, so stock valuation must be viewed as something of an approximation.

Constant Growth Stock Valuation

Often, the projected stream of dividends follows a systematic pattern; hence, it is possible to develop a simplified (i.e., easier to evaluate) version of the general stock valuation model. This section discusses the most common simplifying assumption: *constant growth*.

Although the dividends of only a few firms actually grow at a constant rate, the assumption of constant growth is often made because it makes the forecasting of individual dividends over a long time period unnecessary. Furthermore, many firms come close to meeting constant growth assumptions. For a constant growth company, the expected dividend growth rate is constant for all years, so $E(g_1) = E(g_2) = E(g_3)$ and so on, which implies that $E(g_t)$ becomes merely $E(g)$. Under this assumption, the dividend in any future Year t may be forecast as $E(D_t) = D_0 \times [1 + E(g)]^t$, where D_0 is the last dividend paid, and hence is known with certainty, and $E(g)$ is the constant expected rate of growth. Alternatively, each year's dividend is $E(g)$ percent greater than the previous dividend, so $E(D_t) = E(D_{t-1}) \times [1 + E(g)]$.

To illustrate, if Minnesota Health Systems, Inc., (MHS) just paid a dividend of $1.82 (i.e., $D_0 = \$1.82$) and if investors expect a 10 percent constant dividend growth rate, the dividend expected in one year will be $E(D_1) = \$1.82 \times 1.10 = \$2.00$; $E(D_2)$ will be $\$1.82 \times (1.10)^2 = \$2.20$; the dividend expected in five years will be $E(D_5) = D_0 \times [1 + E(g)]^5 = \$1.82 \times (1.10)^5 = \$2.93$. This method of estimating future dividends can be used to estimate MHS's expected future cash flow stream (i.e., the dividends) for some time into the future, say, 50 years. Then, the present values of this stream can be summed to find the value of MHS's stock.

If $E(g)$ is assumed to be constant, however, a stock can be valued using a simplified model called the *constant growth model*:

$$E(P_0) = \frac{D_0 \times [1 + E(g)]}{R(R_i) - E(g)} = \frac{E(D_1)}{R(R_i) - E(g)}$$

where $R(R_i)$ is the required rate of return on the stock. If $D_0 = \$1.82$, $E(g) = 10\%$, and $R(R_i) = 16\%$ for MHS, the value of its stock would be $33.33:

$$E(P_0) = \frac{\$1.82 \times 1.10}{0.16 - 0.10} = \frac{\$2.00}{0.06} = \$33.33.$$

A necessary condition for the derivation of the constant growth model is that the required rate of return on the stock is greater than its constant dividend growth rate, that is, $R(R_i)$ is greater than $E(g)$. If the constant growth model is used when $R(R_i)$ is not greater than $E(g)$, the results will be meaningless. However, to qualify as a constant growth stock, dividends must be expected to grow at the constant growth rate forever, or at least for a long time. Although stocks can have $E(g)$ greater than $R(R_i)$ for short periods, $E(g)$ cannot exceed $R(R_i)$ over the long run because $E(g)$ measures long-term growth. Although the constant growth model is applied here to stock valuation, it can be used in any situation in which cash flows are growing at a constant rate.

How does an investor determine his or her required rate of return on a particular stock, $R(R_i)$? One way is to use the Security Market Line (SML) of the Capital Asset Pricing Model as discussed in Chapter 10. Assume that MHS's market beta, as reported by a financial advisory service, is 1.5. Assume also that the risk-free rate (the interest rate on long-term Treasury bonds) is 7 percent and the required rate of return on the market is 13 percent. According to the SML, the required rate of return on MHS's stock is 16.0 percent:

$$R(R_{MHS}) = RF + [R(R_M) - RF] \times b_{MHS}$$
$$= 7\% + (13\% - 7) \times 1.5$$
$$= 7\% + (6\% \times 1.5)$$
$$= 7\% + 9\% = 16\%.$$

Remember, in the SML, RF is the riskfree rate, $R(R_M)$ is the required rate of return on the market, or the required rate of return on a b = 1.0 stock, and b_{MHS} is MHS's market beta.

Growth in dividends occurs primarily as a result of growth in earnings per share (EPS). Earnings growth, in turn, results from a number of factors including the general inflation rate in the economy and the amount of earnings the company retains and reinvests. Regarding inflation, if output in units is stable and if both sales prices and input costs increase at the inflation rate, EPS also will grow at the inflation rate. EPS will also grow as a result of the reinvestment, or plowback, of earnings. If the firm's earnings are not all paid out as dividends (i.e., if a fraction of earnings is retained), the dollars of investment behind each share will rise over time, which should lead to growth in productive assets, and hence growth in earnings and dividends.

When using the constant growth model, the most critical input is E(g), the expected constant growth rate in dividends. Investors can make their own E(g) estimates on the basis of historical dividend growth, but E(g) estimates are also available from brokerage and investment advisory firms.

Expected Rate of Return on a Constant Growth Stock   The constant growth model can be rearranged to solve for $E(R_i)$, the *expected rate of return*. In the model's normal form, $R(R_i)$ is the required rate of return, but when the model is transformed, the expected rate of return, $E(R_i)$, is found. This transformation requires that the required rate of return equal the expected rate of return, or $R(R_i) = E(R_i)$. This equality holds if the stock is in equilibrium, which will be discussed later in the chapter. After solving the constant growth model for $E(R_i)$, this expression is obtained:

$$E(R_i) = \frac{D_0 \times [1 + E(g)]}{P_0} + E(g) = \frac{E(D_1)}{P_0} + E(g).$$

If an investor buys MHS's stock today for $P_0 = \$33.33$, and expects the stock to pay a dividend $E(D_1) = \$2.00$ one year from now and for dividends to grow at a constant rate $E(g) = 10\%$ in the future, the expected rate of return on that stock is 16 percent:

$$E(R_i) = \frac{\$2.00}{\$33.33} + 10.0\% = 6.0\% + 10.0\% = 16.0\%.$$

In this form, $E(R_i)$, the expected total return on the stock, consists of an expected dividend yield, $E(D_1)/P_0 = 6.0\%$, plus an expected growth rate or capital gains yield, $E(g) = 10\%$.

Suppose this analysis had been conducted on January 1, 1998, so $P_0 = \$33.33$ is MHS's January 1, 1998, stock price and $E(D_1) = \$2.00$ is the dividend expected at the end of 1998. What is the value of $E(P_1)$, the company's stock price expected at the end of 1998 (the beginning of 1999)? The constant growth model would again be applied, but this time the 1999 dividend, $E(D_2) = E(D_1) \times [1 + E(g)] = \$2.00 \times 1.10 = \$2.20$, would be used:

$$E(P_1) = \frac{E(D_2)}{R(R_i) - E(g)} = \frac{\$2.20}{0.06} = \$36.67.$$

Notice that $E(P_1) = \$36.67$ is 10 percent greater than $P_0 = \$33.33$: $\$33.33 \times 1.10 = \$36.67$. Thus, a capital gain of $\$36.67 - \$33.33 = \$3.34$ would be expected during 1998, which results in a capital gains yield of 10 percent:

$$\text{Capital gains yield} = \frac{\text{Capital gain}}{\text{Beginning price}} = \frac{\$3.34}{\$33.33} = 0.100 = 10.0\%.$$

If the analysis were extended, in each future year the expected capital gains yield would always equal $E(g)$ because the stock price would grow at the 10 percent constant dividend growth rate. The expected dividend yield in 1999 (Year 2) could be found as follows:

$$\text{Dividend yield} = \frac{E(D_2)}{E(P_1)} = \frac{\$2.20}{\$36.67} = 0.060 = 6.0\%.$$

The dividend yield for 2000 (Year 3) could also be calculated and again it would be 6 percent. Thus, for a constant growth stock, the following conditions must hold:

- The dividend is expected to grow forever (or at least for a long time) at a constant rate, $E(g)$.
- The stock price is expected to grow at this same rate.
- The expected dividend yield is a constant.
- The expected capital gains yield is also a constant and is equal to $E(g)$.
- The expected total rate of return in any Year t, which is equal to the expected dividend yield plus the expected growth rate (expected capital gains yield), is expressed by this equation: $E(R_t) = [E(D_{t+1}) / E(P_t)] + E(g)$.

The term *expected* should be clarified—it means expected in a statistical sense. Thus, if MHS's dividend growth rate is expected to remain constant at 10 percent, the growth rate in each year can be represented by a probability distribution with an expected value of 10 percent and not that the growth rate is expected to be exactly 10 percent in each future year. In this sense, the constant growth assumption is reasonable for many large, mature companies.

Nonconstant Growth Stock Valuation

What happens when a company does not meet the constant growth assumption? For example, what if MHS's dividend was expected to grow at 30 percent for three years and then to settle down to a constant growth rate of 10 percent? Under these nonconstant growth conditions, the value of MHS's stock would be $53.86, which is significantly higher than the $33.33 value of the stock assuming 10 percent constant growth. Dividend growth of 30 percent for three years followed by 10 percent constant growth creates a more valuable expected dividend stream than straight constant growth at 10 percent. In this situation, the constant growth model does not apply, so it was necessary to apply a nonconstant growth model to value the stock. Although nonconstant stock valuation models are not very complicated, they are beyond the scope of an introductory text on healthcare finance.[8]

Self-Test Questions

1. What is the basis for valuing common stocks? Does the holding period matter?
2. Write out and explain the valuation model for a constant growth stock.
3. What are the assumptions of the constant growth model?
4. Show the constant growth model in its expected rate of return form.
5. What are the key features of constant growth regarding dividend yield and capital gains yield?

Security Market Equilibrium

Investors will want to buy a security if its expected rate of return exceeds its required rate of return or, put another way, when its value exceeds its current price. Conversely, investors will want to sell a security when its required rate of return exceeds its expected rate of return (i.e., when its current price exceeds its value). When more investors want to buy a security than to sell it, its price is bid up. When more investors want to sell a security than to buy it, its price falls. In *equilibrium*, these two conditions must hold:

1. The expected rate of return on a security must equal its required rate of return to the marginal investor. This means that no investor who owns the stock believes that its expected rate of return is less than its required rate of return, and no investor who does not own the stock believes that its expected rate of return is greater than its required rate of return.
2. The market price of a security must equal its value to the marginal investor.

If these conditions do not hold, trading will occur until they do. Of course, security prices are not constant. A security's price can swing wildly as new information becomes available to the market that changes investors' expectations concerning the security's cash flow stream, or risk, or when the general level of returns (i.e., interest rates) change. However, evidence suggests that securities prices, especially of securities that are actively traded, such as those issued by the U. S. Treasury or by large companies, adjust rapidly to disequilibrium situations. Thus, most people believe that the bonds of the U. S. Treasury and the bonds and stocks of major corporations are generally in equilibrium. The key to the rapid movement of security prices toward equilibrium is informational efficiency, which is discussed in the next section.

1. What is meant by security market equilibrium?
2. What securities are most likely to be in equilibrium?

Self-Test Questions

Informational Efficiency

A securities market, say the market for long-term U. S. Treasury bonds, is informationally efficient if all information relevant to the values of the securities traded can be obtained easily and at low cost, and the market contains many buyers and sellers who act rationally on this information. If these conditions hold, current market prices will have embedded in them all information of possible relevance; hence, future price movements will be based solely on **new** information as it becomes known.

The *Efficient Markets Hypothesis (EMH)*, which is an important concept in financial market analysis, hypothesizes that current market prices reflect all publicly available information.[9] Therefore, spending hours on analyzing past price movements, economic data, or financial reports makes no sense because any information found, whether good or bad, is already embedded in current prices.

The EMH is a hypothesis, not a proven fact. However, hundreds of empirical tests have been conducted to try to prove or disprove the EMH, and the results are relatively consistent. Most tests support the EMH for well-developed markets, such as the U. S. markets for large firms' stocks and bonds, and for Treasury securities. Supporters of the EMH contend that there are some 100,000 or so full-time, highly trained professional analysts and traders who operate in these markets. Furthermore, most of the analysts and traders work for companies such as Citibank, Fidelity Investments, Merrill Lynch, and Prudential, which have billions of dollars available to take advantage of undervalued securities. Finally, as a result of disclosure requirements and electronic information networks, new information about widely followed securities is almost instantaneously available. With immediate information and many analysts processing the information and passing it to traders who have the funds to act on it, security prices in major markets adjust almost immediately as new developments occur.

The EMH has important implications both for securities investment decisions and for business financing decisions. Because security prices appear to generally reflect all public information, most actively followed and traded securities are in equilibrium and fairly valued. This does not mean that new information could not cause a security's price to soar or to plummet, but it does mean that most securities are neither undervalued nor overvalued. Therefore, over the long run, an investor with no inside information can only expect to earn a return on a security that compensates him or her for the amount of risk assumed. In the short run (for example, a year) an investor can only expect to earn a return that is the same as the average for securities of equal risk. In other words, investors should not expect to "beat the market" after adjusting for risk. Also, because the EMH applies to most bond markets, bond prices, and hence interest rates, reflect all current public information. Consistently forecasting future interest rates is impossible because interest rates change in response to new information, and this information could either lower or raise rates.

For managers, the EMH indicates that managerial decisions generally should not be based on perceptions about the market's ability to properly price the firm's securities or on perceptions about which way interest rates will go. In other words, managers should not try to time security issues to try to catch stock prices while they are high or interest rates while they are low. However, in some situations, managers may have information about their own firms that is unknown to the public. This condition is called *asymmetric information*, which can affect managerial decisions. For example, suppose a drug manufacturer has made a breakthrough in AIDS research, but does not want to announce the development until it completes the final series of FDA tests. The firm may want to delay any new securities offerings because securities could probably be sold under more favorable terms once the announcement is made. Managers can and should act on inside information for the benefit of their firms, but inside information cannot legally be used for personal profit.

Are markets really efficient? If markets were not efficient, the better managers of stock and bond mutual funds and pension plans would be able to consistently outperform the broad averages over long periods of time. In fact, very few managers can consistently better the broad averages, and during most years, mutual fund managers, on average, underperform the market. In any year, some mutual fund managers will outperform the market and others will underperform the market—this is known with certainty. But, for an investor to beat the market by investing in mutual funds, he or she must identify the successful managers beforehand, which seems very difficult, if not impossible, to do.

In spite of the evidence, many theorists, and even more Wall Street experts, believe that pockets of inefficiency do exist. In some cases, entire markets may be inefficient. For example, the markets for the securities issued by small companies may be inefficient because there are neither enough analysts ferreting out information on these companies nor sufficient numbers of investors trading these securities. Many people even believe that individual securities traded in efficient markets are occasionally priced inefficiently, or that investor emotions can drive prices too high during raging bull markets or too low during whimpering bear markets. Still, it is wise for both investors and managers to consider the implications of market efficiency when making investment and financing decisions.

1. What two conditions must hold for markets to be efficient?
2. Briefly, what is the Efficient Markets Hypothesis (EMH)?
3. What are the implications of the EMH for investors and managers?

The Risk/Return Trade-Off

Most financial decisions involve alternative courses of action. For example, should a hospital invest its excess funds in Treasury bonds that yield 5 percent or in Revlon bonds that yield 10 percent? Should a group practice buy a replacement piece of equipment now or wait until next year? Should a joint venture outpatient diagnostic center purchase a small, limited-use MRI system or a large, and more expensive, multipurpose system?

Generally, the alternative courses of action will have different expected rates of return, and one may be tempted to automatically accept the alternative with the higher expected return. However, this approach to financial decision making would be incorrect. In efficient markets, those alternatives that offer higher returns will also entail higher risk. The correct question to ask when making financial decisions is not which alternative has the higher expected rate of return, but which alternative has the higher return **after adjusting for risk**. In other words, which alternative has the higher return over and above the return commensurate with that alternative's riskiness?

To illustrate the *risk/return trade-off*, suppose Columbia/HCA Healthcare's stock has an expected rate of return of 14 percent, while its bonds yield 9 percent. Does this mean that investors should flock to buy the company's stock and ignore the bonds? Of course not—the higher expected rate of return on the stock merely reflects the fact that the stock is riskier than the bonds. Those investors who are not willing to assume much risk will buy Columbia's bonds, while those that are less risk averse will buy the stock. From the perspective of Columbia's managers, financing with stock is less risky than using debt, so the firm is willing to pay the higher cost of equity to limit the firm's risk exposure.

In spite of the efficiency of major securities markets, the markets for products and services (i.e., the markets for real assets such as MRI systems) are usually not efficient; hence, returns are not necessarily related to risk. Thus, hospitals, group practices, and other healthcare businesses can make real asset investments and achieve returns in excess of those required by the riskiness of the investment. Furthermore, the market for *innovation* (i.e., the market for ideas) is not efficient. Thus, it is possible for people like Bill Gates, the founder of Microsoft, to become multibillionaires at a relatively young age. However, when excess returns are found in the product, service, or idea markets, new entrants quickly join the innovators, and competition over time will usually force rates of return down to efficient market levels. The result is that later entrants can only expect returns that are commensurate with the risks involved.

Self-Test Questions

1. Explain the meaning of the term *risk/return trade-off*.
2. In what markets does this trade-off hold?

Key Concepts

This chapter contains a wealth of material on equity financing including valuation, plus information on investment banking and market efficiency. The key concepts of this chapter are:

- The most important *common stockholder* rights are a claim on the firm's residual earnings, control, and the preemptive right.
- New common stock may be sold by for-profit corporations in six ways: on a pro rata basis to existing stockholders through a *rights offering;* through investment bankers to the general public in a *public offering*; to a single buyer, or small number of buyers, in a *private placement;* to employees through an *employee stock purchase plan;* to shareholders through a *dividend reinvestment plan;* and to individual investors by *direct purchase.*
- A *closely held corporation* is one that is owned by a few individuals who are typically associated with the firm's management.
- A *publicly owned corporation* is one that is owned by a relatively large number of individuals who are not actively involved in its management.
- Securities markets are regulated at the national level by the *Securities and Exchange Commission (SEC)* and at the state level by state agencies, which are often called *corporation commissions.*
- An *investment banker* assists in the issuing of securities by helping the business determine the size of the issue and the type of securities to be used, by establishing the selling price, by selling the issue, and in some cases, by maintaining an after-market for the securities.
- Not-for-profit firms do not have access to the equity markets. However, *charitable contributions*, which are tax deductible to the donor, and *governmental grants* constitute unique equity sources for not-for-profit firms.
- The *value* of a share of stock is found by *discounting* the stream of *expected dividends* by the stock's required rate of return.
- The value of a stock whose dividends are expected to grow at a constant rate for many years is found by applying the *constant growth model*:

$$E(P_0) = \frac{D_0 \times [1 + E(g)]}{R(R_i) - E(g)} = \frac{E(D_1)}{R(R_i) - E(g)}.$$

- The *expected rate of return* on a stock consists of an *expected dividend yield* plus an *expected capital gains yield.* For a constant growth stock, both the expected dividend yield and the expected capital gains yield are constant over time, and the expected rate of return can be found by this equation:

$$E(R_i) = \frac{D_0 \times [1 + E(g)]}{P_0} + E(g) = \frac{E(D_1)}{P_0} + E(g).$$

- The *Efficient Markets Hypothesis (EMH)* holds that stocks are always in equilibrium and fairly valued, it is impossible for an investor to consistently beat the market, and managers should not try to forecast future interest rates or time security issues.
- In efficient markets, alternatives that offer higher returns must also have higher risk; this is called the *risk/return trade-off*. The implication is that investments must be evaluated on the basis of both risk and return.

The coverage of long-term financing continues in Chapter 13 with a discussion of how managers choose between debt and equity financing. Additionally, Chapter 13 also covers the cost of capital, which is an important concept that provides the benchmark required rate of return used in capital investment analyses.

Questions

12.1 a. What is the preemptive right?
   b. Why is it important to shareholders?
12.2 Why might an investor-owned firm choose to issue different classes of common stock?
12.3 Describe the primary means by which investor-owned firms raise new equity capital.
12.4 What are the similarities and differences between equity capital in investor-owned firms and fund capital in not-for-profit firms?
12.5 What is the general approach for valuing a share of stock?
12.6 Two investors are evaluating the stock of Beverly Enterprises for possible purchase. They agree on the stock's risk and on expectations about future dividends. However, one investor plans to hold the stock for 5 years, while the other plans to hold the stock for 20 years. Which of the two investors would be willing to pay more for the stock? Explain your answer.
12.7 Evaluate the following statement: One of the assumptions of the constant growth model is that the required rate of return must be greater than the expected dividend growth rate. Because of this assumption, the constant growth model is of limited use in the real world.
12.8 a. What is the Efficient Markets Hypothesis (EMH)?
   b. What are its implications for investors and managers?
12.9 a. What is meant by the term *risk/return trade-off*?
   b. Does this trade-off hold in all markets?

Problems

12.1 A person is considering buying the stock of two home health companies that are similar in all respects except for the proportion of earnings paid out as dividends. Both companies are expected to earn $6 per share in the coming year, but Company D (for dividends) is expected to pay out the entire amount as dividends, while Company G (for growth) is expected to pay out only one-third of its earnings or $2 per share. The companies are equally risky, and their required rate of return is 15 percent. D's constant growth rate is zero and G's is 8.33 percent. What are the intrinsic values of Stocks D and G?

12.2 Medical Corporation of America (MCA) has a current stock price of $36 and its last dividend (D_0) was $2.40. In view of MCA's strong financial position, its required rate of return is 12 percent. If MCA's dividends are expected to grow at a constant rate in the future, what is the firm's expected stock price in five years?

12.3 A broker offers to sell a person shares of Bay Area Healthcare, which just paid a dividend of $2 per share. The dividend is expected to grow at a constant rate of 5 percent per year. The stock's required rate of return is 12 percent.

a. What is the expected dollar dividend over the next three years?

b. What is the current value of the stock and the expected stock price at the end of each of the next three years?

c. What is the expected dividend yield and capital gains yield for each of the next three years?

d. (1) What is the expected total return for each of the next three years?

(2) How does the expected total return compare with the required rate of return on the stock? Does this make sense? Explain your answer.

12.4 Assume the risk-free rate is 6 percent and the market risk premium is 6 percent. The stock of Physicians Care Network (PCN) has a beta of 1.5. The last dividend paid by PCN was $2 per share.

a. What would PCN's stock value be if the dividend was expected to grow at a constant:

(1) −5 percent?

(2) 0 percent?

(3) 5 percent?

(4) 10 percent?

b. What would be the stock value if the growth rate is 10 percent, but PCN's beta falls to:

(1) 1.0?

(2) 0.5?

12.5 Better Life Nursing Home, Inc., has maintained a dividend payment of $4 per share for many years. The same dollar dividend is expected to be paid in future years. If investors require a 12 percent rate of return on investments of similar risk, determine the value of the company's stock.

12.6 Jane's sister-in-law, a stockbroker at Invest, Inc., is trying to get Jane to buy the stock of HealthWest, a regional HMO. The stock has a current market price of $25, its last dividend ($D_0$) was $2.00, and the company's earnings and dividends are expected to increase at a constant growth rate of

10 percent. The required return on this stock is 20 percent. From a strict valuation standpoint, should Jane buy the stock?

12.7 Lucas Clinic's last dividend (D_0) was $1.50. Its current equilibrium stock price is $15.75 and its expected growth rate is a constant 5 percent. If the stockholders' required rate of return is 15 percent, what is the expected dividend yield and expected capital gains yield for the coming year?

12.8 St. John Medical, a surgical equipment manufacturer, has been hit hard by increased competition. Analysts predict that earnings and dividends will decline at a rate of 5 percent annually into the foreseeable future. If the firm's last dividend (D_0) was $2.00 and the investors' required rate of return is 15 percent, what will be the company's stock price in **three** years?

12.9 California Clinics, an investor-owned chain of ambulatory care clinics, just paid a dividend of $2 per share. The firm's dividend is expected to grow at a constant rate of 5 percent per year and investors require a 15 percent rate of return on the stock.

a. What is the stock's value?

b. Suppose the riskiness of the stock decreases, which causes the required rate of return to fall to 13 percent. Under these conditions what is the stock's value?

c. Return to the original 15 percent required rate of return. Assume that the dividend growth rate estimate is increased to a constant 7 percent per year. What is the stock's value?

Notes

1. Some for-profit firms use *preferred stock*, which is a form of equity financing that combines some features of both debt and common stock. However, few healthcare providers use preferred stock financing, so this source of financing will not be covered in this book.

2. If a firm is experiencing temporary financial difficulties, it may even borrow the funds necessary to pay the dividend expected by stockholders rather than lower or omit the payment.

3. For more details on the mechanics of a rights offering, see E. F. Brigham and L. C. Gapenski, *Intermediate Financial Management* (Fort Worth, TX: Dryden Press, 1996), 488–492.

4. Large security issues are announced in the *Wall Street Journal* and other publications by advertisements placed by the underwriters called *tombstones*. Check several recent issues of the *Wall Street Journal* to see if any healthcare issues are advertised.

5. Some types of not-for-profit corporations can sell shares to raise capital. However, such "stock" does not pay dividends and cannot be sold for a profit. Because such not-for-profit "stock" corporations are rare, they will not be covered in this text.

6. Stocks generally pay dividends quarterly, so theoretically they should be evaluated on a quarterly basis. However, in stock valuation, most analysts work on an annual basis because the data are not precise enough in most situations to warrant the refinement of a quarterly model.

7. Some stocks, especially those of start-up companies, currently pay no dividends. Furthermore, the owners of such companies often do not expect to ever receive dividends, but rather plan to cash out by selling the company either to another company or to another group of investors. The values of the stocks of such companies are not derived from dividends, but from other sources of cash flow. In the discussion here, the focus is on those companies whose cash flows to shareholders, and hence values, stem exclusively from dividend payments.

8. For more details on the valuation of nonconstant growth stocks, see E. F. Brigham and L. C. Gapenski, *Financial Management: Theory and Practice* (Fort Worth, TX: Dryden Press, 1997), 312–315.

9. For more information on the efficient markets hypothesis, see E. F. Brigham and L. C. Gapenski, *Financial Management: Theory and Practice* (Fort Worth, TX: Dryden Press, 1997), 319–322.

References

Dunn, K. C., G. B. Shields, and J. B. Stern. 1991. "The Dynamics of Leveraged Buy-Outs, Conversions, and Corporate Reorganizations of Not-For-Profit Health Care Institutions." *Topics in Health Care Financing* (Spring): 5–20.

Flaherty, M. P. 1991. "Planned Giving Programs as a Source of Financing: Creating a 'Win-Win' Situation for a Health Care Organization and Its Donors." *Topics in Health Care Financing* (Fall): 70–81.

Shields, G. B. and G. C. McKann. 1991. "Raising Health Care Capital Through the Public Equity Markets." *Topics in Health Care Financing* (Fall): 21–36.

Sykes, C. S., Jr. 1991. "The Role of Equity Financing in Today's Health Care Environment." *Topics in Health Care Financing* (Fall): 1–4.

Wallace, C. 1985. "Not-For-Profits Competing for Capital by Selling Stock in Alternative Ventures." *Modern Healthcare* (August): 32–38.

CHAPTER 13

CAPITAL STRUCTURE AND
THE COST OF CAPITAL

Learning Objectives

After studying this chapter, readers will be able to:

- Explain the effects of debt financing on a business' risk and return.
- Discuss the factors that influence the choice between debt and equity financing.
- Describe the general process for estimating a business' corporate cost of capital.
- Estimate the component costs as well as the overall (corporate) cost of capital for any healthcare business.
- Explain the economic interpretation of the corporate cost of capital and how it is used in capital investment decisions.

Introduction

In Chapter 1, the general concept of a business was described. In this discussion, it was noted that businesses have two basic sources of financing—debt and equity. Furthermore, Chapters 11 and 12 provided detailed information about specific features of such financing and how these securities are valued. Because there are two basic types of financing, managers must determine the best financing mix. The first part of Chapter 13 addresses this issue.

Another primary business decision is the selection of capital investments (i.e., real assets). From a financial perspective, businesses should choose those investments that promise a return at least as great as the cost of the funds needed to make the investment. Thus, an important element in the capital investment decision is the business' cost of funds. The second part of this chapter discusses the procedures for estimating the overall cost of a business' financing.

Capital Structure Basics

All firms, whether investor owned or not for profit, have to raise funds to buy the assets required to meet their strategic objectives. Hospitals, nursing homes, clinics, group practices, and so on, all need assets to provide services. The funds to acquire the assets come in many shapes and forms including contributions, profit retentions, equity sales to stockholders, and debt capital supplied by creditors such as banks, bondholders, lessors, and suppliers, but, in general, capital sources can be classified as either debt or equity.

The mix of debt and equity financing used by a business is called its *capital structure*, which is basically the structure of the right (liabilities and equity) side of the business' balance sheet. One of the most perplexing issues that health services managers must grapple with is how much debt financing, as opposed to equity (or fund) financing, should a business use? Is there an optimal mix of debt and equity (i.e., is there an *optimal capital structure*)? If optimal capital structures do exist, do hospitals have different optimal structures than home health agencies or ambulatory surgery centers? If so, what are the factors that lead to these differences? These questions, although difficult to answer, are important to the financial well-being of any business.[1]

Self-Test Questions

1. What is a business' capital structure?
2. What is meant by the term *capital structure decision*?

Impact of Debt Financing on Risk and Return

To fully understand the consequences of capital structure decisions, it is essential to understand the effects of debt financing on a business' risk and return. To help gain this understanding, consider the situation facing Super Health, Inc., a for-profit (investor-owned) company that is just being formed. The company requires $200,000 in assets to get into operation, and for simplicity, assume there are only two financing alternatives available: all equity (all common stock) and 50 percent equity/50 percent debt.

Table 13.1 contains the business' projected financial statements under the two financing alternatives. To begin, consider the balance sheets shown in the top portion of the table. The business will require $100,000 in current assets and $100,000 in fixed assets to get started. The asset requirement depends on the nature and size of the business rather than on how the business will be financed, so the asset side of the balance sheet is unaffected by the financing mix. However, the type of financing does affect the liabilities and equity side. Under the all-equity alternative, Super Health's owners will put up the entire $200,000 needed to purchase the assets. If 50 percent debt financing is used, the owners will contribute only $100,000, with the remaining $100,000 obtained from creditors, say, a bank loan with a 10 percent interest rate.

What is the impact of the two financing alternatives on Super Health's projected income statement? Revenues are projected to be $150,000 and operating costs are forecasted at $100,000, so the firm's operating income is expected to be $50,000. Because a business' capital structure does not affect revenues and operating costs, the operating income projection is the same under both financing alternatives.

However, interest expense must be paid if debt financing is used. Thus, the stock/debt alternative results in a $0.10 \times $100,000 = $10,000$ annual interest

	Stock	Stock/Debt
Balance Sheets		
Current assets	$ 100,000	$ 100,000
Fixed assets	100,000	100,000
Total assets	$200,000	$200,000
Bank loan (10% cost)	$ 0	$ 100,000
Common stock	200,000	100,000
Total claims	$200,000	$200,000
Income Statements		
Revenues	$ 150,000	$ 150,000
Operating costs	100,000	100,000
Operating income	$ 50,000	$ 50,000
Interest expense	0	10,000
Taxable income	$ 50,000	$ 40,000
Taxes (40%)	20,000	16,000
Net income	$ 30,000	$ 24,000
ROE	15%	24%
Total dollar return to investors	$ 30,000	$ 34,000

TABLE 13.1

Super Health, Inc.: Projected Financial Statements Under Two Financing Alternatives

charge, while no interest expense occurs if the firm is financed entirely by stock. The result is taxable income of $50,000 under the all-equity alternative and a lower taxable income of $40,000 under the stock/debt alternative. Because the business anticipates being taxed at a 40 percent federal-plus-state rate, the expected tax liability is $0.40 \times \$50,000 = \$20,000$ under the all-equity alternative, and $0.40 \times \$40,000 = \$16,000$ for the stock/debt alternative. Finally, when taxes are deducted from the income stream, the business projects $30,000 in net income if it is all-equity financed, and $24,000 in net income if 50 percent debt financing is used.

At first glance, the use of debt financing appears to be the **inferior** alternative. After all, if 50 percent debt financing is used, the business' projected net income will fall by $30,000 − $24,000 = $6,000. But the conclusion that debt financing is bad requires closer examination. What is most important to the owners of Super Health is not the business' net income, but rather the return expected on their equity investment. Perhaps the most meaningful measure of return to a firm's owners is the *rate of return on equity (ROE)*—defined as net income divided by the book value of common equity—which tells the owners the percentage return on their investment. Under all-equity financing, the projected ROE is $30,000 / $200,000 = 0.15 = 15%, but with 50 percent debt financing, the projected ROE increases to $24,000 / $100,000 = 24\%$. The key to the increased ROE is that although net income decreases when debt financing is used, so does the amount of equity capital needed, and the capital requirement decreases proportionally more than does net income.

The bottom line of this preliminary analysis is that debt financing can increase the owners' expected rate of return. Because the use of debt financing increases, or leverages up, the return to equityholders, such financing is often called *financial leverage*. Hence, the use of financial leverage is merely the use of debt financing.

To view the impact of financial leverage from a different perspective, take another look at the Table 13.1 income statements. The total dollar return to all investors, including **both** the owners and the bank, is $30,000 in net income if all-equity financed, but $24,000 in net income plus $10,000 of interest = $34,000 when 50 percent debt financing is used. Where did the extra $4,000 come from? The answer is from the tax man. Taxes are $20,000 if the business is all-equity financed, but only $16,000 when debt financing is used, and $4,000 less in taxes means $4,000 more for investors. Because the use of debt financing reduces taxes, more of a firm's operating income is now available for distribution to investors.[2]

At this point, it appears that Super Health's financing decision is a "no brainer." Given only these two financing alternatives, 50 percent debt financing should be used because it provides owners with a higher rate of return. Unfortunately, like the proverbial no free lunch, there is a catch. The use of financial leverage not only increases the owners' return, it also increases their risk.

To demonstrate the risk-increasing characteristics of debt financing, consider Table 13.2, which recognizes that Super Health, like all businesses, is risky. The first year's revenues and operating costs listed in Table 13.1 are **not** known with certainty, but rather are expected values taken from probability distributions. Super Health's founders believe that operating income could be as low as zero or as high as $100,000 in the business' first year of operation. Furthermore, there is a 25 percent chance of the worst and the best cases occurring, and a 50 percent chance that the Table 13.1 forecast, with an operating income of $50,000, will be realized.

The assumptions regarding uncertainty in the future profitability of the business lead to three different ROEs for each financing alternative. The expected ROEs are the same as when uncertainty was ignored (i.e., 15 percent if the firm is all-equity financed and 24 percent when 50 percent debt financing is used). For example, the expected ROE under all-equity financing is $(0.25 \times 0\%) + (0.50 \times 15\%) + (0.25 \times 30\%) = 15.0\%$. However, the uncertainty in operating income produces uncertainty, and hence risk, in the owners' returns. If owners' risk is measured by the standard deviation of ROE (stand-alone risk), the return is more risky when 50 percent debt financing is used. To be precise, the owners' risk is twice as much in the 50 percent debt financing alternative: 21.2 percent standard deviation of ROE versus 10.6 percent standard deviation in the zero debt alternative.[3]

	Stock			Stock/Debt			TABLE 13.2
Probability	0.25	0.50	0.25	0.25	0.50	0.25	Super Health, Inc.: Partial Income
Operating income	$0	$50,000	$100,000	$ 0	$50,000	$100,000	Statements in an
Interest expense	0	0	0	10,000	10,000	10,000	Uncertain World
Taxable income	$0	$50,000	$100,000	($10,000)	$40,000	$ 90,000	
Taxes (40%)	0	20,000	40,000	(4,000)	16,000	36,000	
Net income	$0	$30,000	$ 60,000	($ 6,000)	$24,000	$ 54,000	
ROE	0%	15%	30%	−6%	24%	54%	
Expected ROE		15%			24%		
Standard deviation of ROE		10.6%			21.2%		

The increase in risk is apparent without even calculating standard deviations of ROE. If only stock financing is used, the worst return that can occur is a ROE of zero. However, with 50 percent debt financing, a ROE of −6 percent can occur. In fact, with no operating income to pay the $10,000 interest to the bank in the worst case scenario, the owners would either have to put up additional funds to pay the interest due (assuming insufficient deprecation cash flow) or declare the business bankrupt. Clearly, the use of 50 percent debt financing has increased the riskiness of the owners' investment.

This simple example illustrates two key points about the use of debt financing:

- A business' use of debt financing increases the percentage return (ROE) to owners.[4]
- At the same time that return is increased, the use of debt financing also increases owners' risk. In the Super Health example, 50 percent debt financing doubled the owners' risk as measured by standard deviation of ROE.

When risk is considered, the ultimate decision on which financing alternative should be chosen is not so clear cut. The zero debt alternative has a lower expected ROE, but also lower risk. The 50 percent debt alternative offers a higher expected ROE, but carries with it more risk. Thus, the decision is a classic risk/return trade-off; higher returns can be obtained only by assuming greater risk. What Super Health's founders need to know is whether or not the higher return is **enough** to compensate them for the higher risk assumed. To complicate the decision even more, there is actually an almost unlimited number of debt level choices available, not just the 50/50 mix used in the illustration. This example vividly illustrates that health services managers face a difficult decision in setting a business' optimal capital structure.

1. What is the impact of debt financing on owners' rate of return?
2. What is the impact of debt financing on owners' risk?
3. What is the basis for choosing the level of debt financing?

Capital Structure Theory

At the end of the previous section, Super Health's founders were left in a quandary because debt financing brings with it both higher returns and higher risk. *Capital structure theory*, which was developed for investor-owned businesses, attempts to resolve their dilemma. If the relationship between the use of debt financing and equity value (stock price) were known, then the optimal capital structure could be identified.

There are many competing theories of capital structure, but one theory—the *trade-off theory*—is most widely accepted. In general, this theory tells managers that an optimal capital structure does exist for every firm. Furthermore, the optimal structure balances the tax advantages of debt financing against the increased risk that arises when debt financing is used. The trade-off theory is summarized in Figure 13.1. Here, the proportion of debt in a firm's capital structure is plotted on the X axis, while the Y axis plots the costs of debt and equity, as well as the combined cost of both financing sources. The focus in Figure 13.1 is not on the absolute level of debt financing—larger firms have higher dollar values of debt than do smaller firms. Rather, the X axis variable is the **proportion** of debt—0 percent (i.e., no debt), 10 percent, 20 percent, and so on, up to 100 percent (i.e., all debt).

First, consider the relationship between the cost of debt and proportion of debt financing. As a business uses a greater proportion of debt financing, the risk to creditors increases because the greater the debt service requirement, the higher the probability that default will occur. In essence, the greater the proportion of debt financing, the riskier the lender's position. Thus, the cost of debt (i.e., the interest rate) increases as the proportion of debt increases. However, the cost of debt increases slowly at low and moderate proportions of debt because the incremental risk to lenders is relatively small, but then increases at a faster rate as even more debt is used. Thus, the cost of debt line first rises slowly and then, as even more debt is used, rises at an even faster rate.

As discussed in the Super Health illustration, the use of debt financing also increases the risk to equityholders. Furthermore, the greater the proportion of debt, the greater the risk. Thus, the cost of equity also increases with the proportion of debt financing, just as does the cost of debt. The primary difference between the cost of debt and the cost of equity curves is not their shape, but rather where they are located on the graph. The cost of equity is higher because owners face more risk than creditors. (Equityholders have a residual claim on the

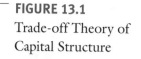

FIGURE 13.1

Trade-off Theory of Capital Structure

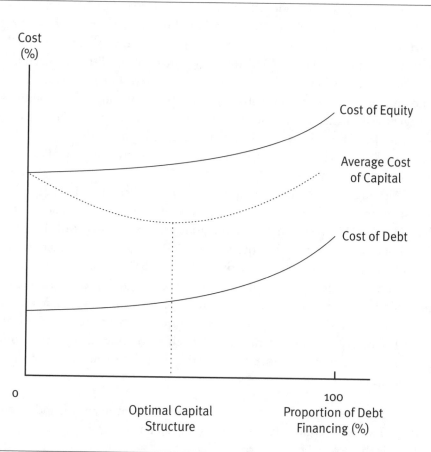

earnings of the firm, while creditors' claims are fixed by contract.) Furthermore, the cost of debt is lowered even more relative to equity because interest payments are tax deductible, while returns to equityholders are not. Thus, as shown in Figure 13.1, the cost of equity is appreciably greater than the cost of debt at any level of debt.

In practice, firms tend to use some, but not all, debt financing, so firms actually use a blend of the two major sources of financing. Under these conditions, what is most relevant to financing decisions is not just the cost of debt or just the cost of equity, but rather the weighted average (blended) cost of the two components. The weighted average cost is shown on the graph as a dotted line labeled average cost of capital. At zero debt (the Y axis), the firm is all-equity financed, so its average cost of capital is simply its cost of equity. When a business first starts using debt financing, it adds a lower cost component to its capital structure, and hence the average cost of financing decreases. However, as the proportion of debt financing increases, both the cost of equity and the cost of debt increase at an increasing rate. At some point, the increasing component costs outweigh the fact that more of the lower cost debt component is being used and the average cost of capital bottoms out. Beyond this point, the average cost of capital begins to increase.

According to the trade-off theory of capital structure, the point at which the firm's average cost of capital is minimized defines the firm's *optimal capital structure*. At this structure, overall financing costs are minimized. Capital, like labor, is an input to the firm and the firm's financial condition is maximized at any given output when its input costs are minimized. Once the optimal capital structure, or perhaps an optimal range, has been identified for a business, its managers will finance asset acquisitions in a way that keeps the firm at its optimal structure. Thus, the optimal capital structure becomes the target for future financing. For this reason, a firm's optimal capital structure is also called its *target capital structure*.

Although theory indicates that every business has an optimal capital structure, it turns out that it is not easy in practice to identify this structure for any given business. However, there is some good news associated with Figure 13.1. Empirical studies confirm that the average cost of capital curve, similar to the one plotted in the figure, has a relatively shallow shape. Thus, variations in debt usage from the optimal structure do not have a significant impact on capital costs, and hence it is not essential to financial performance that managers be able to identify a business' precise optimal structure. Furthermore, even if a precise optimal structure could be identified, relatively large movements away from this structure, which commonly occur in practice, will not materially affect financial performance.

Self-Test Questions

1. What is the relationship between a firm's use of debt financing and its cost of debt? Its cost of equity? Its overall cost of capital?
2. How is the optimal capital structure defined?
3. Is it critical that the precise structure be identified and followed?

Identifying the Optimal Capital Structure in Practice

Unfortunately, as stated in the previous section, theory does not tell us the precise optimal capital structure for any business. That is, a graph such as the one in Figure 13.1 cannot be created for a particular firm and then used to identify the firm's optimal capital structure. The problem is that the component costs, particularly the cost of equity, cannot be estimated with any confidence at different capital structures.

Because the optimal capital structure cannot be determined precisely, managers must apply a great deal of judgment in the capital structure decision. The judgmental analysis involves several different factors, and in one situation a particular factor may have great importance, while the same factor may be relatively unimportant in another situation. Here are some of the more important judgmental issues that managers consider in setting a firm's target capital structure.

Business Versus Financial Risk

Businesses have a certain amount of risk, called *business risk*, inherent in operations even when no debt financing is used. This risk is associated with the ability of managers to forecast future profitability. The more difficult the forecasting process, the greater the inherent risk of the business. To illustrate, refer to Table 13.2. Super Health's business risk can be measured by the standard deviation of ROE **assuming the firm uses zero debt financing**. Thus, the business risk of Super Health is 10.6 percent. If no debt financing is used, return on equity is also return on assets, so business risk is measured by the inherent uncertainty in the return on a business' assets.

When debt financing is used, equityholders must bear additional risk. In a capital structure context, the risk added when debt financing is used is called *financial risk*. For Super Health, the standard deviation of ROE when 50 percent debt financing is used is 21.1 percent. The difference between the standard deviations of ROE with debt financing and without debt financing measures the amount of financial risk. Thus, for Super Health, the financial risk at 50 percent debt financing is 21.1% − 10.6% = 10.6%. Using a mix of half debt and half equity doubles the risk to the owners of a business.

In general, managers will place some limit on the total amount of risk, including **both** business and financial, undertaken by a business. Thus, the greater the inherent business risk, the less "room" available for the use of financial leverage, and hence the lower the proportion of debt used. As an example, pharmaceutical firms generally are regarded as having a great deal of business risk, and hence they tend to use a relatively low proportion of debt financing.

Lender and Rating Agency Attitudes

Regardless of a manager's own analysis of the proper capital structure for his or her firm, there is no question that lenders' and rating agencies' attitudes are frequently important determinants of financial structures. In the majority of situations, corporate managers discuss the business' financial structure with lenders and rating agencies and give much weight to their advice. Often, managers want to maintain some target debt rating, say, single A. Furthermore, rating agencies, such as S&P, publish guidelines that link firm's capital structures within an industry to specific bond ratings, so guidance is readily available.

In addition, if a particular firm's management is so confident of the future that it seeks to use debt financing beyond the norms of its industry, lenders may be unwilling to accept such debt increases or may do so only at a high price. In effect, lenders and rating agencies set an absolute limit on the proportion of debt financing that can be used by any business.

Reserve Borrowing Capacity

Firms generally maintain a *reserve borrowing capacity* that preserves the ability to issue debt when conditions so dictate. In essence, managers want to maintain financial flexibility, that is, they want to ensure, to the extent possible, that the firm always has access to alternative forms of capital under reasonable terms. For example, suppose Merck had just successfully completed an R&D program on a new drug and its internal projections forecast much higher earnings in the future.

However, the new earnings are not yet anticipated by investors, and hence are not reflected in the price of its stock. Merck's managers would not want to issue stock; they would prefer to finance with debt until the higher earnings materialized and were reflected in the stock price, at which time the firm could sell an issue of common stock, retire the debt, and return to its target capital structure. To maintain this reserve borrowing capacity, firms generally use less debt than other factors may indicate should be used.

Industry Averages

Presumably, managers act rationally, so the capital structures of other firms in the industry, particularly the industry leaders, should provide insights about the optimal structure. In general, there is no reason to believe that the managers of one firm are better than the managers of any other firm. Thus, if one firm has a capital structure that is significantly different from other firms in its industry, the managers of that firm should identify the unique circumstances that contribute to the anomaly. If unique circumstances cannot be identified, then it is doubtful that the firm has identified the correct target structure.

Asset Structure

Firms whose assets are suitable as security for loans pay lower interest rates on debt financing than do other firms, and hence tend to use debt heavily. Thus, hospitals tend to be highly leveraged, but companies involved in technological research use relatively little debt. Both the ability to use assets as collateral and low inherent business risk give a firm more *debt capacity*, and hence a target capital structure that includes a relatively high proportion of debt.

Self-Test Questions
1. Is the capital structure decision mostly objective or subjective?
2. What is the difference between business and financial risk?
3. What are some of the factors that managers must consider when setting the target capital structure?

Not-for-Profit Firms

The discussion of capital structure has focused on investor-owned firms. What about not-for-profit firms? The same general concepts apply; namely, some debt financing is good, but too much is bad. However, not-for-profit firms have a unique problem—they cannot go to the capital markets to raise equity capital. If an investor-owned firm has more capital investment opportunities than it can finance with retained earnings and debt financing, it can always raise the needed funds by a new stock issue. It may be costly, but it can be done. Additionally, it is quite easy for investor-owned firms to adjust their capital structures. If they are financially underleveraged (i.e., using too little debt), they can simply issue more debt and use the proceeds to repurchase stock. On the other hand, if they are financially overleveraged (i.e., using too much debt), they can issue additional shares and use the proceeds to refund debt.

Not-for-profit firms do not have access to the equity markets, their sources of equity capital consist of government grants, private contributions, and excess revenues (i.e., retained earnings). Managers of not-for-profit organizations do not have the same degree of flexibility in either capital investment or capital structure decisions as do their proprietary counterparts. Thus, it is sometimes necessary for not-for-profit firms to delay new projects, even profitable ones, because of funding insufficiencies, or to use more than the theoretically optimal amount of debt because that is the only way that needed services can be financed.

Although such actions may be required in certain situations, not-for-profit managers must recognize that these strategies increase costs. Project delays mean that needed services are not being provided on a timely basis. Using more debt than optimal pushes the firm beyond the point of the greatest net benefit of debt financing, and hence capital costs are increased above the minimum. If a not-for-profit firm is forced into a situation where it is using more than the optimal amount of debt financing, its managers should plan to reduce the firm's level of debt, as soon as the situation permits.

The ability of a not-for-profit firm to garner governmental grants, attract private contributions, and generate earnings plays an important role in establishing its competitive position. A firm that has an adequate amount of equity (fund) capital can operate at its optimal capital structure, and thus minimize capital costs. If insufficient equity capital is available, too much financial leverage is then used and the result is higher capital costs. To illustrate this point, consider two not-for-profit hospitals that are similar in all respects except that one has more equity capital and can operate at its optimal structure, while the other has insufficient equity capital and thus must use more debt financing than optimal. In effect, the hospital with insufficient equity must operate at an inefficient capital structure. The former has a significant competitive advantage because it can either offer more services at the same cost by using additional, nonoptimal debt financing or it can offer matching services at lower costs.

Sufficient equity capital provides not-for-profit businesses with the flexibility to offer all of the necessary services and still operate at the lowest capital cost structure. Like companies that have low operating cost structures, not-for-profit firms that have low capital cost structures (that is, operating at their optimal capital structures) have an advantage over their competitors that have higher capital cost structures.

Self-Test Questions

1. What unique problems do managers of not-for-profit businesses face regarding capital structure decisions?
2. Why is capital structure important to the managers of not-for-profit businesses?

Cost of Capital Basics

In the first part of this chapter, the discussion focused on choosing between debt and equity financing. Once that decision is made, the business will raise capital over time in accordance with its optimal (target) structure. Now, the discussion turns to identifying the specific costs associated with that structure.

The ultimate goal of the cost of capital estimation process is to estimate the business' *corporate cost of capital*, which represents the blended, or average, cost of a business' financing. This cost, in turn, is used as the required rate of return, or hurdle rate, on the business' capital investment opportunities. For example, assume Bayside Memorial Hospital has a corporate cost of capital of 10 percent. If a new MRI investment is expected to return at least 10 percent, then it is financially attractive to the hospital. If the MRI is expected to return less than 10 percent, accepting it will have an adverse effect on the hospital's financial soundness. For now, the illustration assumes that the MRI investment has the same risk as Bayside's average project. As discussed in Chapter 16, the corporate cost of capital must be adjusted to reflect project risk when it differs from the overall risk of the business.

The corporate cost of capital is a weighted average of the *component* (i.e., debt and equity) *costs.* After the component costs have been estimated, they are combined to form the corporate cost of capital. Thus, the first step in the cost of capital estimation process is to estimate both the cost of debt and the cost of equity. However, before the mechanics of cost estimation are discussed, some other points regarding the estimation process should be mentioned.

What Capital Components Should Be Included?

The first task in estimating a business' corporate cost of capital is to determine which sources of capital on the right side of the balance sheet should be included in the estimate. In general, the corporate cost of capital focuses on the cost of *permanent* (long-term) *capital* because these are the sources used to finance capital asset acquisitions. Thus, for most firms, the capital components included in the corporate cost of capital estimate are equity and long-term debt. Typically, short-term debt is used only as temporary financing to support seasonal or cyclical fluctuations in volume, and hence it is not included in the cost of capital estimate. However, if a firm does use short-term debt as part of its permanent financing mix, then such debt should be included in the cost of capital estimate. As discussed in Chapter 16, the use of short-term debt to finance permanent assets is highly risky and is not common under normal conditions.

Do Taxes Need To Be Considered?

In developing component costs, the issue of taxes arises for investor-owned companies. Should the component costs be estimated on a before- or after-tax basis? As discussed in the previous section on capital structure, the use of debt financing creates a tax benefit because interest expense is tax deductible, while the use of equity financing has no impact on taxes. This tax benefit can be handled in several ways when working with capital costs, but the most common way is to include it in the cost of capital estimate. Thus, the tax benefit associated with debt financing will be recognized in the component cost of debt estimate, which results in an after-tax cost of debt. For not-for-profit firms, the benefit that arises from the issuance of tax-exempt debt will be incorporated directly in the cost estimate because investors require a lower interest rate on tax-exempt (i.e., municipal) debt.

Should the Focus Be on Historical or Marginal Costs?

Two very different sets of capital costs can be measured: *historical*, or *embedded*, *costs*, which reflect the cost of funds raised in the past, and *new*, or *marginal*, *costs*, which measure the cost of funds to be raised in the future. Historical costs are important for many purposes. For example, payors that reimburse on a cost basis are concerned with embedded costs. However, the primary purpose in developing a firm's corporate cost of capital is to use it in making capital investment decisions, which involve future asset acquisitions and future financing. Thus, for these purposes, the relevant costs are the marginal costs of new funds to be raised during some future planning period, say, a year, and not the cost of funds raised in the past.

1. What is the basic concept of the corporate cost of capital?
2. What financing sources are typically included in a firm's cost of capital estimate?
3. Should the component costs be estimated on a before-tax or an after-tax basis?
4. Should the component costs reflect historical or marginal costs?

Self-Test Questions

Cost of Debt Capital

It is unlikely that a firm's managers will know at the start of a planning period the exact types and amounts of debt that will be issued in the future. The type of debt actually used will depend on the specific assets to be financed and on market conditions as they develop over time. However, a firm's managers do know what types of debt the firm usually issues. For example, Bayside Memorial Hospital typically uses bank debt to raise short-term funds to finance seasonal or cyclical working capital needs and uses 30-year tax-exempt bonds to raise long-term debt capital. Since Bayside does not use short-term debt to finance permanent assets, its managers include only long-term debt in their corporate cost of capital estimate and they assume that this debt will consist solely of 30-year tax-exempt bonds.

Suppose that Bayside's managers are developing the hospital's corporate cost of capital estimate for the coming year. How should they estimate the hospital's component *cost of debt*? Most managers would begin by discussing current and prospective interest rates with their firms' investment bankers, the institutions that help companies bring security issues to market. Assume that the municipal bond analyst at Suncoast Securities, Inc., Bayside's investment banker, states that a new 30-year tax-exempt healthcare issue would require semiannual interest payments of $30.50 ($61 annually) for each $1,000 par value bond issued. Thus, municipal bond investors currently require a $61 / $1,000 = 0.061 = 6.1% return on Bayside's 30-year bonds.

The true cost of the issue to Bayside would be somewhat higher than 6.1 percent because the hospital must incur issuance expenses, often called *flotation costs*, to sell the bonds. However, such expenses are typically small on bond issues, so their impact on the cost of debt estimate is inconsequential, especially when the uncertainty inherent in the entire cost of capital estimation process is considered. Therefore, it is common practice to ignore flotation costs when estimating the component cost of debt. Bayside follows this practice, so its managers would estimate the component cost of debt as 6.1 percent:

$$\text{Tax-exempt component cost of debt} = R(R_d) = 6.1\%.$$

If Bayside's currently outstanding debt were actively traded, then the current **yield to maturity (YTM)** on this debt could be used to estimate the cost of new debt. For example, assume that Bayside has an actively traded 25-year issue outstanding that has a 7 percent coupon rate (semiannual) and currently sells for $1,114.69. Using a financial calculator, the yield to maturity on this bond is found to be 6.1 percent:

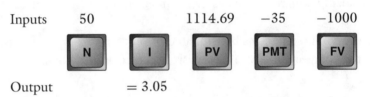

Inputs	50		1114.69	−35	−1000
	N	I	PV	PMT	FV

Output   = 3.05

Because the bond has semiannual coupons, the resulting calculator solution of 3.05 percent must be multiplied by two to get an annual yield to maturity.[5]

Using the yield to maturity on an outstanding issue to estimate the cost of new debt works reasonably well when the remaining life of the old issue approximates the anticipated maturity of the new issue. If this is not the case, then yield curve differentials may cause the estimate to be biased. For example, if the yield curve is upward sloping in the 25- to 30-year range, the yield to maturity on a 25-year outstanding issue would understate the actual cost of a new 30-year issue.

What about smaller businesses that do not have relationships with investment bankers and do not have publicly traded debt? If a business obtains the bulk of its debt financing from banks, then the firm's bankers will be able to provide some insights on the cost of future debt financing. Alternatively, managers can look to marketplace activity for guidance. That is, the interest rate currently being set on the debt issues of similar-risk firms can be used as an estimate of the cost of debt. Here, similar risk can be judged either by debt rating or by subjective analysis (same industry, similar size, similar use of debt, and so on). An awareness of the current interest rate environment generally permits managers to make a reasonable estimate for their own firm's cost of debt.

A taxable healthcare provider would use one or more of the techniques just described to estimate its before-tax cost of debt. However, the tax benefits of interest payments must then be incorporated into the estimate. To illustrate, consider Ann Arbor Health Systems, Inc., an investor-owned company that operates 16 acute care hospitals in Michigan, Indiana, and Ohio. The company's investment bankers indicate that a new 30-year taxable bond issue would require a yield of 11.0 percent. Because the firm's federal-plus-state tax rate is 40 percent, its component cost of debt estimate is 6.6 percent:

$$\text{Taxable component cost of debt} = R(R_d) \times (1 - T)$$

$$= 11.0\% \times (1 - 0.40) = 11.0\% \times 0.60 = 6.6\%.$$

The component cost of debt to an investor-owned firm is an after-tax cost because the effective cost to the firm is reduced by the $(1 - T)$ term. By reducing Ann Arbor's component cost of debt from 11.0 percent to 6.6 percent, the cost of debt estimate has incorporated the benefit associated with interest payment tax deductibility.

In general, the **effective** cost of debt is roughly comparable between investor-owned and not-for-profit firms of similar risk. Investor-owned firms have the benefit of tax deductibility of interest payments, while not-for-profit firms have the benefit of being able to issue tax-exempt debt.

1. What are some methods used to estimate a firm's cost of debt?
2. What is the impact of flotation costs on the cost of debt? Are these costs generally material?
3. For investor-owned firms, how is the before-tax cost of debt converted to an after-tax cost?

**Self-Test
Questions**

Cost of Equity Capital

Investor-owned businesses raise equity capital by selling new common stock and by retaining earnings for use by the firm rather than paying them out as dividends to shareholders. Not-for-profit firms raise equity capital through contributions and grants, and by generating an excess of revenues over expenses, none of which can be paid out as dividends. In the following sections, how to estimate the cost of equity capital, both to investor-owned and not-for-profit firms, is described.[6]

Cost of Equity to Investor-Owned Firms

The cost of debt is based on the return that investors require on debt securities; the *cost of equity* to investor-owned firms can be defined similarly: it is the rate of return that investors require on the firm's common stock. At first glance, it may appear that equity raised through **retained earnings** is a costless source of capital to investor-owned firms. After all, dividend payments must be paid on new shares of stock that are issued, but no such payments are required on funds that are obtained by retaining earnings. The reason why a cost of capital must be assigned to all forms of equity financing involves the *opportunity cost principle*. An investor-owned firm's net income literally belongs to its common stockholders. Employees are compensated by wages, suppliers are compensated by cash payments for supplies, bondholders are compensated by interest payments, governments are compensated by tax payments, and so on. The residual earning of a firm—its net income—belongs to the stockholders and serves to "pay the rent" on stockholder-supplied capital.

Management can either pay out earnings in the form of dividends or retain earnings for reinvestment in the business. If part of the earnings is retained, an opportunity cost is incurred; stockholders could have received these earnings as dividends and then invested this money in stocks, bonds, real estate, commodity futures, and so on. Thus, the firm should earn on its retained earnings at least as much as its stockholders themselves could earn on alternative investments of similar risk. If the firm cannot earn as much as stockholders can in similar risk investments, then the firm's net income should be paid out as dividends rather than retained for reinvestment within the firm. What rate of return can stockholders expect to earn on other investments of equivalent risk? The answer is $R(R_e)$, the required rate of return on equity. Investors can earn this return either by buying more shares of the firm in question or by buying the stock of similar firms.

Whereas debt is a contractual obligation with an easily estimated cost, it is not nearly as easy to estimate $R(R_e)$, the cost of equity. Two primary methods are used: the Capital Asset Pricing Model (CAPM) and the discounted cash flow (DCF) model. These methods should not be regarded as mutually exclusive because neither approach dominates the estimation process. In practice, both approaches should be used to estimate the cost of equity, and then the final value should be chosen on the basis of the managers' confidence in the data at hand.

Capital Asset Pricing Model (CAPM) Approach

The *Capital Asset Pricing Model (CAPM)*, which was introduced in Chapter 10, is a widely accepted finance model that specifies the equilibrium risk/return relationship on common stocks. Basically, the model assumes that investors consider only one risk factor when setting required rates of returns—the volatility of returns on the stock compared with the volatility of returns on a well-diversified portfolio called the *market portfolio*, or just the *market*. The measure of risk in the CAPM is the stock's *market beta*. The market, which is a large collection of stocks, such as the S&P 500 Index, has a beta of 1.0. A stock with a beta of 2.0 has twice the volatility of returns as the market, while a stock with a beta of 0.5 has only half the volatility of returns as the market. Because relative volatility measures market risk, a low beta stock, defined as having a beta less than 1.0, is less risky than the market; while a high beta stock, defined as having a beta more than 1.0, is more risky than the market.

Within the CAPM, the actual equation that relates risk to return is called the *Security Market Line (SML)*:

$$R(R_e) = RF + [R(R_M) - RF] \times b_i$$
$$= RF + (RP_M \times b_i).$$

Here,

RF = risk-free rate.

$R(R_M)$ = required rate of return on the market.

b_i = beta coefficient of the stock in question.

$[R(R_M) - RF)]$ = RP_M = market risk premium, the premium above the risk-free rate

that investors require to buy a stock with average risk.

$(RP_M) \times b_i$ = stock risk premium, the premium above the risk-free rate that

investors require to buy the stock in question.

Managers can estimate the required rate of return on the firm's stock given estimates of the risk-free rate, RF, the beta of the firm's stock, b_i, and the required rate of return on the market, $R(R_M)$. This estimate, in turn, can be used as the estimate for the firm's cost of equity.

The starting point for the CAPM cost of equity estimate is the risk-free rate. Unfortunately, there is no security in the United States that is truly riskless. Treasury securities are essentially free of default risk, but long-term T-bonds will suffer capital losses if interest rates rise, and a portfolio invested in short-term T-bills will provide a volatile earnings stream because the rate paid on T-bills varies over time. Because a truly riskless rate cannot be found in practice, what rate should be used? The preference—shared by most finance professionals—is to use the rate on long-term Treasury bonds.

There are many reasons for favoring the T-bond rate including the fact that T-bill rates are very volatile because they are directly affected by actions taken by the Federal Reserve Board. Perhaps the most persuasive argument is that common stocks are generally viewed as long-term securities, and although a particular stockholder may not have a long investment horizon, the majority of stockholders do invest on a long-term basis. Therefore, it is reasonable to think that stock returns embody long-term inflation expectations similar to those embodied in bonds rather than the short-term inflation expectations embodied in bills. On this account, the cost of equity should be more highly correlated with T-bond rates than with T-bill rates. T-bond rates can be found in local newspapers, in the *Wall Street Journal,* and in the *Federal Reserve Bulletin*. Generally, the yield on 20-year T-bonds is used as the proxy for the risk-free rate.

The required rate of return on the market and its derivative, the market risk premium, $RP_M = R(R_M) - RF$, can be estimated on the basis of either historical returns or expected returns. The most widely used set of historical market returns is provided by Ibbotson Associates. Their data, which are published annually, include annual rates of return on stocks, T-bills, T-bonds, and a set of high-grade corporate bonds.[7] From their most recent data set (1926–1997), Ibbotson Associates estimate that the average historical market risk premium is about 7 percent.

However, the historical market risk premium has a large standard deviation, so one must use it with caution. Also, it should be noted that the choice of the beginning and ending periods has a major impact on the calculated risk premium. Ibbotson Associates used the longest period available to them, but had their data begun some years earlier or later, or had it ended earlier, their results would have been significantly affected. Indeed, in many years their data would indicate a **negative** market risk premium, which would lead to the conclusion that Treasury securities have a higher required return than common stocks—a conclusion that is contrary to both financial theory and common sense. All this suggests that historical risk premiums should be approached with some caution.

In addition to historical estimates for the market risk premium, estimates that focus on future expectations can also be used. Most of the larger financial services companies publish forecasts based on DCF methodology for the expected rate of return on the market. Given this estimate for $R(R_M)$, it is easy to merely subtract the current T-bond rate from the estimate to obtain an estimate of the current market risk premium.

The last parameter needed for a CAPM cost of equity estimate is the firm's beta coefficient. Unfortunately, beta measures how risky a stock was **in the past,** whereas investors are interested in **future** risk. It may be that a given company appeared to be quite safe in the past, but that things have changed and its future risk is judged to be higher than its past risk or vice versa. As a general rule, is future risk sufficiently similar to past risk to warrant the use of historical betas in a CAPM framework? For individual firms, historical betas are often not very stable, so past risk is often **not** a good predictor of future risk.[8]

Furthermore, betas can be calculated over different time periods and different measures for the market return can be used, so different financial advisory services report different betas for the same company. The choice is a matter of judgment and data availability because there is no right beta. With luck, the betas derived from different sources will, for a given company, be close together. If they are not, confidence in the CAPM cost of equity estimate will be diminished.

Table 13.3 contains the betas of some representative investor-owned healthcare firms as provided by Value Line. Value Line uses the New York Stock Exchange Composite Index as its proxy for the market, 260 weekly observations, and it adjusts the betas for their tendency to move toward 1.0 over time (see note 8). On the basis of this very limited selection, it appears that healthcare firms carry above-average market risk for stockholders. Drug producers carry the lowest market risk, while managed care organizations carry the highest.

To illustrate the CAPM approach, consider Ann Arbor Health Systems, which has a beta coefficient, b, of 1.10. Furthermore, assume that the current yield on T-bonds, RF, is 8.5 percent and that the best estimate for the current market risk premium, RP_M, is five percentage points. In words, the current required rate of return on the market, $R(R_M)$, is 13.5 percent. All the required input parameters have been estimated, and the SML equation can be completed as follows:

Company	Primary Line of Business	Beta	TABLE 13.3
			Beta Coefficients
Alza	Drug delivery systems	1.40	for Selected
Ann Arbor Health Systems	Acute care hospitals	1.10	Healthcare
Baxter International	Medical supplies	1.10	Companies
Beverly Enterprises	Nursing homes	1.20	
Bristol-Myers Squibb	Diversified drugs	0.95	
Columbia/HCA	Acute care hospitals	1.10	
Glaxo Wellcome	Diversified drugs	1.00	
HEALTHSOUTH	Outpatient and rehabilitative care	1.35	
Humana	Managed care	1.55	
Lincare	Oxygen and respiratory services	1.15	
Omnicare	Pharmacy management and drug therapy	1.55	
Oxford Health	Managed care	1.30	
PacifiCare Systems	Managed care	1.35	
Phycor	Physician practice management	1.35	
Tenet Healthcare	Acute care hospitals	1.00	
United Healthcare	Managed care	1.70	
U.S. Surgical	Medical equipment	1.30	

Source: Value Line Investment Survey, 1998.

$$R(R_e) = RF + [R(R_M) - RF] \times b_i$$

$$= 8.5\% + (13.5\% - 8.5\%) \times 1.10$$

$$= 8.5\% + (5.0\% \times 1.10)$$

$$= 8.5\% + 5.5\% = 14.0\%.$$

Thus, according to the CAPM, Ann Arbor's required rate of return on equity is 14.0 percent.

In words, what does the 14.0 percent estimate for $R(R_e)$ imply? In essence, equity investors believe that Ann Arbor's stock, with a beta of 1.10, is slightly more risky than the average stock, with a beta of 1.00. With a risk-free rate of 8.5 percent and a market risk premium of five percentage points, an average company, with b = 1.0, has a required rate of return on equity of 8.5% + (5.0% × 1.00) = 8.5% + 5.0% = 13.5%. Thus, according to the CAPM, equity investors require 50 basis points more return for investing in Ann Arbor Health Systems, with b = 1.10, rather than an average stock, with b = 1.0.

There is a great deal of uncertainty in the CAPM estimate of the cost of equity. Some of this uncertainty stems from the fact that there is no assurance that the CAPM is correct (i.e., the CAPM accurately describes the risk/return choices of stock investors). Additionally, there is a great deal of uncertainty in the input parameter estimates, especially the required rate of return on the market and the beta coefficient. Because of these uncertainties, it is highly unlikely that Ann Arbor's true, but unobservable, cost of equity is 14.0 percent. Thus, instead of picking single values for each parameter, it may be better to develop high and low estimates, and then to combine all of the high estimates and all of the low estimates to develop a range, rather than a point estimate, for $R(R_e)$.

Discounted Cash Flow (DCF) Approach

The second procedure for estimating the cost of equity is the *discounted cash flow (DCF) method*. The intrinsic value of a stock can be found as the present value of its expected dividend stream. Furthermore, if the dividend is expected to grow each year at a constant rate, $E(g)$, then the *constant growth model* can be used to estimate the expected rate of return on the stock, $E(R_e)$:

$$E(R_e) = \frac{D_0 \times [1 + E(g)]}{P_0} + E(g) = \frac{E(D_1)}{P_0} + E(g).$$

Because stock prices typically are in equilibrium, the expected rate of return, $E(R_e)$, is also the required rate of return, $R(R_e)$.

As in the CAPM approach, there are three input parameters in the DCF model. Current stock price is readily available for firms that are actively traded. Ann Arbor Health Systems' stock is traded in the over-the-counter (OTC) market, so its stock price generally can be found in the *Wall Street Journal*. At the time of the analysis, Ann Arbor's stock price was $40.

Next year's dividend payment is also relatively easy to estimate. Ann Arbor's managers can obtain this estimate from the firm's five-year financial plan. For an outsider, dividend data on larger, publicly traded firms are available from brokerage houses and investment advisory firms. Also, the current dividend information published in the *Wall Street Journal* can be used as a basis for estimating next year's dividend, $E(D_1)$. Ann Arbor Health Systems is followed by several analysts at major brokerage houses and their consensus estimate for next year's dividend payment is $2.50, so for purposes of this analysis, $E(D_1) = \$2.50$.

The dividend growth rate, $E(g)$, is the most difficult of the DCF model parameters to estimate. Although historical earnings and dividend data can be analyzed directly to estimate growth rates, most finance professionals rely on expert analysts for growth rate estimates. Analysts forecast and then publish growth rate estimates for most of the larger, publicly owned companies. For example, *Value Line* provides such forecasts on about 1,700 companies, and all of the larger brokerage houses provide similar forecasts. Furthermore, several companies compile analysts' forecasts on a regular basis and provide summary information such as the median and range of forecasts on widely followed companies. These growth rate summaries, such as the one compiled by Lynch, Jones & Ryan in its *Institutional Brokers Estimate System (IBES)*, can be ordered for a fee and obtained either in hardcopy format or as online electronic data.

However, analysts' forecasts often assume nonconstant growth. For example, analysts following Ann Arbor Health Systems, on average, forecasted a 12.0 percent annual growth rate in earnings and dividends over the next five years followed by a steady-state growth rate of 6.5 percent. A rough way to handle this situation is to use the nonconstant growth forecast to develop a proxy constant growth rate. Computer simulations indicate that dividends beyond Year 50 contribute very little to the value of any stock—the present value of dividends beyond Year 50 is virtually zero, so for practical purposes, it is safe to ignore anything beyond that point. If only a 50-year horizon is considered, a weighted average growth rate can be developed and used as a constant growth rate for cost of capital purposes. For Ann Arbor Health Systems, the growth rate of 12.0 percent for five years was assumed to be followed by a growth rate of 6.5 percent for 45 years, which produced an arithmetic average annual growth rate of $(0.10 \times 12.0\%) + (0.90 \times 6.5\%) = 7.2\%$. This figure, together with other estimates, leads to the conclusion that Ann Arbor Health System's expected dividend growth rate is in the range of 7.0 to 8.0 percent.[9]

To illustrate the DCF approach, consider the data developed thus far for Ann Arbor Health Systems. The company's current stock price, P_0, is $40 and its next expected annual dividend, $E(D_1)$, is $2.50. Thus, the firm's DCF estimate of $E(R_e)$ according to the DCF model is:

$$R(R_e) = \frac{E(D_1)}{P_0} + E(g)$$

$$= \frac{\$2.50}{\$40} + E(g) = 6.25\% + E(g).$$

With an $E(g)$ estimate range of 7 to 8 percent, the midpoint, 7.5 percent, will be used as the final estimate. Thus, the DCF estimate for Ann Arbor Health System's cost of equity is $6.25\% + 7.5\% = 13.75\% \approx 13.8\%$.

Comparison of the CAPM and DCF Methods

The text has presented two methods for estimating the cost of equity.[10] The CAPM estimate was 14.0 percent and the DCF estimate was 13.8 percent. At this point, most analysts would conclude that there is sufficient consistency in the results to warrant the use of 13.9 percent as the final estimate of the cost of equity for Ann Arbor Health Systems. If the two methods produced widely different estimates, then Ann Arbor's managers would have to use their judgment regarding the relative merits of each estimate and then choose the estimate that seemed most reasonable under the circumstances. In general, this choice would be made on the basis of the managers' confidence in the input parameters of each approach.

Cost of Equity to Not-for-Profit Firms

Not-for-profit firms raise equity (fund) capital two ways: by receiving contributions and grants, and by earning an excess of revenues over expenses (i.e., retained earnings). In recent years, considerable controversy has risen over the cost of this capital to not-for-profit firms. However, for this discussion, the best way to think about the problem is in terms of opportunity costs.[11]

In general, equity capital to not-for-profit firms has about the same opportunity cost as the cost of equity to similar investor-owned firms. The rationale is as follows. Suppose that Bayside Memorial Hospital, a not-for-profit corporation, receives $500,000 in contributions in 1998 and also retains $4,500,000 in earnings, so it has $5 million of new fund capital available for investment. The $5 million could be used to purchase assets related to its core business, such as an outpatient clinic or diagnostic equipment, or it could be temporarily invested in securities with the intent of purchasing healthcare assets some time in the future. The $5 million also could be used to retire debt, pay management bonuses, placed in a non-interest-bearing account at the bank, and so on. By using this capital to invest in real assets, Bayside is deprived of the opportunity to use this capital for other purposes, so an opportunity cost must be assigned.

What opportunity cost should be assigned? The answer is that the hospital's investment in real assets should return at least as much as the return available on securities investments of similar risk. What return is available on securities with similar risk to hospital assets? The answer is the return that is expected from investing in the stock of an investor-owned hospital company such as Ann Arbor Health Systems. Instead of using fund capital to purchase real healthcare assets, Bayside could always use the funds to buy the stock of a hospital company, such as Ann Arbor, and delay the real asset purchase until some time in the future. This does not mean to imply that not-for-profit firms should never invest in a project that will lose money in the opportunity cost sense. Not-for-profit firms do invest in negative profit projects that benefit its stakeholders, but managers must be aware of the financial opportunity costs inherent in such investments. This issue is discussed again in Chapter 14.

The cost of equity capital to not-for-profit firms has been defined as the return available on the stocks of similar investor-owned companies. Thus, Ann Arbor's 13.9 percent cost of equity estimate could be used as the estimate for Bayside's cost of equity capital. However, caution is in order. Although fund capital certainly has an opportunity cost that is similar to the cost of equity to investor-owned firms, there are several problems inherent in implementing this concept. Here are the three most bothersome:

- All else the same, tax and capital structure differences between investor-owned and not-for-profit firms invalidate the direct translation of betas, and hence risk and equity costs.[12]
- The risk to an investor-owned firm's stockholders is not the same as the risk to a not-for-profit firm's stakeholders. In essence, stockholders are well-diversified investors in regards to stock ownership, but stakeholders may not be so well diversified regarding their "investment" in not-for-profit businesses.
- In general, stock betas, and hence required rates of return on equity, are available only for very large companies and the risk inherent in the stock ownership of a large, well-diversified company typically is less than the riskiness of the equity capital of a smaller, less diversified business. For example, stock ownership of HEALTHSOUTH, which owns over 1,000 locations across the United States, even if held in isolation, is less risky that the stakeholder's position in a single outpatient rehabilitation center. In effect, corporate

diversification lowers risk, so the comparison of a widely diversified company with a single enterprise is suspect.

The bottom line here is that the entire process of estimating the cost of equity capital for not-for-profit businesses must be viewed with some skepticism, and hence the value obtained must be regarded as only a very rough estimate. Nevertheless, the estimate is the best that finance theory can muster, and a cost of equity developed in this way is better than ignoring the fact that there is an opportunity cost inherent in such capital.[13]

Accounting for Stock Flotation Costs

In the discussion of the cost of debt, it was specifically stated that flotation (issuance) costs typically are small on debt issues, and hence can be ignored. However, on new stock issues, flotation costs can be significant, and, in theory, such costs should be considered. The effect of these costs is to increase the cost of new common stock above the estimate obtained from the procedures just outlined. Thus, investor-owned firms actually have two costs of equity: one for retained earnings and another higher cost for new common stock sales. Not-for-profit businesses cannot issue new common stock, so the problem of two costs of equity does not arise with such organizations. Because this is an introductory text and because the added complexities associated with differential equity costs do not necessarily result in better managerial decisions, the treatment here will assume a single cost of equity for both investor-owned and not-for-profit businesses.[14]

1. What are the two primary methods for estimating a for-profit firm's cost of equity?
2. What is the best proxy for the risk-free rate in the CAPM method? Why?
3. How would you choose between widely different cost of equity estimates?
4. Why is there a cost associated with fund capital?
5. What is the cost of fund capital?
6. Are flotation costs relevant to the estimate of the cost of equity? Explain your answer.

Self-Test Questions

The Corporate Cost of Capital

The final step in the cost of capital estimation process is to combine the debt and equity cost estimates to form the *corporate cost of capital*. As discussed at the beginning of the chapter, each firm has a target capital structure in mind, which is defined as the particular mix of debt and equity that causes its overall cost of capital to be minimized. Furthermore, when a firm raises new capital, it generally tries to finance in a way that will keep the actual capital structure reasonably close to its target over time. Here is the general formula for the corporate cost of capital for all firms regardless of ownership:

$$\text{Corporate cost of capital} = [w_d \times R(R_d) \times (1 - T)] + [w_e \times R(R_e)].$$

Here w_d and w_e are the target weights for debt and equity, respectively. The cost of the debt component, $R(R_d)$, will be an average if the firm uses several types of debt for its permanent financing. Alternatively, the above equation could be expanded to include multiple debt terms. Investor-owned firms would use their marginal tax rate for T, while T would be zero for not-for-profit firms.

The corporate cost of capital represents the cost of each new dollar of capital raised at the margin. It is **not** the average cost of all the dollars that the firm has raised in the past. The primary interest is in obtaining a cost of capital for use in capital investment analysis; for such purposes, a *marginal cost* is required. The corporate cost of capital formula implies that each new dollar of capital will consist of both debt and equity that is raised, at least conceptually, in proportion to the firm's target capital structure.

The Corporate Cost of Capital for Investor-Owned Firms

To illustrate the corporate cost of capital calculation for investor-owned firms, consider Ann Arbor Health Systems, which has a target capital structure of 60 percent debt and 40 percent equity. As previously estimated, the company's before-tax cost of debt, $R(R_d)$, is 11.0 percent; its tax rate, T, is 40 percent; and its cost of equity, $R(R_e)$ is 13.9 percent, so Ann Arbor's corporate cost of capital estimate is 9.5 percent:

$$\text{Corporate cost of capital} = [w_d \times R(R_d) \times (1 - T)] + [w_e \times R(R_e)]$$
$$= [0.60 \times 11.0\% \times (1 - 0.40)] + [0.40 \times 13.9\%]$$
$$= 9.5\%.$$

In essence, every dollar of new capital that Ann Arbor obtains consists of 60 cents of debt with an after-tax cost of 6.6 percent and 40 cents of equity with a cost of 13.9 percent. The average cost of each new dollar is 9.5 percent. In any one year, Ann Arbor may raise all its required new capital by issuing debt, by retaining earnings, or by selling new common stock. But over the long run, Ann Arbor plans to use 60 percent debt financing and 40 percent equity financing, and these weights must be used in the corporate cost of capital estimate **regardless** of the actual financing plans for the near term.

The Corporate Cost of Capital for Not-for-Profit Firms

The corporate cost of capital for not-for-profit firms is developed in the same way as for investor-owned firms. To illustrate, the corporate cost of capital for Bayside Memorial Hospital, assuming a target capital structure of 50 percent debt and 50 percent equity and using the estimates for the component costs that were developed earlier, is 10 percent:

$$\text{Corporate cost of capital} = [w_d \times R(R_d) \times (1 - T)] + [w_e \times R(R_e)]$$
$$= [0.50 \times 6.1\% \times (1 - 0)] + [0.50 \times 13.9\%]$$
$$= 10.0\%.$$

Businesses, regardless of ownership, cannot raise unlimited amounts of new capital in any given year at a constant cost. Eventually, for several reasons, as more new capital is raised, investors will require higher returns on debt and equity capital, even though the capital is raised in accordance with the firm's target structure. Thus, the corporate costs of capital, as estimated here for Ann Arbor and Bayside, are only valid when the amount required for capital investment falls within the firm's normal range. If capital is required in amounts that far exceed those normally raised, the corporate cost of capital must be subjectively adjusted upward to reflect the higher costs involved.

1. What is the general formula for the corporate cost of capital?
2. What weights should be used in the formula? Why?
3. What is the primary difference between the corporate costs of capital for investor-owned and not-for-profit firms?
4. Is the corporate cost of capital affected by short-term financing plans? Explain your answer.
5. Is the corporate cost of capital constant regardless of the amount of new capital required? Explain your answer.

Self-Test Questions

An Economic Interpretation of the Corporate Cost of Capital

Thus far, the focus of the cost of capital discussion has been on the mechanics of the estimation process. In closing, it is worthwhile to step back from the mathematics of the process and examine the corporate cost of capital's economic interpretation.

The component cost estimates (the costs of debt and equity) that make up a firm's corporate cost of capital are based on the returns that investors require to supply capital to the firm. In turn, investors' required rates of return are based on the opportunity costs borne by investing in the debt and equity of the firm in question rather than in alternative investments of similar risk. These opportunity costs to investors, when combined into the firm's corporate cost of capital, establish the **opportunity cost** to the firm. That is, the corporate cost of capital is the return that the business could earn by investing in alternative investments that have the same risk as its own real assets. From a pure financial perspective, if a business cannot earn its corporate cost of capital on new capital investments, no new investments should be made and no new capital should be raised. If existing investments are not earning the corporate cost of capital, they should be terminated, the assets liquidated, and the proceeds returned to investors for reinvestment elsewhere.

However, the corporate cost of capital is not the appropriate minimum rate of return for all new real asset investments. The required rates of return set by investors on the business' debt and equity are based on perceptions regarding the riskiness of their investments, which, in turn, are based on two factors: the inherent riskiness of the business (i.e., business risk) and the amount of debt financing used (i.e., financial risk). Thus, the firm's inherent business risk and capital structure are embedded in its corporate cost of capital estimate.

Because different firms have different business risk and use different proportions of debt financing, different firms have different corporate costs of capital. Differential capital costs are most pronounced for firms in different industries, as evidenced by the wide variation in beta values contained in Table 13.3. Still, even firms in the same industry can have different business risk, and capital structure differences among such firms can compound corporate cost of capital differences.

The primary purpose of estimating a firm's corporate cost of capital is to help make capital budgeting decisions. That is, the cost of capital will be used as the benchmark capital budgeting *hurdle rate* or the minimum return necessary for a project to be attractive financially. The firm can always earn its cost of capital by investing in selected stocks and bonds that in the aggregate have the same risk as the firm's assets, so it should not invest in real assets unless it can earn at least as much. However, remember that the corporate cost of capital reflects opportunity costs based on the aggregate risk of the firm (i.e., the riskiness of the firm's average project). Thus, the corporate cost of capital can be applied without modification only to those projects under consideration that have average risk, where average is defined as that applicable to the firm's currently held assets in the aggregate. If a project under consideration has risk that differs significantly from that of the firm's average asset, then the corporate cost of capital must be adjusted to account for the differential risk when the project is being evaluated.[15]

To illustrate the concept, Ann Arbor Health System's corporate cost of capital, 10 percent, is probably appropriate for use in evaluating a new outpatient clinic that has risk similar to the hospital's average project, which involves the provision of healthcare services. Clearly, it would **not** be appropriate to apply Ann Arbor's 10 percent corporate cost of capital without adjustment to a new project that involves establishing a managed care subsidiary; this project does not have the same risk as the hospital's average asset. (To confirm the risk differential, refer to Table 13.3. Managed care plans have higher betas, and hence greater risk, than do hospital companies.)

As discussed in Chapter 10, investors require higher returns for riskier investments. Thus, a high-risk project must have a higher *project cost of capital* than a low-risk project. Figure 13.2 illustrates the relationship between project risk, the corporate cost of capital, and project costs of capital. The figure illustrates that Ann Arbor's 10 percent corporate cost of capital is the appropriate hurdle rate **only** for an **average risk** project (Project A), where average means a project that has the same risk as the aggregate business. Project L, which has less risk than Ann Arbor's average project has a project cost of capital, 8 percent, that is less than the corporate cost of capital. Conversely, Project H, with more risk than the average project, has a higher project cost of capital, 12 percent.

The key point here is that the corporate cost of capital is merely a **benchmark** that will be used as the basis for estimating project costs of capital. It is not a one-size-fits-all rate that can be used with abandon whenever an opportunity cost is needed in a financial analysis. This point will be revisited in Chapter 15 when capital investment risk considerations are addressed.

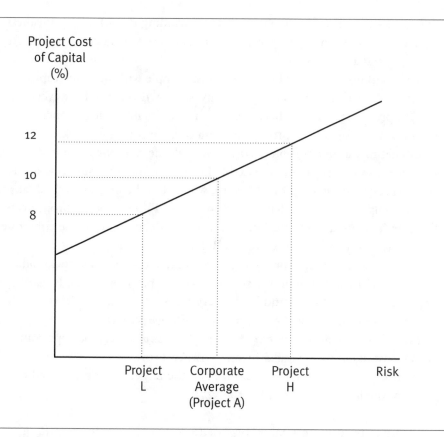

1. Explain the economic interpretation of the corporate cost of capital.
2. Is the corporate cost of capital the appropriate opportunity cost for all projects that a business evaluates?
3. Draw a graph similar to the one shown in Figure 13.2 and explain its implications.

Key Concepts

This chapter discusses optimal capital structure and the corporate cost of capital, two very important concepts in healthcare finance. The key concepts of this chapter are:

- The choice between debt and equity financing is one type of risk/return trade-off. The use of debt financing can *leverage up* the return to owners or, in not-for-profit firms, the return on fund capital, but it also *increases the riskiness* of the business.
- The *optimal*, or *target*, *capital structure* is that structure that minimizes the overall cost of capital to the firm.
- Unfortunately, finance theory is of limited help in actually setting a firm's target structure. Thus, in making the capital structure decision, health services

managers consider a wide range of factors including the following: business risk, lender and rating agency attitudes, reserve borrowing capacity, industry averages, and asset structure.

- Managers of not-for-profit businesses must grapple with the same capital structure decisions as the managers of investor-owned firms. However, not-for-profit firms do not have the same flexibility in making financing decisions because not-for-profit firms cannot issue common stock.

- In estimating a firm's corporate cost of capital, the *component cost of debt* is the *after-tax* cost of new debt. For taxable firms, it is found by multiplying the before-tax cost of new debt by $(1 - T)$, where T is the firm's marginal tax rate, so the component cost of debt is $R(R_d) \times (1 - T)$. For not-for-profit firms, the debt is often tax-exempt, but no other tax effects apply, so the component cost of debt is merely the tax-exempt $R(R_d)$.

- The *cost of equity* to investor-owned firms is the return that its stockholders could obtain by investing in the stocks of similar-risk companies. It usually is estimated by using two methods: the *Capital Asset Pricing Model (CAPM) approach*, and the *discounted cash flow (DCF) approach*.

- For not-for-profit firms, the *cost of equity (fund capital)* can be approximated by the cost of equity of similar investor-owned firms.

- Each firm has a *target capital structure* and the target weights are used to estimate the firm's *corporate cost of capital*:

$$\text{Corporate cost of capital} = [w_d \times R(R_d) \times (1 - T)] + [w_e \times R(R_e)].$$

- When making *capital investment decisions*, the firm will use the corporate cost of capital as the *hurdle rate* for **average-risk** projects.

The concepts developed in this chapter play a vital role in capital investment decision making. They will be revisited in Chapters 14 and 15.

Questions

13.1 Critique this statement: "The use of debt financing lowers the net income of the firm, and hence debt financing should be used only as a last resort."

13.2 Discuss some factors that health services managers must consider when setting a firm's target capital structure. Consider both investor-owned and not-for-profit firms in your answer.

13.3 Is the corporate cost of capital estimate based on historical or marginal costs? Why?

13.4 What capital components are typically included when estimating firm's corporate cost of capital?

13.5 How may a firm's cost of debt be estimated?

13.6 a. Why is there a cost to retained earnings in investor-owned businesses?
   b. What are the two methods commonly used to estimate a for-profit firm's cost of equity?

c. How would you estimate the cost of equity (fund capital) for a not-for-profit business.

13.7 What is the economic interpretation of the corporate cost of capital?

13.8 Is the corporate cost of capital the same for all firms? Explain your answer.

13.9 For any given firm, can the corporate cost of capital be used as the hurdle rate for all projects under consideration? Explain your answer.

Problems

13.1 Seattle Health Plans currently uses zero debt financing. Its operating income (EBIT) is $1 million and it pays taxes at a 40 percent rate. It has $5 million in assets and because it is all-equity financed, $5 million in equity. Suppose the firm is considering replacing half of its equity financing with debt financing bearing an interest rate of 8 percent.
   a. What impact would the new capital structure have on the firm's net income, total dollar return to investors, and ROE?
   b. Redo the analysis, but now assume that the debt financing would cost 15 percent.
   c. Return to the initial 8 percent interest rate. Now assume that EBIT could be as low as $500,000 (with a probability of 20 percent) or as high as $1.5 million (with a probability of 20 percent). There remains a 60 percent chance that EBIT would be $1 million. Redo the analysis for each level of EBIT and find the expected values for the firm's net income, total dollar return to investors, and ROE. What lesson about capital structure and risk does this illustration provide?
   d. Repeat the analysis required for Part a, but now assume that Seattle Health Plans is a not-for-profit corporation, and hence pays no taxes. Compare the results with those obtained in Part a.

13.2 Calculate the after-tax cost of debt for the Wallace Clinic, a for-profit healthcare provider, assuming that the coupon rate set on its debt is 11 percent and its tax rate is:
   a. 0%
   b. 20%
   c. 40%

13.3 St. Vincent's Hospital has a target capital structure of 35 percent debt and 65 percent equity. Its cost of equity (fund capital) estimate is 13.5 percent and its cost of tax-exempt debt estimate is 7 percent. What is the hospital's corporate cost of capital?

13.4 Richmond Clinic has obtained the following estimates for its costs of debt and equity at various capital structures:

Percent Debt	After-Tax Cost of Debt	Cost of Equity
0%	—	16.0%
20	6.6	17.0
40	7.8	19.0

60	10.2	22.0
80	14.0	27.0

What is the firm's optimal capital structure? (Hint: Calculate its corporate cost of capital at each structure. Also, note that data on component costs at alternative capital structures are not reliable in real world situations.)

13.5 Medical Associates is a large for-profit group practice. Its dividends are expected to grow at a constant rate of 7 percent per year into the foreseeable future. The firm's last dividend (D_0) was $2 and its current stock price is $23. The firm's beta coefficient is 1.6, the rate of return on 20-year T-bonds currently is 9 percent, and the expected rate of return on the market, as reported by a large financial services firm, is 13 percent. The firm's target capital structure calls for 50 percent debt financing, the interest rate required on the business' new debt is 10 percent, and its tax rate is 40 percent.

a. What is Medical Associates' cost of equity estimate according to the DCF method?

b. What is the cost of equity estimate according to the CAPM?

c. On the basis of your answers to Parts a and b, what would be your final estimate for the firm's cost of equity?

d. What is your estimate for the firm's corporate cost of capital?

13.6 Morningside Nursing Home, a not-for-profit corporation, is estimating its corporate cost of capital. Its tax-exempt debt currently requires an interest rate of 6.2 percent and its target capital structure calls for 60 percent debt financing and 40 percent equity (fund capital) financing. The estimated costs of equity for selected investor-owned healthcare companies (with betas given in Table 13.3) is given below:

Glaxo Wellcome	15.0%
Beverly Enterprises	16.4
HEALTHSOUTH	17.4
Humana	18.8

a. What is the best estimate for Morningside's cost of equity?

b. What is the firm's corporate cost of capital?

13.7 Golden State Home Health, Inc., is a large, California-based for-profit home health agency. Its dividends are expected to grow at a constant rate of 5 percent per year into the foreseeable future. The firm's last dividend (D_0) was $1 and its current stock price is $10. The firm's beta coefficient is 1.2, the rate of return on 20-year T-bonds currently is 8 percent, and the expected rate of return on the market, as reported by a large financial services firm, is 14 percent. Golden State's target capital structure calls for 60 percent debt financing, the interest rate required on its new debt is 9 percent, and the firm's tax rate is 30 percent.

a. What is the firm's cost of equity estimate according to the DCF method?

b. What is the cost of equity estimate according to the CAPM?

c. On the basis of your answers to Parts a and b, what would be your final estimate for the firm's cost of equity?

d. What is your estimate for the firm's corporate cost of capital?

Notes

1. In this text, we present only an overview of the capital structure decision. For more information, see E. F. Brigham and L. C. Gapenski, *Financial Management: Theory and Practice* (Fort Worth, TX: Dryden Press, 1997), chapters 12 and 13. Also, a secondary capital structure issue involves the appropriate mix of long-term versus short-term debt. This issue is discussed in Chapter 16.

2. The illustration does not address the impact of debt financing on not-for-profit firms. Here are the income statements assuming zero taxes:

	Stock	Stock/Debt
Revenues	$150,000	$150,000
Operating costs	100,000	100,000
Operating income	$ 50,000	$ 50,000
Interest expense	0	10,000
Net income	$ 50,000	$ 40,000
ROE	25%	40%

The use of debt also leverages up the return on ownership capital in not-for-profit firms. Note, however, that the interest rate on tax-exempt debt would be lower than the rate used here, so the advantage of debt financing is actually greater than this illustration suggests.

3. If the impact of debt financing on market risk was examined—as opposed to stand-alone risk—the result will be the same. Namely, the use of debt financing increases the riskiness to Super Health's owners.

4. For debt financing to increase the owners' rate of return, the inherent return on the business must be greater than the interest rate on the debt. The basic return on the business in the Super Health illustration is 25 percent ($50 in operating income divided by $200 in assets) and debt financing costs only 10 percent, so the use of debt financing increases ROE.

5. A question arises here about whether or not the stated rate or the effective annual rate should be used in the cost of debt estimate. In general, the difference will be minimal, so most firms opt for the easier approach, which is simply to use the stated rate. (The effective annual rate in this example is $(1.0305)^2 - 1.0 = 6.19\%$ versus a 6.1 percent stated rate.) More importantly, most capital budgeting analyses use end-of-year cash flows to proxy cash flows that occur throughout the year; in effect understating the value of the cash flows. For consistency, use of a stated cost of debt is preferred; the cash flows will be understated, but so will the cost of capital.

6. Only a few firms in the health services industry use preferred stock financing, so no preferred stock will be included in our cost of capital examples. If preferred stock is used as a source of permanent financing, then it should be included in the cost of capital estimate and its cost would be estimated using procedures similar to those discussed for the cost of debt.

7. See *Stocks, Bonds, Bills and Inflation: 1998 Yearbook* (Chicago: Ibbotson Associates, 1998). Also, note that Ibbotson Associates now recommends using the T-bond rate as the proxy for the risk-free rate when using the CAPM. Before 1988, Ibbotson Associates recommended the use of the T-bill rate.

8. Since historical betas may not be good predictors of future risk, researchers have sought ways to improve them. This has led to the development of two other types of betas: adjusted betas and fundamental betas. *Adjusted betas* recognize the fact that true betas tend to move toward 1.0 over time. Therefore, one can begin with a firm's pure historical statistical beta, make an adjustment for the expected future movement toward 1.0, and produce an adjusted beta that on average will be a better predictor of the future beta than would the unadjusted historical beta. *Fundamental betas* extend the adjustment process to include such fundamental risk variables as the use of debt financing, sales volatility, and the like. These betas are constantly adjusted to reflect changes in a firm's operations and capital structure, whereas with historical betas (including adjusted ones) such changes may not be fully reflected until several years after the company's "true" beta has changed.

9. The *retention growth model* provides another method for estimating the growth rate in dividends:

$$E(g) = \text{Retention ratio} \times \text{Expected ROE}.$$

This model, which produces a constant growth rate, requires four important assumptions: (1) the payout ratio, and thus the retention ratio, is expected to remain constant; (2) the return on equity (ROE) on new investment to equal the firm's current ROE, which implies that the return on equity is expected to remain constant; (3) the firm is not expected to issue new common stock or, if it does, the new stock will be sold at a price equal to its book value; and (4) future projects are expected to have the same degree of risk as the firm's existing assets.

To illustrate the retention growth model, suppose Ann Arbor Health Systems has had an average return on equity of about 14 percent over the past ten years. The ROE has been relatively steady, but even so, it has ranged from a low of 8.9 percent to a high of 17.6 percent during this period. In addition, the firm's dividend payout ratio has averaged 0.45 over the past ten years, so its retention ratio has averaged 1.0 − 0.45 = 0.55. Using these data, the retention growth method gives an E(g) estimate of 7.7 percent:

$$E(g) = 0.55 \times 14\% = 7.7\%.$$

10. A third method—the bond yield plus risk premium method—can also be used. See E. F. Brigham and L. C. Gapenski, *Intermediate Financial Management* (Fort Worth, TX: Dryden Press, 1996), chapter 6.

11. For one of the classic works on equity costs in not-for-profit organizations, see D. A. Conrad, "Returns on Equity to Not-For-Profit Hospitals: Theory and Implementation," *Health Services Research* (April 1984): 41–63. Also, see the follow-up articles by Pauly, Conrad, and Silvers and Kauer in the April 1986 issue of *Health Services Research*.

12. An adjustment to account for capital structure and tax differences can be made using an equation called *Hamada's equation*. See E. F. Brigham and L. C. Gapenski,

Intermediate Financial Management (Fort Worth, TX: Dryden Press, 1996), chapter 11.

13. An alternative approach for not-for-profit businesses is to use the business' long-run future growth rate as the cost of equity. This approach is based on the fact that equity returns must be at least this value to finance future asset growth.

14. For a discussion of flotation-adjusted equity costs, see E. F. Brigham and L. C. Gapenski, *Intermediate Financial Management* (Fort Worth, TX: Dryden Press, 1996), chapter 6.

15. Debt capacity differences should also be accounted for when applying the corporate cost of capital to individual projects. For example, the target capital structure for the firm as a whole may be 50 percent debt, while a project being evaluated involving a medical office building (i.e., real estate) may have a target capital structure (i.e., debt capacity) of, say, 80 percent debt. However, debt capacity is very difficult to measure for most projects. Furthermore, debt capacity differences have less effect on the cost of capital than do risk differences. For these reasons, capital structure adjustments will not be discussed here.

References

Boles, K. E. 1986a. "Implications of the Method of Capital Cost Payment on the Weighted Average Cost of Capital." *Health Services Research* (June): 191–211.

———. 1986b. "What Accounting Leaves Out of Hospital Financial Management." *Hospital & Health Services Administration* (March/April): 8–27.

Gapenski, L. C. 1993. "Hospital Capital Structure Decisions: Theory and Practice." *Health Services Management Research* (November): 237–247.

Harris, J. P. and V. E. Schimmel. 1987. "Market Value: An Underused Financial Planning Tool." *Healthcare Financial Management* (April): 40–46.

McCue, M. J. and Y. A. Ozcan. 1992. "Determinants of Capital Structure." *Hospital & Health Services Administration* (Fall): 333–346.

Sloan, F. A., J. Valvona, and M. Hassan. 1988. "Cost of Capital to the Hospital Sector." *Journal of Health Economics* (March): 25–45.

Smith, D. G. and J. R. C. Wheeler. 1989. "Accounting Based Risk Measures for Not-for-Profit Hospitals." *Health Services Management Research* (November): 221–226.

Sterns, J. B. and T. K. Majidzadeh. 1995. "A Framework for Evaluating Capital Structure." *Journal of Health Care Finance* (Winter): 80–85.

Valvona, J. and F. A. Sloan. 1988. "Hospital Profitability and Capital Structure: A Comparative Analysis." *Health Services Research* (August): 343–357.

Vaughan, J. and J. Wise. 1996. "How to Choose the Right Capitalization Option." *Healthcare Financial Management.* (December): 72–74.

Wedig, G. J., F. A. Sloan, M. Hassan, and M. A. Morrisey. 1988. "Capital Structure, Ownership, and Capital Payment Policy: The Case of Hospitals." *Journal of Finance* (March): 21–40.

Wheeler, J. R. C. and D. G. Smith. 1988. "The Discount Rate for Capital Expenditure Analysis in Health Care." *Health Care Management Review* (Spring): 43–51.

CAPITAL INVESTMENT DECISIONS

THE BASICS OF CAPITAL BUDGETING

Learning Objectives

After studying this chapter, readers will be able to:

- Explain how managers use project classifications and post audits in the capital budgeting process.
- Discuss the role of financial analysis in health services capital budgeting decisions.
- Discuss the key elements of cash flow estimation, breakeven analysis, and profitability analysis.
- Conduct basic capital budgeting analyses.

Introduction

Chapter 13 described how health services managers make capital structure decisions and estimate their business' corporate costs of capital. The focus in this chapter is on fixed asset acquisition decisions. Although some investment decisions, such as the decision to expand the operating hours of a walk-in clinic, involve only the expenditure of operating funds, most investment decisions entail the acquisition of new facilities or equipment. Thus, decisions of this type are often called *capital investment*, or *capital budgeting*, *decisions*. Capital budgeting decisions are of fundamental importance to the success or failure of any business because a firm's capital budgeting decisions, more than anything else, shape its future.

The discussion of capital budgeting is divided into two chapters. Chapter 14 provides an overview of the capital budgeting process, a discussion of the key elements of project cash flow estimation, and an explanation of the basic techniques that are used to assess a project's breakeven and profitability. In Chapter 15, capital budgeting risk analysis and the optimal capital budget are considered.

Importance of Capital Budgeting

Capital budgeting decisions are among the most critical ones that health services managers must make. First and most importantly, the results of capital budgeting decisions generally affect the business for an extended period. If a business invests too heavily in fixed assets, it will have too much capacity and its costs will necessarily be too high. On the other hand, a business that invests too little in fixed assets may face two problems: technological obsolescence and inadequate capacity. A healthcare provider without the latest technology will lose patients to its more up-to-date competitors and, further, will deprive its patients of the best healthcare diagnostics and treatments available. A provider with inadequate capacity may lose a portion of its market share to competitors, which would then require it to increase its marketing costs or aggressively reduce prices to regain the lost share.

Effective capital budgeting procedures provide several benefits to businesses. A business that forecasts its needs for capital assets well in advance will have the opportunity to plan the purchases carefully, and thus will be able to negotiate the highest quality assets at the best prices. Additionally, asset expansion typically involves substantial expenditures, and because large amounts of funds are not usually at hand, they must be raised externally. Good capital budgeting practices permit a business to identify its financing needs and sources well in advance, which ensures both the lowest possible procurement costs and the availability of funds as they are needed.

Self-Test Questions

1. Why are capital budgeting decisions so crucial to the success of a business?
2. What are the benefits of effective capital budgeting procedures?

Project Classifications

Although benefits can be gained from the careful analysis of capital investment proposals, such efforts can be costly. For certain types of projects, a relatively detailed analysis may be warranted; for others, cost/benefit studies suggest that simpler procedures should be used. Accordingly, healthcare businesses generally classify projects into categories and then analyze those in each category differently. For example, Bayside Memorial Hospital uses the following classifications:

- *Category 1: Mandatory replacement.* Category 1 consists of expenditures necessary to replace worn out or damaged equipment that are necessary to the operations of the hospital. In general, these expenditures are mandatory, so they are usually made without going through an elaborate decision process.
- *Category 2: Discretionary replacement.* This category includes expenditures to replace serviceable but obsolete equipment. The purpose of these projects generally is to lower costs or to provide more clinically effective services. Because Category 2 projects are not mandatory, a more detailed analysis is generally required to support the expenditure than that needed for Category 1 projects.
- *Category 3: Expansion of existing products, services, or markets.* Expenditures to increase capacity or to expand within markets currently being served by the hospital are included here. These decisions are more complex, so still more detailed analysis is required, and the final decision is made at a higher level within the organization.

- *Category 4: Expansion into new products, services, or markets.* These are projects necessary to provide new products or services, or to expand into geographical areas that are not currently being served. Such projects involve strategic decisions that could change the fundamental nature of the hospital and normally require the expenditure of large sums of money over long periods. Invariably, a particularly detailed analysis is required, and the board of trustees generally makes the final decision as part of the hospital's strategic plan.
- *Category 5: Safety/Environmental projects.* This category consists of expenditures necessary to comply with government orders, labor agreements, accreditation requirements, and so on. Unless the expenditures are large, Category 5 expenditures are treated like Category 1 expenditures.
- *Category 6: Other.* This category is a catchall for projects that do not fit neatly into another category. The primary determinant of how Category 6 projects are evaluated is their size.

1. What is the advantage of classifying capital projects?
2. What are some typical classifications?

Self-Test Questions

The Role of Financial Analysis in Health Services Capital Budgeting

For investor-owned firms that have shareholder wealth maximization as the primary goal, the role of financial analysis in investment decisions is clear. Those projects that contribute to shareholder wealth should be undertaken, while those that do not should be ignored. However, what about not-for-profit firms that do not have shareholder wealth maximization as a goal? In such firms, the appropriate goal is providing quality, cost-effective service to the communities served. (A strong argument could be made that this should also be the goal of investor-owned firms in the health services industry.) In this situation, capital budgeting decisions must consider many factors besides a project's financial implications. For example, the needs of the medical staff and the good of the community must be taken into account. Indeed, in some instances, these noneconomic factors will outweigh financial considerations.

Nevertheless, good decision making, and hence the future viability of health services organizations, requires that the financial impact of capital investments be fully recognized. If a business takes on a series of highly unprofitable projects that meet nonfinancial goals and such projects are not offset by other profitable projects, the firm's financial condition will deteriorate. If this situation persists over time, the business will eventually lose its financial viability and may even be forced into bankruptcy and closure.[1]

Because bankrupt firms obviously cannot meet a community's needs, even managers of not-for-profit businesses must consider a project's potential impact on the firm's financial condition. Managers may make a conscious decision to accept a project with a poor financial prognosis because of its nonfinancial virtues, but it is important that managers know the financial impact up front rather than be surprised when the project drains the firm's financial resources. Financial analysis provides managers with the relevant information about a project's financial impact, and hence helps managers make better decisions, including those decisions based primarily on nonfinancial considerations.

Self-Test Questions

1. What is the role of financial analysis in capital budgeting decision making within for-profit firms?
2. Why is project financial analysis important in not-for-profit businesses?

Overview of Capital Budgeting Financial Analysis

The financial analysis of capital investment proposals typically involves the following five steps:

1. The capital outlay, or cost, of the project must be estimated.
2. The operating and terminal cash flows of the project must be forecasted. Steps 1 and 2 constitute the cash flow estimation phase, which is discussed in the next section.
3. The riskiness of the estimated cash flows must be assessed. Risk assessment will be discussed in Chapter 15.
4. Given the riskiness of the project, the project's cost of capital must be estimated. As discussed in Chapter 13, the firm's corporate cost of capital reflects the aggregate risk of the firm's assets, that is, the riskiness inherent in the firm's average project. If the project being evaluated does not have average risk, the firm's cost of capital must be adjusted.
5. Finally, the financial impact (profitability) of the project is assessed. Several measures can be used for this purpose; two commonly used measures (NPV and IRR) are discussed in this chapter.

Self-Test Question

1. Explain the five steps in capital budgeting financial analysis.

Cash Flow Estimation

The most critical and most difficult step in evaluating capital investment proposals is *cash flow estimation*. This step involves estimating the investment outlays, the annual net operating flows expected when the project goes into operation, and the cash flows associated with project termination. Many variables are involved in cash flow estimation, and many individuals and departments participate in the process. Making accurate projections of the costs and revenues associated with a large, complex project is difficult, so forecast errors can be quite large. Thus, it is essential that risk analyses be performed on prospective projects.

To emphasize the difficulties involved, one manager with a good sense of humor developed the following five principles of capital budgeting cash flow estimation:

1. It is very difficult to forecast cash flows, especially those that occur in the future.
2. Those who live by the crystal ball soon learn how to eat ground glass.
3. The moment someone forecasts cash flows, they know that they are wrong—they just do not know by how much and in what direction.
4. If someone makes a correct forecast, never let the bosses forget.
5. An expert in cash flow estimation is someone who has been right at least once.

Neither the difficulty nor the importance of cash flow estimation can be overstated. However, if the principles discussed in the next sections are observed, errors that often arise in the process can be minimized.

Incremental Cash Flows

The relevant cash flows to consider when evaluating a new capital investment are the project's *incremental cash flows*, which are defined as the difference in the firm's cash flows in each period if the project is undertaken versus the firm's cash flows if the project is not undertaken:

$$\text{Incremental CF}_t = \text{CF}_{t(\text{Firm with project})} - \text{CF}_{t(\text{Firm without project})}.$$

Here the subscript t specifies a time period, normally years. CF_0 is the incremental cash flow during Year 0, which is generally assumed to end today, CF_1 is the incremental cash flow during the first year, CF_2 is the incremental cash flow during Year 2, and so on. In practice, the early incremental cash flows, and Year 0 in particular, are usually cash outflows, which are the costs associated with getting the project up and running. As the project begins to generate revenues, the incremental cash flows normally turn positive.

In practice, it typically is not feasible to forecast the cash flows of a business with and without a new project. Thus, the actual estimation process focuses on the cash flows that are unique to the project being evaluated. However, if a doubt ever arises as to whether or not a particular cash flow is relevant to the analysis, it is often useful to fall back on the basic definition given above.

Cash Flow Versus Accounting Income

As discussed in Chapters 3 and 4, accounting income statements define revenues and costs in terms that do not reflect the actual movement of cash. In capital investment decisions, the decision must be based on the actual dollars that flow into and out of the firm. A firm's true profitability, and hence its future financial condition, depends more on its cash flows than on income as reported in accordance with generally accepted accounting principles. Accounting items can influence cash flows, however, because items like depreciation can affect tax (for investor-owned firms) or reimbursement cash flows.

Cash Flow Timing

Financial analysts must be careful to account properly for the timing of cash flows. Accounting income statements are for periods such as years or quarters, so they do not reflect exactly when, during the period, revenues and expenses occur. In theory, capital budgeting cash flows should be analyzed exactly as they are expected to occur. Of course, there must be a compromise between accuracy and simplicity. A time line with daily cash flows would, in theory, provide the most accuracy, but daily cash flow estimates would be costly to construct, unwieldy to use, and probably no more accurate than annual cash flow estimates. Thus, in most cases, analysts simply assume that all cash flows occur at the end of every year. However, for some projects, it may be useful to assume that cash flows occur every six months or to forecast quarterly or monthly cash flows.

Project Life

One of the first decisions that must be made in forecasting a project's cash flows is the life of the project. Does the forecast for cash flows need to be for 20 years or is five years sufficient? Many projects, such as a new hospital wing or an ambulatory care clinic, potentially have very long lives, perhaps 50 years or more. In theory, a cash flow forecast should extend for the full life of a project, yet most managers would have very little confidence in any cash flow forecasts beyond the near term. Thus, most organizations set an arbitrary limit on the project life assumed in capital budgeting analyses, which is often five or ten years. If the forecasted life is less than the arbitrary limit, the forecasted life is used to develop the cash flows, but if the forecasted life exceeds the limit, project life is truncated and the operating cash flows beyond the limit are ignored.

Although cash flow truncation is a practical solution to a difficult problem, it does create another problem: the value inherent in the cash flows beyond the truncation point is lost to the project. This problem can be addressed either objectively or subjectively. The standard procedure at some organizations is to estimate the project's *terminal value*, which is the estimated value of the cash flows beyond the truncation point. Often, the terminal value is estimated as the *liquidation value* of the project at that point in time. If the terminal value is too difficult to estimate, the fact that some portion of the project's cash flow value is being ignored should, at a minimum, be subjectively recognized by decision makers. The saving grace in all of this is that cash flows that are forecasted to occur well into the future typically contribute a relatively small amount to project profitability. For example, a $100,000 terminal value projected ten years in the future contributes only about $38,500 to the project's value when the cost of capital (discount rate) is 10 percent.

Some projects have short lives, and hence the analysis can extend over the project's entire life. In such situations, the assets associated with the project may still have some value remaining, perhaps only as scrap, when the project is terminated. The scrap or other value of assets at the end of a project's life is called *salvage value*. Even if a project is being terminated for "old age," any cash flow that will arise by virtue of scrap value must be included in the project's cash flows. For investor-owned businesses, such asset sales typically will trigger tax consequences, which are discussed in the cash flow estimation example presented in the next major section.

Sunk Costs

A *sunk cost* refers to an outlay that has already occurred or has been irrevocably committed, so it is an outlay that is unaffected by the current decision to accept or reject a project. To illustrate, suppose that in 1999 Bayside Memorial Hospital is evaluating the purchase of a lithotripter system. To help in the decision, the hospital hired and paid $10,000 to a consultant in 1998 to conduct a marketing study. This 1998 cash flow is **not** relevant to the 1999 capital investment decision. The $10,000 is a sunk cost; Bayside cannot recover it whether or not the lithotripter is purchased. Sometimes a project appears to be unprofitable when **all** of its associated costs, including sunk costs, are considered. However, on an *incremental* basis, the project may be profitable and should be undertaken. Thus, the correct treatment of sunk costs may be critical to the decision.

Assume for a moment that Bayside goes ahead with the lithotripter project. In 2000, when conducting a periodic analysis (i.e., a post audit, which is discussed later in the chapter) of the *historical* profitability of the project, the $10,000 cost of the consultant's report would be included because it is part of the total cash flows attributable to the project. However, when making the 1999 decision regarding project acceptance, the $10,000 consultant's fee is *nonincremental*, and hence not relevant to the decision as to whether or not to go ahead with the project at that time.

Opportunity Costs

All relevant *opportunity costs* must be included in a capital investment analysis. To illustrate, one opportunity cost involves the use of the funds required to finance the project. If the firm uses its capital to invest in Project A, it cannot use the capital to invest in Project B, or for any other purpose. The opportunity cost associated with capital use is accounted for in the project's cost of capital, which is the rate used to discount the project's expected cash flows, and represents the return that the firm could earn by investing in alternative investments of similar risk.

In addition to the opportunity cost of capital, there are other types of opportunity costs. For example, assume that Bayside's lithotripter would be installed in a freestanding facility and that the hospital currently owns the land on which the facility would be constructed. In fact, the hospital purchased the land ten years ago at a cost of $50,000, but the current market value of the property is $130,000, after subtracting both legal and real estate fees. When evaluating the lithotripter, the value of the land cannot be disregarded merely because no cash outlay is necessary. There is an opportunity cost inherent in the use of the property because using the property for the lithotripter facility deprives Bayside of its use for anything else. The property may be used for a walk-in clinic, ambulatory surgery center, or parking garage rather than sold, but the best measure of its value to Bayside, and hence the opportunity cost inherent in its use, is the cash flow that could be realized from selling the property.

By considering the property's current market value, Bayside is letting market forces assign the value for the land's best alternative use. Thus, the lithotripter project should have a $130,000 opportunity cost charged against it. The opportunity cost is the property's $130,000 net market value, irrespective of whether the property was acquired for $50,000 or $200,000.

Effects on Other Parts of the Business

Capital budgeting analyses must consider the effects of the project under consideration on the firm's other projects. Such effects can be either positive or negative; when negative, it is often called *cannibalization*. To illustrate, assume that some of the patients that are expected to use Bayside's new lithotripter would have been treated surgically at Bayside, so these surgical revenues will be lost if the lithotripter facility goes into operation. Thus, the incremental revenues to Bayside are the revenues attributable to the lithotripter, **less** the revenues lost from forgone surgery services.

On the other hand, new patients that use the lithotripter may utilize other services provided by the hospital. In this situation, the incremental cash flows generated by the lithotripter patients' utilization of other services should be credited to the lithotripter project. If possible, both positive and negative effects on other projects should be quantified, but at a minimum they should be noted, so that these effects are considered when the final decision regarding the project is made.

Shipping, Installation, and Related Costs

When a firm acquires fixed assets, it often incurs substantial costs for shipping and installing the equipment or for other related activities. These charges must be added to the invoice price of the equipment to determine the overall cost of the project. Also, the full cost of the equipment, **including** such costs, typically is used as the basis for calculating depreciation charges. Thus, if Bayside Memorial Hospital purchases intensive care monitoring equipment that costs $200,000, but another $20,000 is required for shipping and installation, the full cost of the equipment would be $220,000; this amount would be the starting point for both tax and book depreciation calculations.

Changes in Net Working Capital

Normally, expansion projects require additional inventories; expanded patient volumes also lead to additional accounts receivable. The increase in these current assets must be financed, just as an increase in fixed assets must be financed.

(Increases in the left side of the balance sheet require matching increases on the right side.) However, accounts payable and accruals will probably also increase as a result of the expansion; these current liability funds will reduce the net cash needed to finance the increase in inventories and receivables.

Current assets are often referred to as *working capital*; the difference between current assets and current liabilities is called *net working capital*. Thus, projects that have an impact on current assets and current liabilities create **changes** in net working capital. If this change is positive (i.e., if the increase in current assets exceeds the increase in current liabilities), this amount is as much a cash cost to the project as is the dollar cost of the asset itself. Such projects must be charged an additional amount above the dollar cost of the new fixed asset to reflect the net financing needed for the current asset accounts. Similarly, if the change in net working capital is negative, the project is generating a positive working capital cash flow because the increase in liabilities exceeds the project's current asset requirements and this cash flow partially offsets the cost of the asset being acquired.

As the project approaches termination, inventories will be sold off and not replaced, and receivables will be converted to cash without new receivables being created. In effect, the business will recover its investment in net working capital when the project is terminated. This will result in a cash flow that is equal, but **opposite** in sign, to the change in net working capital cash flow that arises at the beginning of a project.

For healthcare providers, where inventories often represent a very small part of the investment in new projects, the change in net working capital often can be ignored without materially affecting the results of the analysis. However, when a project results in a large positive change in net working capital, failure to consider the net investment in current assets will result in an overstatement of the project's profitability.

Inflation Effects

Inflation seems to be a fact of life, and because inflation effects can have a considerable influence on a project's profitability, inflation must be considered in any sound capital budgeting analysis. As discussed in Chapter 13, a firm's corporate cost of capital is a weighted average of its costs of debt and equity. These costs are estimated on the basis of investors' required rates of return, and investors incorporate an inflation premium into their required returns. For example, a debt investor may require a 5 percent return on a ten-year bond in the absence of inflation. However, if inflation is expected to average 6 percent over the coming ten years, the investor would require an 11 percent return. Thus, investors add an inflation premium to their required rates of return to help protect them against the loss of purchasing power that stems from inflation.

Because inflation effects are already imbedded in the corporate cost of capital and because this cost will be used as the starting point to discount the cash flows in the profitability measures, inflation effects must also be built into the project's estimated cash flows. If cash flow estimates do not include inflation effects, but a discount rate is used that includes inflation effects, the profitability of the project will be understated.

The most effective way to deal with inflation is apply inflation effects to each cash flow element using the best available information about how each element will be affected. Because it is impossible to estimate future inflation rates with much precision, errors will probably be made. Often, inflation is assumed to be neutral (i.e., it is assumed to affect revenues and costs, except depreciation, equally). However, situations can arise where costs may be inflating faster than charges, or vice versa. When such situations are expected to occur, then different inflation rates should be applied to each cash flow element. For example, charges net of bad debt losses and discounts may be expected to increase at a 4 percent rate, while labor costs are expected to increase at an 8 percent rate. Inflation adds to the uncertainty, or riskiness, of capital budgeting analysis, as well as to its complexity. Fortunately, computers and spreadsheet programs are available to help with inflation analysis, so the mechanics of inflation adjustments are not difficult.

Strategic Value

Sometimes, a project will have value in addition to the value inherent in its cash flows. Such hidden value often stems from *strategic value*, which is defined as the value of future investment opportunities that can be undertaken only if the project that is currently under consideration is accepted.

To illustrate this concept, consider a hospital management company that is analyzing a management contract for a hospital in Hungary, which marks its first move into Eastern Europe. On a stand-alone basis, this project may be unprofitable, but the project may provide entry into the Eastern European market, which could unlock the door to a whole range of highly profitable new projects. Or consider Bayside Memorial Hospital's decision to start a kidney transplant program. The financial analysis of this project showed the program to be unprofitable, but Bayside's managers considered kidney transplants to be the first step in an aggressive transplant program that would not only be profitable in itself, but would enhance the hospital's reputation for technological and clinical excellence, and thus would contribute to the hospital's overall profitability.

In theory, the best approach to dealing with strategic value is to forecast the cash flows from the follow-on projects, estimate their probabilities of occurrence, and then add the expected cash flows from the follow-on projects to the cash flows of the project under consideration. In practice, this is usually impossible to do—either the follow-on cash flows are too nebulous to forecast or the potential follow-on projects are too numerous to quantify.[2] At a minimum, decision makers must recognize that some projects have strategic value, and this value should be qualitatively considered when making capital budgeting decisions.

Self-Test Questions

1. Briefly discuss the following concepts associated with cash flow estimation:
   a. Incremental cash flow

    b. Cash flow versus accounting income
    c. Cash flow timing
    d. Project life
       (1) Terminal value
       (2) Salvage value
    e. Sunk costs
    f. Opportunity costs
    g. Effects on other projects
    h. Shipping and installation costs
    i. Changes in net working capital
    j. Inflation effects
    k. Strategic value
2. Evaluate the following statement: Ignoring inflation effects and strategic value can result in **overstating** a project's financial attractiveness.

Cash Flow Estimation Example

Up to this point, several critical aspects of cash flow estimation have been discussed. In this section, an example is presented that illustrates some of the concepts already covered and introduces several others that are important to good cash flow estimation.

The Basic Data

Consider the situation faced by Bayside Memorial Hospital, a not-for-profit hospital, in its evaluation of a new MRI system. The system costs $1.5 million, and the hospital would have to spend another $1 million for site preparation and installation. Because the system would be installed in the hospital, the space to be used has a very low, or zero, market value to outsiders. Furthermore, its value to Bayside for other projects is very difficult to estimate, so no opportunity cost has been assigned to account for the value of the site.

The MRI system is estimated to generate weekly usage (i.e., volume) of 40 scans, and each scan on average would cost the hospital $15 in supplies. The system is expected to operate 50 weeks a year, with the remaining two weeks devoted to maintenance. The estimated average charge per scan is $500, but 25 percent of this amount, on average, is expected to be lost to indigent patients, contractual allowances, and bad debt losses. Bayside's managers developed the project's forecasted revenues by conducting the revenue analysis contained in Table 14.1.

The MRI system would require two technicians, which results in an incremental increase in annual labor costs of $50,000, including fringe benefits. Cash overhead costs would increase by $10,000 annually if the MRI is activated. The equipment would require maintenance, which would be furnished by the manufacturer for an annual fee of $150,000, payable at the end of each year of

TABLE 14.1

Bayside Memorial
Hospital: MRI Site
Revenue Analysis

Payor	Number of Scans per Week	Charge per Scan	Total Charges	Basis of Payment	Net Payment per Scan	Total Payments
Medicare	10	$500	$ 5,000	Fixed fee	$370	$ 3,700
Medicaid	5	500	2,500	Fixed fee	350	1,750
Private insurance	9	500	4,500	Full charge	500	4,500
Blue Cross	5	500	2,500	Percent of charge	420	2,100
Managed care	7	500	3,500	Percent of charge	390	2,730
Self-pay	4	500	2,000	Full charge	55	220
Total	40		$20,000			$15,000
Average			$ 500			$ 375

operation. For book purposes, the MRI will be depreciated by the straight-line method over a five-year life.

The MRI system is expected to be in operation for five years, at which time the hospital's master plan calls for a new imaging facility. The hospital plans to sell the MRI at that time for an estimated $750,000 salvage value, net of removal costs. The inflation rate is estimated to average 5 percent over the period, and this rate is expected to affect all revenues and costs except depreciation. Bayside's managers initially assume that projects under evaluation have average risk, and thus the hospital's 10 percent corporate cost of capital is the appropriate project cost of capital (opportunity cost discount rate). In Chapter 15, a risk assessment of the project may indicate that a different cost of capital is appropriate.

Although the MRI project is expected to take away some patients from the hospital's other imaging systems, the new MRI patients are expected to generate revenues for some of the hospital's other departments. On net, the two effects are expected to balance out. That is, the cash flow loss from other imaging systems is expected to be offset by the cash flow gain from other services utilized by new MRI patients. Also, the project is estimated to have negligible net working capital implications, so changes in net working capital will be ignored in the analysis.

Cash Flow Analysis

The first step in the financial analysis is to estimate the MRI site's net cash flows. This analysis is presented in Table 14.2. Here are the key points of the analysis by line number:

- *Line 1:* Line 1 contains the estimated cost of the MRI system. In general, capital budgeting analyses assume that the first cash flow, normally an outflow, occurs today or at the end of Year 0. Expenses, or cash outflows, are shown in parentheses.
- *Line 2:* The related site construction expense, $1,000,000, is also assumed to occur at Year 0.

TABLE 14.2

Bayside Memorial Hospital: MRI Site Cash Flow Analysis

			Cash Revenues and Costs			
	0	1	2	3	4	5
1. System cost	($1,500,000)					
2. Related expenses	(1,000,000)					
3. Gross revenues		$1,000,000	$1,050,000	$1,102,500	$1,157,625	$1,215,506
4. Deductions		250,000	262,500	275,625	289,406	303,877
5. Net revenues		$ 750,000	$ 787,500	$ 826,875	$ 868,219	$ 911,630
6. Labor costs		50,000	52,500	55,125	57,881	60,775
7. Maintenance costs		150,000	157,500	165,375	173,644	182,326
8. Supplies		30,000	31,500	33,075	34,729	36,465
9. Incremental overhead		10,000	10,500	11,025	11,576	12,155
10. Depreciation		350,000	350,000	350,000	350,000	350,000
11. Operating income		$ 160,000	$ 185,500	$ 212,275	$ 240,389	$ 269,908
12. Taxes		0	0	0	0	0
13. Net operating income		$ 160,000	$ 185,500	$ 212,275	$ 240,389	$ 269,908
14. Depreciation		350,000	350,000	350,000	350,000	350,000
15. Net salvage value						750,000
16. Net cash flow	($2,500,000)	$ 510,000	$ 535,500	$ 562,275	$ 590,389	$1,369,908

Note: Totals are rounded.

- *Line 3:* Annual gross revenues = Weekly volume × Weeks of operation per year × Charge per scan = 40 × 50 × $500 = $1,000,000 in the first year. The 5 percent inflation rate is applied to all charges and costs that would likely be affected by inflation, so the gross revenue amount shown on Line 3 increases by 5 percent over time.

  Although most of the operating revenues and costs would occur more or less evenly over the year, it is very difficult to forecast exactly when the flows would occur. Furthermore, there is significant potential for large errors in cash flow estimation. For these reasons, operating cash flows are often assumed to occur at the end of each year. Also, the assumption is that the MRI system could be placed in operation quickly. If this were not the case, then the first year's operating flows would be reduced. In some situations, it may take several years from the first investment cash flow to get to the point when the project is operational and begins to generate revenues.

- *Line 4:* Deductions from charges are estimated to average 25 percent of gross revenues, so in Year 1, 0.25 × $1,000,000 = $250,000 of gross revenues would be uncollected. This amount increases each year by the 5 percent inflation rate.

- *Line 5:* Line 5 contains the net revenues in each year, Line 3 − Line 4.

- *Line 6:* Labor costs are forecasted to be $50,000 during the first year, but increase over time at the 5 percent inflation rate.

- *Line 7:* Maintenance fees must be paid to the manufacturer at the end of each year of operation. These fees are assumed to increase at the 5 percent inflation rate.

- *Line 8:* Each scan uses $15 of supplies, so supply costs in the first year total 40 × 50 × $15 = $30,000; they are expected to increase each year by the inflation rate.

- *Line 9:* If the project is accepted, overhead cash costs will increase by $10,000 in the first year. Note that the $10,000 are cash costs that are related directly to the acceptance of the MRI project. Existing overhead costs that are arbitrarily allocated to the MRI project are **not** incremental cash flows, and thus should not be included in the analysis. Overhead costs are also assumed to increase over time at the inflation rate.

- *Line 10:* Book depreciation in each year is calculated by the straight-line method, assuming a five-year depreciable life. The depreciable basis is equal to the capitalized cost of the project, which includes the cost of the asset and related construction, less the estimated salvage value. Thus, the depreciable basis is ($1,500,000 + $1,000,000) − $750,000 = $1,750,000. Then, the straight-line depreciation in each year of the project's five-year depreciable life is (1/5) × $1,750,000 = $350,000.

  Note that depreciation is based solely on acquisition costs, so it is unaffected by inflation. Also, note that the Table 14.2 cash flows are presented in a generic format that can be used by both investor-owned and not-for-profit hospitals. Depreciation expense is not a cash flow, but an accounting convention that recognizes the reduction in value of fixed assets caused by wear and tear and obsolescence. Because Bayside Memorial Hospital is tax exempt, and hence depreciation will not affect taxes, and because depreciation is added back to the cash flows on Line 14, depreciation could be totally omitted from the cash flow analysis.

- *Line 11:* Line 11 shows the project's operating income in each year, which is merely net revenues less all operating expenses.
- *Line 12:* Line 12 contains zeros because Bayside is not-for-profit, and hence does not pay taxes.
- *Line 13:* Bayside pays no taxes, so the project's net operating income equals its operating income.
- *Line 14:* Because depreciation, a noncash expense, was included on Line 10, it must be added back to the project's net operating income in each year to obtain each year's net cash flow.
- *Line 15:* The project is expected to be terminated after five years, at which time the MRI system would be sold for an estimated $750,000. This salvage value cash flow is shown as an inflow at the end of Year 5 on Line 15.
- *Line 16:* The project's net cash flows are shown on Line 16. The project requires a $2,500,000 investment at Year 0, but then generates cash inflows over its five-year operating life.

The Table 14.2 cash flows do not include any allowance for interest expense. On average, Bayside hospital will finance new projects in accordance with its target capital structure, which consists of 50 percent debt financing and 50 percent equity (i.e., fund) financing. The costs associated with this financing mix, including both interest costs and the opportunity cost of equity capital, are incorporated into the firm's 10 percent corporate cost of capital. Because the cost of debt financing is included in the discount rate that will be applied to the cash flows, recognition of interest expense in the cash flows would be double counting.

Taxable Organizations

The Table 14.2 cash flow analysis can be easily modified to reflect tax implications if the analyzing firm is taxable. To illustrate, assume that the MRI project is being evaluated by Ann Arbor Health Systems, an investor-owned hospital chain. Assume also that all of the project data presented earlier apply to Ann Arbor, except that the MRI falls into the MACRS five-year class for tax depreciation, and the firm has a 40 percent tax rate.

Table 14.3 contains Ann Arbor's cash flow analysis. Note the following differences from the not-for-profit analysis performed in Table 14.2:

TABLE 14.3
Ann Arbor Health Systems: MRI Site Cash Flow Analysis

		Cash Revenues and Costs				
	0	1	2	3	4	5
1. System cost	($1,500,000)					
2. Related expenses	(1,000,000)					
3. Gross revenues		$1,000,000	$1,050,000	$1,102,500	$1,157,625	$1,215,506
4. Deductions		250,000	262,500	275,625	289,406	303,877
5. Net revenues		$ 750,000	$ 787,500	$ 826,875	$ 868,219	$ 911,630
6. Labor costs		50,000	52,500	55,125	57,881	60,775
7. Maintenance costs		150,000	157,500	165,375	173,644	182,326
8. Supplies		30,000	31,500	33,075	34,729	36,465
9. Incremental overhead		10,000	10,500	11,025	11,576	12,155
10. Depreciation		500,000	800,000	475,000	300,000	275,000
11. Operating income		$ 10,000	($ 264,500)	$ 87,275	$ 290,389	$ 344,908
12. Taxes		4,000	(105,800)	34,910	116,156	137,963
13. Net operating income		$ 6,000	($ 158,700)	$ 52,365	$ 174,233	$ 206,945
14. Depreciation		500,000	800,000	475,000	300,000	300,000
15. Net salvage value						510,000
16. Net cash flow	($2,500,000)	$ 506,000	$ 641,300	$ 527,365	$ 474,233	$ 991,945

Note: Totals are rounded.

- *Line 10:* Depreciation expense must be modified to reflect tax depreciation rather than book depreciation. Tax depreciation is calculated using the *Modified Accelerated Cost Recovery System (MACRS)* as specified in current tax laws. Each year's tax depreciation is found by multiplying the asset's depreciable basis, without considering its estimated salvage value, by the appropriate depreciation factor. In the MRI illustration, the depreciable basis is $2,500,000, and the MRI system falls into the MACRS five-year class, so the MACRS factors specified by the tax code are 0.20, 0.32, 0.19, 0.12, 0.11, and 0.06, in Years 1 to 6, respectively. Thus, the tax depreciation in Year 1 is $0.20 \times \$2,500,000 = \$500,000$, in Year 2 the depreciation is $0.32 \times \$2,500,000 = \$800,000$, and so on.[3]
- *Line 12:* Taxable firms must reduce the operating income on Line 11 by the amount of taxes. Taxes, which appear on Line 12, are computed by multiplying the Line 11 pre-tax operating income by the firm's marginal tax rate. For example, the project's taxes for Year 1 are $0.40 \times \$10,000 = \$4,000$. The taxes shown for Year 2 are a negative $105,800. In this year, the project is expected to lose $264,500, and hence Ann Arbor's taxable income, assuming that its existing projects are profitable, will be reduced by this amount if the project is undertaken. This reduction in taxable income would lower the firm's tax bill by T × Reduction in taxable income = $0.40 \times \$264,500 = \$105,800$.[4]
- *Line 14:* The MACRS depreciation is added back in Line 14.
- *Line 15:* Investor-owned firms will normally incur a tax liability on the sale of a capital asset at the end of the project's life. According to the IRS, the value of the MRI system at the end of Year 5 is the *tax book value*, which is the depreciation that remains on the tax books. For the MRI, five years worth of depreciation would be taken, so only one year of depreciation remains. The MACRS factor for Year 6 is 0.06, so by the end of Year 5, Ann Arbor has expensed 0.94 of the MRI's depreciable basis and the remaining tax book value is $0.06 \times \$2,500,000 = \$150,000$. Thus, according to the IRS, the value of the MRI system is $150,000. When Ann Arbor sells the system for its estimated salvage value of $750,000, it realizes a "profit" of $750,000 − $150,000 = \$600,000$, and it must repay the IRS an amount equal to $0.4 \times \$600,000 = \$240,000$. The $240,000 tax bill recognizes that Ann Arbor took too much depreciation on the MRI system, so it represents a *recapture* of the excess tax benefit taken over the five-year life of the system. The $240,000 in taxes reduces the cash flow received from the sale of the MRI equipment, so the salvage value net of taxes is $750,000 − $240,000 = \$510,000$.

As can be seen by comparing Line 16 in Tables 14.2 and 14.3, with all else the same, the taxes paid by investor-owned firms tend to reduce a project's net operating cash flows and net salvage value, and hence reduce the project's financial attractiveness.

Replacement Analysis

Bayside Hospital's MRI project was used to illustrate how the cash flows from an *expansion project* are analyzed. All firms, including Bayside Memorial Hospital, also make *replacement decisions* in which a new asset is being considered to replace an existing asset which could, if not replaced, continue in operation. The cash flow analysis for a replacement decision is somewhat more complex than for an expansion decision because the cash flows from the existing asset must be considered.

Again, the key to cash flow estimation is to focus on the **incremental cash flows**. If the new asset is acquired, the existing asset can be sold, so the current market value of the existing asset is a cash inflow in the analysis. When considering the operating flows, the incremental flows are the cash flows expected from the replacement asset less the flows that the existing asset would produce if not replaced. By applying the incremental cash flow concept, the correct cash flows can be estimated for replacement decisions.[5]

Self-Test Questions

1. Briefly, how is a project cash flow analysis constructed?
2. Is it necessary to include depreciation expense in a cash flow analysis by a not-for-profit provider? Explain your answer.
3. What are the key differences in cash flow analyses performed by investor-owned and not-for-profit businesses?
4. How do expansion and replacement cash flow analyses differ?

Breakeven Analysis

Breakeven analysis was first introduced in Chapter 5 in conjunction with breakeven volume in an accounting profit analysis. Here, the breakeven concept is reapplied in a project analysis setting. In project analyses, many different types of breakeven can be determined. Rather than discuss all the possible types of breakeven, the focus here is on one type—time breakeven.

Payback is defined as the expected number of years required to recover the investment in a project, so payback, or *payback period*, measures time breakeven. To illustrate, consider the net cash flows for the MRI project contained in Table 14.2. The best way to determine the MRI's payback is to construct the project's *cumulative cash flows* as shown in Table 14.4. The cumulative cash flow at any point in time is merely the sum of all the cash flows (with proper sign indicating an inflow or outflow) that have occurred up to that point. Thus, in Table 14.4, the cumulative cash flow at Year 0 is −$2,500,000, at Year 1 it is −$2,500,000 + $510,000 = −$1,990,000, at Year 2 it is −$2,500,000 + $510,000 + $535,500 = −$1,990,000 + $535,500 = −$1,454,500, and so on.

As shown in Table 14.4, the $2,500,000 investment in the MRI project will be recovered some time during Year 5 if the cash flow forecasts are correct. Furthermore, if the cash flows are assumed to come in evenly during the year,

Year	Annual Cash Flows	Cumulative Cash Flows
0	($2,500,000)	($2,500,000)
1	510,000	(1,990,000)
2	535,500	(1,454,500)
3	562,275	(892,225)
4	590,389	(301,836)
5	1,369,908	1,068,072

TABLE 14.4
Bayside Memorial Hospital: MRI Site Cumulative Cash Flows

breakeven will occur $301,836 / \$1,369,908 = 0.22$ years into Year 5, so the MRI project's payback is 4.22 years.

Initially, payback was used by managers as the primary financial evaluation tool in project analyses. For example, a business may accept all projects with paybacks less than five years. However, payback has two serious deficiencies when it is used as a project selection criterion. First, payback ignores all cash flows that occur after the payback period. To illustrate, Bayside may be evaluating a competing project that has the same cash flows as the MRI project in Years 0 through 5. However, the alternative project may have a cash inflow of $2 million in Year 6. Both projects would have the same payback, 4.22 years, and hence be ranked the same, even though the alternative project clearly is better from a financial perspective. Second, payback ignores the opportunity costs associated with the capital employed. For these reasons, payback generally is no longer used as the primary evaluation tool.[6]

However, payback is useful in capital investment analysis. The shorter the payback, the more quickly the funds invested in a project will become available for other purposes, and hence the more *liquid* the project. Also, cash flows expected in the distant future are generally regarded as being riskier than near-term cash flows, so shorter payback projects generally are less *risky* than those with longer paybacks. Therefore, payback is often used as a rough measure of a project's liquidity and risk.

1. What is payback?
2. What are the benefits of payback?
3. What are its deficiencies when used as the primary evaluation tool?

Self-Test Questions

Profitability Analysis

Up to this point, the chapter has focused on cash flow estimation and breakeven analysis. Perhaps the most important element in a project's financial analysis is its expected profitability. Like all investments, the expected profitability of proposed projects can be measured either in dollars or in percentage rate of return. In the next sections, a dollar measure—net present value (NPV)—and a rate of return measure—internal rate of return (IRR)—are presented.

Net Present Value (NPV)

Net present value (NPV) is a dollar profitability measure that uses discounted cash flow (DCF) techniques, so it is often referred to as a *DCF measure*. To apply the NPV method:

1. Find the present (Time 0) value of each net cash flow, including both inflows and outflows, when discounted at the project's cost of capital.
2. Sum the present values. This sum is defined as the project's net present value.
3. If the NPV is positive, the project is expected to be profitable, and the higher the NPV, the more profitable the project. If the NPV is zero, the project just breaks even in cash flow profitability. If the NPV is negative, the project is expected to be unprofitable.

With a project cost of capital of 10 percent, the NPV of Bayside's MRI project is calculated as follows:

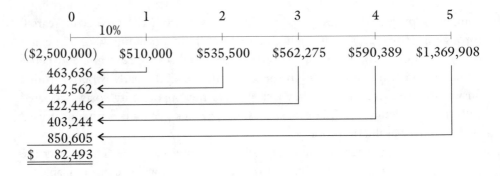

Financial calculators and spreadsheets have NPV functions that easily perform the mathematics if given the cash flows and cost of capital.

The rationale behind the NPV method is straightforward. An NPV of zero signifies that the project's cash inflows are just sufficient to return the capital invested in the project and to provide the required rate of return on that capital. If a project has a positive NPV, it is generating excess cash flows; these excess cash flows are available to management to reinvest in the firm and, for investor-owned firms, to pay dividends. If a project has a negative NPV, its cash inflows are insufficient to compensate the firm for the capital invested, so the project is unprofitable and acceptance would cause the financial condition of the firm to deteriorate. For investor-owned firms, NPV is a direct measure of the contribution of the project to shareholder wealth, so NPV is considered by many academics and practitioners as the best measure of project profitability.

The NPV of the MRI project is $82,493; on a present value basis, the project is expected to generate a cash flow excess of over $80,000 after all costs, including capital costs, have been considered. Thus, the project is profitable and its acceptance would have a positive impact on Bayside's financial condition.

Internal Rate of Return (IRR)

Like NPV, *internal rate of return (IRR)* is also a discounted cash flow (DCF) measure of profitability. However, whereas NPV measures a project's dollar profitability, IRR measures a project's percentage profitability (i.e., its expected rate of return).

Mathematically, the IRR is defined as the discount rate that equates the present value of the project's expected cash inflows to the present value of the project's expected cash outflows, so the IRR is simply that discount rate which forces the NPV of the project to equal **zero**. Financial calculators and spreadsheets have IRR functions that calculate IRRs very rapidly. Simply input the project's cash flows, and the computer or calculator computes the IRR.

For Bayside's MRI project, the IRR is the rate that causes the sum of the present values of the cash inflows to equal the $2,500,000 cost of the project:

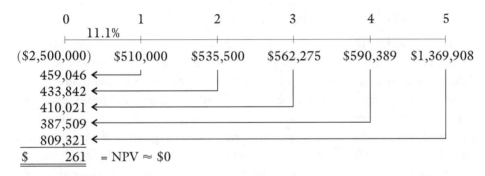

When all of the MRI project's cash flows are discounted at 11.1 percent, the NPV of the project is approximately zero. Thus, the MRI project's IRR is 11.1 percent. Put another way, the project is expected to generate an 11.1 percent rate of return on its $2,500,000 investment. Note that the IRR is like a bond's yield to maturity; it is the rate of return expected on the investment if all the cash flows anticipated actually occur.

If the IRR exceeds the project's cost of capital, a surplus is projected to remain after recovering the invested capital and paying for its use; this surplus accrues to the firm's stockholders (in Bayside's case, to its stakeholders). If the IRR is less than the project's cost of capital, however, taking on the project imposes an expected cost on the firm's stockholders or stakeholders. The MRI project's 11.1 percent IRR exceeds the project's 10 percent cost of capital. Thus, as measured by IRR, the MRI project is profitable and its acceptance would enhance Bayside's financial condition.

Comparison of the NPV and IRR Methods

Consider a project with a zero NPV. In this situation, the project's IRR must equal its cost of capital. The project has zero expected profitability, and acceptance would neither enhance nor diminish the firm's financial condition. To have a positive NPV, the project's IRR must be greater than its cost of capital, and a negative

NPV signifies a project with an IRR less than its cost of capital. Thus, projects that are deemed profitable by the NPV method will also be deemed profitable by the IRR method. In the MRI example, the project would have a positive NPV for all costs of capital less than 11.1 percent. If the cost of capital were greater than 11.1 percent, the project would have a negative NPV. In effect, the NPV and IRR are perfect substitutes for each other in measuring whether or not a project is profitable.[7]

Self-Test Questions
1. Briefly describe how to calculate net present value (NPV) and internal rate of return (IRR).
2. What is the rationale behind each method?
3. Do the two methods lead to the same conclusions regarding project profitability? Explain your answer.

Some Final Thoughts on Breakeven and Profitability Analysis

Three approaches to breakeven and profitability analysis have been presented. However, several additional measures are commonly used in project analysis.[8] Today, virtually all capital budgeting decisions of financial consequence are analyzed by computer, and hence the mechanics of calculating and listing numerous breakeven and profitability measures is easy. Because each measure contributes slightly different information about the financial consequences of a project, managers should not focus on only one or two financial measures. A thorough financial analysis of a new project includes numerous financial measures, and capital budgeting decisions are enhanced if all information inherent in all measures is considered in the process.

Self-Test Questions
1. Evaluate the following statement: The difficulty in calculating numerous breakeven and profitability measures restricts the amount of information available in capital budgeting analyses.
2. Should capital budgeting analyses look at only one breakeven or profitability measure? Explain your answer.

Capital Budgeting in Not-for-Profit Businesses

Although the capital budgeting techniques discussed to this point are appropriate for use by both investor-owned and not-for-profit firms, a not-for-profit firm has the additional consideration of meeting its charitable mission. In this section, two models that extend the capital budgeting decision to not-for-profit firms are discussed.

Net Present Social Value (NPSV) Model[9]

Except for the discussion of strategic value, the financial analysis techniques discussed so far have focused exclusively on the cash flow implications of a proposed project. Some healthcare firms, particularly not-for-profit providers, have the goal of producing social services along with commercial services. For such firms, the proper analysis of proposed projects must systematically consider the *social value* of a project along with its pure financial, or cash flow, value.

When social value is considered, the *total net present value (TNPV)* of a project can be expressed as follows:

$$TNPV = NPV + NPSV.$$

Here, NPV represents the conventional NPV of the project's cash flow stream and *NPSV* is the *net present social value* of the project. The NPSV term, which represents managers' assessment of the social value of the project, clearly differentiates capital budgeting in not-for-profit firms from that in investor-owned firms.

In evaluating each project, a project is acceptable if its TNPV is greater than or equal to zero. This means that the sum of the project's financial and social values is at least zero, so when both facets of value are considered, the project has positive, or at least non-negative, worth. Probably not all projects will have social value, but if a project does, it is considered formally in this decision model. However, no project should be accepted if its NPSV is negative, even if its TNPV is positive. Furthermore, to ensure the financial viability of the firm, the sum of the NPVs of all projects initiated in a planning period must equal or exceed zero.[10] If this restriction were not imposed, social value could displace financial value over time, and a firm cannot continue to provide social value without financial integrity.

NPSV is the sum of the present (Year 0) values of each year's social value. In essence, the suppliers of fund capital to a not-for-profit firm never receive a cash return on their investment. Instead, they receive a return on their investment in the form of social dividends. These dividends take the form of services with social value to the community such as charity care, medical research and education, and a myriad of other services that, for one reason or another, do not pay their own way. Services provided to patients at a price equal to or greater than the full cost of production do not create social value. Similarly, if governmental entities purchase care directly for beneficiaries of a program or support research, the resulting social value is created by that governmental entity and not by the provider of the services.

In estimating a project's NPSV, it is necessary to estimate the social value of the services provided by the project in each year and determine the discount rate to apply to those services. When a project produces services to individuals who are willing and able to pay for those services, the value of those services is captured by the amount that they actually pay. Thus, the value of the services provided to those who cannot pay, or to those who cannot pay the full amount, can be estimated by the average net price paid by those individuals who are able to pay.

This approach to valuing social services has intuitive appeal, but certain points below merit further discussion.

- *Price is a fair measure of value only if the payor has the capacity to judge the true value of the service provided.* Many observers of the health services industry would argue that information asymmetries between the provider and the purchaser inhibit the ability of the purchaser to judge true value.
- *The fact that most payments for healthcare services are made by third-party payors may result in price distortions.* For example, insurers may be willing to pay more for services than an individual would pay in the absence of insurance, or the existence of monopsony power by Medicare may result in a net price that is less than individuals would be willing to pay.
- *A great deal of controversy exists over the true value of treatment in many situations.* Suppose that some people are entitled to whatever healthcare is available, regardless of cost, and are not required to personally pay for the care. Even though society as a whole must cover the bill, people may demand a level of care that is of questionable value. For example, should $500,000 be spent to keep a comatose 92-year old alive for 11 more days? If the true value of such an expenditure is zero, assigning a $500,000 value just because that is its cost makes little sense.

In spite of the potential problems, it still seems reasonable to assign a social value to many, but not all, healthcare services on the basis of the price that others are willing to pay for those services.

The second element required to estimate the NPSV of a project is the discount rate to apply to the annual social value stream. Like the required rate of return on equity for not-for-profit firms, there has been considerable controversy over the proper discount rate to apply to future social values. However, contributors of fund capital clearly can capture social value in two ways. First, as is commonly done, contributions can be made directly to not-for-profit organizations. Second, contributors could always invest the funds in a portfolio of securities and then use the proceeds to purchase the healthcare services directly. In the second situation, there would be no tax consequences on the portfolio's return because the contributed proceeds would qualify for tax exemption, but the contributor would lose the tax exemption on the full amount of the funds placed in the portfolio. Because the second alternative exists, providers should require a return on their social value stream that approximates the return available on the equity investment in for-profit firms offering the same services.

The NPSV model formalizes the capital budgeting decision process applicable to not-for-profit healthcare providers. Although few organizations actually attempt to quantify NPSV, not-for-profit firms should, at a minimum, subjectively consider the social value inherent in projects under consideration.

Project Scoring Approach

Managers of not-for-profit firms, as well as many managers of investor-owned firms, recognize that nonfinancial factors should be considered in any capital budgeting analysis. The NPSV model examines only one other factor, and it is difficult to implement in practice. Thus, many firms use a quasi-subjective project scoring approach to capital budgeting decisions that attempts to capture both financial and nonfinancial factors. Table 14.5, the *project scoring matrix* used by Bayside Memorial Hospital, illustrates one such approach.

Bayside ranks projects on three dimensions: stakeholder factors, operational factors, and financial factors. Within each dimension, multiple factors are examined and assigned scores that range from two points, for very favorable impact, to minus one point, for negative impact. The scores within each dimension are added to obtain scores for stakeholder, operational, and financial factors, and then the dimension scores are aggregated to obtain a total score for the project. The total score gives Bayside's managers a feel for the relative values of projects under consideration when all factors, including financial, are taken into account.

Bayside's managers recognize that the scoring system is completely arbitrary, so a project with a score of ten, for example, is not really twice as good as a project scoring five. Nevertheless, Bayside's project scoring matrix forces its managers to address multiple issues when making capital budgeting decisions. Although Bayside's approach should not be used at other organizations without modification for firm- and industry-unique circumstances, it provides insight into how a firm-unique matrix might be developed.

TABLE 14.5
Project Scoring Matrix

Criteria	Relative Score			
	2	1	0	−1
Stakeholder Factors:				
Physicians	Strongly support	Support	Neutral	Opposed
Employees	Helps morale a lot	Helps morale a little	No effect	Hurts morale
Visitors	Greatly enhances visit	Enhances visit	No effect	Hurts image
Social value	High	Moderate	None	Negative
Operational Factors:				
Outcomes	Greatly improves	Improves	No effect	Hurts outcomes
Length of stay	Documented decrease	Anecdotal decrease	No effect	Increases
Technology	Breakthrough	Improves current	Adds to current	Lowers
Productivity	Large decrease in FTEs	Decrease in FTEs	No change in FTEs	Adds FTEs
Financial Factors:				
Life cycle	Innovation	Growth	Stabilization	Decline
Payback	Less than 2 years	2–4 years	4–6 years	Over 6 years
IRR	Over 20%	15–20%	10–15%	Less than 10%
Correlation	Negative	Uncorrelated	Somewhat positive	Highly positive

Stakeholder factor score _____

Service factor score _____

Financial factor score _____

   Total score ══════

1. Describe the net present social value model of capital budgeting.
2. Describe the construction and use of a project-scoring matrix.

The Post Audit

Capital budgeting is not a static process. If there is a long lag between a project's acceptance and its implementation, any new information concerning either capital costs or the project's cash flows should be analyzed before the final start-up occurs. Furthermore, the performance of each project should be monitored throughout the project's life. The process of formally monitoring project performance over time is called the *post audit*. It involves comparing actual results with those projected by the project's sponsors, explaining why differences occur, and analyzing potential changes to the project's operations, including replacement or termination.

The post audit has several purposes:

1. *Improve forecasts.* When managers systematically compare their projections to actual outcomes, there is a tendency for estimates to improve. Conscious or unconscious biases that occur can be identified and, one hopes, eliminated; new forecasting methods are sought as the need for them becomes apparent; and managers tend to do everything better, including forecasting, if they know that their actions are being monitored.
2. *Develop historical risk data.* Post audits permit managers to develop historical data on new project analyses regarding risk and expected rates of return. These data can then be used to make judgments about the relative risk of future projects as they are evaluated.
3. *Improve operations.* Businesses are run by managers who can perform at higher or lower levels of efficiency. When a forecast is made, for example, by the surgery department, the department director and medical staff are, in a sense, putting their reputations on the line. If costs are above predicted levels and usage is below expectations, the people involved will strive, within ethical bounds, to improve the situation and to bring results into line with forecasts. As one hospital CEO put it, "You academics worry only about making good decisions. In the health services industry, we also have to worry about making decisions good."
4. *Reduce losses.* Post audits monitor the performance of projects over time, so the first indication that termination or replacement should be considered often arises when the post audit indicates that a project is performing poorly.

1. What is a post audit?
2. Why are post audits important to the efficiency of a business?

Using Capital Budgeting Techniques in Other Contexts

The techniques developed in this chapter can help health services managers make a number of different types of decisions in addition to project selection. One example is the use of NPV and IRR to evaluate corporate merger opportunities. Healthcare companies often acquire other companies to increase capacity, to expand into other service areas, or for other reasons. A key element of any merger analysis is the valuation of the target company. Although the cash flows in such an analysis typically are structured differently than in project analysis, the same evaluation tools are applied.[11]

Managers also use capital budgeting techniques when deciding whether or not to divest assets or reduce staffing. Like capital budgeting, these actions require an analysis of the impact of the decision on the firm's cash flows. When cutting personnel, firms typically spend money up-front in severance payments, but then receive benefits in the form of lower wages and benefits in the future. When assets are sold, the pattern of cash flows is reversed. That is, cash inflows occur when the asset is sold, but any future cash inflows associated with the asset are sacrificed. (If future cash flows are negative, the decision, at least from a financial perspective, should be easy.) In both situations, the techniques discussed here, perhaps with modifications, can be applied to assess the financial consequences of the action.

1. Can capital budgeting tools be used in different settings? Explain your answer.   **Self-Test Question**

Key Concepts

This chapter discussed the basics of capital budgeting. The key concepts of this chapter are:

- *Capital budgeting* is the process of analyzing potential expenditures on fixed assets and deciding whether the firm should undertake those investments.
- A capital budgeting financial analysis consists of five steps: (1) estimate the investment outlay on the project; (2) estimate the expected cash inflows from the project; (3) assess the riskiness of those flows; (4) estimate the appropriate cost of capital at which to discount those flows; and (5) determine the project's profitability and breakeven characteristics.
- The most critical and most difficult step in analyzing a project is estimating the *incremental cash flows* that the project will generate.
- In determining incremental cash flows, *opportunity costs* (i.e., the cash flows forgone by using an asset) must be considered, but *sunk costs* (i.e., cash outlays that cannot be recouped) are not included. Further, any impact of the project on the firm's *other projects* must be included in the analysis.
- *Tax laws* generally affect investor-owned firms three ways: (1) taxes reduce a project's operating cash flows; (2) tax laws prescribe the depreciation expense that can be taken in any year; and (3) taxes affect a project's salvage value cash flow.

- Capital projects often require an investment in *net working capital* in addition to the investment in fixed assets. Such increases represent a cash outlay that, if material, must be included in the analysis. The investment in net working capital is recovered when the project is terminated.
- A project may have some *strategic value* that is not accounted for in the estimated cash flows. At a minimum, strategic value should be noted and considered qualitatively in the analysis.
- The *effects of inflation* must be considered in project analyses. The best procedure is to build inflation effects directly into the component cash flow estimates.
- Time breakeven, which is measured by the *payback period,* provides managers with insights concerning a project's liquidity and risk.
- *Net present value (NPV)*, which is simply the sum of the present values of all the project's net cash flows when discounted at the project's cost of capital, measures a project's expected dollar profitability. An NPV greater than zero indicates that the project is expected to be profitable, and the higher the NPV, the more profitable the project.
- *Internal rate of return (IRR)*, which is that discount rate that forces a project's NPV to equal zero, measures a project's expected rate of return. If a project's IRR is greater than its cost of capital, the project is expected to be profitable, and the higher the IRR, the more profitable the project.
- The NPV and IRR profitability measures provide identical indications of profitability, that is, a project that is judged to be profitable by its NPV will also be profitable by its IRR.
- The *net present social value (NPSV) model* formalizes the capital budgeting decision process for not-for-profit firms.
- Firms often use *project scoring matrixes* to subjectively incorporate a large number of factors, including financial and nonfinancial, into the capital budgeting decision process.
- The *post audit* is a key element in capital budgeting. By comparing actual results with predicted results, managers can improve both operations and the cash flow estimation process.
- Capital budgeting techniques are used in a wide variety of settings in addition to project evaluation.

The discussion of capital investment decisions will continue in Chapter 15, which focuses on risk assessment and incorporation.

Questions

14.1 a. What is capital budgeting? Why are capital budgeting decisions so important to businesses?

b. What is the purpose of placing capital projects into categories such as mandatory replacement or expansion of existing products, services, or markets?

    c. Should financial analysis play the dominant role in capital budgeting
       decisions? Explain your answer.

    d. What are the five steps of capital budgeting analysis?

14.2 Briefly define the following cash flow estimation concepts:

    a. Incremental cash flow

    b. Cash flow versus accounting income

    c. Sunk cost

    d. Opportunity cost

    e. Net working capital

    f. Strategic value

    g. Inflation effects

14.3 Describe the following project breakeven and profitability measures. Be
    sure to include each measure's economic interpretation.

    a. Payback

    b. Net present value (NPV)

    c. Internal rate of return (IRR)

14.4 Critique this statement: NPV is a better measure of project profitability
    than IRR because it leads to better capital investment decisions.

14.5 a. Describe the net present social value (NPSV) model.

    b. What is a project scoring matrix?

14.6 What is a post audit? Why is the post audit critical to good investment
    decision making?

14.7 From a purely financial perspective, are there situations in which a business
    would be better off choosing a project with a shorter payback over one that
    has a larger NPV?

Problems

14.1 Winston Clinic is evaluating a project that costs $52,125 and has expected
    net cash inflows of $12,000 per year for eight years. The first inflow occurs
    one year after the cost outflow, and the project has a cost of capital of 12
    percent.

    a. What is the project's payback?

    b. What is the project's NPV? Its IRR?

    c. Is the project financially acceptable? Explain your answer.

14.2 Better Health, Inc., is evaluating two investment projects, each of which
    requires an up-front expenditure of $1.5 million. The projects are expected
    to produce the following net cash inflows:

Year	Project A	Project B
1	$ 500,000	$2,000,000
2	1,000,000	1,000,000
3	2,000,000	600,000

a. What is each project's IRR?

b. What is each project's NPV if the cost of capital is 10 percent? 5 percent? 15 percent?

14.3 Capitol Healthplans, Inc., is evaluating two different methods for providing home health services to its members. Both methods involve contracting out for services, and the health outcomes and revenues are not effected by the method chosen. Therefore, the incremental cash flows for the decision are all outflows. Here are the projected flows:

Year	Method A	Method B
0	($300,000)	($120,000)
1	(66,000)	(96,000)
2	(66,000)	(96,000)
3	(66,000)	(96,000)
4	(66,000)	(96,000)
5	(66,000)	(96,000)

a. What is each alternative's IRR?

b. If the cost of capital for both methods is 9 percent, which method should be chosen? Why?

14.4 Great Lakes Clinic has been asked to provide exclusive healthcare services for the 2002–2003 World Exposition. Although flattered by the request, the clinic's managers want to conduct a financial analysis of the project. There will be an up-front cost of $160,000 to get the clinic in operation. Then, a net cash inflow of $1 million is expected from operations in each of the two years of the Exposition. However, the clinic has to pay the organizers of the exposition a fee for the marketing value of the opportunity. In essence, the clinic can call itself "The Healthcare Provider to the 2002–2003 World Expo." This fee, which must be paid at the end of the second year, is $2 million.

a. What are the cash flows associated with the project?

b. What is the project's IRR?

c. Assuming a project cost of capital of 10 percent, what is the project's NPV?

14.5 Assume that you are the chief financial officer at Porter Memorial Hospital. The CEO has asked you to analyze two proposed capital investments, Project X and Project Y. Each project requires a net investment outlay of $10,000, and the cost of capital for each project is 12 percent. The projects' expected net cash flows are:

Year	Project X	Project Y
0	($10,000)	($10,000)
1	6,500	3,000

2	3,000	3,000
3	3,000	3,000
4	1,000	3,000

a. Calculate each project's payback period, net present value (NPV), and internal rate of return (IRR).

b. Which project (or projects) is financially acceptable? Explain your answer.

14.6 The director of capital budgeting for Big Sky Health Systems, Inc., has estimated the following cash flows in thousands of dollars for a proposed new service:

Year	Expected Net Cash Flow
0	($100)
1	70
2	50
3	20

The project's cost of capital is 10 percent.

a. What is the project's payback period?

b. What is the project's NPV?

c. What is the project's IRR?

14.7 California Health Center, a for-profit hospital, is evaluating the purchase of new diagnostic equipment. The equipment, which costs $600,000, has an expected life of five years and an estimated pre-tax salvage value of $200,000 at that time. The equipment is expected to be used 15 times a day for 250 days a year for each year of the project's life. On average, each procedure is expected to generate $80 in collections, which is net of bad debt losses and contractual allowances, in its first year of use. Thus, net revenues for Year 1 are estimated at $15 \times 250 \times \$80 = \$300,000$.

Labor and maintenance costs are expected to be $100,000 during the first year of operation, while utilities will cost another $10,000 and cash overhead will increase by $5,000 in Year 1. The cost for expendable supplies is expected to average $5 per procedure during the first year. All costs and revenues, except depreciation, are expected to increase at a 5 percent inflation rate after the first year.

The equipment falls into the MACRS five-year class for tax depreciation, and hence is subject to the following deprecation allowances:

Year	Allowance
1	0.20
2	0.32
3	0.19
4	0.12

5	0.11
6	0.06
	1.00

The hospital's tax rate is 40 percent and its corporate cost of capital is 10 percent.

a. Estimate the project's net cash flows over its five-year estimated life. (Hint: Use the following format as a guide.)

	Year					
	0	1	2	3	4	5
Equipment cost						
Net revenues						
Less: Labor/maintenance costs						
Utilities costs						
Supplies						
Incremental overhead						
Depreciation						
Income before taxes						
Taxes						
Project net income						
Plus: Depreciation						
Plus: Equipment salvage value						
Net cash flow						

b. What are the project's NPV and IRR? (Assume for now that the project has average risk.)

14.8 You have been asked by the president and CEO of Kidd Pharmaceuticals to evaluate the proposed acquisition of a new labeling machine for one of the firm's production lines. The machine's price is $50,000 and it would cost another $10,000 for transportation and installation. The machine falls into the MACRS three-year class, and hence the tax depreciation allowances are 0.33, 0.45, and 0.15 in Years 1, 2, and 3, respectively. The machine would be sold after three years because the production line is being closed at that time. The best estimate of the machine's salvage value after three years' use is $20,000. The machine would have no effect on the firm's sales or revenues, but it is expected to save Kidd $20,000 per year in before-tax operating costs. The firm's tax rate is 40 percent and its corporate cost of capital is 10 percent.

a. What is the project's net investment outlay at Year 0?

b. What are the project's operating cash flows in Years 1, 2, and 3?

c. What are the terminal cash flows at the end of Year 3?

d. If the project has average risk, is it expected to be profitable?

14.9 The staff of Jefferson Memorial Hospital has estimated the following net cash flows for a satellite food services operation that it may open in its outpatient clinic:

Year	Expected Net Cash Flow
0	($100,000)
1	30,000
2	30,000
3	30,000
4	30,000
5	30,000
5 (salvage value)	20,000

The Year 0 cash flow is the investment cost of the new food service, while the final amount is the terminal cash flow (the clinic is expected to move to a new building in five years.) All other flows represent net operating cash flows. Jefferson's corporate cost of capital is 10 percent.

a. What is the project's IRR?

b. Assuming the project has average risk, what is its NPV?

c. Now, assume that the operating cash flows in Years 1–5 could be as low as $20,000 or as high as $40,000. Furthermore, the salvage value cash flow at the end of Year 5 could be as low as $0 or as high as $30,000. What is the worst case and best case IRR? The worst case and best case NPV?

Notes

1. Within not-for-profit providers, project losses can be offset by contributions and grants. However, long-run survival is best assured by striving for operating profitability.

2. In most situations, the strategic value of a project stems from managerial *options* brought about by the project that may or may not be used (exercised). One way to assess the value of these options is to use option pricing techniques that were first developed to value stock options, which confer upon their holders the right, but not the obligation, to buy or sell a particular stock at a specified price. The Spring 1987 edition of the *Midland Corporate Finance Journal* contains several articles related to the use of stock option concepts in capital budgeting analyses. For an overview, see S. C. Myers, "Finance Theory and Financial Strategy," 6–13.

3. As stated in Chapter 2, tax laws are complex and change often. Therefore, this book does not include a complete discussion of the MACRS system. For more information, see either the IRS publication pertaining to depreciation or any of the tax guidebooks available at local bookstores.

4. If Ann Arbor did not have taxable income to offset in Year 2 and had no taxable income to offset in the three previous years, the loss would have to be carried forward, and hence the tax benefit would not be immediately realized. In this situation, the *tax shield* value of the loss would be reduced because it would be pushed into the future rather than recognized immediately.

5. For a more complete discussion of replacement analysis, see E. F. Brigham and L. C. Gapenski, *Intermediate Financial Management* (Fort Worth, TX: Dryden Press, 1996), 256–259.

6. The *discounted payback* is a breakeven measure similar to the conventional payback, except that the cash flows in each year are discounted to Year 0 by the project's cost of capital prior to calculating the payback. Thus, the discounted payback solves the conventional payback's problem of not considering the project's cost of capital in the payback calculation.

7. However, when mutually exclusive projects are being analyzed (i.e., two or more projects are being investigated, but only one can be chosen), NPV and IRR rankings can conflict. That is, Project A could have the higher NPV, but Project B could have the higher IRR. In such situations, the NPV method is generally considered to be the best measure of profitability. See E. F. Brigham and L. C. Gapenski, *Intermediate Financial Management* (Fort Worth, TX: Dryden Press, 1996), chapter 7.

8. For example, the *modified IRR (MIRR)* has advantages over the straight IRR, and the *profitability index (PI)* gives decision makers information about a project's cost effectiveness (i.e., the project's bang for the buck). For more information on these profitability measures, see E. F. Brigham and L. C. Gapenski, *Intermediate Financial Management* (Fort Worth, TX: Dryden Press, 1996), chapter 7.

9. This section is drawn primarily from an article by J. R. C. Wheeler and J. P. Clement. See "Capital Expenditure Decisions and the Role of the Not-for-Profit Hospital: An Application of the Social Goods Model," *Medical Care Review* (Winter 1990): 467–486.

10. As noted in endnote 1, contributions and grants can be used to offset project losses.

11. For a complete discussion of merger analysis, see L. C. Gapenski, *Understanding Health Care Financial Management* (Chicago: Health Administration Press, 1996), chapter 17.

References

Allen, R. J. 1989. "Proper Planning Reduces Risk in New Technology Acquisitions." *Healthcare Financial Management* (December): 48–56.

Bergman, J. T. and B. J. McIntyre. 1989. "Valuation Analysis." *Topics in Health Care Financing* (Summer): 32–40.

Campbell, C. 1994. "Hospital Plant and Equipment Replacement Decisions: A Survey of Hospital Financial Managers." *Hospital & Health Services Administration* (Winter): 538–556.

Carroll, J. J. and G. D. Newbold. 1986a. "Inflation, Risk, Replacement, Closure: Concerns in Capital Budgeting." *Healthcare Financial Management* (December): 64–68.

———. 1986b. "NPV versus IRR: With Capital Budgeting, Which Do You Choose?" *Healthcare Financial Management* (November): 62–68.

Chow, C. W. and A. H. McNamee. 1991. "Watch for Pitfalls of Discounted Cash Flow Techniques." *Healthcare Financial Management* (April): 34–43.

Chow, C. W., K. M. Haddad, and A. Wong-Boren. 1991. "Improving Subjective Decision Making in Health Care Administration." *Hospital & Health Services Administration* (Summer): 191–210.

Cleverley, W. O. and J. G. Felkner. 1984. "The Association of Capital Budgeting Techniques with Hospital Financial Performance." *Health Care Management Review* (Summer): 45–55.

Gapenski, L. C. 1989a. "A Better Approach to Internal Rate of Return." *Healthcare Financial Management* (April): 93–99.

———. 1989b. "Analysis Provides Test for Profitability of New Services." *Healthcare Financial Management* (November): 48–58.

———. 1993. "Capital Investment Analysis: Three Methods." *Healthcare Financial Management* (August): 60–66.

Gordon, D. C. and D. F. Londal. 1989. "Guidelines to Capital Investment." *Topics in Health Care Financing* (Summer): 9–17.

Horowitz, J. L. and P. F. Straley. 1988. "Developing Investment Criteria: There is More to it than Financial Criteria Alone." *Topics in Health Care Financing* (Fall): 23–31.

Horowitz, J. L. 1993. "Contribution Margin Analysis: A Case Study." *Healthcare Financial Management* (June): 129–133.

Kamath, R. R. and J. Elmer. 1989. "Capital Investment Decisions in Hospitals: Survey Results." *Health Care Management Review* (Spring): 45–56.

Kennedy, W. F. and D. A. Plath. 1994. "A Return-Based Alternative to IRR Evaluations." *Healthcare Financial Management* (March): 38–49.

Manecke, S. R. 1993. "Practice Acquisition: Buy or Build." *Healthcare Financial Management* (December): 33–41.

Mellen, C. M. 1992. "Valuing a Long-Term Care Facility." *Healthcare Financial Management* (October): 20–25.

Meyer, A. D. 1985. "Hospital Capital Budgeting: Fusion of Rationality, Politics and Ceremony." *Health Care Management Review* (Spring): 17–27.

Ryan, J. B., M. E. Ward, and D. S. Kolb. 1990. "Capital Management Balances Charitable, Financial Goals." *Healthcare Financial Management* (March): 32–40.

Ryan, J. B. and M. E. Ward, editors. 1992. "Capital Management." *Topics in Health Care Financing* (Fall): 1–88.

Schramm, C. J. and G. D. Pillari. 1987. "Investing in the Wrong Future for Hospitals." *Health Care Management Review* (Fall): 31–37.

Straley, P. F. and C. R. Swaim. 1993. "Financial Analysis of Medical Office Buildings." *Topics in Health Care Financing* (Spring): 76–85.

Watts, D., D. L. Finney, and B. Louie. 1993. "Integrating Technology Assessment into the Capital Budgeting Process." *Healthcare Financial Management* (February): 21–29.

RISK ASSESSMENT AND INCORPORATION

Learning Objectives

After studying this chapter, readers will be able to:

- Describe the three types of risk relevant to capital budgeting decisions.
- Discuss the techniques used in project risk assessment.
- Conduct a project risk assessment.
- Explain how risk is incorporated into the capital budgeting process.

Introduction

Chapter 14 covered the basics of capital budgeting including cash flow estimation, breakeven analysis, and profitability measures. This chapter extends the discussion of capital budgeting to include risk analysis, which is composed of three elements: defining the type of risk relevant to the project, measuring the project's risk, and incorporating that risk assessment into the capital budgeting decision process. Although risk analysis is a key element in all financial decisions, the importance of capital investment decisions to a healthcare provider's success or failure makes risk analysis vital in such decisions.

The higher the risk associated with an investment, the higher its required rate of return. This principle is just as valid for healthcare businesses that make capital expenditure decisions as it is for individuals who make personal investment decisions. Thus, the ultimate goal in project risk analysis is to ensure that the cost of capital used as the discount rate in a project's profitability analysis properly reflects the riskiness of that project. The corporate cost of capital, which was covered in detail in Chapter 13, reflects the cost of capital to the organization based on its aggregate risk, that is, based on the riskiness of the firm's average project. In project risk analysis, a project's risk is assessed relative to the firm's average project: Does the project have average risk, below-average risk, or above-average risk? The corporate cost of capital is then adjusted to reflect any differential risk, which results in a *project cost of capital*. In general, high-risk projects are assigned a project cost of capital that is higher than the corporate cost of capital, average risk projects are evaluated at the corporate cost of capital, and low-risk projects are assigned a discount rate that is less than the corporate cost of capital.

Types of Project Risk

Three separate and distinct types of financial risk can be defined in a capital budgeting context:

- Stand-alone risk, which views the risk of a project as if it were held in isolation, and hence ignores portfolio effects both within the firm and among equity investors
- Corporate risk, which views the risk of a project within the context of the firm's portfolio of projects
- Market risk, which views a project's risk from the perspective of a shareholder who holds a well-diversified portfolio of stocks[1]

The type of risk that is most relevant to a particular capital budgeting decision depends on the number of projects that the firm holds and the business' form of ownership.

Stand-Alone Risk

Conceptually, *stand-alone risk* is only relevant in one situation: when a not-for-profit firm, which has no shareholders, is evaluating its first project. In this situation, the project will be operated in isolation and no portfolio diversification is present—the business does not have a collection of different projects nor does the firm have stockholders who hold portfolios of stocks of different companies. Although stand-alone risk is generally not relevant in real-world decision making, the other types of risk, which are more relevant, are very difficult (if not impossible) to measure. In practice, most project risk analyses measure stand-alone risk and then apply subjective adjustments to convert the project's assessed stand-alone risk to either corporate risk or market risk.

Stand-alone risk is present in a project whenever there is a chance of a return that is less than the expected return. In effect, a project is risky whenever its cash flows are not known with **certainty**. Furthermore, the greater the probability of a return far below the expected return, the greater the risk. In this context, stand-alone risk can be measured by the *standard deviation* of the project's profitability, as measured typically by net present value (NPV) or internal rate of return (IRR). Because standard deviation measures the dispersion of a distribution about its expected value, the larger the standard deviation, the greater the dispersion, and hence the greater the probability of the project's profitability (NPV or IRR) being far below that expected.

Corporate Risk

The previous section discussed stand-alone risk, which is measured by the standard deviation of a project's profitability and which is relevant only when a not-for-profit firm is considering its first project. In reality, firms usually offer a myriad of different products or services, and thus can be thought of as having a large number (i.e., hundreds or even thousands) of individual projects. For example, MinuteMan Healthcare, a New England HMO, offers healthcare services to a large number of diverse employee groups in numerous service areas; each different group could be considered to be a separate project. In this situation, the stand-alone risk of a project under consideration by MinuteMan is not relevant because the project will not be held in isolation. The relevant risk of a new project to MinuteMan is its contribution to the HMO's overall risk or the impact of the project on the variability of the overall profitability of the business. This type of risk, which is relevant when the project is part of a not-for-profit firm's portfolio of projects, is called *corporate risk*.

Conceptually, a project's corporate risk is measured by its *corporate beta*, which reflects the volatility of the project's profitability relative to that of the firm as a whole, which has a corporate (aggregate) beta of 1.0. A project with a corporate beta of 1.5 has returns that are more volatile than the firm's average project, and hence has high corporate risk. Similarly, a project with a corporate beta of 0.5 has returns that are less volatile than the aggregate business, and hence has low corporate risk. A project's corporate risk depends on the context (i.e., the firm's other projects), so a project may have high corporate risk to one firm, but low corporate risk to another, particularly when the two firms operate in widely different industries.

Market Risk

Market risk is generally viewed as the relevant risk for projects being evaluated by investor-owned businesses. The goal of shareholder wealth maximization implies that a project's returns, as well as its risk, should be defined and measured from the shareholders' perspective. The riskiness of an individual project, as seen by a well-diversified shareholder, is not the riskiness of the project as if it were owned and operated in isolation (which is defined as stand-alone risk), nor is it the contribution of the project to the riskiness of the firm (which is defined as corporate risk). Most shareholders hold a large diversified portfolio of stocks of many firms, which can be thought of as a very large diversified portfolio of individual projects. Thus, the risk of any single project as seen by a firm's stockholders is its contribution to the riskiness of a well-diversified stock portfolio, which is measured by the project's *market beta*.

A project's market beta measures the volatility of the project's returns relative to the returns on a well-diversified portfolio of stocks. To managers of investor-owned firms, a project's market risk relative to the market risk of the firm's other projects is measured by comparing the project's market beta to the firm's market beta. A project with a market beta higher than the firm's market beta has higher-than-average market risk, where average is defined as the market risk of the firm's stock. Note that a project's absolute market risk, as measured by its market beta, is independent of the context. That is, a project's market beta does not depend on the characteristics of the business, assuming the project's cash flows are the same to all firms. However, the market risk of a project, **relative to the market risk of the firm's other projects**, depends on the aggregate market risk of the firm.

1. What are the three types of project risk?
2. How is each type of project risk measured, both in absolute and relative terms?

Relationships Among Stand-Alone, Corporate, and Market Risks

After discussing the three different types of project risk and the situations in which each is relevant, it is tempting to say that stand-alone risk is almost never important because not-for-profit firms should focus on a project's corporate risk and investor-owned firms should focus on a project's market risk. Unfortunately, the situation is not that simple.

First, it is almost impossible in practice to quantify a project's corporate or market risk because it is extremely difficult—some practitioners would say impossible—to estimate the prospective returns distributions for given economic states for either the project, the firm as a whole, or for the market. If these distributions cannot be estimated, then it is impossible to precisely quantify a project's corporate or market risk.

Fortunately, as will be demonstrated in the next section, it is possible to get a rough idea of the relative stand-alone risk of a project. Thus, managers can make statements such as Project A has above-average risk, Project B has below-average risk, or Project C has average risk, all in the stand-alone sense. After a project's stand-alone risk has been assessed, the primary factor in converting stand-alone risk to either corporate or market risk is correlation. If a project's returns are expected to be highly positively correlated with the firm's returns, high stand-alone risk translates to high corporate risk. Similarly, if the firm's returns are expected to be highly correlated with the stock market's returns, high corporate risk translates to high market risk. The same analogies hold when the project is judged to have average or low stand-alone risk.

Most projects will be in a firm's primary line of business, and hence will be in the same line of business as the firm's average project. Because all projects in the same line of business are generally affected by the same economic factors, such projects' returns are usually highly correlated. When this situation exists, a project's stand-alone risk is a good proxy for its corporate risk. Furthermore, most projects' returns are also positively correlated with the returns on other assets in the economy—most assets have high returns when the economy is strong and low returns when the economy is weak. When this situation holds, a project's stand-alone risk is a good proxy for its market risk.

Thus, for most projects, the stand-alone risk assessment also gives good insights into a project's corporate and market risk. The only exception is when a project's returns are expected to be independent of or negatively correlated to the firm's average project. In these situations, considerable judgment is required because the stand-alone risk assessment will overstate the project's corporate risk. Similarly, if a project's returns are expected to be independent of or negatively correlated to the market's returns, the project's stand-alone risk overstates its market risk.

A second risk assessment problem arises with investor-owned healthcare firms. Finance theory specifies that investor-owned firms should focus on market risk when making capital budgeting decisions. However, most healthcare businesses, even proprietary ones, have corporate goals that focus on the provision of quality healthcare services in addition to shareholder wealth maximization. Furthermore, a proprietary healthcare firm's stability and financial condition, which primarily depend on corporate risk, is important to all the firm's other stakeholders: its managers, physicians, patients, community, and so on. Some financial theorists even argue that stockholders, including those that are well diversified, consider factors other than market risk when setting required returns. Considering all this, it may be reasonable for managers of investor-owned healthcare providers to be just as concerned about corporate risk as are managers of not-for-profit providers. Fortunately, in most real-world situations, a project's risk in the corporate sense will be the same as its risk in the market sense.[2]

Self-Test Questions

1. Name and define the three types of risk relevant to capital budgeting.
2. How are these risks related?
3. Should managers of investor-owned providers focus exclusively on a project's market risk?

Risk Analysis Illustration

To illustrate project risk analysis, consider Bayside Memorial Hospital's evaluation of a new MRI system that was first presented in Chapter 14. Table 15.1 contains the project's cash flow analysis. If all of the project's component cash flows were known with certainty, the project's projected profitability would be known with certainty, and hence the project would have no risk. However, in most project analyses, future cash flows, and hence profitability, are uncertain, and in many cases, highly uncertain, so risk is present.

The starting point for analyzing a project's risk involves estimating the uncertainty inherent in the project's cash flows. Most of the individual cash flows in Table 15.1 are subject to uncertainty. For example, volume was projected at 40 scans per week. However, utilization would almost certainly be higher or lower than the 40 scan forecast. In effect, the volume estimate is really an expected value taken from some probability distribution of potential utilization, as are many of the other values listed in Table 15.1. The distributions of the variables could be relatively tight, which reflect small standard deviations and low risk, or they could be relatively flat, which denote a great deal of uncertainty about the variable in question, and hence a high degree of risk.

TABLE 15.1
Bayside Memorial Hospital: MRI Site Cash Flow Analysis

	0	1	2	3	4	5
				Cash Revenues and Costs		
1. System cost	($1,500,000)					
2. Related expenses	(1,000,000)					
3. Gross revenues		$1,000,000	$1,050,000	$1,102,500	$1,157,625	$ 1,215,506
4. Deductions		250,000	262,500	275,625	289,406	303,877
5. Net revenues		$ 750,000	$ 787,500	$ 826,875	$ 868,219	$ 911,630
6. Labor costs		50,000	52,500	55,125	57,881	60,775
7. Maintenance costs		150,000	157,500	165,375	173,644	182,326
8. Supplies		30,000	31,500	33,075	34,729	36,465
9. Incremental overhead		10,000	10,500	11,025	11,576	12,155
10. Depreciation		350,000	350,000	350,000	350,000	350,000
11. Operating income		$ 160,000	$ 185,500	$ 212,275	$ 240,389	$ 269,908
12. Taxes		0	0	0	0	0
13. Net operating income		$ 160,000	$ 185,500	$ 212,275	$ 240,389	$ 269,908
14. Depreciation		350,000	350,000	350,000	350,000	350,000
15. Net salvage value						750,000
16. Net cash flow	($2,500,000)	$ 510,000	$ 535,500	$ 562,275	$ 590,389	$ 1,369,908

Profitability Measures:
Net present value (NPV) @ 10% = $82,493.
Internal rate of return (IRR) = 11.1%.

The nature of the component cash flow distributions and their correlations with one another determine the nature of the project's profitability distribution, and thus the project's risk. In the following sections, three techniques for assessing a project's risk are discussed: sensitivity analysis, scenario analysis, and Monte Carlo simulation.[3]

1. What condition creates project risk?
2. What makes one project riskier than another?

Self-Test Questions

Sensitivity Analysis

Many of the variables that determine a project's cash flows are subject to some type of probability distribution rather than known with certainty. If the realized value of such a variable is different from its expected value, the project's profitability will differ from its expected value. *Sensitivity analysis* is a technique that indicates exactly how much a project's profitability (NPV or IRR) will change in response to a given change in a single input variable, with other things held constant.

Sensitivity analysis begins with a *base case* developed using **expected values** (in the statistical sense) for all uncertain variables. To illustrate, assume that Bayside's managers believe that all of the MRI project's component cash flows are known with certainty except for weekly volume and salvage value. The expected values for these variables (volume = 40 and salvage value = $750,000) were used in Table 15.1 to obtain the base case NPV of $82,493. Sensitivity analysis is designed to provide managers the answers to such questions as these: What if volume is more or less than the expected level? What if salvage value is more or less than expected?

In a sensitivity analysis, each uncertain variable is usually changed by a fixed percentage amount above and below its expected value, while all other variables are held constant at their expected values. Thus, all input variables except one are held at their base case values. The resulting NPVs (or IRRs) are recorded and plotted. Table 15.2 contains the NPV sensitivity analysis for the MRI project assuming that there are two uncertain variables: volume and salvage value.

Note that the NPV is a constant $82,493 when there is no change in any of the variables. This situation occurs because a zero percent change recreates the base case. Also, managers can examine the Table 15.2 values to get a feel for which input variable has the greatest impact on the MRI project's NPV—the larger the NPV change for a given percentage input change, the greater the impact. Clearly, NPV is most affected by changes in volume.

Often, the results of sensitivity analyses are shown in graphical form. For example, the Table 15.2 sensitivity analysis is graphed in Figure 15.1. Here, the slopes of the lines show how sensitive the MRI project's NPV is to changes in each of the uncertain input variables—the steeper the slope, the more sensitive NPV is to a change in the variable. Note that the sensitivity lines intersect at the base case values—0 percent change from base case level and $82,493. Also, spreadsheet

TABLE 15.2
MRI Project
Sensitivity Analyses

Change from	Net Present Value (NPV)	
Base Case Level	Volume	Salvage Value
−30%	($814,053)	($ 57,215)
−20	(515,193)	(10,646)
−10	(216,350)	35,923
0	82,493	82,493
+10	381,335	129,062
+20	680,178	175,631
+30	979,020	222,200

models are ideally suited for performing sensitivity analyses because such models both automatically recalculate NPV when an input value is changed and facilitate graphing.[4]

Figure 15.1 vividly illustrates that the MRI project's NPV is very sensitive to volume and mildly sensitive to changes in salvage value. If a sensitivity plot has a negative slope, it indicates that **increases** in the value of that variable **decrease** the project's NPV. If two projects were being compared, the one with the steeper sensitivity lines would be regarded as riskier because a relatively small error in estimating a variable, for example, volume, would produce a large error in the project's projected NPV. If information was available on the sensitivity of NPV to input changes for Bayside's average project, similar judgments regarding the riskiness of the MRI project could be made, but now relative to the firm's average project.

Although sensitivity analysis is widely used in project risk analysis, it has severe limitations. For example, suppose that Bayside Memorial Hospital had a contract with a HMO that guaranteed a minimum MRI usage at a fixed reimbursement rate. In that situation, the project would not be very risky at all, in spite of the fact that the sensitivity analysis showed NPV to be highly sensitive to changes in volume. In general, a project's **stand-alone** risk, which is what is being measured by sensitivity analysis, depends on both the sensitivity of its profitability to changes in key input variables as well as the ranges of likely values of these variables. Because sensitivity analysis considers only the first factor, it can give misleading results. Furthermore, sensitivity analysis does not consider any interactions among the uncertain input variables, it considers each variable independently of the others.

In spite of the shortcomings of sensitivity analysis as a risk measure, it does provide managers with valuable information. First, it provides profitability breakeven information for the project's uncertain variables. For example, Table 15.2 and Figure 15.1 show that just a few percent decrease in expected volume makes the project unprofitable, whereas the project remains profitable even if

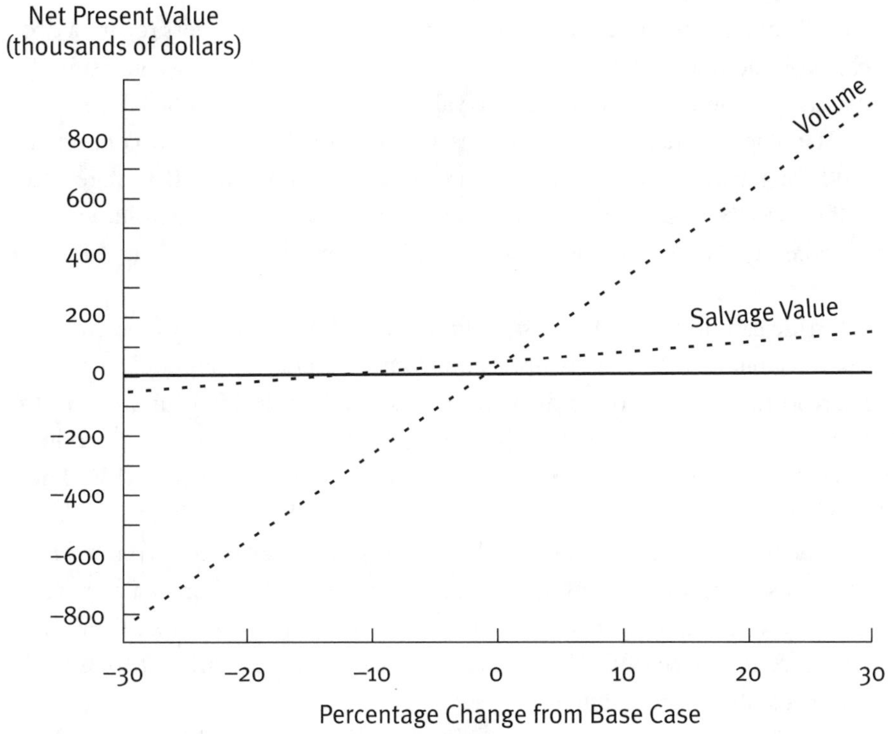

FIGURE 15.1
Sensitivity Analysis
Graphs

Net Present Value
(thousands of dollars)

salvage value falls by more than 10 percent. Although somewhat rough, this breakeven information is clearly of value to Bayside's managers.

Second, sensitivity analysis tells managers which input variables are most critical to the project's profitability, and hence to the project's financial success. In this MRI example, volume is clearly the key input variable of the two that were examined, so Bayside's managers should ensure that the volume estimate is the best possible. The concept here is that Bayside's managers have a limited amount of time to spend on analyzing the MRI project, so the resources expended should be as productive as possible.

1. Briefly describe sensitivity analysis?
2. What type of risk does it attempt to measure?
3. What are its strengths and weaknesses?

**Self-Test
Questions**

Scenario Analysis

Scenario analysis is a stand-alone risk analysis technique that considers the sensitivity of NPV to changes in key variables, the likely range of variable values, and the interactions among variables. To conduct a scenario analysis, the managers pick a "bad" set of circumstances (i.e., low volume, low salvage value, and so on), an average or "most likely" set, and a "good set." The resulting input values are then used to create a probability distribution of NPV.

To illustrate scenario analysis, assume that Bayside's managers regard a drop in weekly volume below 30 scans as very unlikely and a volume above 50 is also improbable. On the other hand, salvage value could be as low as $500,000 or as high as $1 million. The most likely values are 40 scans per week for volume and $750,000 for salvage value. Thus, volume of 30 and a $500,000 salvage value define the lower bound, or pessimistic, worst case scenario; while volume of 50 and a salvage value of $1 million define the upper bound, or optimistic, best case scenario.

Bayside can now use the *worst, most likely*, and *best case* values for the input variables to obtain the NPV corresponding to each scenario. Bayside's managers used a spreadsheet model to conduct the analysis and Table 15.3 summarizes the results. The most likely case results in a positive NPV; the worst case produces a negative NPV; and the best case results in a very large, positive NPV. These results can now be used to determine the expected NPV and standard deviation of NPV. For this, an estimate is needed of the probabilities of occurrence of the three scenarios. Suppose that Bayside's managers estimate that there is a 20 percent chance of the worst case occurring, a 60 percent chance of the most likely case, and a 20 percent chance of the best case. Of course, it is very difficult to estimate scenario probabilities accurately.

Table 15.3 contains a discrete distribution of returns, so the expected NPV can be found as follows:

$$\text{Expected NPV} = (0.20 \times [-\$819,844]) + (0.60 \times \$82,493) + (0.20 \times \$984,829)$$

$$= \$82,493.$$

The expected NPV in the scenario analysis is the same as the base case NPV, $82,493. The consistency of results occurs because the values of the uncertain variables used in the scenario analysis—30, 40, and 50 scans for volume and $500,000, $750,000, and $1,000,000 for salvage value—produce the same expected values that were used in the Table 15.1 base case analysis. If inconsistencies exist between the base case NPV and the expected NPV in the scenario analysis, the two analyses

TABLE 15.3
MRI Project
Scenario Analyses

Scenario	Probability of Outcome	Volume	Salvage Value	NPV
Worst case	0.20	30	$ 500,000	($819,844)
Most likely case	0.60	40	750,000	82,493
Best case	0.20	50	1,000,000	984,829
Expected value		40	$ 750,000	$ 82,493
Standard deviation				$570,688

have inconsistent input assumptions. Such inconsistencies should be identified and removed to ensure that common assumptions are used throughout the project risk analysis.

The standard deviation of NPV, as shown here, is $570,688:

$$\sigma_{NPV} = [0.20 \times (-\$819,844 - \$82,493)^2 + 0.60 \times (\$82,493 - \$82,493)^2$$
$$+ 0.20 \times (\$984,829 - \$82,493)^2]^{1/2}$$
$$= \$570,688.$$

The standard deviation of NPV measures the MRI project's stand-alone risk. Bayside's managers can compare the standard deviation of NPV of this project with the uncertainty inherent in Bayside's aggregate cash flows, or average project. (Perhaps they would scale the standard deviation to account for project size by dividing it by the cost of the project or by the expected NPV.)[5] On the basis of this judgmental comparison of stand-alone risk, Bayside's managers may conclude that the MRI project is riskier than the firm's average project, so it would be classified as a high-risk project.

Scenario analysis can also be interpreted in a less mathematical way. The worst case NPV, a loss of about $800,000 for the MRI project, represents an estimate of the worst possible financial consequences of the project. If Bayside can absorb such a loss in value without much impact on its financial condition, the project does not represent a significant financial danger to the hospital. Conversely, if such a loss would mean financial ruin for the hospital, its managers may be unwilling to undertake the project regardless of its profitability under the most likely and best case scenarios.

While scenario analysis provides useful information about a project's stand-alone risk, it is limited in two ways. First, it only considers a few discrete states of the economy, and hence provides information on only a few potential profitability outcomes for the project. In reality, an almost infinite number of possibilities exist. Although the illustrative scenario analysis contained only three scenarios, it could be expanded to include more states of the economy, say, five or seven. However, there is a practical limit on how many scenarios can be included in a scenario analysis.

Second, scenario analysis—at least as normally conducted—implies a very definite relationship among the uncertain variables. That is, the analysis assumed that the worst value for volume (30 scans per week) would occur at the same time as the worst value for salvage value ($500,000) because the worst case scenario was defined by combining the worst possible value of each uncertain variable. Although this relationship (all worst values occurring together) may hold in some situations, it may not hold in others. For example, if volume is low, maybe the MRI will have less wear and tear, and hence be worth more after five years of use. The worst value for volume, then, should be coupled with the best salvage value. Conversely, poor volume may be symptomatic of poor medical effectiveness of the

MRI, and hence lead to limited demand for used equipment and a low salvage value. Scenario analysis tends to create extreme profitability values for the worst and best cases because it automatically combines all worst and best input values, even if these values actually have only a remote chance of occurring together. The next section describes a method of assessing a project's stand-alone risk that deals with these two problems.

Self-Test Questions
1. Briefly describe scenario analysis.
2. What type of risk does it attempt to measure?
3. What are its strengths and weaknesses?

Monte Carlo Simulation

Monte Carlo simulation, so named because it grew out of work on the mathematics of casino gambling, describes uncertainty in terms of *continuous* probability distributions, which have an infinite number of outcomes, rather than just a few *discrete* values. Thus, Monte Carlo simulation provides a better view of a project's risk than does scenario analysis.

Although the use of Monte Carlo simulation in capital investment decisions was first proposed over 25 years ago, it had not been used extensively in practice primarily because it required a mainframe computer along with relatively powerful financial planning or statistical software. Recently, however, Monte Carlo simulation software has become available for personal computers as an add-in to the spreadsheet software. Because most financial analysis today is being done with spreadsheets, Monte Carlo simulation is now accessible to virtually all health services organizations.

The first step in a Monte Carlo simulation is to create a model that calculates the project's net cash flows and profitability measures as was done for Bayside's MRI project. The relatively certain variables are estimated as single, or point, values in the model; continuous probability distributions are used to specify the uncertain cash flow variables. After the model has been created, the simulation software automatically executes the following steps:

1. The Monte Carlo program chooses a single random value for each uncertain variable on the basis of its specified probability distribution.
2. The value selected for each uncertain variable, along with the point values for the relatively certain variables, are combined in the model to estimate the net cash flow for each year.
3. Using the net cash flow data, the model calculates the project's profitability, say, as measured by NPV. A single completion of Steps 1, 2, and 3 constitutes one iteration, or "run," in the Monte Carlo simulation.
4. The Monte Carlo software repeats the above steps many times, say, 5,000. Because each run is based on different input values, each run produces a different NPV.

The ultimate result of the simulation is an NPV (or IRR) probability distribution based on 5,000 individual scenarios, and hence which encompasses almost all of the likely financial outcomes. Monte Carlo software usually displays the results of the simulation in both tabular and graphical forms, and automatically calculates summary statistical data such as expected value, standard deviation, and skewness.[6]

To illustrate Monte Carlo simulation, again, consider Bayside Hospital's MRI project. As in the scenario analysis, the illustration has been simplified by specifying the distributions for only two key variables: weekly volume and salvage value. Weekly volume is not expected to vary by more than ±10 scans from its expected value of 40 scans. Because this is a symmetrical situation, the normal (bell shaped) distribution can be used to represent the uncertainty inherent in volume. In a normal distribution, the expected value plus or minus three standard deviations will encompass almost the entire distribution. Thus, a normal distribution with an expected value of 40 scans and a standard deviation of 10 / 3 = 3.33 scans is a reasonable description of the uncertainty inherent in weekly volume.

A triangular distribution was chosen for salvage value because it specifically fixes the upper and lower bounds, whereas the tails of a normal distribution are, in theory, limitless. The triangular distribution is also used extensively when the input distribution is nonsymmetrical because it can easily accommodate skewness. Salvage value uncertainty was specified by a triangular distribution with a lower limit of $500,000, a most likely value of $750,000, and an upper limit of $1,000,000.

The basic MRI model containing these two continuous distributions was used, plus a Monte Carlo add-in to the spreadsheet program, to conduct a simulation with 5,000 iterations. The output is summarized in Table 15.4, and the resulting probability distribution of NPV is plotted in Figure 15.2. The mean, or expected, NPV, $82,498, is about the same as the base case NPV and expected NPV indicated in the scenario analysis, $82,493. In theory, all three results should be the same because the expected values for all input variables are the same in the three analyses. However, there is some randomness in the Monte Carlo simulation, which leads to an expected NPV that is slightly different from the others. The more iterations that are run, the more likely the Monte Carlo NPV will be the same as the base case NPV.

The standard deviation of NPV is lower in the simulation analysis because the NPV distribution in the simulation contains values within the entire range of possible outcomes, while the NPV distribution in the scenario analysis contains only the most likely value and best and worst case extremes.

In this illustration, one value for volume uncertainty was specified for all five years. That is, the value chosen by the Monte Carlo software for volume in Year 1, for example, 40 scans, was used as the volume input for the remaining four years in that iteration of the simulation analysis. As an alternative, the normal distribution for Year 1 could be applied to each year separately, and hence specify individual volumes for each year. Then, the Monte Carlo software may choose 35 as the value for Year 1, 43 as the Year 2 input, 32 for Year 3, and so on. This

TABLE 15.4
Simulation Results
Summary

Expected NPV	$82,498
Minimum NPV	($951,760)
Maximum NPV	$970,191
Probability of a positive NPV	62.8%
Standard deviation	$256,212
Skewness	0.002

FIGURE 15.2
NPV Probability
Distribution

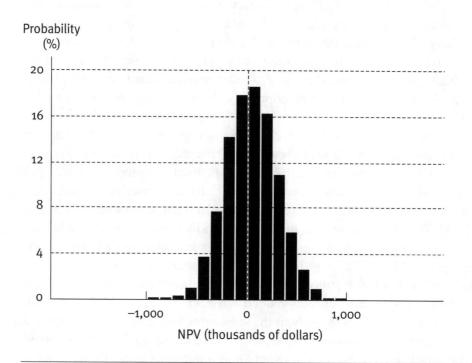

approach, however, probably does not do a good job of describing real world behavior; high usage in the first year presumably means strong acceptance of the MRI system, and hence high usage in the remaining years. Similarly, low usage in the first year probably portends low usage in future years.

The volume and salvage value variables were treated as independent in the simulation; that is, the value chosen by the Monte Carlo software from the salvage value distribution was not related to the value chosen from the volume distribution. Thus, in any run, a low volume could be coupled with a high salvage value and vice versa. If Bayside's managers believed that high usage at the hospital indicates a strong national demand for MRI systems, they could specify a positive correlation between these variables. This would tend to increase the riskiness of the project because a low volume pick in one iteration could not be offset by a high salvage value pick. Conversely, if the salvage value is more a function of the technological advances that occur over the next five years than local usage, then it may be best to specify the variables as being independent.

As in scenario analysis, the project's simulation results must be compared with a similar analysis of the firm's average project. If Bayside's average project was considered to have less stand-alone risk when a Monte Carlo simulation was conducted, then the MRI project would be judged to have above-average (i.e., high) stand-alone risk.

Monte Carlo simulation has two primary advantages over scenario analysis: all possible input variable values are considered, and correlations among the uncertain inputs can be incorporated in the analysis. However, these two advantages lead to the primary disadvantage. Although it is mechanically easy to input the probability distributions for uncertain variables and their correlations into a Monte Carlo simulation, it is much more difficult to realistically specify what those distributions and correlations should be. The problem is that the more information a risk analysis technique requires, the harder it is to develop the data with any confidence, and hence managers can be left with a very elegant result of questionable value.

1. Briefly, what is Monte Carlo simulation?
2. What type of risk does it attempt to measure?
3. What are its strengths and weaknesses?

Self-Test Questions

Incorporating Risk into the Decision Process

Thus far, the MRI illustration has demonstrated that it is difficult to quantify a project's riskiness. It may be possible to reach the general conclusion that one project is more or less risky than another, or to compare the riskiness of a project with the firm as a whole, but it is difficult to develop a really good measure of project risk. This lack of precision in measuring project risk adds to the difficulties involved in incorporating differential risk into the capital budgeting decision.

There are two methods for incorporating project risk into the capital budgeting decision process: the certainty equivalent method, in which a project's expected cash flows are adjusted to reflect project risk, and the risk-adjusted discount rate method, in which differential risk is dealt with by changing the cost of capital. Although the risk-adjusted discount rate method is used by most businesses, the certainty equivalent method does have some theoretical advantages. Furthermore, it raises some interesting issues related to the risk-adjustment process.

The Certainty Equivalent Method

The *certainty equivalent (CE) method* follows directly from the economic concept of *utility*.[7] Under the CE approach, managers must first evaluate a cash flow's risk and then specify how much money, with certainty, would be required to be indifferent between the riskless (certain) sum and the risky cash flow's expected value. To illustrate, suppose that a rich eccentric offered someone the following two choices:

- *Flip a coin:* If it is head, the person receives $1 million; if it is tail, the person gets nothing. The expected value of the gamble is $(0.5 \times \$1,000,000) + (0.5 \times \$0) = \$500,000$, but the actual outcome will be either zero or $1 million, so the gamble is quite risky.
- *Do not flip the coin:* Simply pocket $400,000 in cash.

If the person is indifferent to the two alternatives, $400,000 is defined to be his or her *certainty equivalent* amount for this particular risky expected $500,000 cash flow. The riskless $400,000 provides that individual with the same satisfaction (utility) as the risky $500,000 expected return.

In general, investors are risk averse, so the certainty equivalent amount for this gamble will be something less than the $500,000 expected value. But, each individual would have his or her own certainty equivalent value—the greater the individual's degree of risk aversion, the lower the certainty equivalent amount.

The CE concept can be applied to capital budgeting decisions, at least in theory, in this way:

1. Convert each net cash flow of a project to its certainty equivalent value. Here, the riskiness of **each cash flow** is assessed, and a certainty equivalent cash flow is chosen on the basis of that risk. The greater the risk, the greater the difference between the expected value and its lower certainty equivalent value. (If a cash outflow is being adjusted, the certainty equivalent value is higher than the expected value. The unique risk adjustments required on cash outflows will be discussed in a later section.)
2. Once each cash flow is expressed as a certainty equivalent, discount the project's certainty equivalent cash flow stream by the **risk-free rate** to obtain the project's *differential risk-adjusted* NPV.[8] Here, the term "differential risk-adjusted" implies that the unique riskiness of the project, as compared to the overall riskiness of the business, has been incorporated into the decision process. The risk-free rate is used as the discount rate because certainty equivalent cash flows are analogous to risk-free cash flows.
3. A positive differential risk-adjusted NPV indicates that the project is profitable even after adjusting for differential project risk.

The CE method is simple and neat. Furthermore, it can easily handle differential risk among the **individual** net cash flows. For example, the final year's certainty equivalent cash flow may be adjusted downward an additional amount to account for salvage value risk if that risk is considered to be greater than the risk inherent in the operating cash flows.

Unfortunately, there is no practical way to estimate a risky cash flow's certainty equivalent value. There are no benchmarks available to help make the estimate, so each individual would have his or her own estimate, which could vary significantly. Also, the risk assessment techniques (for example, scenario analysis) focus on profitability, and hence measure the stand-alone risk of a project in its entirety. This process provides no information about the riskiness of individual cash flows, so there is no basis for adjusting each cash flow for its own unique risk.

The Risk-Adjusted Discount Rate Method

In the *risk-adjusted discount rate (RADR) method*, expected cash flows are used in the valuation process and the risk adjustment is made to the discount rate (the opportunity cost of capital). All average-risk projects are discounted at the firm's corporate cost of capital, which represents the opportunity cost of capital for average-risk projects; high-risk projects are assigned a higher cost of capital; and low-risk projects are discounted at a lower cost of capital.

One advantage of the RADR method is that the process has a starting benchmark: the firm's corporate cost of capital. This discount rate reflects the riskiness of the business in the aggregate or the riskiness of the firm's average project. Another advantage is that project risk assessment techniques identify a project's aggregate risk—the combined risk of all of the cash flows—and the RADR applies a single adjustment to the cost of capital rather than attempting to adjust individual cash flows. However, the disadvantage is that, typically, there is no theoretical basis for setting the size of the RADR adjustment, so the amount of adjustment remains a matter of judgment.

The RADR method has one additional disadvantage. RADR combines the factors that account for time value (the risk-free rate) and the adjustment for risk (the risk premium): Project cost of capital = Differential risk-adjusted discount rate = Risk-free rate + Risk premium. The CE approach, on the other hand, keeps risk adjustment and time value separate—time value in the discount rate and risk in the cash flows. By lumping together risk and time value, the RADR method compounds the risk premium over time—just as interest compounds over time, so does the risk premium. This compounding of the risk premium means that the RADR method automatically assigns more risk to cash flows that occur in the distant future, and the farther into the future, the greater the implied risk. Because the CE method assigns risk to each cash flow individually, it does not impose any assumptions regarding the relationship between risk and time.

Consciously or unconsciously, the RADR method as it is normally used, with a constant discount rate applied to all cash flows of a project, implies that risk increases with time. This imposes a greater burden on long-term projects, so short-term projects will tend to look better financially than long-term projects. For most projects, the assumption of increasing risk over time is probably reasonable because cash flows are more difficult to forecast the farther one moves into the future. However, managers should be aware that the RADR approach automatically penalizes distant cash flows, so an additional explicit penalty based solely on cash flow timing is probably not warranted unless some specific additional risk can be identified.

Applying the RADR Method to the MRI Project

In most project risk analyses, it is impossible to assess quantitatively the project's corporate or market risk, and, similar to Bayside's MRI project, managers are left with only an assessment of the project's stand-alone risk. However, like the MRI project, most projects that are evaluated are in the same line of business as the firm's other projects, and the profitability of most firms is highly correlated with the national economy. Thus, stand-alone, corporate, and market risk are usually highly correlated. This suggests that managers can get a feel for the relative risk of most projects on the basis of the scenario and/or simulation analyses conducted to assess the project's stand-alone risk. In Bayside's case, its managers concluded that the MRI project has above-average risk, and hence the project was categorized as a high-risk project.

The business' corporate cost of capital provides the basis for estimating a project's differential RADR—average-risk projects are discounted at the corporate cost of capital, high-risk projects are discounted at a higher cost of capital, and low-risk projects are discounted at a rate below the cost of capital. Unfortunately, there is no good way of specifying exactly how much higher or lower these discounts rates should be; given the present state of the art, risk adjustments are necessarily judgmental and somewhat arbitrary.

Bayside Hospital's standard procedure is to add four percentage points to its 10 percent corporate cost of capital when evaluating high-risk projects, and to subtract two percentage points when evaluating low-risk projects. Thus, to estimate the high-risk MRI project's differential risk-adjusted NPV, the project's expected (base case) cash flows shown in Table 15.1 are discounted at $10\% + 4\% = 14\%$. This rate is called the *project cost of capital*, as opposed to the corporate cost of capital, because it reflects the risk characteristics of a specific project rather than the aggregate risk characteristics of the business (or average project). The resultant NPV is −$200,017, so the project becomes unprofitable when the analysis is adjusted to reflect its high risk. Bayside's managers may still decide to go ahead with the MRI project, but at least they know that its expected profitability is not sufficient to make up for its riskiness.

Self-Test Questions

1. What are the differences between the certainty equivalent (CE) and risk-adjusted discount rate (RADR) methods for risk incorporation?
2. What assumptions about time and risk are inherent in the RADR method?
3. How do most firms incorporate differential risk in the capital budgeting decision process?

Adjusting Cash Outflows for Risk

Some projects are evaluated on the basis of minimizing the present value of future costs rather than on the basis of the projects' NPVs. This is done because it is often impossible to allocate revenues to a particular project, and it is easier to focus on comparative costs when two projects will produce the same revenue stream. For example, suppose that Bayside Memorial Hospital must choose one of two ways for disposing its medical wastes. There is no question about the need for the project, and the hospital's revenue stream is unaffected by which method is chosen. In this case, the decision will be based on the present value of expected future costs—the method with the lower present value of costs will be chosen.

Table 15.5 contains the projected annual costs associated with each method. The in-house system would require a large expenditure at Year 0 to upgrade the hospital's current disposal system, but the yearly operating costs are relatively low. Conversely, if Bayside contracts for disposal services with an outside contractor, it will only have to pay $25,000 up front to initiate the contract. However, the annual contract fee would be $200,000 a year.[9]

If both methods were judged to have average risk, then Bayside's corporate cost of capital, 10 percent, would be applied to the cash flows to obtain the present value (PV) of costs for each method. Because the PVs of costs for the two waste disposal systems ($784,309 for the in-house system and $783,157 for the contract method) are roughly equal, on the basis of financial considerations only, Bayside's managers are indifferent to which method should be chosen.

However, Bayside's managers believe that the contract method is much riskier than the in-house method. The cost of modifying the current system is known almost to the dollar, and operating costs can be predicted fairly well. Furthermore, with the in-house system, operating costs are under the control of Bayside's management. Conversely, if Bayside relies on the contractor for waste disposal, the hospital is more or less stuck with continuing the contract because it will not have the in-house capability. Because the contractor was only willing to quote a price for the first year, perhaps the bid was low balled and large price increases will occur in future years. The two methods have about the same PV of costs when both are considered to have average risk, so which method should be chosen if the contract method is judged to have high risk? Clearly, if the costs are

Year	In-House System	Outside Contract
Cash Flows:		
0	($500,000)	($ 25,000)
1	(75,000)	(200,000)
2	(75,000)	(200,000)
3	(75,000)	(200,000)
4	(75,000)	(200,000)
5	(75,000)	(200,000)
Present Value of Costs at a Discount Rate of:		
10%	($784,309)	($783,157)
14%	—	($711,616)
6%	—	($867,473)

TABLE 15.5
Bayside Memorial Hospital: Waste Disposal Analysis

the same under a common discount rate, the lower-risk, in-house project should be chosen.

Now, try to incorporate this intuitive differential risk conclusion into the quantitative analysis. Conventional wisdom is to increase the corporate cost of capital for high-risk projects, so the contract cash flows would be discounted using a project cost of capital of 14 percent, which is the rate that Bayside applies to high-risk projects. But, at a 14 percent discount rate, the contract method has a PV of costs of only $711,616, which is about $70,000 lower than that for the in-house method. If the discount rate was increased to 20 percent on the contract method, it would appear to be $161,000 cheaper than the in-house method. Thus, the riskier the contract method is judged to be, the better it looks.

Something is obviously wrong here. To penalize a cash outflow for higher-than-average risk, that outflow must have a **higher** present value, not a **lower** one. Therefore, a cash outflow that has higher-than-average risk must be evaluated with a lower-than-average cost of capital. Recognizing this, Bayside's managers actually applied a 10% − 4% = 6% discount rate to the high-risk contract method's cash flows. This produces a PV of costs for the contract method of $867,473, which is about $83,000 more than the PV of costs for the average-risk, in-house method.

The appropriate risk adjustment for cash outflows is also applicable to other situations. For example, the City of Detroit offered Ann Arbor Health Systems the opportunity to use a city-owned building in one of the city's blighted areas for a walk-in clinic. The city offered to pay to refurbish the building, and all profits made by the clinic would accrue to Ann Arbor. However, after ten years, Ann Arbor would have to buy the building from the city at the then current market value. The market value estimate that Ann Arbor used in its analysis was $2,000,000, but the realized cost could be much greater, or much less, depending on the economic condition of the neighborhood at that time. The project's other cash flows were of average risk, but this single outflow had high risk, so Ann Arbor lowered the discount rate that it applied to this one cash flow. This action created a higher present value on a cost (outflow), and hence lowered the project's NPV.

Self-Test Questions

1. Is there any difference between the risk adjustments applied to cash inflows and cash outflows? Explain your answer.
2. Can differential risk adjustments be made to single cash flows or must the same adjustment be made to all of a project's cash flows?

Subsidiary Costs of Capital

In theory, project costs of capital should reflect both a project's differential risk and its differential *debt capacity*. The logic here is that if a project's optimal financing mix is significantly different from the business in the aggregate, then the weights used in estimating the corporate cost of capital do not reflect the weights appropriate to the project. Because of the difficulties encountered in estimating a project's debt capacity (its optimal capital structure), such adjustments are rarely made in practice.

Even though it is not common to make capital structure adjustments for individual projects, firms often make both capital structure and risk adjustments when developing subsidiary costs of capital. To illustrate, a for-profit healthcare system may have one subsidiary that invests primarily in real estate for medical uses and another subsidiary that runs a HMO. Clearly, each subsidiary has its own unique business risk and optimal capital structure. The low-risk, high debt capacity real estate subsidiary could have a cost of capital of 10 percent, while the high-risk, low debt capacity HMO subsidiary could have a cost of capital of 14 percent. The health system itself, which consists of 50 percent real estate assets and 50 percent HMO assets, would have a corporate cost of capital of 12 percent.

If all capital budgeting decisions within the system were made on the basis of the overall system's 12 percent cost of capital, the process would be biased in favor of the higher-risk HMO subsidiary. The cost of capital would be too low for the HMO subsidiary and too high for the real estate subsidiary. Over time, this cost of capital bias would result in too many HMO projects being accepted and too few real estate projects, which would skew the business line mix toward HMO assets, and hence increase the overall riskiness of the firm. The solution to the cost of capital bias problem is to use *subsidiary costs of capital*, rather than the overall corporate cost of capital, in the capital budgeting decision process.

Unlike individual project costs of capital, subsidiary costs of capital often can be estimated with some confidence because it is usually possible to identify publicly traded firms that are predominantly in the same line of business as the subsidiary. For example, the cost of capital for the HMO subsidiary could be estimated by looking at the debt and equity costs and capital structures of the major for-profit HMOs such as Humana and United Healthcare. With such market data at hand, it is relatively easy to develop subsidiary costs of capital. As a final check, the weighted average of the subsidiary costs of capital should **equal** the firm's corporate cost of capital.

Self-Test Questions

1. In theory, should project cost of capital estimates include capital structure effects?
2. Should all subsidiaries of a firm use the firm's corporate cost of capital as the benchmark rate in making capital budgeting decisions?
3. How might a business go about estimating its subsidiary costs of capital?

An Overview of the Capital Budgeting Decision Process

The discussion of capital budgeting thus far has focused on how managers evaluate individual projects. For capital planning purposes, health services managers also need to forecast the total number of projects that will be undertaken and the dollar amount of capital needed to fund these projects. The list of projects to be undertaken is called the *capital budget*, and the optimal selection of new projects is called the *optimal capital budget*.

While every healthcare provider estimates its optimal capital budget in its own unique way, some procedures are common to all firms. The procedures followed by Bayside Memorial Hospital are used to illustrate the process:

1. The chief financial officer (CFO) estimates the hospital's corporate cost of capital. As discussed in Chapter 13, this estimate depends on market conditions, the business risk of the hospital's assets in the aggregate, and the hospital's capital structure.
2. The CFO then scales the corporate cost of capital up or down to reflect the unique risk and capital structure features of each division. To illustrate, assume that Bayside has three divisions. For simplicity, the divisions are identified as LRD, ARD, and HRD, which stand for low-risk, average-risk, and high-risk divisions.
3. Managers within each of the hospital's divisions evaluate the riskiness of the proposed projects within their divisions and categorize each project as having low risk (LRP), average risk (ARP), or high risk (HRP). These project risk classifications are based on the riskiness of each project relative to the **other projects in the division**, not to the hospital in the aggregate.
4. Each project is then assigned a project cost of capital that is based on the **divisional cost of capital** and the project's relative riskiness. As discussed previously, this *project cost of capital* is then used to discount the project's expected net cash flows. From a financial standpoint, all projects with positive NPVs are acceptable, while those with negative NPVs should be rejected. Subjective factors are also considered, and these factors may result in an optimal capital budget that differs from the one established solely on the basis of financial considerations.

Figure 15.3 summarizes Bayside's overall capital budgeting process. Here, the corporate cost of capital is adjusted upward to 14 percent in the high-risk division and downward to 8 percent in the low-risk division. The same adjustment—four percentage points upward for high-risk projects and two percentage points downward for low-risk projects—is applied to differential risk projects within each division. The end result is a range of project costs of capital within Bayside that runs from 18 percent for high-risk projects in the high-risk division to 6 percent for low-risk projects in the low-risk division.

The final result is a capital budget that incorporates each project's debt capacity (at least at the divisional level) and riskiness. However, managers also must consider other possible risk factors that may not have been included in the quantitative analysis. For example, could the MRI project that was previously considered significantly increase Bayside's liability exposure? Conversely, does the project have any strategic value or social value or other attributes that could impact its profitability or riskiness? Such additional factors must be considered, at least subjectively, before a final decision can be made. Typically, if the project involves new products or services and is large (in capital requirements), relative

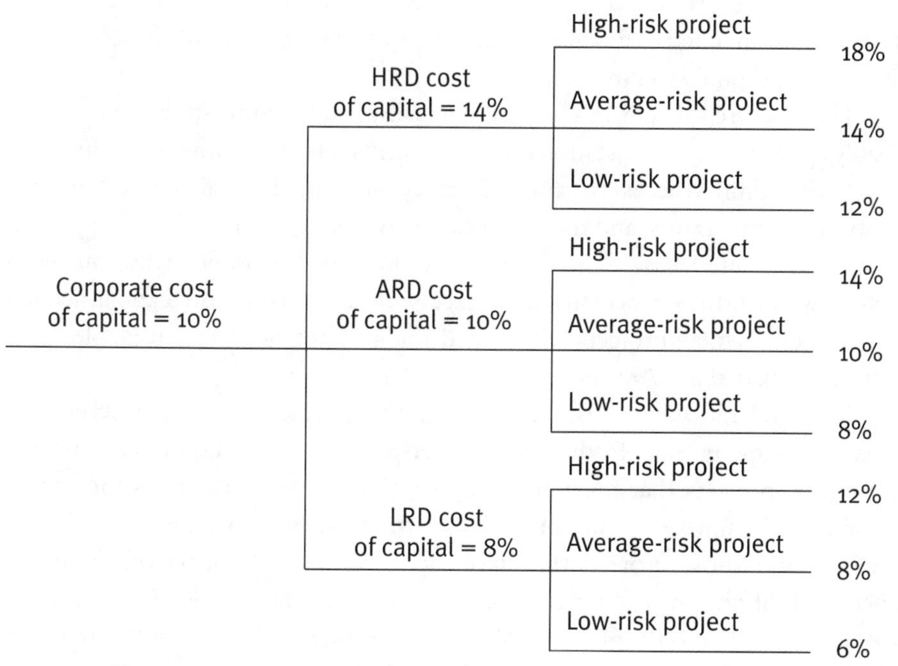

FIGURE 15.3
Bayside Memorial
Hospital: Project
Costs of Capital

to the size of the firm's average project, then the additional subjective factors will be very important to the final decision; one large mistake can bankrupt a firm, so "bet the company" decisions are not made lightly. On the other hand, the decision on a small replacement project would be made mostly on the basis of numerical analysis.

Ultimately, capital budgeting decisions require an analysis of a mix of objective and subjective factors such as risk, debt capacity, profitability, medical staff needs, and social value. The process is not precise and often there is a temptation to ignore one or more important factors because they are so nebulous and difficult to measure. Despite the imprecision and subjectiveness, a project's risk, as well as its other attributes, should be assessed and incorporated into the capital budgeting decision process.

1. Describe a typical capital budgeting decision process.
2. Are decisions made solely on the basis of quantitative factors? Explain your answer.

**Self-Test
Questions**

Capital Rationing

Standard capital budgeting procedures assume that businesses can raise virtually unlimited amounts of capital to meet capital budgeting needs. Presumably, as long as a business is investing the funds in profitable (i.e., positive NPV) projects, it should be able to raise the debt and equity needed to fund all projects that come along. Additionally, standard capital budgeting procedures assume that a business raises the capital needed to finance its optimal capital budget roughly in accordance with its target capital structure.

This picture of a firm's capital financing/capital investment process is probably appropriate for most investor-owned firms. However, not-for-profit firms do not have unlimited access to capital. Their equity capital is limited to retentions, contributions, and grants, and their debt capital is limited to the amount supported by the equity capital base. Thus, it is likely that not-for-profit firms, and even investor-owned firms on occasion, will face periods in which the capital needed for investment in new projects will exceed the amount of capital available. This situation is called *capital rationing*.

If capital rationing exists, and hence the business has more acceptable projects than capital, then, from a financial perspective, the firm should accept that set of capital projects that maximizes aggregate NPV and still meets the capital constraint. This approach could be called "getting the most bang from the buck" because it picks those projects that have the most positive impact on the firm's financial condition. In healthcare businesses, priority may be assigned to some low or even negative NPV projects. This is fine as long as these projects are offset by the selection of profitable projects, which would prevent the low-profitability, priority projects from eroding the firm's financial condition.

Self-Test Questions
1. What is capital rationing?
2. From a financial perspective, how are projects chosen when capital rationing exists?

Key Concepts

This chapter, which continued the discussion of capital budgeting started in Chapter 14, focused on risk assessment and incorporation. The key concepts of this chapter are:

- Three separate and distinct types of *project risk* can be identified and defined: (1) stand-alone risk, (2) corporate risk, and (3) market risk.
- A project's *stand-alone risk* is the risk the project would have if it were the sole project of a not-for-profit firm. It is a function of the project's profit uncertainty, and is generally measured by the *standard deviation* of NPV. Stand-alone risk is often used as a proxy for both corporate and market risk because (1) corporate and market risk are often impossible to measure and (2) the three types of risk are usually highly correlated.
- *Corporate risk* reflects the contribution of a project to the overall riskiness of the business. Corporate risk ignores stockholder diversification, so it is the relevant risk for most not-for-profit firms.

- *Market risk* reflects the contribution of a project to the overall riskiness of stockholders' well-diversified portfolios. In theory, market risk is the relevant risk for investor-owned firms, but many people argue that corporate risk is also relevant to stockholders and is certainly relevant to a firm's other stakeholders.
- Three techniques are commonly used to *assess* a project's stand-alone risk: (1) sensitivity analysis, (2) scenario analysis, and (3) Monte Carlo simulation.
- *Sensitivity analysis* shows how much a project's profitability, for example, as measured by NPV, changes in response to a given change in an input variable, such as volume, while other things are held constant.
- *Scenario analysis* defines a project's best, most likely, and worst cases, and then uses these data to measure its stand-alone risk.
- Whereas scenario analysis focuses on only a few possible outcomes, *Monte Carlo simulation* uses continuous distributions to reflect the uncertainty inherent in a project's component cash flows. The result is a probability distribution of NPV (or IRR) that provides a great deal of information about the project's riskiness.
- Projects are generally classified as high risk, average risk, or low risk on the basis of their stand-alone risk assessment. High-risk projects are evaluated at a *project cost of capital* greater than the firm's corporate cost of capital. Average-risk projects are evaluated at the firm's corporate cost of capital, while low-risk project's are evaluated at a rate less than the corporate cost of capital.
- When evaluating *risky cash outflows*, the risk adjustment process is reversed, that is, lower rates are used to discount more risky cash flows.
- Ultimately, capital budgeting decisions require an analysis of a mix of objective and subjective factors such as risk, debt capacity, profitability, medical staff needs, and service to the community. The process is not precise, but good managers do their best to ensure that none of the relevant factors is ignored.

This chapter concludes the discussion of capital investment decisions. The remaining chapters cover two diverse topics: current asset management and financing, and analyzing financial performance.

Questions

15.1 a. Why is risk analysis so important to the capital budgeting process?
   b. Describe the three types of project risk. Under what situation is each of the types most relevant to the capital budgeting decision?
   c. Which type of risk is easiest to measure in practice?
   d. Are the three types of project risk usually highly correlated? Explain your answer.
   e. Why is the correlation among project risk measures important?
15.2 a. Briefly describe sensitivity analysis.
   b. What are its strengths and weaknesses?
15.3 a. Briefly describe scenario analysis.

b. What are its strengths and weaknesses?

15.4 a. Briefly describe Monte Carlo simulation.

b. What are its strengths and weaknesses?

15.5 a. How is project risk incorporated into a capital budgeting analysis?

b. Suppose that two mutually exclusive projects are being evaluated on the basis of cash costs. How would risk adjustments be applied in this situation?

15.6 What is the difference between the corporate cost of capital and a project cost of capital?

15.6 What is meant by the term *capital rationing*? From a purely financial standpoint, what is the optimal capital budget under capital rationing?

15.7 Reading Healthcare, Inc., is evaluating two projects. One project involves spending $5 million to open a satellite hospital in an adjacent town, while the other involves spending $500,000 to expand the outpatient pharmacy. On which project would the firm's managers be most likely to use Monte Carlo simulation? Explain your answer.

15.8 Santa Roberta Clinic has estimated its corporate cost of capital to be 11 percent. What are reasonable values for the project costs of capital for low-risk, average-risk, and high-risk projects?

Problems

15.1 The managers of Merton Medical Clinic are analyzing a proposed project. The project's most likely NPV is $120,000, but, as evidenced by the following NPV distribution, there is considerable risk involved:

Probability	NPV
0.05	($700,000)
0.20	(250,000)
0.50	120,000
0.20	200,000
0.05	300,000

a. What are the project's expected NPV and standard deviation of NPV?

b. Should the base case analysis use the most likely NPV or expected NPV? Explain your answer.

15.2 Heywood Diagnostic Enterprises is evaluating a project with the following net cash flows and probabilities:

Year	Prob = 0.2	Prob = 0.6	Prob = 0.2
0	($100,000)	($100,000)	($100,000)
1	20,000	30,000	40,000
2	20,000	30,000	40,000
3	20,000	30,000	40,000
4	20,000	30,000	40,000
5	30,000	40,000	50,000

The Year 5 values include salvage value. Heywood's corporate cost of capital is 10 percent.

a. What is the project's expected (i.e., base case) NPV assuming average risk? (Hint: The base case net cash flows are the expected cash flows in each year.)

b. What are the project's most likely, worst, and best case NPVs?

c. What is the project's expected NPV on the basis of the scenario analysis?

d. What is the project's standard deviation of NPV?

e. Assume that Heywood's managers judge the project to have lower-than-average risk. Furthermore, the company's policy is to adjust the corporate cost of capital up or down by three percentage points to account for differential risk. Is the project financially attractive?

15.3 Consider the project contained in Problem 14.7 in Chapter 14.

a. Perform a sensitivity analysis to see how NPV is affected by changes in the number of procedures per day, average collection amount, and salvage value.

b. Conduct a scenario analysis. Suppose that the hospital's staff concluded that the three most uncertain variables were number of procedures per day, average collection amount, and the equipment's salvage value. Furthermore, the following data were developed:

Scenario	Probability	Number of Procedures	Average Collection	Equipment Salvage Value
Worst	0.25	10	$ 60	$100,000
Most likely	0.50	15	80	200,000
Best	0.25	20	100	300,000

c. Finally, assume that California Health Center's average project has a coefficient of variation of NPV in the range of 1.0–2.0. (Hint: Coefficient of variation is defined as the standard deviation of NPV divided by the expected NPV.) The hospital adjusts for risk by adding or subtracting three percentage points to its 10 percent corporate cost of capital. After adjusting for differential risk, is the project still profitable?

d. What type of risk was measured and accounted for in the preceding Parts b and c? Should this be of concern to the hospital's managers?

15.4 The managers of United Medtronics are evaluating the following four projects for the coming budget period. The firm's corporate cost of capital is 14 percent.

Project	Cost	IRR
A	$15,000	17%
B	15,000	16
C	12,000	15
D	20,000	13

a. What is the firm's optimal capital budget?

b. Now suppose Medtronics' managers want to consider differential risk in the capital budgeting process—Project A has average risk, B has below-average risk, C has above-average risk, and D has average risk. What is the firm's optimal capital budget when differential risk is considered? (Hint: The firm's managers **lower** the IRR of high-risk projects by 3 percentage points and **raise** the IRR of low-risk projects by the same amount.)

15.5 Allied Managed Care Company is evaluating two different computer systems for handling provider claims. There are no incremental revenues attached to the projects, so the decision will be made on the basis of the present value of costs. Allied's corporate cost of capital is 10 percent. Here are the net cash flow estimates in thousands of dollars:

Year	System X	System Y
0	($500)	($1,000)
1	(500)	(300)
2	(500)	(300)
3	(500)	(300)

a. Assume initially that the systems both have average risk. Which one should be chosen?

b. Assume that System X is judged to have high risk. Allied accounts for differential risk by adjusting its corporate cost of capital up or down by two percentage points. Which system should be chosen?

Notes

1. The three types of risk relevant to capital budgeting decisions were first discussed in Chapter 10. A review of the applicable sections may be useful for some readers.

2. For an algebraic representation of the relationships among stand-alone, corporate, and market risk, see L. C. Gapenski, "Project Risk Definition and Measurement in a Not-For-Profit Setting," *Health Services Management Research* (November 1992): 216–224.

3. A fourth method, *decision tree analysis*, also is used to assess project risk. This method is particularly useful when a project is structured with a series of decision points (i.e., stages) that allow cancellation prior to full implementation. For more information, see L. C. Gapenski, *Understanding Health Care Financial Management* (Chicago: Health Administration Press, 1996), 463–67.

4. Spreadsheet programs have Data Table functions that automatically perform sensitivity analyses. After the table is roughed in, the spreadsheet automatically calculates and records the NPV (or some other profitability measure) values in the appropriate locations on the table.

5. One measure of risk that is commonly used in making stand-alone risk comparisons is the *coefficient of variation (CV)*, which is defined as the standard deviation divided by the expected value. In the scenario analysis, the MRI project's CV of NPV is $570,688 / $82,493 = 6.9. The CV measures the risk per unit of return, and hence is a better

measure of comparative risk than is the standard deviation of NPV, especially when projects have widely differing NPVs.

6. *Skewness* measures the degree of symmetry of a distribution. A skewness of zero indicates a symmetric distribution, positive skewness indicates a distribution that is skewed to the right (i.e., its right tail is longer than its left), and negative skewness indicates a distribution that is skewed to the left.

7. Utility theory is used by economists to explain how individuals make choices among risky alternatives.

8. The risk-free rate does **not** incorporate the tax advantages of debt financing, so such benefits to taxable firms should be incorporated in the cash flows when the certainty equivalent method is used.

9. For the sake of simplicity, inflation effects are ignored in this illustration.

References

Allen, R. J. 1989. "Proper Planning Reduces Risk in New Technology Acquisitions." *Healthcare Financial Management* (December): 48–56.

Ang, J. S. and W. G. Lewellen. 1982. "Risk Adjustment in Capital Investment Project Evaluations." *Financial Management* (Summer): 5–14.

Capettini, R., C. W. Chow, and J. E. Williamson. 1990. "Breakdown Approach Helps Managers Select Projects." *Healthcare Financial Management* (November): 48–56.

Gapenski, L. C. 1992a. "Accuracy of Investment Risk Models Varies." *Healthcare Financial Management* (April): 40–52.

———. 1992b. "Project Risk Definition and Measurement in a Not-for-Profit Setting." *Health Services Management Research* (November): 216–224.

———. 1990. "Using Monte Carlo Simulation to Help Make Better Capital Investment Decisions." *Hospital & Health Services Administration* (Summer): 207–219.

Gup, B. E. and S. W. Norwood, III. 1981. "Divisional Cost of Capital: A Practical Approach." *Financial Management* (Spring): 20–24.

Hastie, K. L. 1974. "One Businessman's View of Capital Budgeting." *Financial Management* (Winter): 36–43.

Hertz, D. B. 1964. "Risk Analysis in Capital Investments." *Harvard Business Review* (January–February): 96–106.

Lewellen, W. G. and M. S. Long. 1972. "Simulation versus Single-Value Estimates in Capital Expenditure Analysis." *Decision Sciences* (October): 19–33.

Ryan, J. B. and J. L. Gocke. 1988. "Incorporating Risk Into the Investment Decision." *Topics in Health Care Financing* (Fall): 49–65.

Ryan, J. B. and M. E. Ward, editors. 1992. "Capital Management." *Topics in Health Care Financing* (Fall): 1–88.

Weaver, S. C., P. J. Clemmens, III, J. A. Gunn, and B. D. Danneburg. 1989. "Divisional Hurdle Rates and the Cost of Capital." *Financial Management* (Spring): 18–25.

OTHER TOPICS

CURRENT ASSET MANAGEMENT
AND FINANCING

Learning Objectives

After studying this chapter, readers will be able to:

- Describe alternative current asset investment and financing policies.
- Discuss in general terms how businesses manage cash and marketable securities.
- Discuss the key elements of receivables and inventory management.
- Explain the alternatives available for short-term financing including the use of security.

Introduction

In the discussion of financial analysis that led to this chapter, the general focus has been on long-term strategic decisions. The topic of this chapter is another important element of healthcare finance: management of short-term (current) assets and their financing. The chapter begins with an overview of short-term financial management, as well as a discussion of the policy decisions that health services managers must make regarding the level of current assets and how those assets are financed. A brief discussion of the management of each current asset account is then provided. The chapter closes with a discussion of the various types of short-term financing available to healthcare providers.

An Overview of Short-Term Financial Management

Short-term financial management involves all current assets and most current liabilities. The primary goal of short-term financial management is to support the operations of the business at the lowest possible cost. This goal involves two separate elements. First, the business must have the current assets necessary to meet operational requirements. However, it is imprudent to hold too high a level of current assets because of the costs of carrying them. Second, the business must be *liquid*, which means that it can meet its cash obligations as they become due. A firm that is liquid has the funds that are needed to pay salaries, taxes, interest, supplies invoices, and so on. Conversely, a firm that is illiquid cannot easily generate the cash needed to make these payments, and thus its operations suffer.

To both illustrate the requirement for short-term financing and to review the current asset and current liability accounts, consider the situation facing Sun Coast Clinics, a for-profit operator of four ambulatory care clinics in South Florida. Table 16.1 contains the firm's December 1998 and April 1999 balance sheets. The provision of ambulatory care services in this part of Florida is a seasonal business. The peak season for Sun Coast is December through April, when the population of the area soars because of tourism. Even more important to Sun Coast's peak level of operations is the arrival of the "snow birds" (i.e., the retired individuals who typically live in the north during the summer and fall months, but move to residences in Florida for the winter).

In December of each year, Sun Coast finishes its slow season and prepares for its busy season. Thus, the firm's accounts receivables are relatively low, but its cash and marketable securities and inventories are relatively high. By the end of April, Sun Coast has completed its busy season, so its accounts receivable are relatively high, but its cash and marketable securities and inventories are relatively low in preparation for the slow summer season. On the current liabilities side, Sun Coast's accounts payable and accruals are relatively high at the end of April, just after the busy season.

Consider what happens to Sun Coast's total current assets and total current liabilities over the December to April period. Current assets increase from $200,000 to $240,000, so the firm must raise $40,000—an increase on the left side of the balance sheet must be financed by an increase on the right side. However, the higher volume of both purchases and labor expenditures associated with increased services causes accounts payable and accruals to increase *spontaneously* by $20,000,

TABLE 16.1
Sun Coast Clinics, Inc.: End-of-Month Balance Sheets (in thousands of dollars)

	December 1998	April 1999
Cash and marketable securities	$ 30	$ 20
Accounts receivable	155	210
Inventories	15	10
Total current assets	$200	$240
Net fixed assets	500	500
Total assets	$700	$740
Accounts payable	$ 30	$ 40
Accruals	15	25
Notes payable	85	105
Current portion of long-term debt	20	20
Total current liabilities	$150	$190
Long-term debt	150	140
Common equity	400	410
Total liabilities and equity	$700	$740

from $30,000 + $15,000 = $45,000 in December to $40,000 + $25,000 = $65,000 in April. The net result is an additional $40,000 − $20,000 = $20,000 current asset financing requirement in April, which Sun Coast obtained from the bank as a short-term loan. Therefore, at the end of April, Sun Coast showed notes payable of $105,000, up from $85,000 in December.

These fluctuations for Sun Coast resulted from seasonal factors. Similar fluctuations in current asset requirements, and hence in financing needs, can occur because of business cycles; typically, current asset requirements and financing needs contract during recessions and expand during good times. In the next section, two policy issues regarding current assets and financing are discussed.

1. What is the goal of short-term financial management?
2. What is liquidity and why is it important to businesses?
3. Describe how seasonal volume fluctuations influence both current asset levels and financing requirements.

Self-Test Questions

Current Asset Investment and Financing Policies

Current asset financial policy involves two basic questions:

- What is the appropriate level for current assets, both in total and by specific accounts?
- How should current assets be financed?

In this section, these two questions are discussed in detail.

Current Asset Investment Policies

Figure 16.1 shows three alternative policies regarding the total amount of current assets carried. Essentially, *current asset investment policies* differ in that different amounts of current assets are carried to support a given volume level. The line with the steepest slope represents a *high* current asset investment policy. Here, relatively large amounts of cash, marketable securities, and inventories are carried; utilization is stimulated by the use of a credit policy that provides liberal financing to customers and a corresponding high level of receivables. Conversely, with the *low* current asset investment policy, the holdings of cash, securities, inventories, and receivables are minimized at each volume level.

Under conditions of certainty (i.e., when utilization, operating costs, collection times, and so on, are known) all healthcare providers would hold only minimal levels of current assets, and hence follow a low current asset investment policy. Any larger amounts would increase the need for current asset financing, and hence increase costs, without a corresponding increase in profits. Any smaller holdings would involve late payments to labor and suppliers, operating inefficiencies because of inventory shortages, and lower utilization caused by an overly restrictive credit policy.

FIGURE 16.1

Alternative Working
Capital Investment
Policies (in
thousands of
dollars)

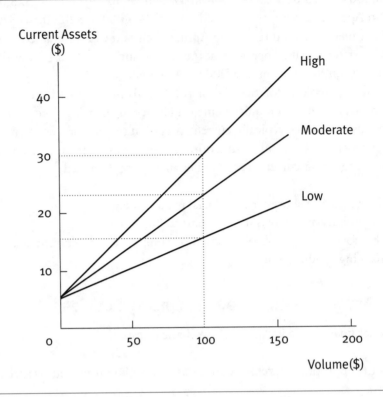

However, the picture changes when uncertainty is introduced. Now, the provider must carry the minimum amounts of cash and inventories to meet expected needs **plus** additional amounts, or *safety stocks,* which enable it to deal with realizations that differ from expectations. Similarly, accounts receivable levels are determined by credit terms (i.e., payor mix and collections policy), and the tougher the credit terms, the lower the receivables for any given level of sales. With a low current asset investment policy, the business would hold minimal levels of safety stocks for cash and inventories and would have a tight credit policy. A low policy generally provides the highest expected return on the business' investment in current assets, but it entails the greatest risk, while the converse is true under a high current asset investment policy. The moderate policy falls in between the two extremes in terms of expected risk and return.

The profit penalty for holding excess current assets is very much dependent on the cost of financing current asset holdings. Therefore, corporate policy regarding the level of current assets is never set in isolation. It is always established on the basis of current financing costs and in conjunction with the firm's current asset financing policy.

Current Asset Financing Policies

Most businesses experience seasonal fluctuations as illustrated previously with Sun Coast Clinics. Similarly, most businesses must build up current assets when the economy is strong, but they then sell off inventories and have reductions in receivables when the economy slacks off. Still, current assets **never** drop to zero—this realization has led to the concept of permanent versus temporary assets.

To illustrate the concept of permanent versus temporary assets, consider Sun Coast Clinics. Table 16.1 suggests that, at this stage in its life, seasonality causes the firm's total assets to fluctuate between $700,000 and $740,000. Thus, Sun Coast has $700,000 in *permanent assets*, which is defined as the amount of total assets required to sustain operations during seasonal (or cyclical) lows. Sun Coast's permanent assets are composed of $500,000 of fixed assets and $200,000 in *permanent current assets*. In addition, Sun Coast carries *seasonal*, or *temporary, current assets*, which fluctuate from zero to a maximum of $40,000. The manner in which the permanent and temporary current assets are financed defines the firm's *current asset financing policy*.

One policy, *maturity matching*, which is sometimes called a *moderate financing policy*, calls for the firm to match asset and liability maturities as shown in Panel (a) of Figure 16.2. That is, permanent assets are financed with permanent capital (i.e., equity and long-term debt) and temporary assets are financed with temporary capital (i.e., short-term debt). This strategy limits the risk that a business will be unable to pay off its maturing obligations. To illustrate, suppose Sun Coast borrows on a one-year basis and uses the funds obtained to build and equip a new clinic. Cash flows from the clinic (i.e., profits plus depreciation) would almost never be sufficient to pay off the loan at the end of only one year, so the loan must be renewed at that time. If interest rates increase during the year, Sun Coast's new debt would cost more. Even worse, if the lender refused to renew the loan, Sun Coast would have problems. Had the clinic been financed with long-term financing, however, the required loan payments would have been better matched with cash flows from profits and depreciation, and the problem of loan renewal would not have arisen.

At the limit, a business could attempt to match exactly the maturity structure of its assets and liabilities. Inventory expected to be sold in 30 days could be financed with a 30-day bank loan, a machine expected to last for five years could be financed by a five-year loan, a 20-year building could be financed by a 20-year mortgage bond, and so forth. Actually, three factors make this exact maturity matching strategy both unpractical and wrong: there is uncertainty about the lives of assets; some common equity (or fund capital) must be used, and this capital has no maturity; and to develop a meaningful current asset financing policy, it is necessary to consider whether an asset is permanent or temporary.

The proper framework for evaluating current asset financing policies requires the use of the concept of permanent and temporary assets. Thus, for financing purposes, assets are not classified by their accounting definitions of current and long term, but either as permanent or temporary. In this framework, maturity matching calls for the permanent portion of cash, receivables, and inventories (i.e., permanent current assets) to be financed with permanent capital (i.e., long-term debt and equity). The key is that each dollar of cash, each individual receivable, and each dollar of inventory may well be short term in that these items will be quickly turned over or converted to cash. However, as each individual current asset item

FIGURE 16.2
Alternative Working
Capital Financing
Policies

(a) Moderate Approach (Maturity Matching)

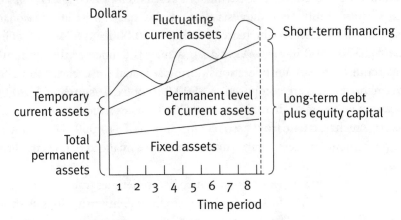

(b) Relatively Aggressive Approach

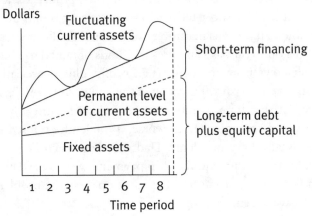

(c) Conservative Approach

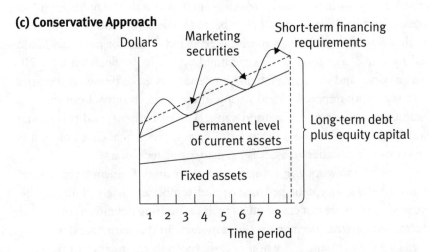

is converted, it will be replaced by a like item if it is permanent in nature, and hence such short-term assets are actually carried permanently over the long term. The implication is that the accounting definition of current assets, although useful for many purposes, does not provide managers with the correct guidance regarding the financing of such assets.

Panel (b) of Figure 16.2 illustrates an *aggressive financing policy*. Here, the firm finances all of its fixed assets with long-term capital, but part of its permanent current assets with short term, nonspontaneous credit. A look back at Table 16.1 will show that Sun Coast actually follows this strategy. Assuming that the $20,000 current portion of long-term debt will be refinanced with new long-term debt, Sun Coast has $500,000 in net fixed assets and $570,000 of long-term capital, which leaves only $70,000 of long-term capital to finance $200,000 in permanent current assets. Additionally, Sun Coast has a minimum of $45,000 of costless, spontaneous short-term credit (accounts payable and accruals). Thus, Sun Coast uses $85,000 of short-term notes payable to help finance its permanent level of current assets.

Returning to Figure 16.2, the term *relatively* is used in the title for Panel (b) because there can be different *degrees* of aggressiveness. For example, the dashed line in Panel (b) could have been drawn *below* the line designating fixed assets, which indicates that all of the permanent current assets and part of the fixed assets were financed with short-term credit. Such a policy would be a highly aggressive, extremely unconservative position, and the firm would be very much subject to dangers from rising interest rates as well as to loan renewal problems. However, short-term debt is often cheaper than long-term debt, and some businesses are willing to sacrifice safety for the chance of higher profits.

As shown in Panel (c) of Figure 16.2, the dashed line could also be drawn above the line designating permanent current assets, which indicates that permanent capital is being used to finance all permanent asset requirements and also to meet some, or all, of the temporary demands. In the situation depicted in the graph, the firm uses a small amount of short-term, nonspontaneous credit to meet its peak requirements, but it also meets a part of its seasonal needs by storing liquidity in the form of marketable securities during the off season. The humps above the dashed line represent short-term financing, and the troughs below the dashed line represent short-term security holdings. Panel (c) represents a very safe, *conservative financing policy*.

As with current asset investment policy, the choice among alternative financing policies involves a risk/return trade-off. The aggressive policy's use of generally lower cost, short-term debt has the highest expected return and the highest risk, while the conservative policy has the lowest expected return and lowest risk. The maturity matching policy falls between the extremes. Unfortunately, there is no underlying finance theory that managers can use to pick the "correct" financing policy. Often, firms that have low business risk elect to take on higher-than-average financial risk. Thus, such firms tend to have more debt in their target capital structures and are more likely to use an aggressive current asset financing policy. Conversely, firms with high business risk usually take a conservative view regarding added financial risk, whether that risk arises from a high level of debt or an aggressive current asset financing policy.

Self-Test Questions

1. What two key issues does current asset policy involve?
2. What is involved in the current asset investment decision?
3. What is involved in the current asset financing decision?
4. What is meant by the term *permanent assets*?
5. What is meant by the term *temporary assets*?

Cash Management

Businesses need *cash*, which includes both actual cash and funds held in commercial checking accounts, to pay for labor and materials, to buy fixed assets, to pay taxes, to service debt, and so on. However, cash is a nonrevenue producing asset, it earns no return. Thus, the goal of cash management is to minimize the amount of cash that the business must hold to conduct its normal activities, but at the same time, have sufficient cash on hand to support operations.

Cash Management Techniques

A key element in a business' cash management process is the cash budget, which is discussed in Chapter 8. In essence, the cash budget tells managers how effective they are in applying the cash management techniques discussed in the following sections.[1]

Cash Flow Synchronization

If a person received income once a year, he or she would probably put it in the bank, draw down the account during the year as cash is needed, and have an average balance over the year equal to about half the annual income. If the person received income monthly instead of once a year, he or she would operate similarly, but the average balance would be much smaller. If the person could arrange to receive income daily to pay for rent, food, and other charges on a daily basis, and was quite confident of the forecasted inflows and outflows, he or she could hold a very small cash balance.

Exactly the same situation applies to businesses—by improving cash flow forecasts and by taking steps to match cash receipts with required cash outflows, firms can reduce their cash balances to a minimum. Recognizing this point, some companies bill customers on a regular billing cycle throughout the month that matches their own outflows. This improves the *synchronization of cash flows,* which in turn enables a business to reduce its cash balances, decrease its bank loans, lower interest expenses, and boost profits.

Using Float

Float is defined as the difference between the balance shown on a firm's or individual's checkbook and the balance on the bank's records. Suppose that on the average, a business writes checks in the amount of $5,000 each day, and it takes six days for these checks to clear and to be deducted from the firm's bank account. This will cause the firm's own checkbook to show a balance that is $6 \times \$5,000 = \$30,000$ smaller than the balance on the bank's records—this difference is called *disbursement float.*

Suppose that the firm also receives checks in the amount of $5,000 daily, but it loses four days while they are being deposited and cleared. This will result in $4 \times \$5,000 = \$20,000$ of *collections float.* In total, the firm's *net float,* the difference between the $30,000 disbursement float and the $20,000 collections float, will be $10,000.

If the firm's own collection and clearing process is more efficient than that of the recipients of its checks—which is generally true of larger, more efficient firms—the firm could actually show a *negative* balance on its own books, but have a *positive* balance on the records of its bank. Some firms indicate that they *never* have positive book cash balances. One medical equipment manufacturer stated that its bank's records show an average cash balance of about $200,000, while its own *book* balance is *minus* $200,000—it has $400,000 of net float. Obviously the firm must be able to forecast its disbursements and collections accurately in order to make such heavy use of float.

Basically, a firm's net float is a function of its ability to speed up collections on checks received and to slow down collections on checks written. Efficient firms go to great lengths to speed up the processing of incoming checks, thus putting the funds to work faster, and they try to stretch their own payments out as long as possible without engaging in unethical or illegal practices.

Acceleration of Receipts

Managers have searched for faster ways to collect receivables since the day that credit transactions began. Although cash collection is the responsibility of a firm's managers, the speed with which checks are cleared is dependent on the banking system. Several techniques are now used both to speed collections and to get funds where they are needed, but the three most popular are: lockbox services, concentration banking, and electronic claims processing. Here are some points to note about lockbox services and concentration banking. The discussion of electronic claims processing occurs later in this chapter.

Lockboxes are one of the oldest cash management tools—virtually all banks that offer cash management services also offer lockbox services. In a lockbox system, incoming checks are sent to post office boxes rather than to corporate headquarters. For example, Health SouthWest, a regional HMO headquartered in Oklahoma City, has its Texas members send their payments to a box in Dallas, while its New Mexico members send their checks to Albuquerque, and so on, rather than having all checks sent to Oklahoma City. Several times a day, a local bank collects the contents of each lockbox and deposits the checks into the company's local account. The bank then provides the HMO with daily records of the receipts collected, usually via an electronic data transmission system in a format that permits online updating of the firm's receivables accounts.

A lockbox system reduces the time required for a firm to receive incoming checks, to deposit them, and to get them cleared through the banking system, so that the funds are available for use more quickly. This time reduction occurs because mail time and check collection time are both reduced if the lockbox is located in the geographic area where the customer is located. Lockbox services can often increase the availability of funds by one to four days over the regular system for firms with customers over a large geographical area.

Lockbox systems, although efficient in speeding up collections, result in the firm's cash being spread around among many banks. The primary purpose of *concentration banking* is to mobilize funds from decentralized receiving locations, whether they are lockboxes or decentralized company locations, into one or more central cash pools. In a typical concentration system, the firm's collection banks record deposits received each day. Based on disbursement needs, the funds are then transferred from these collection points to a concentration bank. Concentration accounts allow firms to take maximum advantage of economies of scale in cash management and investment. Health SouthWest uses an Oklahoma City bank as its concentration bank. The HMO cash manager then uses this pool for short-term investing or reallocation among its other banks.

One of the keys to concentration banking is the ability to quickly transfer funds from collecting banks to concentration banks—electronic systems make such transfers easy. *Automated clearinghouses* are communication networks that provide a means of sending data from one financial institution to another. Instead of using paper checks, computer files are created and all entries for a particular bank are placed on a single file that is sent to that bank. Some banks send and receive their data on tapes, while others have direct computer links to the clearinghouse. In addition to automated clearinghouses, the *Federal Reserve wire system* can be used for cash concentration or for other cash transfers. This system is used to move large sums that occur on a sporadic basis, which would occur if Humana borrowed $10 million in the commercial paper market.

Disbursement Control

Accelerated collections represent one side of using float; controlling funds outflows is the flip side of the coin. Efficient cash management can only result if both inflows and outflows are effectively managed.

No single action controls disbursements more effectively than *payables centralization*. This permits the firm's managers to evaluate the payments coming due for the entire firm and to schedule cash transfers to meet these needs on a company-wide basis. Centralized disbursement also permits more efficient monitoring of payables and float balances. However, centralized disbursement can have a downside: centralized offices may not be able to make prompt payment for services rendered, which can create ill will with suppliers.

Zero-balance accounts (ZBAs) are special disbursement accounts that have a zero-dollar balance on which checks are written. Typically, a firm establishes several ZBAs in the concentration bank and funds them from a *master account*. As checks are presented to a ZBA for payment, funds are automatically transferred from the master account. If the master account goes negative, it is replenished by borrowing from the bank against a line of credit or by selling some securities from the firm's marketable securities portfolio. Zero-balance accounts simplify the control of disbursements and cash balances, and hence reduce the amount of idle (i.e., non-interest-bearing) cash.

Whereas ZBAs are typically established at concentration banks, *controlled disbursement accounts* can be set up at any bank. In fact, controlled disbursement accounts were initially used only in relatively remote banks, so this technique was originally called *remote disbursement*. The basic technique is simple: controlled disbursement accounts are not funded until the day's checks are presented against the account. The key to controlled disbursement is the ability of the bank that has the account to report the total amount of checks received for clearance each day by 11 A.M., eastern standard time. This early notification gives a firm's managers sufficient time to wire funds to the controlled disbursement account to cover the checks presented for payment and to invest excess cash at midday when money market trading is at a peak.

Matching the Costs and Benefits of Cash Management

Although a number of techniques have been discussed to reduce cash balance requirements, implementing these procedures is not a costless operation. How far should a firm go in making its cash operations more efficient? As a general rule, the firm should incur these expenses only so long as the marginal returns exceed the marginal costs.

The value of careful cash management depends on the opportunity costs of funds invested in cash, which in turn depends on the current rate of interest. For example, in the early 1980s, with interest rates at relatively high levels, firms were devoting a great deal of care to cash management. Today, with interest rates much lower, the value of cash management is reduced. Clearly, larger firms, with larger cash balances, can better afford to hire the personnel necessary to maintain tight control over their cash positions. Cash management is one element of business operations in which economies of scale are present. Banks also have placed considerable emphasis on developing and marketing cash management services. Because of scale economies, banks can generally provide these services to smaller companies at lower costs than companies can achieve by operating in-house cash management systems.

1. What is float?
2. How do firms use float to increase cash management efficiency?
3. What are some methods that firms can use to accelerate receipts?
4. What are some methods that firms can use to control disbursements?
5. How should cash management actions be evaluated?

**Self-Test
Questions**

Marketable Securities Management

Many firms hold large portfolios of temporary financial investments called *marketable securities*. There are two underlying reasons for these holdings: they serve as an interest earning substitute for cash balances, and they are used to hold funds that are being accumulated for a specific purpose. Although discussed in separate sections, cash and marketable securities management cannot be separated in practice because management of one implies management of the other.

Specific Rationales for Holding Marketable Securities

Many businesses hold portfolios of marketable securities in lieu of larger cash balances. Then, part of the portfolio is liquidated periodically to increase the cash account when cash outflows exceed inflows. Most businesses also rely on bank credit to meet unforeseen needs, but they may still hold some marketable securities to guard against a possible shortage of bank credit. Not-for-profit providers, and hospitals in particular, often have large marketable securities holdings compared with similar sized businesses in other industries. The reasons that not-for-profit hospitals typically carry large marketable securities portfolios are:

- Not-for-profit hospitals often set aside funds for future fixed asset replacement rather than acquire the funds at time of replacement.
- Many hospitals self-insure at least part of their professional liability exposure, and hence establish an investment pool to meet actuarial needs.
- Many hospitals have defined benefit pension plans, which require a firm-sponsored pension fund.
- Not-for-profit hospitals receive endowment gifts that must be managed over time.
- Recent turbulence in the industry has created uncertainty, and large holdings of liquid assets are a prudent hedge against a potentially harsh future.

Criteria for Selecting Marketable Securities

In general, the key characteristic sought in marketable securities investments is safety. Thus, most health services managers are willing to give up some return to ensure that funds are available, in the amounts expected, when needed.

Large businesses, with large amounts of surplus cash, often directly own Treasury bills, commercial paper, negotiable certificates of deposit, and even Euromarket securities (i.e., dollar denominated loans held outside the United States). In addition, large taxable firms often hold preferred stock because of its 70 percent dividend exclusion from federal income taxes. Conversely, smaller firms are more likely to invest with a bank or with a money market or preferred stock mutual fund because a small firm's volume of investment simply does not warrant its hiring specialists to manage a marketable securities portfolio. Small businesses often use a mutual fund and then literally write checks on the fund to bolster the cash account as the need arises.[2] Interest rates on mutual funds are somewhat lower than rates on direct investments of equivalent risk because of management fees. However, for smaller companies, net returns may well be higher on mutual funds because no in-house management expense is required.

1. Why do firms hold marketable securities portfolios?
2. What are some securities that are commonly held as marketable securities?
3. Why are these the securities of choice?

Receivables Management

Generally, businesses would rather sell for cash than on credit, but competitive pressures force most firms to offer credit. The problem is most acute in the health services industry where the third-party payment system forces providers to extend credit to most patients. In a credit sale, goods are shipped or services are provided, inventories are reduced, and an account receivable is created. Eventually, the customer or third-party payor will pay the account, at which time the business will receive cash and its receivables will decline.

The Accumulation of Receivables

The total amount of accounts receivable outstanding at any given time is determined by two factors: the volume of credit sales and the average length of time between sales and collections. For example, suppose Home Infusion, Inc., a home health care firm, begins operations on January 1, and on the first day starts to provide services to patients billed at $1,000 each day. For simplicity, assume that all patients have the same insurance, that it takes Home Infusion 10 days to submit patients' bills, and it takes the insurer another ten days to make the payments. Thus it takes 20 days from delivery of service to receipt of payment.

At the end of the first day, Home Infusion's accounts receivable will be $1,000; they will rise to $2,000 by the end of the second day; by January 20, they will have risen to $20,000. On January 21, another $1,000 will be added to receivables, but, assuming that the insurer pays the full amount for services provided 20 days earlier, payments for services provided on January 1 will reduce receivables by $1,000, so total accounts receivable will remain constant at $20,000. If either the volume of credit sales or the collection period changes, such changes will be reflected in amount of receivables.

What is the cost implication of carrying $20,000 in receivables? The $20,000 on the left side of the balance sheet must be financed by a like amount on the right side.[3] Home Infusion uses a bank loan to finance its receivables, which has an interest rate of 12 percent. Thus, over a year, the firm must pay the bank $0.12 \times \$20,000 = \$2,400$ in interest to carry its receivables balance. The cost associated with carrying other current assets can be thought of in a similar way.

Monitoring the Receivables Position

If a sale is made for cash, the profit is definitely earned, but if the sale is on credit, the profit is not actually earned until the account is collected. If the account is never collected, the profit is never earned. Thus, health services managers must monitor receivables to ensure that they are being collected in a timely manner and to uncover any deterioration in the "quality" of receivables. Early detection can help managers take corrective action before the situation has a significant negative impact on the organization's financial condition.

Average Collection Period (ACP)

Suppose Adolph Weiss & Sons, a manufacturer of surgical instruments, manufactures and sells 200,000 instruments each year at an average sales price of $198 each. Furthermore, assume that all sales are on credit, with terms of 2/10, net 30. Finally, assume that 70 percent of the firm's customers take discounts and pay on Day 10, while the other 30 percent pay on Day 30.

Weiss's *average collection period (ACP)*, often called *days sales outstanding (DSO)* or *days in receivables*, is 16 days:

$$\text{ACP} = (0.7 \times 10 \text{ days}) + (0.3 \times 30 \text{ days}) = 16 \text{ days}.$$

Weiss's *average daily sales (ADS)*, assuming a 360-day year, is $110,000:

$$\text{ADS} = \frac{\text{Annual sales}}{360} = \frac{\text{Units sold} \times \text{Sales price}}{360} = \frac{200,000 \times \$198}{360}$$

$$= \frac{\$39,600,000}{360} = \$110,000.$$

If the company had made cash as well as credit sales, the analysis would focus on credit sales only, and the calculated amount would have been average daily *credit* sales.

Weiss's accounts receivable, assuming a constant, uniform rate of sales all during the year, will at any point in time be $1,760,000[4]:

$$\text{Receivables balance} = \text{ADS} \times \text{ACP}$$

$$= \$110,000 \times 16 = \$1,760,000.$$

The ACP is a measure of the average length of time it takes Weiss's customers to pay off their credit purchases; the ACP is often compared to the industry average ACP. For example, if all surgical instrument manufacturers sell on the same credit terms and if the industry average ACP is 25 days versus Weiss's 16-day ACP, then Weiss either has a higher percentage of discount customers or else its credit department is exceptionally good at ensuring prompt payment.

The ACP can also be compared with the firm's own credit terms. For example, suppose Weiss's ACP had been running at a level of 35 days versus its 2/10, net 30 credit terms, which means that customers must pay within 30 days but receive a 2 percent discount if they pay within 10 days. With a 35-day ACP, some customers would obviously be taking more than 30 days to pay their bills. In fact, if some customers were paying within ten days to take advantage of the discount, the others would, on average, have to be taking much longer than 35 days. One way to check this possibility is to use an aging schedule.

An *aging schedule* breaks down a firm's receivables by age of account. Table 16.2 contains the December 31, 1998 aging schedules of two surgical instrument manufacturers: Weiss and Cutright. Both firms offer the same credit terms, 2/10, net 30, and both show the same total receivables balance. However, Weiss's aging schedule indicates that all of its customers pay on time: 70 percent pay on Day 10, while 30 percent pay on Day 30. Cutright's schedule, which is more typical, shows that many of its customers are not abiding by its credit terms—27 percent of its receivables are more than 30 days past due, even though Cutright's credit terms call for full payment by Day 30. *Aging Schedules*

Aging schedules cannot be constructed from the type of summary data that are reported in a firm's financial statements, they must be developed from the firm's accounts receivable ledger. However, well-run businesses have computerized accounts receivable records. Thus, it is easy to determine the age of each invoice, sort electronically by age categories, and thus generate an aging schedule.

Unique Problems Faced by Healthcare Providers

Although the general principles of receivables management discussed up to this point are applicable to all businesses, healthcare providers face some unique problems. The most obvious problem is the complexities in billing created by the third-party payor system. For example, rather than having a single billing system which applies to all customers, providers have to deal with the rules and regulations of many different governmental and private insurers using different payment methodologies. Thus, providers have to maintain large staffs of specialists that operate under the firm's *patient accounts manager*.

To illustrate the problem, consider Table 16.3, which contains the receivables mix for the hospital industry. There are multiple payors within many of the categories listed in the table, so the actual number of different payors can easily run into the hundreds or thousands.

Table 16.4 provides information on how long it takes hospitals to collect receivables. Because of the large number of payors and the complexities involved with billing and follow-up actions, which lead to high error rates, hospitals clearly

TABLE 16.2
Aging Schedules for Two Firms

| Age of Account (Days) | Weiss | | Cutright | |
	Value of Account	Percentage of Total Value	Value of Account	Percentage of Total Value
0–10	$1,232,000	70%	$ 825,000	47%
11–30	528,000	30	460,000	26
31–45	0	0	265,000	15
46–60	0	0	179,000	10
Over 60	0	0	31,000	2
Total	$1,760,000	100%	$1,760,000	100%

TABLE 16.3

Hospital Industry's
Receivables Mix

Payor	Percentage of Total Accounts Receivable
Medicare	30.2%
Commercial insurers	19.5
Medicaid	14.0
Self-pay	13.4
HMO/PPO	9.7
Blue Cross	8.1
CHAMPUS	5.1
	100.0%

Source: Aspen Publishers, *Hospital Accounts Receivable Analysis (HARA),* published quarterly.

TABLE 16.4

Hospital Industry's
Collection
Performance

Aggregate Aging Schedule:

Age of Account (Days)	Percentage of Total Accounts Receivable
0–30	42.5%
31–60	21.4
61–90	11.2
91–120	7.8
Over 120	17.1
	100.0%

Average Collection Period:

Percentile Values	Average Collection Period (Days)
10th	44.0 days
25th	52.5
Median	62.1
75th	73.0
90th	85.1

Sources: Aspen Publishers, *Hospital Accounts Receivable Analysis (HARA),* published quarterly.
Center for Healthcare Industry Performance Studies, *1997–98 Almanac of Hospital Financial and Operating Indicators.*

have a great deal of difficulty in collecting bills in a timely manner. On average, collecting a receivable takes 62.1 days. However, this number has decreased in recent years as hospital managers have become increasingly aware of the costs associated with carrying receivables, and as automated systems have made the collections process more efficient. In spite of the positive trend, 24.9 percent of receivables still were over 90 days old. In addition, 5.2 percent of patient bills were never paid at all, 3.4 percent were charged off as bad debt losses, and 1.8 percent went to charity care.

One development of note in provider collections is the movement toward electronic claims processing. In 1991, new standards were promulgated for the *electronic data interchange (EDI)* of healthcare claims, which will facilitate widespread adoption of electronic claims processing and payment systems over time. In such a system, claims information is electronically transmitted over telephone lines in a standard format that can be processed by receiving firms without human intervention. Because the health services reimbursement system is paper intensive, mountains of paper claims are currently produced, which lead to high error rates and numerous delays. Although some Medicare intermediaries, as well as other third-party payors, are currently passing information to providers on magnetic tape, these systems tend to be payor unique and require providers to have relatively sophisticated computer systems.[5]

Self-Test Questions

1. Explain how a firm's receivables balance is built up over time and why there are costs associated with carrying receivables.
2. Briefly discuss two means by which a firm can monitor its receivables position.
3. What are some of the unique problems faced by healthcare providers in managing receivables?
4. What trends are occurring in billing and collections?

Inventory Management

Inventories are an essential part of virtually all business operations. As is the case with accounts receivable, inventory levels depend heavily upon sales volume. However, whereas receivables build up after sales have been made, inventories must be acquired *ahead* of sales. This is a critical difference, and the necessity of forecasting sales before establishing target inventory levels makes inventory management a difficult task. Also, because errors in the establishment of inventory levels quickly lead either to lost sales or to excessive carrying costs, inventory management is as important as it is difficult. In the health services industry, inventory management is even more critical because an inventory shortage could lead to catastrophic consequences for patients.

Proper inventory management requires close coordination among the marketing, purchasing, patient services, and finance departments. The marketing department is generally the first to spot changes in demand. These changes must be worked into the company's purchasing and operating schedules, and the financial manager must arrange any financing that will be needed to support the inventory buildup. Improper communication among departments, poor sales forecasts, or both, can lead to disaster.

Larger businesses employ *computerized inventory control systems*. The computer starts with an inventory count in memory. As withdrawals are made, they are recorded in the computer, and the inventory balance is revised. When the order point is reached, the computer automatically places an order, and when the order is received, the recorded balance is increased.

A good inventory control system must be dynamic. A large provider may stock thousands of different items. The usage of these various items can rise or fall quite separately from rising or falling aggregate utilization. As the usage rate for an individual item begins to rise or fall, the inventory manager must adjust its balance to avoid running short or ending up with obsolete items. If the change in the usage rate appears to be permanent, then the *base inventory* level should be recomputed, the *safety stock* should be reconsidered, and the computer model used in the control process should be reprogrammed.

A relatively new approach to inventory control called *just-in-time (JIT)* is gaining popularity in all industries, including health services. To illustrate the use of just-in-time systems among providers, consider St. Luke's Episcopal Hospital in Houston, which consumes large quantities of medical supplies each year. A few years ago, the hospital maintained a 25,000 square foot warehouse to hold its medical supplies. However, as cost pressures mounted, the hospital closed its warehouse and sold the inventory to Baxter International, a major hospital supplier. Now, Baxter is a full-time partner of St. Luke's in ordering and delivering Baxter's hospital supplies, as well as the products of some 400 other companies.

The inventory streamlining process began with daily deliveries to the hospital's loading dock, but soon expanded to a JIT system called stockless inventory. Now, Baxter fills orders in exact, sometimes small, quantities and delivers them directly to departments, including the operating rooms and nursing floors, inside St Luke's. St. Luke's managers estimate that the stockless system has saved the hospital about $1.5 million a year since it was instituted, which includes savings of $350,000 from staff reductions and $650,000 from inventory reductions. Additionally, the hospital has converted space that was previously used as storerooms to patient care and other cash-generating uses. The distributors that offer stockless inventory systems typically add 3 to 5 percent service fees, but many hospitals still can realize savings on total inventory costs.

The stockless inventory concept has its own set of problems. The major concern is that a *stock out,* which occurs when an inventory item is not in stock, will cause a serious problem. "We walk very carefully and slowly because we can't afford a glitch," said a Baxter spokesperson. "The first morning that an operating room doesn't open, we've got a problem." Some hospital managers are concerned that such systems create too much dependence on a single supplier, and eventually the cost savings will disappear as prices are increased.

As stockless inventory systems become more prevalent in hospitals, more and more hospitals are decreasing their in-house inventory management, or *materials management,* as it is often called, in favor of outside contractors who assume both inventory management and supplier roles. In effect, hospitals are beginning to outsource inventory management. For example, some hospitals are experimenting with an inventory management program known as *point-of-service distribution,* which is one generation ahead of stockless systems. Under point-of-service programs, the supplier delivers supplies, intravenous solutions, medical forms, and so on, to the supply rooms. The supplier owns the products in the supply rooms until used by the hospital, at which time the hospital pays for the items. This system has been used by Owens & Minor, a medical supplier, to deliver supplies to 200 inventory locations at UCLA Medical Center.

In addition to reducing inventories, outside inventory managers are often better at ferreting out waste that are their in-house counterparts. For example, an inventory management company recently found that one hospital was spending $600 for products used in open-heart surgery, while another was spending only $420. Because there was no meaningful difference in the procedure or its outcomes, the higher-cost hospital was able to change the medical devices used in the surgery and pocket the difference.

In an even more advanced form of inventory management, some hospitals are just beginning to negotiate with suppliers to furnish materials on the basis of how much medical care is delivered rather than the type and number of products used. In such agreements, providers pay suppliers a set fee for each unit of patient service provided, for example, $125 for each case-mix-adjusted patient day. Under this type of system, a hospital ties its supplies expenditures to its revenues, which, at least for now, are for the most part tied to the number of units of patient service. The end of the evolution of inventory management techniques for healthcare providers is expected to be some form of capitated payment, whereby providers will pay suppliers a previously agreed-upon fee regardless of actual future patient usage, and hence regardless of the amount of materials actually consumed.

1. Why is good inventory management important to a firm's success?
2. Describe some recent trends in inventory management by healthcare providers.

**Self-Test
Questions**

Short-Term Financing

Chapters 11, 12, and 13 focused on long-term financing decisions. However, as pointed out in the introduction to Chapter 11, healthcare providers use 5 percent short-term debt in their total financing mix. This section provides some of the details associated with short-term financing.

Advantages and Disadvantages of Short-Term Credit

Short-term credit has three primary advantages over long-term debt. First, a short-term loan can be obtained much faster than long-term credit. Lenders will insist on a more thorough financial examination before extending long-term credit, and the loan agreement will have to be spelled out in considerable detail because a lot can happen during the life of a 10- or 20-year loan. Thus, if a business requires funds in a hurry, it should look to the short-term markets.

Second, if needs for funds are seasonal or cyclical, a firm may not want to commit itself to long-term debt for three reasons:

• First, issuance costs are generally high when raising long-term debt, but trivial for short-term credit. Although long-term debt can be repaid early, provided the loan agreement includes a prepayment provision, prepayment penalties can be expensive. Accordingly, if a firm thinks its need for funds may diminish in the near future, it should choose short-term debt for the flexibility it provides.

- Second, long-term loan agreements always contain restrictive covenants that constrain the firm's future actions. Short-term credit agreements are generally much less onerous in this regard.
- Third, the interest rate on short-term debt generally is lower than the rate on long-term debt because the yield curve normally is upward sloping. Thus, when coupled with lower issuance costs, short-term debt can have a significant total cost advantage over long-term debt.

In spite of these advantages, short-term credit has one serious disadvantage: it subjects the firm to more risk than does long-term financing. The increased risk occurs for two reasons. First, if a firm borrows on a long-term basis, its interest costs will be relatively stable over time, but if it uses short-term credit, its interest expense can fluctuate widely, and at times possibly going quite high. For example, the short-term rate banks charge (the prime rate) to large corporations more than tripled over a two-year period in the early 1980s, rising from 6.25 to 21 percent. Many firms that had borrowed heavily on a short-term basis simply could not meet their rising interest costs, and as a result, bankruptcies hit record levels during that period.

Second, the principal amount on short-term debt comes due on a regular basis. If the financial condition of business temporarily deteriorates, it may find itself unable to repay this debt when it matures. Furthermore, it may be in such a weak financial position that the lender will not extend the loan. Such a scenario can result in severe problems for the borrower, which, like unexpectedly high interest rates, could force the business into bankruptcy.

Sources of Short-Term Financing

Statements about the flexibility, cost, and riskiness of short-term versus long-term debt depend, to a large extent, on the type of short-term credit that is actually used. Three major types of short-term financing—accruals, accounts payable, and bank loans—are discussed in the following sections.[6]

Accruals Firms generally pay employees on a weekly, biweekly, or monthly basis, so the balance sheet will typically show some accrued wages. Similarly, the firm's own estimated income taxes (if applicable), the social security and income taxes withheld from employee payrolls, and the sales taxes collected are generally paid on a weekly, monthly, or quarterly basis. Thus, as discussed in Chapter 4, the balance sheet accruals account typically includes both taxes and wages.

Accruals increase automatically, or spontaneously, as a firm's operations expand. Furthermore, this type of debt is free in the sense that no explicit interest is paid on funds raised through accruals. However, a firm cannot ordinarily control its accruals because the timing of wage payments is set by economic forces and industry custom, while tax payment dates are established by law. Thus, businesses should use all the accruals they can because they represent free financing, but managers have little control over the levels of such accounts.

Accounts Payable (Trade Credit)

Firms often make purchases from other firms on credit. Such debt is recorded on the balance sheet as an *accounts payable*. Accounts payable, or *trade credit*, is the largest single category of short-term debt for many businesses. Because small companies often do not qualify for financing from other sources, they rely especially heavily on trade credit.[7]

Trade credit is another spontaneous source of financing in the sense that it arises from ordinary business transactions. For example, suppose that a hospital purchases an average of $2,000 a day of supplies on terms of net 30, which means that it must pay for goods 30 days after the invoice date. On average, the hospital will owe 30 times $2,000, or $60,000, to its suppliers, assuming that the hospital's managers act rationally and do not pay before the credit is due. If the hospital's volume, and consequently its purchases, were to double, its accounts payable would also double to $120,000. Simply by growing, the hospital would have spontaneously generated an additional $60,000 of financing. Similarly, if the terms under which it bought supplies were extended from 30 to 40 days, the hospital's accounts payable would expand from $60,000 to $80,000. Thus, a supplier lengthening the credit period, as well as expanding volume, and hence purchases, generates additional financing for a business.

Firms that sell on credit have a *credit policy* that includes certain *terms of credit*. For example, Midwestern Medical Supply Company sells on terms of 2/10, net 30, meaning that a 2 percent discount is given if payment is made within ten days of the invoice date, with the full invoice amount being due and payable within 30 days if the discount is not taken. Suppose that Chicago Health System, Inc., buys an average of $12 million of medical and surgical supplies from Midwestern each year, less a 2 percent discount, for net purchases of $11,760,000 / 360 = $32,666.67 per day. For the sake of simplicity, suppose that Midwestern is Chicago Health System's only supplier. If Chicago Health System takes the discount and pays at the end of the tenth day, its payables will average 10 × $32,666.67 = $326,667, so Chicago Health System, on average, will be receiving $326,667 of credit from its only supplier, Midwestern Medical Supply Company.

Suppose now that the health system's managers decide not to take the discount. What effect will this decision have on the system's financial condition? First, Chicago Health System will begin paying invoices after 30 days, so its accounts payable will increase to 30 × $32,666.67 = $980,000.[8] Midwestern will now be supplying Chicago Health System with $980,000 − $326,667 = $653,333 of **additional** trade credit. The health system could use this additional credit to pay off bank loans, to expand inventories, to increase fixed assets, to build up its cash account, or even to increase its own accounts receivable.

Chicago Health System's additional credit from Midwestern has a cost—it is foregoing a 2 percent discount on its $12 million of purchases, so its costs will rise by $240,000 per year. Dividing this $240,000 dollar cost by the amount of additional credit provides the implicit approximate percentage cost of the added trade credit:

$$\text{Approximate percentage cost} = \frac{\$240,000}{\$653,333} = 36.7\%.$$

Assuming that Chicago Health System can borrow from its bank or from other sources at an interest rate less than 36.7 percent, it should not expand its payables by foregoing discounts.

The following equation can be used to calculate the approximate percentage cost, on an annual basis, of not taking discounts:

$$\text{Approximate \% cost} = \frac{\text{Discount percent}}{100 - \text{Discount percent}}$$

$$\times \frac{360}{\text{Days credit received} - \text{Discount period}}.$$

The numerator of the first term, Discount percent, is the cost per dollar of credit, while the denominator in this term, $100 - \text{Discount percent}$, represents the funds made available by not taking the discount. Thus, the first term is the periodic cost rate of the trade credit; in this example, Chicago Health System must spend $2 to gain $98 of credit, for a cost rate of $2 / 98 = 0.0204 = 2.04\%$. The second term shows how many times each year this cost is incurred; in this example, $360 / (30 - 10) = 360 / 20 = 18$ times. When the two terms are put together, the approximate cost of not taking the discount when the terms are 2/10, net 30, is computed as follows[9]:

$$\text{Approximate \% cost} = \frac{2}{98} \times \frac{360}{20} = 0.0204 \times 18$$

$$= 0.367 = 36.7\%.$$

The cost of trade credit can be reduced by paying late, that is, by paying beyond the date that the credit terms allow. Such a strategy is called *stretching*. If Chicago Health System could get away with paying Midwestern in 60 days rather than in the specified 30, the effective credit period would become $60 - 10 = 50$ days, and the approximate cost would drop from 36.7 percent to $(2 / 98) \times (360 / 50) = 14.7\%$. In recessionary periods, businesses may be able to get away with late payments to suppliers, but they will also suffer a variety of problems associated with stretching accounts payable and being branded a slow payor account.

On the basis of the preceding discussion, it is clear that trade credit often consists of two distinct components:

- *Free trade credit*. This involves credit received during the discount period and which for Chicago Health System amounts to ten days' net purchases, or $326,667.
- *Costly trade credit*. This involves credit in excess of the free credit, and whose cost is an implicit one based on the foregone discount.

From a finance perspective, managers should view trade credit in this way. First, the actual price of supplies is the discounted price, that is, the price that would be paid on a cash purchase. Any credit that can be taken without an increase in price is free credit that should be taken. Second, if the discounted price is the actual price, then the added amount that must be paid if the discount is not taken is, in reality, a *finance charge* for granting additional credit. A business should take the additional credit only if the finance charge is less than the cost of alternative credit sources.

In the example, Chicago Health System should take the $326,667 of free credit offered by Midwestern Medical Supply Company. Free credit is good credit. However, the cost rate of the additional $653,333 of costly trade credit is approximately 37 percent. The health system has access to bank loans at a 9.5 percent rate, so it does not take the additional credit. Under the terms of trade found in most industries, the costly component will involve a relatively high percentage cost, so stronger firms will avoid using it.

Commercial banks, whose short-term loans generally appear on firms' balance sheets as notes payable, are another important source of short-term financing.[10] The banks' influence is actually greater than it appears from the dollar amounts they lend because banks provide *nonspontaneous* funds. As a business' financing needs increase, it requests its bank to provide the additional funds. If the request is denied, the firm may be forced to abandon attractive growth opportunities.

Bank Loans

Although banks make longer-term loans, the bulk of their lending is on a short-term basis (about two-thirds of all bank loans mature in a year or less). Bank loans to businesses are frequently written as 90-day notes, so the loan must be repaid or renewed at the end of 90 days. When a bank loan is approved, the agreement is executed by signing a *promissory note*, which is similar to a bond indenture or loan agreement but much less detailed. The note specifies:

- the amount borrowed;
- the percentage interest rate;
- the repayment schedule, which can involve either a lump sum or a series of installments;
- any collateral that may have to be put up as security for the loan; and
- any other terms and conditions to which the bank and the borrower may have agreed.

When the note is signed, the bank credits the borrower's checking account with the amount of the loan, while both cash and notes payable increase on the borrower's balance sheet.

Banks sometimes require borrowers to maintain a checking account balance equal to 10 to 20 percent of the face amount of the loan. This requirement is called a *compensating balance,* and such balances raise the effective interest rate on the loan. For example, suppose that Pine Garden nursing home needs an $80,000 bank loan to pay off maturing obligations. If the loan requires a 20 percent compensating balance, then the nursing home must borrow $100,000 to obtain a usable $80,000, assuming that the business does not have an "extra" $20,000 around to use as a compensating balance. If the stated interest rate is 8 percent, the effective cost rate is actually 10 percent: $0.08 \times \$100,000 = \$8,000$ in interest expense divided by $80,000 of usable funds equals 10 percent.

A *line of credit*, sometimes called a *revolving credit agreement* or just *revolver*, is a formal understanding between the bank and the borrower, which indicates the maximum credit the bank will extend to the borrower over some specified period of time. For example, on December 31 a bank loan officer may indicate to Pine Garden's manager that the bank regards the nursing home as being good for up to $80,000 during the forthcoming year. If on January 10, Pine Garden's manager signs a promissory note for $15,000 for 90 days, this would be called *taking down* $15,000 of the credit line. This take down would be credited to the nursing home's checking account at the bank, and before repayment of the $15,000, Pine Garden could borrow additional amounts up to a total of $80,000 outstanding at any one time. Lines of credit are generally for one year or less, and borrowers typically have to pay an up-front commitment fee of about 0.5 to 1 percent of the total amount of the line.

Revolvers typically involve large sums over longer periods. To illustrate, in 1998 Colorado Healthcare negotiated a revolving credit agreement for $100 million with a group of banks. The banks were formally committed for four years to lend the firm up to $100 million if the funds were needed. Colorado Healthcare, in turn, paid an annual commitment fee of one-quarter of 1 percent on the unused credit to compensate the banks for making the commitment. Thus, if Colorado Healthcare did not take down any of the $100 million commitment during a year, it would still be required to pay a $250,000 annual fee in monthly installments of $20,833.33. If it borrowed $50 million on the first day of the agreement, the unused portion of the credit line would fall to $50 million and the annual fee would fall to $125,000. But, interest would have to be paid on the money Colorado Healthcare actually borrowed. As a general rule, the rate of interest on credit lines is pegged to the prime rate, so the cost of the loan varies over time as interest rates change.[11] Colorado Healthcare's rate was set at prime plus 0.5 percentage points.

Secured Short-Term Loans

Thus far, the question of whether or not short-term loans are *secured* has not been addressed. Given a choice, it is ordinarily better to borrow on an unsecured basis because the administrative costs associated with secured loans are often high. However, weak businesses may find that they can borrow only if they put up some form of security to protect the lender, or that by using security they can borrow at a much lower rate.

Several kinds of *collateral*, or security, can be employed including marketable securities, land or buildings, equipment, inventory, and accounts receivable. Marketable securities make excellent collateral, but generally, businesses that need short-term credit do not hold large marketable securities portfolios. Both real property (i.e., land and buildings) and equipment are good forms of collateral. However, because of maturity matching, such assets are generally used as security for long-term loans rather than for short-term credit. Therefore, most secured short-term business borrowing involves the use of accounts receivable or inventories as collateral.[12]

Accounts receivable financing involves either the pledging of receivables or the selling of receivables. Such financing is provided by commercial banks or by one of the large industrial finance companies such as GE Capital Corporation. The *pledging* of accounts receivable is characterized by the fact that the lender not only has a claim against the dollar amount of the receivables, but also has recourse against the pledging firm. This means that if the person or firm that owes the receivable does not pay, the business that borrows against the receivable must take the loss. Therefore, the risk of default on the accounts receivable pledged remains with the borrowing firm. When receivables are pledged, the payor is not ordinarily notified about the pledging, and payments are made on the receivables in the same way as when receivables are not used as loan security.

The second form of receivables financing is *factoring,* or *selling accounts receivable.* In this type of secured financing, the receivables account is actually "purchased" by the lender, generally, without recourse to the borrowing business. In a typical factoring transaction, the buyer of the receivables pays the seller about 90 to 95 percent of the face value of the receivables. When receivables are factored, the person or firm that owes the receivable is often notified of the transfer and is asked to make payment directly to the company that bought the receivables. Because the factoring firm assumes the risk of default on bad accounts, it must perform a credit check on the receivables prior to the purchase. Accordingly, *factors,* which are the firms that buy receivables, can provide not only money but also a credit department for the borrower. Incidentally, the same financial institutions that make loans against pledged receivables also serve as factors. Thus, depending on the circumstances and the wishes of the borrower, a financial institution will provide either form of receivables financing.

Because healthcare providers tend to carry relatively large amounts of receivables, such firms are prime candidates for receivables financing. For example, hospitals alone have accounts receivable that total nearly $15 billion. The selling of these receivables, especially by hospitals that are experiencing liquidity problems, represents one way to reduce carrying costs and stimulate cash flow.[13]

To illustrate receivables financing for hospitals, consider the program recently instituted between Chase Manhattan Bank and Presbyterian Hospital, New York City's largest hospital. This program provides $15 million in advance funding of receivables over a three-year period. Presbyterian sells its accounts receivable to Chase for cash. In turn, Chase obtains the cash it needs by selling commercial paper. The payors of the receivables technically make payments directly to Chase, although Chase actually pays Presbyterian a fee to service the receivables accounts. Chase charges an up-front fee for the program and then charges an interest rate of about 1 to 1.5 percent above the prime rate on the amount advanced.

Interestingly, the expanding volume of healthcare receivables financing has created a new class of receivables-backed securities. For example, Prudential Securities recently placed $40 million in medium-term, taxable, AAA-rated notes issued by NPF III, a company created solely to buy receivables from cash-strapped providers. The notes are backed by the Medicare, Medicaid, and commercial insurance receivables of 21 hospitals nationwide. Under the plan, the hospitals sell their receivables to NPF III each week, and hence get cash in less than ten days versus the 60 to 70 days commonly required to collect from third-party payors.

Although receivables financing is a way to reduce current assets, and hence financing costs, critics contend that such programs are too expensive. Because of costs involved, most receivables financing programs are used by providers that have serious liquidity problems, although programs are being developed that can provide benefits even to well-run companies that are not facing a liquidity crunch. Although the illustrations here have focused on the use of receivables financing by hospitals, readers should note that such financing is also used by medical group practices and other healthcare providers.

Receivables financing dominates healthcare providers' use of secured financing, but other healthcare businesses, such as equipment manufacturers and pharmaceutical firms, are more likely to obtain credit secured by business inventories. If a firm is a relatively good credit risk, the mere existence of the inventory may be sufficient to obtain an unsecured loan. However, if the firm is a relatively poor risk, the lending institution may insist upon security, which can take the form of a blanket lien against all inventory or either trust receipts or warehouse receipts against specific inventory items. The *inventory blanket lien* gives the lending institution a lien against all the borrower's inventories. However, the borrower is free to sell inventories, so the value of the collateral can be reduced below the level that existed when the loan was granted.

Because of the inherent weakness of the blanket lien, another procedure for inventory financing was developed. The *security instrument*, also called a *trust receipt*, is an instrument acknowledging that the goods are held in trust for the lender. When trust receipts are used, the borrowing firm, upon receiving funds from the lender, signs and delivers a trust receipt for the goods. The goods can be stored in a public warehouse or held on the premises of the borrower. The trust receipt acknowledges that the goods are held in trust for the lender and that any proceeds from the sale of trust goods must be transmitted to the lender at the end of each day.

Self-Test Questions

1. What are accruals and what is their role in short-term financing?
2. What is the difference between free and costly trade credit?
3. How might a hospital that expects to have a cash shortage sometime during the coming year make sure that needed funds will be available?
4. What are some types of current assets that might be pledged as security for short-term loans?

Key Concepts

This chapter examined current asset management and financing. The key concepts of this chapter are:

- The essence of current asset management and financing is to *support the business' operations* and to ensure *liquidity*.
- Under a *high current asset investment policy*, a firm holds relatively large amounts of each type of current asset. A *low policy* entails holding minimal amounts of these items, whereas a *moderate policy* falls between the two extremes.
- *Permanent assets* are those assets that the firm holds even during slack times, whereas *temporary assets* are the additional assets, usually current assets, that are needed during seasonal or cyclical peaks. The method used to finance permanent and temporary assets defines the firm's *current asset financing policy*.
- A *moderate* approach to current asset financing involves matching, to the extent possible, the maturities of assets and liabilities, so that temporary current assets are financed with temporary financing and permanent assets are financed with permanent financing. Under an *aggressive* approach, some permanent current assets and perhaps some fixed assets are financed with short-term debt. A *conservative* approach would be to use long-term capital to finance all permanent assets and some temporary current assets.
- The *primary goal of cash management* is to reduce the amount of cash held to the minimum necessary to conduct business.
- *Cash management techniques* generally fall into four categories: *synchronizing cash flows, using float, accelerating collections*, and *controlling disbursements*.
- *Lockboxes* are used to accelerate collections. A *concentration banking system* consolidates the collections into a centralized pool that can be managed more efficiently than a large number of individual accounts.
- Three techniques for controlling disbursements are *payables centralization, zero-balance accounts*, and *controlled disbursement accounts*.
- The implementation of a sophisticated cash management system is costly, and all cash management actions must be *evaluated* to ensure that the benefits exceed the costs.
- Firms can reduce their cash balances by holding *marketable securities*. Marketable securities serve both as a *substitute* for cash and as a *temporary investment* for funds that will be needed in the near future. Safety is the primary consideration when selecting marketable securities.
- When a firm sells goods to a customer on credit, an *account receivable* is created.
- Firms can use an *aging schedule* and the *average collection period (ACP)* to help keep track of their receivables position and to help avoid the buildup of possible bad debts.

- Proper *inventory management* requires close coordination among the marketing, purchasing, patient services, and finance departments. Because the cost of holding inventory can be high, inventory management is important.
- *Just-in-time (JIT)* systems are used to minimize inventory costs and, simultaneously, to improve operations.
- The advantages of short-term credit are the *speed* with which short-term loans can be arranged, increased *flexibility*, and that short-term *interest rates* are generally *lower* than long-term rates. The principal disadvantage of short-term credit is the *extra risk* that borrowers must bear because lenders can demand payment on short notice, and the cost of the loan will increase if interest rates rise.
- *Accruals*, which are continually recurring short-term liabilities, represent free spontaneous credit.
- *Accounts payable*, or *trade credit*, arises spontaneously as a result of purchases on credit. Businesses should use all the *free trade credit* they can obtain, but they should use *costly trade credit* only if it is less expensive than alternative sources of short-term debt.
- *Bank loans* are an important source of short-term credit. When a bank loan is approved, a *promissory note* is signed.
- Banks sometimes require borrowers to maintain *compensating balances*, which are deposit requirements set at between 10 and 20 percent of the loan amount. Compensating balances raise the effective rate of interest on bank loans.
- *Lines of credit*, or *revolving credit agreements*, are formal understandings between the bank and the borrower in which the bank agrees to extend some maximum amount of credit to the borrower over some specified period.
- Sometimes a borrower will find that it is necessary to borrow on a *secured basis* in which case the borrower uses assets such as real estate, securities, equipment, inventories, or accounts receivable as collateral for the loan.

Questions

16.1 Describe three alternative current asset investment policies. Explain each policy's risk and return characteristics.

16.2 a. What is the difference between permanent assets and temporary assets?
   b. If a firm uses the maturity matching approach to current asset financing, how will its temporary assets be financed?
   c. Describe three alternative current asset financing policies. Explain each policy's risk and return characteristics.

16.3 a. What is the goal of cash management?
   b. Briefly describe the following cash management techniques:
      (1) Cash flow synchronization
      (2) Float
      (3) Receipt acceleration
      (4) Disbursement control

16.4 a. Give two reasons why firms would hold marketable securities.

   b. Which types of securities are most suitable for holding as marketable securities?

   c. Suppose Southwest Regional Medical Center has just raised $6 million in new capital that it plans to use to build three freestanding clinics, one each year over the next three years. (For the sake of simplicity, assume that equal payments have to be made at the end of each of the next three years.) What securities should be bought for the firm's marketable securities portfolio, assuming that the firm has no other excess cash? (Hint: Consider both the type and maturity of the securities.)

   d. Now consider the situation faced by the Huntsville Physical Therapy Group. It has accumulated $20,000 in cash above its target cash balance and it has no immediate needs for this excess cash. However, the firm may at any time need some part or all of the $20,000 to meet unforeseen cash needs. What securities should be bought for the firm's marketable securities portfolio?

16.5 a. Define average collection period.

   b. How is it used to monitor a firm's accounts receivable?

   c. What is an aging schedule?

   d. How is it used to monitor a firm's accounts receivable?

16.6 a. What is a just-in-time (JIT) inventory system?

   b. What are the advantages and disadvantages of JIT systems?

   c. Can JIT inventory systems be used by healthcare providers? Explain your answer.

16.7 Describe the three major sources of short-term financing.

16.8 a. What is the difference between free trade credit and costly trade credit?

   b. Should firms use all the free trade credit that they can get? Explain your answer.

   c. Should firms use all the costly trade credit they can get? Explain your answer.

16.9 Explain briefly how businesses can obtain secured short-term financing.

Problems

16.1 On a typical day, Park Place Clinic writes $1,000 in checks. It generally takes four days for those checks to clear. Each day the clinic typically receives $1,000 in checks that take three days to clear. What is the clinic's average net float?

16.2 Drugs 'R Us operates a mail order pharmaceutical business on the West Coast. The firm receives an average of $325,000 in payments per day. On average, it takes the firm four days from the time customers mail their checks until it receives and processes them. A lockbox system that consists of ten local depository banks and a concentration bank in San Francisco would cost $6,500 per month. Under this system, customers' checks would be received at the lockbox locations one day after they are mailed, and the daily total would be wired to the concentration bank at a cost of $9.75 each. Assume that the firm could earn 10 percent on marketable securities and that there are 260 working days, and hence 260 transfers from each lockbox location per year.

a. What is the total annual cost of operating the lockbox system?

b. What is the dollar benefit of the system to Drugs 'R Us?

c. Should the firm initiate the lockbox system?

16.3 Suppose one of the suppliers to Seattle Health Systems offers terms of 3/20, net 60.

a. When does Seattle Health Systems have to pay its bills from this supplier?

b. What is the approximate cost of the costly trade credit offered by this supplier? (Assume 360 days per year.)

16.4 Langley Clinics, Inc., buys $400,000 in medical supplies a year (at gross prices) from its major supplier, Consolidated Services, which offers Langley terms of 2.5/10, net 45. Currently, Langley is paying the supplier the full amount due on Day 45, but it is considering taking the discount, paying on Day 10, and replacing the trade credit with a bank loan that has a 10 percent annual cost.

a. What is the amount of free trade credit that Langley obtains from Consolidated Services? (Assume 360 days per year throughout this question.)

b. What is the amount of costly trade credit?

c. What is the approximate annual cost of the costly trade credit?

d. Should Langley replace its trade credit with the bank loan? Explain your answer.

e. If the bank loan is used, how much of the trade credit should be replaced?

16.5 Milwaukee Surgical Supplies, Inc., sells on terms of 3/10, net 30. Gross sales for the year are $1,200,000 and the collections department estimates that 30 percent of the customers pay on the tenth day and take discounts, 40 percent pay on the 30th day, and the remaining 30 percent pay, on average, 40 days after the purchase. (Assume 360 days per year.)

a. What is the firm's average collection period?

b. What is the firm's current receivables balance?

c. What would be the firm's new receivables balance if Milwaukee Surgical toughened up on its collection policy, with the result that all nondiscount customers paid on the 30th day?

d. Suppose that the firm's cost of carrying receivables was 8 percent annually. How much would the toughened credit policy save the firm in annual receivables carrying expense? (Assume that the entire amount of receivables had to be financed.)

16.6 Fargo Memorial Hospital has annual net patient service revenues of
$14,400,000. It has two major third-party payors, plus some of its patients
are self-payors. The hospital's patient accounts manager estimates that 10
percent of the hospital's paying patients (its self-payors) pay on Day 30, 60
percent pay on Day 60 (Payor A), and 30 percent pay on Day 90 (Payor
B). (Five percent of total billings end up as bad debt losses, but that is not
relevant for this problem.)
  a. What is Fargo's average collection period? (Assume 360 days per year
     throughout this problem.)
  b. What is the firm's current receivables balance?
  c. What would be the firm's new receivables balance if a newly proposed
     electronic claims system resulted in collecting from third-party payors in
     45 and 75 days, instead of 60 and 90 days?
  d. Suppose the firm's annual cost of carrying receivables was 10 percent. If
     the electronic claims system costs $30,000 a year to lease and operate,
     should it be adopted? (Assume that the entire receivables balance has to
     be financed.)

Notes

1. This discussion of cash management is necessarily brief. For a much more detailed
   discussion of cash management within the health services industry, see A. G. Seidner
   and W. O. Cleverley, *Cash and Investment Management for the Health Care Industry*
   (Rockville, MD: Aspen, 1990).
2. Mutual funds cannot be used as a replacement for commercial checking accounts
   because the number of checks that can be written against such accounts is normally
   limited to a few per month.
3. To be precise, the full amount of the receivables account does **not** require financing.
   The cash costs associated with producing the $20,000 in revenues do need to be
   financed, but the profit component does not. For example, assume that Home
   Infusion has cash costs of $800 to support each day's sales of $1,000. Then, 20 days of
   receivables would actually require financing of 20 × $800 = $16,000. The remaining
   $4,000 in the receivables account would be offset on the balance sheet by $4,000
   profit placed in the retained earnings account.
4. The ACP can be calculated, given a firm's accounts receivable balance and its average
   daily credit sales (ADS), as follows:

$$ \text{ACP} = \frac{\text{Receivables}}{\text{ADS}} = \frac{\$1,760,000}{\$110,000} = 16 \text{ days.} $$

5. Medicare spent over $100 million in preliminary work to develop an all-encompassing
   electronic payment system that was supposed to be in operation in 2000. However,
   the effort has been plagued with problems. In 1997, Medicare was forced to cancel
   the ongoing work and to go back to the drawing board.
6. The fourth major type of short-term financing is *commercial paper*, which is a type
   of unsecured business debt sold primarily to other businesses, insurance companies,
   pension funds, and money market mutual funds. Commercial paper is issued with

maturities less than 270 days and, generally, carries an interest rate below the prime rate but above the rate on short-term Treasury securities. The catch is that commercial paper only can be issued by very large companies with excellent credit standing, so most healthcare providers are not large enough to use this source of financing.

7. In a credit sale, the seller records the transaction as a receivable, while the buyer records it as a payable. If a firm's payables exceed its receivables, it is said to be *receiving net trade credit*, whereas if its receivables exceed its payables, it is *extending net trade credit*. Smaller firms frequently receive net credit, while larger firms generally extend it.

8. A question arises here as to whether accounts payable should reflect gross purchases or purchases net of discounts. Although the GAAP permit either treatment on the grounds that the difference is not material, most accountants prefer to record payables net of discounts and to report the higher payments that result from not taking discounts as an additional expense, which is called "discounts lost."

9. This cost has purposely been labeled as the **approximate** percentage cost. The true effective cost, which recognizes intra-year compounding, is 43.8 percent, which is found as follows:

$$(1 + 0.0204)^{18} - 1.0 = (1.0204)^{18} - 1.0 = 0.438 = 43.8\%.$$

10. Although commercial banks remain the primary source of short-term loans, other sources are available. For example, in 1998, GE Capital Corporation had over $2 billion in commercial loans outstanding. Firms such as GE Capital, which was initially established to finance consumers' purchases of GE's appliances, often find business loans to be more profitable than consumer loans.

11. The *prime rate* is the interest rate charged to a bank's very best customers. Each bank sets its own prime rate, but because of competition, most banks' prime rates are identical. Furthermore, most banks follow the lead of the large New York City banks. In late 1998, the prime rate was 8.0 percent.

12. In addition to business assets, owners of small businesses are often required to pledge personal assets as collateral for bank business loans.

13. For more information on the use of receivables financing by healthcare providers, see T. J. Kincaid, "Selling Accounts Receivable to Fund Working Capital," *Healthcare Financial Management* (May 1993): 27–32.

References

Anderson, A. M. 1993. "Enhancing Hospital Cash Reserves Management." *Healthcare Financial Management* (July): 91–95.

Anderson, H. J. 1989. "Patient Accounts Managers Share Views on Receivables." *Healthcare Financial Management* (December): 42–46.

Berling, R. J., Jr. and J. T. Geppi. 1989. "Hospitals Can Cut Materials Costs by Managing Supply Pipeline." *Healthcare Financial Management* (April): 19–26.

Bruch, N. M. and L. L. Lewis. 1994. "Using Control Charts to Help Manage Accounts Receivable." *Healthcare Financial Management* (July): 44–48.

Clarkin, J. F. 1990. "Managing Accounts Receivable." *Topics in Health Care Financing* (Fall): 1–93.

Coyne, J. S. 1987. "Corporate Cash Management in Health Care: Can We do Better?" *Healthcare Financial Management* (September): 76–79.

Dias, K. and D. Stockamp. 1992. "Nursing Process Approach Improves Receivables Management." *Healthcare Financial Management* (September): 55–64.

Dixon, L. H. and S. K. Bossert. 1993. "The Commercial Bank as Investment Advisor for Hospital Investable Assets." *Topics in Health Care Financing* (Summer): 58–68.

Edwards, D. E., W. C. Hamilton, and R. Hauser. 1991. "Financial Reserve: Hospitals Leery of Credit Lines, Factoring Receivables." *Healthcare Financial Management* (October): 82–88.

Ferconio, S. and M. R. Lane. 1991. "Financing Maneuvers: Two Opportunities to Boost a Hospital's Working Capital." *Healthcare Financial Management* (October): 74–80.

Folk, M. D. and P. R. Roest. 1995. "Converting Accounts Receivable into Cash." *Healthcare Financial Management* (September): 74–78.

Frohlich, R. M., Jr. 1994. "Effective Reassignment of Accounts Can Decrease Bad Debt." *Healthcare Financial Management* (July): 37–42.

Funsten, R. S. 1993. "Accounts Receivable Management." *Topics in Health Care Financing* (Fall): 1–91.

Green, L. A. 1993. "Cash Management: Acceleration and Information Strategies." *Topics in Health Care Financing* (Summer): 44–57.

Groenevelt, C. J. 1990. "Applying Japanese Management Tips to Patient Accounts." *Healthcare Financial Management* (April): 46–55.

Hauser, R. C., D. E. Edwards, and J. T. Edwards. 1991. "Cash Budgeting: An Underutilized Resource Management Tool in Not-for-Profit Health Care Entities." *Hospital & Health Services Administration* (Fall): 439–446.

Kelly, V. K. 1993. "Banks As a Source of Capital." *Topics in Health Care Financing* (Summer): 21–34.

Kincaid, T. J. 1993. "Selling Accounts Receivable to Fund Working Capital." *Healthcare Financial Management* (May): 27–32.

Kowalski, J. C. 1991a. "Materials Management Crucial to Overall Efficiency." *Healthcare Financial Management* (January): 40–44.

———. 1991b. "Inventory to Go: Can Stockless Deliver Efficiency." *Healthcare Financial Management* (November): 21–34.

Ladewig, T. L. and B. A. Hecht. 1993. "Achieving Excellence in the Management of Accounts Receivable." *Healthcare Financial Management* (September): 25–32.

Marshall, S. 1993. "Cost Justifying the Electronic Billing Decision." *Healthcare Financial Management* (June): 68–72.

Masonson, L. N. 1992. "Banks Aggressively Marketing Cash Management Services." *Healthcare Financial Management* (December): 59–60.

McFadden, D. R. 1989. "How to Gain Maximum Returns Through Cash Management." *Healthcare Financial Management* (October): 44–53.

Melson, L. M. and M. K. Schultz. 1989. "Overcoming Barriers to Operating Room Inventory Control." *Healthcare Financial Management* (April): 28–34.

Moynihan, J. J. 1993. "Improving the Claims Process with EDI." *Healthcare Financial Management* (January): 48–52.

Newton, R. L. 1993. "Measuring Accounts Receivable Performance: A Comprehensive Method." *Healthcare Financial Management* (May): 33–36.

Prince, T. R. and R. Ramanan. 1992. "Collection Performance: An Empirical Analysis of

Not-for-Profit Community Hospitals." *Hospital & Health Services Administration* (Summer): 181–196.

Reiss, J. B. and S. J. Di Cioccio. 1991. "Where There's a Will: How to Finance Medicare Receivables—Legally." *Healthcare Financial Management* (October): 90–96.

Robinson, E. F. 1989. "Automated Collection Systems Improve Cash Flow." *Healthcare Financial Management* (December): 31–40.

Seidner, A. G. 1987. "Reviewing the Basics of Investment Management." *Healthcare Financial Management* (October): 68–72.

Sen, S. and J. P. Lawler. 1995. "Securitizing Receivables Offers Low-Cost Financing Option." *Healthcare Financial Management* (May): 32–37.

Slater, R. M., R. Corti, and J. Privitera. 1991. "Giving Receivables an 'Outside' Chance." *Healthcare Financial Management* (October): 56–66.

Smith, D. and L. C. McPherson. 1988. "Improving Hospital Investments Using a Disciplined Approach." *Healthcare Financial Management* (July): 32–41.

Souders, R. V. 1990. "Electronic Claims Can be a Remedy for Cash Flow Troubles." *Healthcare Financial Management* (June): 62–68.

Spiegel, M. 1989. "Selling Accounts Receivable Can Improve Cash Flow." *Healthcare Financial Management* (September): 40–46.

Swarzman, G. F. 1994. "Does Your Patient Accounting System Pass the Systems Test?" *Healthcare Financial Management* (July): 27–34.

Zimmerman, D. 1993. *Cash is King*. Franklin, WI: Eagle Press.

ANALYZING FINANCIAL PERFORMANCE

Learning Objectives

After studying this chapter, readers will be able to:

- Explain the purposes of financial statement and operating analyses.
- Describe the primary techniques used in financial statement and operating analyses.
- Conduct basic financial and operating statement analyses to assess the financial condition of a business.
- Describe the problems associated with financial statement and operating analyses.

Introduction

One of the most important characteristics of a business is its *financial performance*. Financial performance has many dimensions, but to health services managers the most relevant feature of performance is the business' *financial condition*: Does the business have the financial capacity to perform its mission? Often, judgments about financial condition are made on the basis of *financial statement analysis*, which focuses on the data contained in a firm's financial statements. Financial statement analysis is applied both to historical data, which reflect the results of past managerial decisions, and to forecasted data, which comprise the roadmap for the business' future. Therefore, managers use financial statement analysis both to assess current condition and as a springboard to predicting and planning for the future.

Although financial statement analysis provides a great deal of important information regarding financial condition, it often fails to provide much insight into the operational causes of that condition. Thus, financial statement analysis is often supplemented by *operating analysis*, which uses operating data not usually found in a firm's financial statements, such as occupancy, patient mix, length of stay, and productivity measures, to help identify those factors that contributed to the assessed financial condition. Through operating analyses, managers are better able to identify and implement strategies that ensure a sound financial condition in the future.

Financial statement and operating analyses involve a number of techniques that extract information contained in a firm's financial statements and elsewhere, and combine it in a form that facilitates making judgments about the business' financial condition and operations. Often, the end result of such analyses is a list of corporate strengths and weaknesses. In this chapter, several analytical techniques used in financial statement and operating analyses, some related topics, and the problems inherent in such analyses are discussed.

In much of the chapter, Riverside Memorial Hospital, a 450-bed, not-for-profit facility, is used to illustrate financial performance analysis. Although a hospital is being used to illustrate the techniques, they can be applied to any health services setting. Simplified versions of Riverside's primary financial statements are contained in Tables 17.1, 17.2, and 17.3.

The Statement of Cash Flows

The statement of cash flows was first described in Chapter 4. Specifically, this statement tells such things as whether or not the firm's core operations are profitable, how much capital the firm raised and how this capital was used, and what impact operating and financing decisions had on the firm's cash position.

Table 17.3 contains Riverside's statement of cash flows, which focuses on the overall sources and uses of cash in 1998. The top part shows cash generated by and used in operations. For Riverside, operations provided $11,196,000 in net cash flow. The income statement reported net income plus depreciation of $8,572,000 + $4,130,000 = $12,702,000, but as part of its operations Riverside invested $1,297,000 in current assets (receivables and inventories) and

TABLE 17.1
Riverside Memorial Hospital: Statements of Operations (Income Statements), Years Ended December 31, 1998 and 1997 (in thousands)

	1998	1997
Net patient service revenue	$108,600	$ 97,393
Premium revenue	5,232	4,622
Other revenue	3,644	6,014
Total revenue	$117,476	$108,029
Expenses:		
Nursing services	$ 58,285	$ 56,752
Dietary services	5,424	4,718
General services	13,198	11,655
Administrative services	11,427	11,585
Employee health and welfare	10,250	10,705
Provision for uncollectibles	3,328	3,469
Provision for malpractice	1,320	1,204
Depreciation	4,130	4,025
Interest expense	1,542	1,521
Total expenses	$108,904	$105,634
Net income	$ 8,572	$ 2,395

TABLE 17.2
Riverside Memorial
Hospital: Balance
Sheets, December
31, 1998 and 1997
(in thousands)

	1998	1997
Cash and equivalents	$ 4,263	$ 5,095
Short-term investments	2,000	0
Accounts receivable	21,840	20,738
Inventories	3,177	2,982
Total current assets	$ 31,280	$ 28,815
Gross plant and equipment	$ 145,158	$ 140,865
Accumulated depreciation	25,160	21,030
Net plant and equipment	$ 119,998	$ 119,835
Total assets	$ 151,278	$ 148,650
Accounts payable	$ 4,707	$ 5,145
Accrued expenses	5,650	5,421
Notes payable	825	4,237
Current portion of long-term debt	2,150	2,000
Total current liabilities	$ 13,332	$ 16,803
Long-term debt	$ 28,750	$ 30,900
Capital lease obligations	1,832	2,155
Total long-term liabilities	$ 30,582	$ 33,055
Net assets (equity)	$ 107,364	$ 98,792
Total liabilities and net assets	$ 151,278	$ 148,650

lost $209,000 in spontaneous liabilities (payables and accruals). The end result, *net cash flow from operations*, was $12,702,000 − $1,297,000 − $209,000 = $11,196,000.

The next section of the statement of cash flows focuses on investments in fixed assets. Riverside spent $4,293,000 on capital expenditures in 1998.

Riverside's financing activities, as shown in the third section, highlight the fact that the hospital used cash to pay off previously incurred debt and to invest in marketable securities. The net effect of the hospital's financing activities was a *net cash outflow from financing* of $7,735,000.

When the three major sections are totaled, Riverside had a $11,196,000 − $4,293,000 − $7,735,000 = $832,000 *net decrease in cash* (i.e., net cash outflow) during 1998. The very bottom of Table 17.3 reconciles the 1998 net cash flow with the 1998 ending cash balance shown on the balance sheet. Riverside began 1998 with $5,095,000, experienced a cash outflow of $832,000 during the year, and ended the year with $5,095,000 − $832,000 = $4,263,000 in its cash and equivalents account, as verified by the value reported on Table 17.2.

TABLE 17.3

Riverside Memorial
Hospital: Statement
of Cash Flows, Year
End December 31,
1998
(in thousands)

Cash Flows from Operating Activities:	
Change in net assets (net income)	$ 8,572
Adjustments:	
Depreciation	4,130
Increase in accounts receivable	(1,102)
Increase in inventories	(195)
Decrease in accounts payable	(438)
Increase in accrued expenses	229
Net cash flow from operations	$11,196
Cash Flows from Investing Activities:	
Investment in plant and equipment	($ 4,293)
Cash Flows from Financing Activities:	
Investment in short-term securities	($ 2,000)
Repayment of long-term debt	(2,150)
Repayment of notes payable	(3,412)
Capital lease principal repayment	(323)
Change in current portion of LT debt	150
Net cash flow from financing	($ 7,735)
Net increase (decrease) in cash	($ 832)
Beginning cash and equivalents	$ 5,095
Ending cash and securities	$ 4,263

Riverside's statement of cash flows shows nothing unusual or alarming. It does show that the hospital's operations are inherently profitable, at least in 1998. Had the statement showed an operating cash drain, Riverside's managers would have had something to worry about; if it continued, such a drain could bleed the hospital to death. The statement of cash flows also provided easily interpreted information about Riverside's financing and fixed asset investing activities for the year. For example, Riverside's cash flow from operations was used primarily to purchase new fixed assets, to invest in short-term securities, and to pay off notes payable and long-term debt. Again, such uses of operating cash flow do raise any red flags regarding the hospital's financial actions.

Managers and investors must pay close attention to the statement of cash flows. Financial condition is driven by cash flows, and the statement gives a good picture of the annual cash flows generated by the business.[1] An examination of Table 17.3 (or, better yet, a series of such tables going back the last five years and projected five years into the future) would give Riverside's managers and creditors an idea of whether or not the hospital's operations are self-sustaining. That is, does the business generate the cash flows necessary to pay the expenses, including those associated with raising capital? Although the statement of cash flows is filled with valuable information, the bottom line tells little about the business' financial condition because operating losses can be covered by financing transactions such as borrowing or selling new common stock (if investor owned), at least in the short run.

Self-Test Questions

1. What type of financial performance information is provided in the statement of cash flows?
2. What is the difference between net income and cash flow, and which is more meaningful to a business' financial condition?
3. Does the fact that a business' cash position has improved provide much insight into the year's financial results?

Ratio Analysis

Although a firm's balance sheet and income statement contain a wealth of financial information, it is often difficult to make meaningful judgments about financial performance by merely examining the raw data. To illustrate, one managed care plan may have $5,248,760 in long-term debt and interest charges of $419,900, while another may have $52,647,980 in debt and interest charges of $3,948,600. The true burden of these debts, and each managed care plan's ability to pay the interest and principal due on them, cannot be easily assessed without additional comparisons, such as those provided by *ratio analysis*. In essence, ratio analysis combines data from the balance sheet and the income statement to create single numbers that have easily interpreted financial significance (i.e., numbers that measure various aspects of financial performance). In the case of debt and interest payments, ratios could be constructed that relate each plan's debt to its assets and the interest it pays to the income it has available for payment.

Unfortunately, an almost unlimited number of financial ratios can be constructed and the choice of ratios depends, in large part, on the nature of the business being analyzed, the purpose of the analysis, and the availability of comparative data. Generally, ratios are grouped into categories to make them easier to interpret. In the paragraphs that follow, the data presented in Tables 17.1 and 17.2 are used to calculate an illustrative sampling of 1998 financial ratios for Riverside Memorial Hospital, which are then compared with hospital industry average ratios.[2] Note that in a real analysis, many more ratios would be calculated and analyzed. Also, although a hospital is used to illustrate ratio analysis, the specific ratios used in any analysis depend on the type of healthcare provider. Some ratios are more meaningful for hospitals, some ratios are more meaningful for managed care organizations, some for group practices, and so on.

Profitability Ratios

Profitability is the net result of a large number of managerial policies and decisions, so *profitability ratios* provide one measure of the aggregate financial performance of a business.

Total Margin The *total margin*, often called the *total profit margin*, or just *profit margin*, is defined as net income divided by total revenue:

$$\text{Total margin} = \frac{\text{Net income}}{\text{Total revenue}} = \frac{\$8,572}{\$117,476} = 0.073 = 7.3\%.$$

Industry average = 5.0%.

Riverside's total margin of 7.3 percent shows that the hospital makes 7.3 cents on every dollar of total revenue. The total margin measures the ability of the organization to control expenses. With all else the same, the higher the total margin, the lower the expenses relative to revenues. Riverside's total margin is above the industry average of 5.0 percent, which indicates relatively good expense control. How good? The industry data source also reports quartiles; for total margin, the upper quartile was 8.4 percent, which means that 25 percent of hospitals had total margins higher than 8.4 percent. Thus, although Riverside's total margin was better than average, it was not as good as the top hospitals.

Riverside's relatively high total margin could mean that the hospital's gross charges are relatively high, its allowances are relatively low, its costs are relatively low, it has relatively high nonoperating income, or a combination of these factors. A thorough operating analysis would help pinpoint the cause, or causes, of Riverside's high total margin.

When data are available, another useful margin ratio is the *operating margin*, which is defined as operating income divided by operating revenues. (Operating revenues are patient service revenue plus premium revenue.) The advantage of this margin measure is that it focuses on core business operations, and hence removes the influence of nonoperating gains and losses, which often are transitory and unrelated to core operations. However, the current format of healthcare financial statements makes this ratio difficult to determine without additional information.

With only the data given in the financial statements, Riverside's operating margin can be estimated as follows. First, Riverside's operating revenue for 1998 was $108,600,000 + $5,232,000 = $113,832,000. If the assumption is that all expenses were operating expenses, Riverside's 1998 operating margin would be ($113,832 − $108,904) / $113,832 = $4,928 / $113,832 = 0.043 = 4.3%. Removing nonoperating revenue from the calculation lowers the profit margin.

Return on Total Assets (ROA) The ratio of net income to total assets measures the *return on total assets*, often just called *return on assets* (*ROA*):

$$\text{Return on assets} = \frac{\text{Net income}}{\text{Total assets}} = \frac{\$8,572}{\$151,278} = 0.057 = 5.7\%.$$

Industry average = 4.8%.

Riverside's 5.7 percent ROA, which means that each dollar of total assets generated 5.7 cents in profit, is well above the 4.8 percent average for the hospital industry. ROA tells managers how productively, in a financial sense, a business is using its assets. The higher the ROA, the greater the net income for each dollar invested in assets, and hence the more productive the assets. ROA measures both a company's ability to control expenses, as expressed by the total margin, and its ability to use its assets to generate revenue.

The ratio of net income to total equity (net assets) measures the *return on equity* (ROE):

Return on Equity (ROE)

$$\text{Return on equity} = \frac{\text{Net income}}{\text{Total equity}} = \frac{\$8,572}{\$107,364} = 0.080 = 8.0\%.$$

Industry average $= 8.4\%$.

Riverside's 8.0 percent ROE is slightly below the 8.4 percent industry average. The hospital was able to generate 8.0 cents of income for each dollar of equity investment, while the average hospital produced 8.4 cents. ROE is especially meaningful for investor-owned businesses. Owners are concerned with how well the business' managers are utilizing owner-supplied capital, and ROE gives one answer to this question. For not-for-profit businesses such as Riverside, ROE tells its board of trustees and managers how well, in financial terms, its community-supplied capital is being utilized.

Riverside's 1998 total margin and return on assets were above the industry averages, yet the hospital's ROE is below the average. As will be shown when Du Pont analysis is discussed, this apparent inconsistency is caused by the hospital's relatively low use of debt financing.

Liquidity Ratios

One of the first concerns of most managers, and the major concern of a firm's creditors, is the business' *liquidity*. Will the business be able to meet its obligations in a timely manner as they become due? Riverside has debts totaling over $13 million (i.e., its current liabilities) that must be paid off within the coming year. Will the hospital be able to make these payments? A full liquidity analysis requires the use of a cash budget, which was discussed in Chapter 8. However, by relating the amount of cash and other current assets to current obligations, ratio analysis provides a quick, easy-to-use, rough measure of liquidity.

The *current ratio* is computed by dividing current assets by current liabilities:

Current Ratio

$$\text{Current ratio} = \frac{\text{Current assets}}{\text{Current liabilities}} = \frac{\$31,280}{\$13,332} = 2.3, \text{ or } 2.3 \text{ times.}$$

Industry average $= 2.0$.

The current ratio tells managers that the liquidation of Riverside's current assets at book value would provide 2.3 dollars of cash for every $1 of current liabilities. If a business is getting into financial difficulty, it will begin paying its accounts payable more slowly, building up short-term bank loans (i.e., notes payable), and so on. If these current liabilities rise faster than current assets, the current ratio will fall, which could spell trouble. Because the current ratio is an indicator of the extent to which short-term claims are covered by assets that are expected to be converted to cash in the near term, it is one commonly used measure of liquidity.

Riverside's current ratio is slightly above the average for the hospital industry. Because current assets should be converted to cash in the near future, it is highly probable that these assets could be liquidated at close to their stated values. With a current ratio of 2.3, the hospital could liquidate current assets at only 43 percent of book value and still pay off current creditors in full.[3]

Although industry average figures are discussed in detail later, it should be stated here that the industry average is not a magic number that all businesses should strive to achieve. In fact, some very well managed businesses will be above the average, while other good firms will be below it. However, if a firm's ratios are far removed from the average for the industry, its managers should be concerned about why this difference occurs.

Days Cash on Hand

The current ratio measures liquidity on the basis of balance sheet accounts as opposed to income statement items. However, the true measure of a business' liquidity is whether or not it can meet its payments as they become due, so liquidity is more related to cash flows than it is to assets and liabilities. The *days cash-on-hand ratio* moves closer to those factors that truly determine liquidity:

$$\text{Days cash on hand} = \frac{\text{Cash} + \text{Marketable securities}}{(\text{Expenses} - \text{Depreciation} - \text{Provision for uncollectibles})/365}$$

$$= \frac{\$4,263 + \$2,000}{(\$108,904 - \$4,130 - \$3,328)/365} = \frac{\$6,263}{\$277.93} = 22.5 \text{ days.}$$

Industry average $= 30.6$ days.

The denominator of the equation **estimates** average daily cash expenses by stripping out noncash expenses from reported total expenses. The numerator is the cash and securities that are available to make those cash payments. Because Riverside's days cash on hand is lower than the industry average, its liquidity position as measured by days cash on hand is worse than that of the average hospital.

For Riverside, the two measures of liquidity—current ratio and days cash on hand—give conflicting results. Perhaps the average hospital has a greater proportion of cash and marketable securities in its current assets than does Riverside. More analysis would be required to make a supportable judgment concerning Riverside's liquidity position. Remember, though, that the cash budget is the primary tool used by managers to ensure liquidity.

Debt Management (Capital Structure) Ratios

The extent to which a firm uses debt financing, or *financial leverage,* is an important measure of financial performance for several reasons. First, by raising funds through debt, owners of for-profit firms can maintain control of the firm with a limited investment. For not-for-profit firms, debt financing allows the organization to provide more services than it could if it were solely financed with contributed and earned capital. Next, creditors look to owner-supplied funds to provide a margin of safety; if the owners have provided only a small proportion of total financing, the risks of the enterprise are borne mainly by its creditors. Finally, if the firm earns more on investments financed with borrowed funds than it pays in interest, the return on equity capital is magnified or leveraged up.

Two types of ratios are used to assess debt management:

- Balance sheet data are used to determine the extent to which borrowed funds have been used to finance assets. Such ratios are called *capitalization ratios*.
- Income statement data are used to determine the extent to which fixed financial charges are covered by reported profits. Such ratios are called *coverage ratios*.

The two sets of ratios are complementary, so most financial statement analyses examine both types.

The ratio of total debt to total assets, generally called the *debt ratio*, measures the percentage of total funds provided by creditors:

Capitalization Ratio 1: Total Debt to Total Assets (Debt Ratio)

$$\text{Debt ratio} = \frac{\text{Total debt}}{\text{Total assets}} = \frac{\$43,914}{\$151,278} = 0.290, \text{ or } 29.0\%.$$

Industry average $= 43.3\%$.

In this case, debt is defined as **all debt** and includes current liabilities, long-term debt, and capital lease obligations—everything but equity. However, this ratio has many variations, all of which use different definitions of what constitutes debt. Creditors prefer low debt ratios because the lower the ratio, the greater the cushion against creditors' losses in the event of bankruptcy and liquidation. Conversely, owners of for-profit firms may seek high leverage either to leverage up returns or because selling new stock would mean giving up some degree of control. In not-for-profit firms, managers may seek high leverage to offer more services.

Riverside's debt ratio is 29.0 percent. This means that its creditors have supplied somewhat less than one-third of the firm's total financing. Put another way, each dollar of assets was financed with 29 cents of debt, and consequently, 71 cents of equity. (The *equity ratio* is 1 − Debt ratio, so Riverside's equity ratio is 71 percent.) Because the average debt ratio for the hospital industry is over 40 percent, Riverside uses significantly less debt than the average hospital. The low debt ratio indicates that the hospital would find it relatively easy to borrow additional funds, presumably at favorable rates.

Another commonly used capitalization ratio is the *debt to equity ratio*. The debt ratio and debt to equity ratios are transformations of each other, and hence provide the same information, but with a slightly different twist:

Capitalization Ratio 2: Debt to Equity Ratio

$$\text{Debt to equity ratio} = \frac{\text{Total debt}}{\text{Total equity}} = \frac{\$43,914}{\$107,364} = 0.409, \text{ or } 40.9\%.$$

Industry average $= 73.3\%$.

This ratio tells analysts that Riverside's creditors have contributed 40.9 cents for each dollar of equity capital, while the industry average is 73.3 cents per dollar. Both the debt ratio and debt to equity ratio increase as a business of a given size uses a greater proportion of debt financing, but the debt ratio rises linearly and approaches a limit of 100 percent, while the debt to equity ratio rises exponentially and approaches infinity.

Lenders, in particular, prefer the debt to equity ratio to the debt ratio. Their preference is based on the fact that it tells them how much capital creditors have provided to the business **per dollar of equity capital**. The higher this ratio, the riskier the creditors' position.

Coverage Ratio 1: Times-Interest-Earned Ratio

The *times-interest-earned (TIE) ratio* is determined by dividing earnings before interest and taxes (EBIT) by the interest charges. EBIT is used in the numerator because it represents the amount of income that is available to pay interest expense. For a not-for-profit business, which does not pay taxes, EBIT = Net income + Interest expense. For Riverside:

$$\text{TIE ratio} = \frac{\text{EBIT}}{\text{Interest expense}} = \frac{\$8,572 + \$1,542}{\$1,542} = \frac{\$10,114}{\$1,542} = 6.6 \text{ times.}$$

Industry average $= 4.0$.

The TIE ratio measures the number of dollars of income available to pay each dollar of interest expense. In essence, it is an indicator of the extent to which income can decline before the business' earnings are less than its annual interest costs. Failure to pay interest can bring legal action by the firm's creditors, which could possibly result in bankruptcy.

Riverside's interest is covered 6.6 times, so it has 6.6 dollars of accounting income to pay each dollar of interest expense. Because the industry average TIE ratio is four times, the hospital is covering its interest charges by a relatively high margin of safety. Thus, the TIE ratio reinforces the previous conclusion based on the debt ratio, namely, that the hospital could easily expand its use of debt financing.

Coverage ratios are often better measures of a firm's debt utilization than capitalization ratios because coverage ratios discriminate between low interest rate debt and high interest rate debt. For example, a group practice may have $10 million of 4 percent debt on its balance sheet, while another may have $10 million of 8 percent debt. If both practices have the same income and assets, both would have the same debt ratio. However, the group paying 4 percent interest would have the lower interest charges, and hence would be in a better financial position than the group paying 8 percent. Such improved financial performance is captured by the TIE ratio.

Although the TIE ratio is easy to calculate, it has two major deficiencies. First, leasing has become widespread in recent years. Also, many debt contracts require that principal payments be made over the life of the loan rather than only at maturity. Thus, most businesses must meet fixed financial charges other than interest payments. Second, the TIE ratio ignores the fact that accounting income, whether measured by EBIT or net income, does not indicate the actual cash flow available to meet fixed charge payments. These deficiencies are corrected in the *cash flow coverage (CFC) ratio*, which shows the margin by which cash flow covers fixed financial requirements:

Coverage Ratio 2: Cash Flow Coverage Ratio

$$
\text{CFC ratio} = \frac{\text{EBIT} + \text{Lease payments} + \text{Depreciation expense}}{\text{Interest expense} + \text{Lease payments} + \text{Debt principal}/(1-T)}
$$

$$
= \frac{\$10,114 + \$1,368 + \$4,130}{\$1,542 + \$1,368 + \$2,000/(1-0)} = \frac{\$15,612}{\$4,910} = 3.2 \text{ times.}
$$

Industry average = 2.3.

Although not shown directly on Riverside's financial statements, the hospital had $1,368,000 of lease payments and $2,000,000 of debt principal repayments in 1998.

What is the purpose of the $(1-T)$ term applied to the debt principal? For investor-owned firms, the debt principal repayments, because they are paid with after-tax dollars, must be *grossed up* by dividing by $1-T$. This gives the amount of pre-tax dollars, which is what is contained in the numerator, that are required to cover the principal repayments.

Like its TIE ratio, Riverside's CFC ratio exceeds industry standard, indicating that Riverside is better at covering total fixed payments with cash flow than the average hospital. This fact should reassure both creditors and management and should reinforce the view that Riverside has untapped debt capacity.

Asset Management (Activity) Ratios

The next group of ratios, the *asset management ratios*, is designed to measure how effectively the business' assets are being managed. These ratios help to answer whether or not the total amounts of each type of asset, as reported on the balance sheet, seem reasonable, too high, or too low in view of current and projected operating levels. Riverside and other hospitals must borrow or raise equity capital to acquire assets. If they have too many assets, then their capital costs will be too high and their profits will be depressed. Conversely, if assets are too low, then profitable sales may be lost or vital services not offered.

The *fixed asset turnover ratio*, also called the *fixed asset utilization ratio*, measures the utilization of plant and equipment, and it is the ratio of total revenues to fixed assets:

Fixed Asset Turnover Ratio

$$\text{Fixed asset turnover} = \frac{\text{Total revenue}}{\text{Net fixed assets}} = \frac{\$117,476}{\$119,998} = 0.98 \text{ times.}$$

Industry average $= 2.2.$

Riverside's ratio of 0.98 indicates that each dollar of fixed assets generated 98 cents in revenue. This value compares poorly with the industry average of 2.2 times which indicates that Riverside is not using its fixed assets as productively as the average hospital. (The lower quartile value for the industry is 1.8; thus, Riverside falls in the bottom 25 percent of all hospitals in its fixed asset utilization.)

Before condemning Riverside's management for poor performance, it should be pointed out that a major problem exists with the use of the fixed asset turnover ratio for comparative purposes. Recall that all assets, except cash and accounts receivable, reflect historical costs rather than current value. Inflation and depreciation have caused the values of many assets that were purchased in the past to be seriously understated. Therefore, if an old hospital that had acquired much of its plant and equipment years ago is compared to a new hospital with the same physical assets, the old hospital, because of a much lower book value, would report a much higher turnover ratio. This difference in fixed asset turnover is more reflective of the inability of financial statements to deal with inflation than of any inefficiency on the part of the new hospital's managers.

Total Asset Turnover Ratio

The *total asset turnover ratio* measures the turnover, or utilization, of all of the firm's assets. It is calculated by total revenue divided by total assets:

$$\text{Total asset turnover} = \frac{\text{Total revenue}}{\text{Total assets}} = \frac{\$117,476}{\$151,278} = 0.78 \text{ times.}$$

Industry average $= 0.97.$

Thus, each dollar of total assets generated 78 cents in total revenue. Riverside's total asset ratio is below the industry average, but not as far below as its fixed asset turnover ratio. Thus, the hospital is utilizing its current assets better than its fixed assets, relative to the industry. Such judgments could be confirmed by examining Riverside's current asset turnover.[4]

Days in Patient Accounts Receivable

Days in patient accounts receivable is used to measure effectiveness in managing receivables. This measure of financial performance, which is sometimes classified as a liquidity ratio rather than an asset management ratio, has many names including *average collection period (ACP)* and *days' sales outstanding (DSO)*. It is computed by dividing net patient accounts receivable by average daily patient revenue to find the number of days that it takes an organization, on average, to collect its receivables[5]:

$$\text{Days in patient accounts receivable} = \frac{\text{Net patient accounts receivable}}{\text{Net patient service revenue}/365}$$

$$= \frac{\$21,840}{\$108,600/365} = 73.4 \text{ days.}$$

Industry average $\quad = 64.0$ days.

In the calculation for Riverside, premium revenue has not been included because such revenue is collected before services are provided, and hence does not affect receivables.

Riverside is not doing as well as the average hospital in collecting its receivables. The lower quartile value is 78.7 days, so a relatively large number of hospitals are doing worse. Still, as was discussed in Chapter 16, it is important that businesses collect their receivables as soon as possible. Clearly, Riverside's managers should strive to increase the hospital's performance in this key area.

Other Ratios

The final group of ratios examines other facets of a business' financial condition. For investor-owned firms, at least those with publicly traded stock, some ratios can be developed that relate the firm's stock price to its earnings and book value per share. Such *market value ratios* give managers an indication of what investors think of the company's past performance and future prospects. If the firm's liquidity, asset management, debt management, and profitability ratios are all good, its stock price, and hence market value ratios, will be high.

The *average age of plant* gives a rough measure of the average age in years of a business' fixed assets: **Average Age of Plant**

$$\text{Average age of plant} = \frac{\text{Accumulated depreciation}}{\text{Depreciation expense}} = \frac{\$25,160}{\$4,130} = 6.1 \text{ years.}$$

Industry average $\quad = 9.1$ years.

Riverside's physical assets are newer than those of the average hospital. Thus, the hospital is offering more up-to-date facilities than average, and hence it will probably have fewer capital expenditures in the near future. On the other hand, Riverside's net fixed asset valuation will be relatively high, which biases the hospital's fixed asset and total asset turnover ratios downward. This fact raises serious questions about the validity of the turnover ratios calculated previously.

For investor-owned firms, the *price/earnings (P/E) ratio* shows how much investors are willing to pay per dollar of reported profits. Suppose that the stock of General Home Care, an investor-owned home health care company, sells for $28.50, while the firm had 1998 earnings per share (EPS) of $2.20. Then, its P/E ratio would be 13.0: **Price/Earnings Ratio**

$$\text{P/E ratio} \quad = \frac{\text{Price per share}}{\text{Earnings per share}} = \frac{\$28.50}{\$2.20} = 13.0 \text{ times.}$$

Industry average $= 15.2$.

P/E ratios are higher for firms with high growth prospects, with other things held constant, but they are lower for riskier firms. General's P/E ratio is slightly below the average of other investor-owned home health care companies, which suggests that the company is regarded as being somewhat riskier than most, as having poorer growth prospects, or both.

Market/Book Ratio The ratio of a stock's market price to its book value gives another indication of how investors regard the company. Companies with relatively high rates of return on equity generally sell at higher multiples of book value than those with low returns. General reported $80 million in total equity on its 1998 balance sheet, and the firm had five million shares outstanding, so its book value per share is $80 / 5 = $16.00. Dividing the price per share by the book value per share gives a *market/book (M/B) ratio* of 1.8 times:

$$\text{M/B ratio} = \frac{\text{Price per share}}{\text{Book value per share}} = \frac{\$28.50}{\$16.00} = 1.8 \text{ times.}$$

Industry average = 2.1.

Investors are willing to pay slightly less for each dollar of General's book value than for that of an average home health care company.

Comparative and Trend Analysis

When conducting ratio analysis, the value of a particular ratio, in the absence of other information, tells almost nothing. For example, if it is known that a nursing home company had a current ratio of 2.5, it is virtually impossible to say whether this is good or bad. Additional data are needed to help interpret the results of this ratio analysis. In the discussion of Riverside's ratios, the focus was on *comparative analysis,* that is, the hospital's ratios were compared with the average ratios for the industry. Another useful ratio analysis tool is *trend analysis* in which the trend of a single ratio is analyzed over time. Trend analysis gives clues about whether a firm's financial situation is improving, holding constant, or deteriorating.

It is easy to combine comparative and trend analyses in a single graph, such as the one shown in Figure 17.1. Here, Riverside's ROE (the solid line) and industry average ROE data (the dashed lines) are plotted for the past five years. The graph shows that the hospital's ROE has been declining faster than the industry average from 1994 through 1997, but that it rose above the industry in 1998. Other ratios can be analyzed in a similar manner.

Self-Test Questions
1. What is the purpose of ratio analysis?
2. What are two ratios that measure profitability?
3. What are two ratios that measure liquidity?
4. What are two ratios that measure debt management?
5. What are two ratios that measure asset management?
6. What are two ratios that measure market value?
7. How can comparative and trend analyses be used to help interpret ratio results?

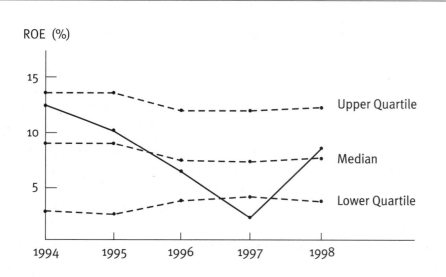

FIGURE 17.1
Riverside Memorial
Hospital: ROE
Analysis,
1994–1998

Return on Equity (ROE)

		Industry		
Year	Riverside	Lower Quartile	Median	Upper Quartile
1994	12.5%	2.6%	8.6%	13.3%
1995	10.0	2.5	8.6	13.3
1996	6.7	2.8	7.2	12.1
1997	2.4	4.1	7.2	12.1
1998	8.0	3.8	7.4	12.3

Tying the Ratios Together: Du Pont Analysis

Ratio analysis provides a detailed picture of a business' financial condition, but it does not provide an overview of a firm's condition nor does it tie any of the ratios together. *Du Pont analysis* provides an overview of a business' financial condition and helps managers and investors understand the relationships among several ratios. Essentially, Du Pont analysis, so named because managers at the Du Pont Company developed it, combines basic financial ratios in a way that provides valuable insights into a firm's financial performance. The analysis decomposes return on equity (ROE), one of the most important measures of a business' profitability, into the product of three other ratios, each of which has an important economic interpretation. The result is the *Du Pont equation*:

$$ROE = \text{Total margin} \times \text{Total asset turnover} \times \text{Equity multiplier}$$

$$\frac{\text{Net income}}{\text{Total equity}} = \frac{\text{Net income}}{\text{Total revenue}} \times \frac{\text{Total revenue}}{\text{Total assets}} \times \frac{\text{Total assets}}{\text{Total equity}}.$$

Riverside's 1998 data is used to illustrate the Du Pont equation:

$$\frac{\$8,572}{\$107,364} = \frac{\$8,572}{\$117,476} \times \frac{\$117,476}{\$151,278} \times \frac{\$151,278}{\$107,364}$$

$$7.98\% = \quad 7.30\% \quad \times \quad 0.78 \quad \times \quad 1.41$$

$$= \quad 5.69\% \quad \times \quad 1.41.$$

In the Du Pont equation, the product of the first two terms on the right side is return on assets (ROA), so the equation can also be written as ROE = ROA × Equity multiplier. Riverside's 1998 total margin was 7.3 percent, so the hospital made 7.3 cents profit on each dollar of total revenue. Furthermore, assets were turned over (or created revenues) 0.78 times during the year, so the hospital earned a return of 7.30% × 0.78 = 5.69% on its assets. This value for ROA, when rounded, is the same as was calculated previously in the discussion of ratio analysis.

If the hospital used only equity financing, its 5.69 percent ROA would equal its ROE. However, creditors supplied 29 percent of Riverside's capital, while the equityholders (i.e., the community) supplied the rest. Because the 5.69 percent ROA belongs exclusively to the suppliers of equity capital, which makes up only 29 percent of total capital, Riverside's ROE is higher than 5.69 percent. Specifically, ROA must be multiplied by the *equity multiplier*, which shows the total assets working for each dollar of equity capital, to obtain the ROE of 7.98 percent. This 7.98 percent ROE could be calculated directly: ROE = Net income / Total equity = $8,572 / $107,364 = 7.98%. However, the Du Pont equation shows how total margin, which measures expense control; total asset turnover, which measures asset utilization; and financial leverage, which measures debt utilization, interact to determine ROE.

Riverside's managers use the Du Pont equation to analyze ways of improving the hospital's financial performance. To influence the profit margin (i.e., expense control), the hospital's marketing staff can study the effects of raising charges or lowering them to increase volume, moving into new services or markets with higher margins, entering into new contracts with managed care plans, and so on. Furthermore, management accountants can study the expense items and, while working with department heads and clinical staff, can seek ways to reduce costs.

Regarding total asset turnover (i.e., asset utilization), Riverside's analysts, while working with both clinical and marketing staffs, can investigate ways of reducing investments in various types of assets. Finally, the hospital's financial staff can analyze the effects of alternative financing strategies on the equity multiplier (i.e., debt utilization), seeking to hold down interest expenses and the risks of debt, while still using debt to leverage up ROE.

The Du Pont equation provides a useful comparison between a business' performance, as measured by ROE, and the performance of an average hospital. For example, here is the comparative analysis for 1998:

Riverside : $\quad$ ROE $= 7.3\% \times 0.78 \times 1.41$

$$= \quad 5.69\% \quad \times 1.41 \approx 8.0\%.$$

Industry average : $\;$ ROE $= 5.0\% \times 0.97 \times 1.73$

$$4.85\% \quad \times 1.73 \approx 8.4\%.$$

The Du Pont analysis tells managers and creditors that Riverside has a significantly higher profit margin, and thus better control over expenses than does the average hospital. However, the average hospital has a better total asset turnover, and thus Riverside is getting below-average utilization from its assets. In spite of the average hospital's advantage in asset utilization, Riverside's superior expense control outweighs its utilization disadvantage because its ROA of 5.69 percent is higher than the industry average ROA of 4.85 percent. Finally, the average hospital has offset Riverside's advantage in ROA by using more financial leverage, although Riverside's lower use of debt financing decreases its risk. The end result is that Riverside gets somewhat less return on its equity capital than does the average hospital.

One potential problem with Du Pont and ratio analyses that is applied to not-for-profit organizations, especially hospitals, is that a large portion of their net income may come from nonoperating gains rather than from operations. If such nonoperating gains are highly variable and unpredictable, as they are often, return on equity and the ratios, as previously defined, may be a poor measure of the hospital's inherent profitability. All applicable ratios, as well as the Du Pont analysis, could be recast to focus on operations by using operating revenue in lieu of total revenue.

1. Explain how the Du Pont equation combines several ratios to obtain an overview of a business' financial condition.
2. Why may a focus on operating revenue be preferable to a focus on total revenue?

Self-Test Questions

Other Analytical Techniques

Two additional financial statement analysis techniques are common size analysis and percentage change analysis. In *common size analysis*, all income statement items are divided by revenues and all balance sheet items are divided by total assets. Thus, a common size income statement shows each item as a percentage of revenues, and a common size balance sheet shows each account as a percentage of total assets. The advantage of common size statements is that they facilitate comparisons of income statements and balance sheets over time and across companies because they remove the influence of company size.

Another frequently used technique when analyzing financial statements is *percentage change analysis*. Here, the percentage changes in the balance sheet accounts and income statement items from year to year are calculated and compared.

In this format, it is easy to see what items are growing faster or slower than others, and thus to identify which are under control and which are out of control.

The conclusions reached in common size and percentage change analyses generally parallel those derived from ratio analysis. However occasionally, a serious deficiency is highlighted only by one of the three analytical techniques, while the other two techniques fail to bring the deficiency to light. Thus, a thorough financial statement analysis usually consists of a Du Pont analysis to provide an overview, and then includes several different techniques such as ratio, common size, and percentage change analyses.

Self-Test Questions
1. How are common size statements created?
2. What advantage do common size statements have over regular statements when conducting a financial analysis?
3. What is percentage change analysis and why is it useful?
4. Which analytical techniques should be used in a complete financial statement analysis?

Market Value Added and Economic Value Added

Two financial performance measures that are being used by managers with increasing frequency focus directly on management's success or failure in creating value; they are Market Value Added (MVA) and Economic Value Added (EVA). These measures are especially useful in investor-owned businesses because of their direct link with shareholder wealth maximization. However, EVA can be used with not-for-profit firms, so the discussion to follow is relevant to both forms of ownership.

Market Value Added (MVA)

A primary financial goal of any investor-owned firm is shareholder wealth maximization. This goal obviously benefits shareholders, and it also ensures that scarce resources are allocated as efficiently as possible. However, managerial zeal to enhance shareholder wealth does not mean that other stakeholders, including creditors, employees, patients, and so on, should be treated unfairly because such actions are both unethical and will ultimately be detrimental to shareholders.

Although the fundamental goal of shareholder wealth maximization is widely accepted, managers sometimes confuse shareholder wealth maximization with maximizing the total market value of the firm's stock. A firm's total market value—its stock price multiplied by the number of shares outstanding—can be increased by raising and investing as much equity capital as possible, which increases the size and aggregate value of the firm. Although size increasing actions often result in higher managerial salaries and benefits, such a strategy rarely benefits shareholders because it ignores the fact that what is most relevant to shareholders is not the size of the firm, but rather the return that it earns on shareholder supplied capital.

Individual shareholder's wealth is actually maximized when a firm's managers maximize the **difference** between the market value of the firm's stock and the amount of capital that equity investors have supplied to the firm. This difference is called *Market Value Added (MVA)*:

$$MVA = \text{Market value of equity} - \text{Book value of equity}.$$

To illustrate the MVA concept, consider Columbia/HCA Healthcare. In August 1998, its total market value of equity was 643 million shares outstanding × $25 stock price = $16.1 billion, while its shareholders had supplied about $7.5 billion in equity capital. Thus, Columbia/HCA's MVA was $16.1 − $7.5 = $8.6 billion. This amount represents the difference between the funds, including retained earnings, that Columbia/HCA's equity investors have put into the corporation since its founding, and the value of the cash they could get by selling the business. In other words, Columbia/HCA's managers have created $8.6 billion of wealth for the company's shareholders. (Columbia/HCA's MVA had been significantly higher prior to the summer of 1997 when the company became the target of a federal probe looking into Medicare fraud.)

In spite of recent problems, the managers of Columbia/HCA have done a good job of creating shareholder wealth. However, the managers of HEALTH-SOUTH have done even better. In August 1998, HEALTHSOUTH's total market value of equity was 401 million shares outstanding × $24 stock price = $9.6 billion, while its shareholders had supplied about $3.3 billion in equity capital. Thus, HEALTHSOUTH's MVA was $9.6 − $3.3 = $6.3 billion. While Columbia/HCA's managers created $16.1 / $7.5 = $2.15 of wealth for every dollar supplied by its stockholders, HEALTHSOUTH's managers created $9.6 / $3.3 = $2.91 of wealth for every stockholder dollar.

Clearly, the MVA concept is applicable only to investor-owned firms because it focuses on how well managers have done in creating value for shareholders, and hence equity market value is needed for its calculation. However EVA, which is discussed in the next section, applies to both investor-owned and not-for-profit businesses.

Economic Value Added (EVA)

Whereas MVA measures the combined effect of managerial actions to create shareholder wealth since the inception of the company, *Economic Value Added (EVA)* focuses on managerial effectiveness in a given year. The basic formula for EVA is:

$$EVA = \text{After-tax operating profit} - (\text{Total capital} \times \text{Cost of capital}).$$

In the EVA equation, operating profit is revenues minus all operating costs including taxes, if applicable, but excluding interest expense; total capital supplied is the sum of the book values of debt and equity, and hence total assets; and cost of capital is the corporate cost of capital. Also, in the EVA context, after-tax operating profit is often called *net operating profit after taxes (NOPAT)*, and it is calculated as EBIT $(1 - T)$. Unlike MVA, EVA does not focus directly on market values, and hence EVA can be applied to not-for-profit firms.[6]

To illustrate the EVA concept, consider Birmingham Health Providers, a medical group practice. The group had $1 million in NOPAT in 1998, generated from $5 million of investor-supplied debt and equity capital. The firm's corporate cost of capital was 10 percent. With these assumptions, Birmingham Health Providers' 1998 EVA was $500,000:

$$\text{EVA} = \$1 - (\$5 \times 0.10) = \$1 - \$0.5 = \$0.5 \text{ million.}$$

EVA is an estimate of a business' true economic profit for the year, and it differs substantially from accounting profitability measures such as net income. EVA represents the residual income that remains after **all** costs have been recognized, including the opportunity cost of the employed equity capital. Conversely, accounting profit is formulated without imposing a charge for equity capital. EVA depends on both operating efficiency and balance sheet management. Without operating efficiency, profits will be low, and without efficient balance sheet management, there will be too many assets, and hence too much capital, which results in higher than necessary dollar capital costs.

For not-for-profit firms, equity capital is a scarce resource that must be managed well to ensure the financial viability of the organization, and hence its ability to continue to perform its stated mission. EVA lets managers know how well they are doing in managing this scarce resource because the higher the EVA in any year, the better the job that managers are doing in using the organization's contributions and earnings to create value for the community. Of course, EVA measures only economic value; any social value created by the equity capital is ignored and, therefore, must be subjectively considered.

EVA, not MVA, can be applied to divisions as well as to entire companies, and the charge for capital should reflect the riskiness and capital structure of the business unit, whether it is the whole company or an operating division. The specific calculation of EVA for a company or division is much more complex than presented here because many accounting issues, such as inventory valuation, depreciation, amortization of research and development costs, and the like, must be addressed properly when estimating a firm's after-tax operating profit.[7]

Self-Test Questions

1. What is Market Value Added (MVA) and how is it measured?
2. What is Economic Value Added (EVA) and how is it measured?
3. Can MVA and EVA be applied to not-for-profit firms?
4. Why is EVA a better measure of financial performance than are accounting measures, such as earnings per share and return on equity?

Benchmarking

Ratio analysis, as well as other financial performance evaluation techniques, requires comparisons to make meaningful judgments. In the previous examination of selected ratios, Riverside's ratios were compared to industry average ratios. However, similar to most businesses, Riverside's managers go one step further—they compare their ratios not only with industry averages, but also with the industry leaders, as well as their primary competitors. The technique of comparing ratios against selected standards is called *benchmarking*, while the comparative ratios are called *benchmarks*. Riverside's managers benchmark against industry averages; against National/GFB Healthcare and Pennant Healthcare, which are two leading for-profit hospital companies; and which are against Woodbridge Memorial Hospital and St. Anthony's, its primary local competitors.

To illustrate, consider how Riverside's analysts present total margin data to the firm's board of trustees:

	1998		1997
National/GFB	9.8%	National/GFB	9.6%
Industry top quartile	*8.4*	*Industry top quartile*	*8.0*
St. Anthony's	8.0	St. Anthony's	7.9
Riverside	**7.3**	Pennant Healthcare	5.0
Industry median	5.0	Industry median	4.7
Pennant Healthcare	4.8	**Riverside**	**2.2**
Industry lower quartile	*1.8*	*Industry lower quartile*	*2.1*
Woodbridge Memorial	0.5	Woodbridge Memorial	(1.3)

Benchmarking permits Riverside's managers to easily see exactly where the firm stands relative to its competition, both in any given year and over time. As the data show, Riverside was roughly in the middle of the pack in 1998 with respect to its primary competitors and two large investor-owned hospital chains, although its showing was better than the average hospital. Its 1997 performance was significantly worse, so Riverside improved substantially from 1997 to 1998. Although benchmarking is illustrated with one ratio, other ratios could be analyzed similarly. Also, for presentation purposes, comparative data can be color coded for ease of recognition and interpretation.

All comparative analyses require comparative data. Such data are available from a number of sources including commercial suppliers, federal and state governmental agencies, and various industry trade groups. Each of these data suppliers uses a somewhat different set of ratios designed to meet its own needs. Thus, when a comparative data source is selected, in a very real sense the ratios that will be used in the analysis are being chosen. Also, there are minor and sometimes major differences in ratio definitions between data sources; for example, one source may use a 365-day year while another uses a 360-day year. There are also numerous differences on using operating values versus total values when constructing ratios. It is **very important** to know the specific definitions used in the comparative data because definitional differences between the ratios being calculated and comparative ratios can lead to erroneous interpretations and conclusions. Thus, the first task in a ratio analysis is to make sure that the definitions used to develop the comparative data are understood.

Self-Test   1. What is benchmarking?
Questions   2. Why is it important to be familiar with the comparative data set?

Operating Analysis

Operating analysis goes one step beyond financial statement analysis in that operating analysis examines operating variables with the goal of **explaining** a business' financial performance. Like ratios, operating analysis *indicators* are typically grouped into major categories to make interpretation easier. For hospitals, some common categories of indicators are:

- profit;
- net price;
- volume;
- length of stay;
- service intensity;
- efficiency; and
- unit cost indicators.

Because of the number of indicators used in a typical operating analysis, it cannot be discussed in detail here. However, to give readers an appreciation for this type of analysis, six commonly used hospital operating analysis indicators are defined and illustrated. Note that much of the data needed to calculate operating analysis indicators are not contained in a business' financial statements. Thus, more complete data are required for this type of analysis, and hence it is used more by managers than by outside analysts.

Net Price Per Discharge

Net price per discharge measures the average revenue collected on each inpatient discharge. In 1998, Riverside reported $93,740,000 in inpatient service revenues and discharged 18,281 patients:

$$\text{Net price per discharge} = \frac{\text{Net inpatient revenue}}{\text{Total discharges}} = \frac{\$93,740,000}{18,281} = \$5,128.$$

$$\text{Industry average} = \$5,510.$$

Riverside collects less per discharge than the average hospital, which ignores bad debt losses. However, if Riverside's case mix, which measures the average intensity of services provided, were lower than average, perhaps its net price per discharge is appropriate, even though it is below the industry average. In fact, Riverside's case mix is slightly higher than average.

Medicare Payment Percentage

Medicare payment percentage measures the exposure of a hospital to Medicare patients, and hence to payments set by political rather than economic processes:

$$\text{Medicare payment percentage} = \frac{\text{Medicare discharges}}{\text{Total discharges}} = \frac{7,642}{18,281} = 41.8\%.$$

Industry average $= 43.5\%.$

Riverside has a somewhat lower percentage of Medicare patients than the average hospital. To the extent that Medicare payments are less than payments from other third-party payors, a higher Medicare payment percentage puts pressure on operating revenues. Conversely, if Medicare payments are higher than reimbursements by managed care plans, then, in some situations, a higher Medicare payment percentage may be good. Similar operating indicators could be constructed for Medicaid, managed care plan, and bad debt and charity care patients.

Outpatient Revenue Percentage

The *outpatient revenue percentage* measures the mix between outpatient and inpatient revenues:

$$\text{Outpatient revenue percentage} = \frac{\text{Net outpatient revenue}}{\text{Net patient service revenue}} = \frac{\$20,092,000}{\$113,832,000} = 17.6\%.$$

Industry average $= 34.5\%.$

Riverside has a much smaller outpatient program, relative to its size, than the average hospital. During the 1990s, most hospitals significantly expanded their outpatient programs based on the belief that such services were more profitable because Medicare paid for outpatient services on a charge basis, whereas inpatient services were paid for on a prospective basis. However, the claims of increased profitability were never proved, and Medicare is in the process of changing to a prospective payment system for outpatient services.

Occupancy Percentage (Rate)

Occupancy rate measures the extent of utilization of a hospital's beds, and hence fixed assets. As discussed in Chapter 5, because overhead costs are incurred on all assets, whether used or not, higher occupancy spreads fixed costs over more patients, and hence increases per patient profitability. Based on 95,061 inpatient days in 1998, Riverside's occupancy rate was 57.9 percent:

$$\text{Occupancy percentage} = \frac{\text{Inpatient days}}{\text{Number of staffed beds} \times 365} = \frac{95,061}{450 \times 365} = 57.9\%.$$

Industry average $= 44.9\%.$

Riverside has a higher occupancy rate, and hence is using its fixed assets more productively that the average hospital. It is interesting to note that this conclusion is contrary to the financial analysis interpretation of the hospital's 1998 fixed asset turnover ratio. While that ratio is affected by inflation and accounting convention, the occupancy percentage is not. Hence, it is a superior measure of pure asset utilization, at least regarding inpatient utilization. On this basis, it appears that

Riverside's managers are doing a good job, relative to the industry, of utilizing the hospital's inpatient fixed assets.

Average Length of Stay (ALOS)

Average length of stay (ALOS), or just *length of stay (LOS)*, is the number of days that an average inpatient is hospitalized with each admission.

$$\text{ALOS} = \frac{\text{Inpatient days}}{\text{Total discharges}} = \frac{95{,}061}{18{,}281} = 5.2 \text{ days.}$$

Industry average = 4.1 days.

On average, Riverside keeps its patients in the hospital longer than the average hospital does. Riverside has a *case-mix index* of 1.28, compared with an average for the industry of 1.14. The case-mix index is a weighted average of DRG weights, so the higher the index, the more intense the services provided. Thus, the hospital's patients, on average, require more intensive treatment than patients in the average hospital.

Cost Per Discharge

So far, the operating analysis illustration has focused on revenue and volume measures. *Cost per discharge* measures the dollar amount of resources, on average, expended on each discharge. Because Riverside's inpatient operating expenses for 1998 were $84,865,000, its cost per discharge was $4,642:

$$\text{Cost per discharge} = \frac{\text{Inpatient operating expenses}}{\text{Total discharges}} = \frac{\$84{,}865{,}000}{18{,}281} = \$4{,}642.$$

Industry average = $5,446.

Even though Riverside's price per discharge is below average, its cost per discharge is even more so. Thus, the hospital's average margin on each discharge is more than that for the hospital industry. Another operating indicator that would be useful here is the *cost per visit*, which measures the cost per outpatient visit.

As is apparent from the six operating indicators presented, operating analysis goes beyond financial analysis in an attempt to identify the operating strengths and weaknesses that underlie a firm's financial performance. Although operating analysis has been illustrated using the hospital industry, the concepts can be applied to any healthcare business, although the ratios selected would differ. Also, operating indicators are interpreted in the same way as financial ratios (i.e., by using comparative and trend analysis).

Self-Test Questions

1. What is the difference between financial and operating analyses?
2. Why is operating analysis important?
3. Describe four indicators commonly used in operating analysis.

Limitations of Financial Performance Analysis

While financial performance analysis can provide a great deal of useful information concerning a company's operations and financial condition, such analyses have limitations that necessitate care and judgment. In this section, some of the problem areas are highlighted:

- Many large healthcare businesses operate a number of different divisions in quite different lines of business, and in such cases, it is difficult to develop meaningful comparative data. This problem tends to make financial statement and operating analyses somewhat more useful for businesses with single product or service lines than for large, multiservice companies.

- Most businesses want to be better than average, although half will be above and half will be below average. Merely attaining average performance is not necessarily good. However, as was demonstrated earlier, compilers of industry data often report ratios in quartiles or other percentiles. Also, it is useful for managers to compare their firms not only with the industry average, but also with the top companies in the industry as well as their leading competitors. In the end, it is extremely important that senior managers establish their own standards of performance and ensure that all other managers are aware of those goals and are taking actions on a daily basis to achieve them. That is the purpose of the financial planning and control process.

- Generalizing about whether or not a particular ratio or indicator is good or bad is often difficult. For example, a high current ratio may show a strong liquidity position, which is good, or an excessive amount of receivables, which is bad. Similarly, a high asset turnover ratio may denote either a business that uses its assets efficiently or one that is undercapitalized and simply cannot afford to buy enough assets.

- Firms often have some ratios and indicators that look good and others that look bad, which make the firm's financial position—strong or weak—difficult to determine. For this reason, significant judgment is required when analyzing financial and operating performance. Several methodologies have been proposed to reduce the information contained in a financial statement analysis to a single value, and hence make interpretation much easier. One method applied is *multiple discriminant analysis*, which attempts to divide companies into two groups on the basis of their probabilities of going bankrupt. Another method merely combines ratios selected judgmentally into a composite index, which is then compared to the industry average index. Therefore, to distill the wide variety of information contained in a ratio analysis into a single measure of financial condition is very difficult.[8]

- Different accounting practices can distort financial statement ratio comparisons. For example, firms can use different accounting conventions to value cost of goods sold and ending inventories. During inflationary periods these differences can lead to ratio distortions. Other accounting practices, such as those related to leases, can also create distortions.

- Inflation effects can distort both firms' balance sheets and income statements. Numerous reporting methods have been proposed to adjust accounting statements for inflation, but no consensus has been reached either on how to do this or even on the practical usefulness of the resulting data. Nevertheless, accounting standards encourage, but do not require, businesses to disclose supplementary data to reflect the effects of general inflation. Inflation effects tend to make ratio comparisons over time for a given company, and across companies at any point in time, less reliable than would be the case in the absence of inflation.

Self-Test Questions

1. Briefly describe some of the problems encountered when performing financial statement and operating analyses.
2. Explain how inflation effects created problems in the Riverside illustration.

Key Concepts

The primary purpose of this chapter is to present the techniques used by managers and investors to assess a business' financial performance. The main focus is on financial performance as reflected in a business' financial statements, although operating data was also introduced to try to explain financial performance. The key concepts of this chapter are:

- *Financial statement analysis*, which is designed to identify a firm's financial condition, focuses on the firm's financial statements. *Operating analysis* provides insights into why a firm is in a strong or weak financial condition.
- *Ratio analysis* is designed to reveal the relative strengths and weaknesses of a company, as compared to other companies in the same industry, and to show whether the firm's position has been improving or deteriorating over time.
- The *Du Pont equation* indicates how the total margin, the total asset turnover ratio, and the use of debt interact to determine the rate of return on equity. It provides a good overview of a business' financial performance.
- *Liquidity ratios* indicate the business' ability to meet its short-term obligations.
- *Asset management ratios* measure how effectively managers are utilizing the business' assets.
- *Debt management ratios* reveal the extent to which the firm is financed with debt, and the extent to which operating cash flows cover debt service and other fixed charge requirements.
- *Profitability ratios* show the combined effects of liquidity, asset management, and debt management on operating results.
- Ratios are analyzed using *comparative analysis*, in which a firm's ratios are compared with industry averages, or those of another firm, and *trend analysis*, in which a firm's ratios are examined over time.

- In a *common size analysis,* a business' income statement and balance sheet are expressed in percentages. This facilitates comparisons between firms of different sizes and for a single firm over time.
- In *percentage change analysis,* the differences in income statement items and balance sheet accounts from one year to the next are expressed in percentages. In this way, it is easy to identify those items and accounts that are growing appreciably faster or slower than average.
- *Market Value Added (MVA)* and *Economic Value Added (EVA)* are two measures of firm performance that focus directly on management's ability to enhance shareholder wealth. Although MVA is not applicable to not-for-profit businesses, EVA can be used to assess the performance of any business regardless of ownership.
- *Benchmarking* is the process of comparing the performance of a particular company with a group of benchmark companies, often industry leaders and primary competitors, as well as with industry averages.
- Financial performance analysis is hampered by some serious problems including *development of comparative data, interpretation of results,* and *inflation effects.*

Financial performance analysis has its limitations, but if used with care and judgment, these analyses can provide a sound picture of a healthcare business' financial condition, as well as identify those operating factors that contribute to that condition.

Questions

17.1 a. What is the primary difference between financial statement analysis and operating analysis?

b. Why are both types of analyses useful to health services managers and investors?

17.2 Should financial statement and operating analyses be conducted only on historical data? Explain your answer.

17.3 One asset management ratio, the inventory turnover ratio, is defined as sales (i.e., revenues) divided by inventories. Why would this ratio be more important for a medical device manufacturer than for a hospital management company?

17.4 a. Assume that Beverly Enterprises and Manor Care, two operators of nursing homes, have fiscal years that end at different times, say, one in June and one in December. Would this fact cause any problems when comparing ratios between the two companies?

b. Assume that two companies operating walk-in clinics both had the same December year end, but one was based in Aspen, Colorado, a winter resort, while the other operated in Cape Cod, Massachusetts, a summer resort. Would this lead to problems in a comparative analysis?

17.5 a. How does inflation distort ratio analysis comparisons both for one company over time and when different companies are compared?

b. Are only balance sheet accounts or both balance sheet accounts and income statement items affected by inflation?

17.6 a. What is the difference between trend analysis and comparative analysis?

b. Which one is more important?

17.7 Assume that a large managed care company has a low return on equity (ROE). How could Du Pont analysis be used to identify possible actions to help boost ROE?

17.8 Regardless of their specific line of business, should all healthcare businesses use the same set of ratios when conducting a financial statement analysis? Explain your answer.

Problems

17.1 a. Modern Medical Devices has a current ratio of 0.5. Which of the following actions would improve (i.e., increase) this ratio?

(1) Use cash to pay off current liabilities.

(2) Collect some of the current accounts receivable.

(3) Use cash to pay off some long-term debt.

(4) Purchase additional inventory on credit (i.e., accounts payable).

(5) Sell some of the existing inventory at cost.

b. Assume that the company has a current ratio of 1.2. Now, which of the above actions would improve this ratio?

17.2 Southwest Physicians, a medical group practice, is just being formed. It will need $2 million of total assets to generate $3 million in revenues. Furthermore, the group expects to have a profit margin of 5 percent. The group is considering two financing alternatives. First, it can use all-equity financing by requiring each physician to contribute his or her pro rata share. Alternatively, the practice can finance up to 50 percent of its assets with a bank loan. Assuming that the debt alternative has no impact on the expected profit margin, what is the difference between the expected ROE if the group finances with 50 percent debt versus the expected ROE if it finances entirely with equity capital?

17.3 Riverside Memorial's financial statements are presented in Tables 17.1, 17.2, and 17.3.

a. Calculate Riverside's financial ratios for 1997. Assume that Riverside has $1,000,000 in lease payments and $1,400,000 in debt principal repayments in 1997. (Hint: Use the text discussion to identify the applicable ratios.)

b. Interpret the ratios. Use both trend and comparative analysis. For the comparative analysis, assume that the industry average data presented in the text is valid for both 1997 and 1998.

17.4 Consider the following financial statements for BestCare HMO, a not-for-profit managed care plan:

BestCare HMO
Statement of Operations and Change in Net Assets
Year Ended June 30, 1998
(in thousands)

Revenue:	
Premiums earned	$26,682
Co-insurance	1,689
Interest and other income	242
Total revenue	$28,613
Expenses:	
Salaries and benefits	$15,154
Medical supplies and drugs	7,507
Insurance	3,963
Provision for bad debts	19
Depreciation	367
Interest	385
Total expenses	$27,395
Net income	$ 1,218
Net assets, beginning of year	$ 900
Net assets, end of year	$ 2,118

BestCare HMO
Balance Sheet
June 30, 1998
(in thousands)

Assets	
Cash and cash equivalents	$ 2,737
Net premiums receivable	821
Supplies	387
Total current assets	$ 3,945
Net property and equipment	$ 5,924
Total assets	$ 9,869
Liabilities and Net Assets	
Accounts payable–medical services	$ 2,145
Accrued expenses	929
Notes payable	141
Current portion of long-term debt	241
Total current liabilities	$ 3,456
Long-term debt	$ 4,295
Total liabilities	$ 7,751

Net assets–unrestricted (equity)	$ 2,118
Total liabilities and net assets	$ 9,869

a. Perform a Du Pont analysis on BestCare. Assume that the industry average ratios are as follows:

Total margin	3.8%
Total asset turnover	2.1
Equity multiplier	3.2
Return on equity (ROE)	25.5%

b. Calculate and interpret the following ratios for BestCare:

	Industry Average
Return on assets (ROA)	8.0%
Current ratio	1.3
Days cash on hand	41 days
Average collection period	7 days
Debt ratio	69%
Debt to equity ratio	2.2
Times-interest-earned (TIE) ratio	2.8
Fixed asset turnover ratio	5.2

17.5 Consider the following financial statements for Green Valley Nursing Home, Inc., a for-profit, long-term care facility:

Green Valley Nursing Home, Inc.
Statement of Income and Retained Earnings
Year Ended December 31, 1998

Revenue:	
Net patient service revenue	$ 3,163,258
Other revenue	106,146
Total revenues	$ 3,269,404
Expenses:	
Salaries and benefits	$ 1,515,438
Medical supplies and drugs	966,781
Insurance and other	296,357
Provision for bad debts	110,000
Depreciation	85,000
Interest	206,780
Total expenses	$ 3,180,356
Operating income	$ 89,048
Provision for income taxes	31,167
Net income	$ 57,881
Retained earnings, beginning of year	$ 199,961

Retained earnings, end of year	$ 257,842

Green Valley Nursing Home, Inc.
Balance Sheet
December 31, 1998

Assets
Current Assets:

Cash and cash equivalents	$ 105,737
Investments	200,000
Net patient accounts receivable	215,600
Supplies	87,655
Total current assets	$ 608,992
Property and equipment	$ 2,250,000
Less accumulated depreciation	356,000
Net property and equipment	$ 1,894,000
Total assets	$ 2,502,992

Liabilities and Shareholders' Equity
Current Liabilities:

Accounts payable	$ 72,250
Accrued expenses	192,900
Notes payable	100,000
Current portion of long-term debt	80,000
Total current liabilities	$ 445,150
Long-term debt	$ 1,700,000

Shareholders' Equity:

Common stock, $10 par value	$ 100,000
Retained earnings	257,842
Total shareholders' equity	$ 357,842
Total liabilities and shareholders' equity	$ 2,502,992

a. Perform a Du Pont analysis on Green Valley. Assume that the industry average ratios are as follows:

Total margin	3.5%
Total asset turnover	1.5
Equity multiplier	2.5
Return on equity (ROE)	13.1%

b. Calculate and interpret the following ratios:

	Industry Average
Return on assets (ROA)	5.2%
Current ratio	2.0
Days cash on hand	22 days
Average collection period	19 days

Debt ratio	71%
Debt to equity ratio	2.5
Times-interest-earned (TIE) ratio	2.6
Fixed asset turnover ratio	1.4

    c. Assume that there are 10,000 shares of Green Valley's stock outstanding, and that some was sold on January 5, 1999 at $45 per share.

      (1) What was the firm's price/earnings ratio?

      (2) What was its market/book ratio?

17.6 Examine the industry average ratios given in Problems 17.4 and 17.5 above. Explain why the ratios are different between the managed care and nursing home industries?

Notes

1. A business' cash flows are particularly important to takeover specialists at investment banking firms. For them, cash flows are the primary determinant of a business' value.

2. Industry average ratios are available from many sources. For example, the Center for Healthcare Industry Performance Studies (CHIPS) publishes an annual almanac that provides hospital industry data on 33 financial ratios and 43 operating ratios. The ratios are reported in several groupings such as by hospital size and geographic location. See W. O. Cleverley, *Almanac of Hospital Financial & Operating Indicators* (Columbus, OH: CHIPS, published annually). The industry average ratios presented in this chapter are for illustrative use only, and hence should not be used for making real-world comparisons.

3. To determine the minimum proportional value that must be obtained from current assets to meet current obligations, divide the number 1 by the current ratio. For Riverside, $1 / 2.3 = 0.43$, or 43%. If liquidated at 43 cents on the dollar, the hospital's current assets would provide $0.43 \times \$31,280,000 \approx \$13,332,000$ in cash, which equals the amount of current liabilities.

4. Riverside's 1998 current asset turnover ratio (i.e., total revenue divided by total current assets) was 3.8, compared to an industry average of 3.6, so the hospital is slightly above average regarding current asset utilization.

5. Because information on credit sales is generally unavailable, total sales must be used. Although almost all hospital services are provided on credit because of the third-party payor system, other healthcare businesses may not have the same percentage of credit sales. As the proportion of cash sales increases, the days in patient accounts receivable measure loses its usefulness. Also, it would be better to use **average** receivables in the ratio, either calculated as an average of monthly figures or as (Beginning receivables + Ending receivables) / 2.

6. For an excellent example of the application of EVA in setting managerial compensation within not-for-profit firms, see W. O. Cleverley and R. K. Harvey, "Economic Value Added—A Framework for Health Care Executive Compensation," *Hospital & Health Services Administration* (Summer 1993): 215–228.

7. The EVA concept was first developed in detail by the consulting firm of Stern Stewart Management Services. For a more complete discussion, see G. B. Stewart, III, *The Quest for Value* (New York: HarperBusiness, 1991).

8. For a general discussion of multiple discrimimant analysis, see E. F. Brigham and L. C. Gapenski, *Intermediate Financial Management* (Fort Worth, TX: Dryden Press, 1996), chapter 26. See W. O. Cleverley, "Predicting Hospital Failure with the Financial Flexibility Index," *Healthcare Financial Management* (May 1985): 29–37, for a discussion of the financial flexibility index.

References

Beaver, W. H. and J. E. Horngren. 1991. "Ten Commandants of Financial Statement Analysis." *Financial Analysts Journal* (January–February): 9.

Boles, K. E. 1992. "Insolvency in Managed Care Organizations: Financial Indicators." *Topics in Health Care Financing* (Winter): 40–57.

Cleverley, W. O. and R. K. Harvey. 1990. "Profitability: Comparing Hospital Results with Other Industries." *Healthcare Financial Management* (March): 42–52.

———. 1995. "Understanding Your Hospital's True Financial Position and Changing It." *Health Care Management Review* (Spring): 62–73.

———. 1994. "Trends in the Hospital Financial Picture." *Healthcare Financial Management* (February): 56–63.

Coyne, J. S. 1985. "Measuring Hospital Performance in Multi-Institutional Organizations Using Financial Ratios" *Health Care Management Review* (Fall): 35–42.

———. 1990. "Analyzing the Financial Performance of Hospital-Based Managed Care Programs: The Case of Humana." *Journal of Health Administration Education* (Fall): 571–642.

Eastaugh, S. R. 1992. "Hospital Strategy and Financial Performance." *Health Care Management Review* (Summer): 19–32.

Finkler, S. A. 1982. "Ratio Analysis: Use with Caution." *Health Care Management Review* (Spring): 65–72.

Harkey, J. and R. Vraciu. 1992. "Quality of Health Care and Financial Performance: Is There a Link?" *Health Care Management Review* (Fall): 55–61.

Lynn, M. L. and P. Wertheim. 1993. "Key Financial Ratios Can Foretell Hospital Closures." *Healthcare Financial Management* (November): 66–70.

McCue, M. J. 1991. "The Use of Cash Flow to Analyze Financial Distress in California Hospitals." *Hospital & Health Services Administration* (Summer): 223–241.

Prince, T. R. 1991. "Assessing Financial Outcomes of Not-for-Profit Community Hospitals." *Hospital & Healthcare Administration* (Fall): 331–349.

Sherman, B. 1990. "How Investors Evaluate the Creditworthiness of Hospitals." *Healthcare Financial Management* (March): 25–31.

Sylvestre, J. and F. R. Urbancic. 1994. "Effective Methods for Cash Flow Analysis." *Healthcare Financial Management* (July): 62–72.

INDEX

ABOUT THE AUTHOR

Louis C. Gapenski, Ph.D., is a professor in both health services administration and finance at the University of Florida. He is the author or coauthor of over twenty textbooks on corporate and healthcare finance. Dr. Gapenski's books are used world wide, with Canadian and international editions, as well as translations into Russian, Bulgarian, Chinese, Indonesian, and Spanish. In addition, he has published numerous journal articles related to corporate and healthcare finance.

Dr. Gapenski received a B.S. degree from the Virginia Military Institute, a M.S. degree from the U.S. Naval Postgraduate School, and M.B.A. and Ph.D. degrees from the University of Florida.

Dr. Gapenski is an active member of the Association of University Programs in Health Administration, the American College of Healthcare Executives, and the Healthcare Financial Management Association. He has acted as academic advisor, chaired sessions, and presented papers at numerous national meetings. Additionally, Dr. Gapenski has acted as a reviewer for eleven academic and professional journals.